Anti-ageing nutrients

Anti-ageing nutrients

Evidence-based prevention of age-associated diseases

EDITED BY

Delminda Neves

Universidade do Porto

WILEY Blackwell

Registered Office
John Wiley & Sons, Ltd, The Atrium, Southern Gate, Chichester, West Sussex, PO19 8SQ, UK

Editorial Offices
9600 Garsington Road, Oxford, OX4 2DQ, UK
The Atrium, Southern Gate, Chichester, West Sussex, PO19 8SQ, UK
111 River Street, Hoboken, NJ 07030-5774, USA

For details of our global editorial offices, for customer services and for information about how to apply for permission to reuse the copyright material in this book please see our website at www.wiley.com/wiley-blackwell.

Library of Congress Cataloging-in-Publication Data applied for.

ISBN: 9781118733271

A catalogue record for this book is available from the British Library.

Wiley also publishes its books in a variety of electronic formats. Some content that appears in print may not be available in electronic books.

Cover image: © iStockphoto.com

Set in 9.5/12pt Meridien by SPi Publishers Services, Pondicherry, India
Printed and bound in Malaysia by Vivar Printing Sdn Bhd

1 2015

Contents

Part III – Evidence-based retardation of ageing

List of contributors

Henrique Almeida
Department of Experimental Biology, Faculty of Medicine, Instituto de Biologia Molecular e Celular (IBMC), and Instituto de Investigação e Inovação em Saúde, University of Porto, Porto, Portugal

José Paulo Andrade
Department of Anatomy, Faculty of Medicine, University of Porto, Porto, Portugal

Carmen Brás Silva
Department of Physiology and Cardiothoracic Surgery, Faculty of Medicine, and Faculty of Nutrition and Food Sciences, University of Porto, Porto, Portugal

Ângela Carneiro
Department of Ophthalmology of Hospital de São João and Department of sense organs, Faculty of Medicine, University of Porto, Porto, Portugal

Joana Carvalho
Research Centre in Physical Activity, Health and Leisure, Faculty of Sport Science, University of Porto, Porto, Portugal

Emilio Jirillo
Department of Basic Medical Sciences Neuroscience and Sensory Organs, University of Bari, Bari, Italy

Jean Krutmann
IUF - Leibniz Research Institute for Environmental Medicine, Heinrich-Heine-University Düsseldorf, Düsseldorf, Germany

Ana Paula de Melo Loureiro
Department of Clinical and Toxicological Analyses, Faculty of Pharmaceutical Sciences, University of São Paulo, São Paulo, Brazil

Thea Magrone
Department of Basic Medical Sciences Neuroscience and Sensory Organs, University of Bari, Bari, Italy

Alessandra Marini
IUF - Leibniz Research Institute for Environmental Medicine, Heinrich-Heine-University Düsseldorf, Düsseldorf, Germany

Elisa Marques
Research Centre in Physical Activity, Health and Leisure, Faculty of Sport Science, University of Porto, Porto, Portugal

Maria João Martins
Department of Biochemistry, Faculty of Medicine, and Instituto de Investigação e Inovação em Saúde, University of Porto, Porto, Portugal

Liliana Matos
Department of Experimental Biology, Faculty of Medicine, Instituto de Biologia Molecular e Celular (IBMC), Instituto de Investigação e Inovação em Saúde, and Faculty of Nutrition and Food Sciences (FCNAUP), University of Porto, Porto, Portugal

Jill Ann McKay
Sir James Spence Institute, Royal Victoria Infirmary, Queen Victoria Road, Newcastle upon Tyne, UK

Pedro Moreira
Faculty of Nutrition and Food Sciences, University of Porto, Research Center in Physical Activity, Health and Leisure, Faculty of Sport Science, University of Porto, Porto, Portugal

Delminda Neves
Department of Experimental Biology, Faculty of Medicine, and Institute for Molecular and Cell Biology, University of Porto, Porto, Portugal

Thomas Prates Ong
Laboratory of Nutrigenomics and Programming, Food and Experimental Nutrition Department, Faculty of Pharmaceutical Sciences, and Food and Nutrition Research Center, University of São Paulo, São Paulo, Brazil

Emanuel dos Passos
Department of Biochemistry, Faculty of Medicine, and CIAFEL – Research Centre in Physical Activity, Health and Leisure, Faculty of Sport, University of Porto, Porto, Portugal

Inês Tomada
Department of Experimental Biology, Faculty of Medicine, and Institute for Molecular and Cell Biology, University of Porto, Porto, Portugal

Luisa Anne Wakeling
School of Dental Sciences, Newcastle University, Newcastle upon Tyne, UK

Preface

Ageing is a complex time-related biological phenomenon that is genetically determined and environmentally modulated, and that leads to a progressive loss of function in an adult individual, and ultimately to death. According to all projections, even the most pessimistic, life expectancy will increase worldwide in the next two decades, greatly increasing the number of aged individuals. In parallel with the main causes of death in the elderly in developed and high-outcome countries, such as cancer and cardiovascular diseases, other pathologies frequently afflict aged people, including cognitive decline, sarcopenia, osteroporosis, skin fragility, loss of vision acuity and decay of immunity, indicating that organs are differentially affected by chronological ageing.

Actually, while specific features characterize senescent cells, growing evidence demonstrates that the ageing phenotype varies among tissues. Furthermore, during chronological ageing, the transcriptoma of tissues and organs change in a time-dependent fashion and these changes, mostly owing to epigenetic modifications, provide a link between genes and environment and thus enable cells to respond quickly to internal or environmental factors. An increasing body of literature supports the hypothesis that some of these age-related phenotypic changes could be avoided by specific nutritional patterns. One that has been known for over 500 years is restriction of energy intake. Lifelong energy restriction may extend life by up to 50% in rodents and significantly reduces the incidence of age-associated diseases, which according to gene expression profiling may be achieved through alterations in chromatin structure and a shift in transcription of specific genes. Interestingly, an equivalent effect to that obtained by energy restriction could be achieved by oral intake of resveratrol, a polyphenol found largely in the skins of red grapes and also in red wine. Further evidence that other specific oligonutrients contribute to the avoidance of age-related cellular and organ modifications has generated a promising opportunity to make an entirely natural intervention in elderly people, just like an "elixir of youth" that comes from food.

This book is written by a group of researchers who are all interested in nutritional modulation of ageing mechanisms. They come from different areas of research, such as basic science, food science and study of organ-specific ageing, or are physicians. The book is aimed at health professionals, undergraduates and graduates who have a basic grounding in biological sciences and who are interested in learning about nutrition and healthy lifestyles, and in addition updates and reviews the available literature about anti-ageing nutrients.

The book is divided into three parts. Part 1 includes Chapters 1–3 and covers cellular modifications that underlie the senescence of cells and the ageing of organisms, the effects of energy restriction on cellular and molecular mechanisms and the whole organism, the epigenetic modifications associated with ageing, and nutritional interventions targeted to epigenetic markers. Part 2 includes Chapters 4–10, and discusses the nutritional modulation of age-associated pathologies and the functional decline of organs, considering those primarily affected by chronological ageing, and aims to explain the scientific fundamentals of anti-ageing organ-oriented nutritional interventions.

Part 3 is constituted by the last chapter of the book, which puts together all of the knowledge presented in the previous chapters and discusses in a science-based fashion the best diet pattern for aged people.

Until now, most of the knowledge concerning the molecular effects of specific nutrients was restricted to researchers and the scientific community, and only rarely spread to the general public or health professionals who contact and advise their elderly patients every day. This book reflects the most recent advances in nutrition science, and the authors hope that it will strongly help elucidate for readers the best choices in anti-ageing nutrition.

Delminda Neves

Acknowledgment

I am profoundly grateful to all the authors who, besides their many duties in universities, research institutes and medical centers, contributed to this book. Without their contribution it would not have been possible. Also, I would like to thank Sérgio Evangelista and Tiago Franco de Oliveira for artwork in figures included in this book.

This project would not have been possible without the support of David McDade, senior editor of IFT press series books at Wiley-Blackwell. I thank him for his enthusiasm, which greatly inspired me.

Finally, I am indebted to my husband Alexandre, and to my daughters, Teresa and Leonor, who gave me all the emotional support that was essential to conclude this project.

PART I

Ageing of cells and organisms

CHAPTER 1
Human ageing, a biological view

Henrique Almeida[1] and Liliana Matos[2]

[1]*Department of Experimental Biology, Faculty of Medicine, Instituto de Biologia Molecular e Celular (IBMC) and Instituto de Investigação e Inovação em Saúde, University of Porto, Porto, Portugal*

[2]*Department of Experimental Biology, Faculty of Medicine, Instituto de Biologia Molecular e Celular (IBMC), Instituto de Investigação e Inovação em Saúde and Faculty of Nutrition and Food Sciences (FCNAUP), University of Porto, Porto, Portugal*

1.1 Introduction

The relentless increase in number of aged people might be perceived as an opportunity for a wiser society, should that be the sole consequence of old age. Instead, it carries a worrisome prospect because of the perception that such demographic change brings with it societal stresses and disturbing medical conditions. Owing to the improbability of such trends changing favorably in the near or mid future, most middle-aged populations see the problem with growing concern.

Every aspect of human life from biological to sociological, including economical and cultural, takes part in and interacts with this ageing process, which appears to worsen them all. However, as the major concern of most humans is likely to be physical or mental disability, the biological dimension of ageing stands out as the crucial one, because its resolution or mitigation is decisive in improving all of the others. Therefore, in-depth knowledge of ageing as a biological issue is necessary.

In the early 1950s, in an influential lecture, Sir Peter Medawar pointed out that ageing is a "problem of conspicuous sociological importance" but still a biologically unsolved one (Medawar, 1952). This lecture probably attracted attention to the subject in a time of remarkable achievements in life science knowledge and technology. However, much of the study of ageing in the succeeding years has remained quite descriptive until the last quarter of a century. In fact, only recently has the gerontology established in the modern laboratory became experimental and investigated the causes of ageing so that the process has become no longer an unsolved entity (Holliday, 2006). The field has been opened to state-of-the-art life science techniques, including recombinant DNA technology, which has produced a vast amount of information, and whose insights and applications foresee the ability to modulate ageing in a predictable way. As an important consequence, the possibility of extending the healthy human lifespan is now in sight. We refer to Kirkwood (1999) for an elegant comprehensive overview and Macieira-Coelho (2003) and Finch (2007) for an extended synthesis of the most relevant data on the subject.

In the following sections, we will address ageing, focusing on human or other mammalian biological aspects. We will start with a demographic approach, before moving into

Anti-Ageing Nutrients: Evidence-Based Prevention of Age-Associated Diseases, First Edition. Edited by Delminda Neves.

cells and tissues, where the realm of functional involution is likely to be found, and finish by going back to the whole organism.

1.2 Human ageing and frailty

1.2.1 Mortality curves

In contrast to their young counterparts, old people are at higher risk of dying, irrespective of the cause. This simple fact of observation received the attention of Alex Comfort. While discussing a way to measure the "decrease in viability and an increase in vulnerability", which he referred as the properties of senescence (i.e. ageing), he defined this process as a "progressive increase throughout life, or after a given stadium, in the likelihood that a given individual will die, during the next succeeding unit of time, from randomly distributed causes" (Comfort, 1956; the sentence was maintained in the following editions of the book).

Such a strict definition of ageing is in fact a description of the mortality rate, as a function of the final event of the ageing process but not a description of the conditions underlying this rate. However, the elucidation and quantitative assessment of the progress of these conditions are critical.

To measure and analyze the mortality rate, one should have access to a cohort of people and verify the lifespan of each cohort member; the ensuing mathematical analysis would then produce a theoretical model for the interpretation of the data. The first record of such analysis, perhaps the first scientific assessment related to ageing, was made in the 19th century by the English actuary Benjamin Gompertz. He found that, after a considerable risk of death during early infancy, there was a reduction that extended through to young adulthood; from then onwards, the risk increased progressively, doubling every 8 years. This finding, later adapted to become known as the Gompertz–Makeham law, is thus a measurement of the risk of death and is usually depicted as a curve, where the mortality rates, or probabilities of death, are plotted against age. It is objective, as it relates to a clear event of the organism's life, and harmonizes with the common intuition concerning the progressive nature of the ageing process that causes the elderly to die at a faster rate than the youth. Recognition of the Gompertz–Makeham law in other human populations and other species, including invertebrates, was important for further support for its biological value (Gavrilov & Gavrilova, 2006; Olshansky, 2010).

However, it should be pointed out that the data were collected in populations in specific environments. In fact, humans do not live in the wild as they have regular access to food and are medicated when ill; the other studied animals were confined to protected laboratory environments, therefore avoiding exposure to the hazards of wild-living, where death by accident, famine or predation is common.

The improvement of human living standards observed throughout the first half of the 20th century changed the Gompertz curves because of the decline in mortality rates in infancy. In more recent decades, however, continued sanitary improvements have modified the mortality rates of the remaining members of the cohort. Consequently, while the curves established in the 19th century fit well to mortality trends of the adult human population until the age of around 80 years old, they fail to do so after that because the logarithmic increase in the death rate tends to level off and even decelerate (Vaupel *et al.*, 1998; Rau *et al.*, 2008). As a result, postponement of mortality has continued and the number of centenarians has increased in all developed countries. Another consequence, more subtle and assuming that improvements in public health as a whole will continue, is the upward shift in the limits of human longevity (Vaupel, 2010). Surprising as it may be, estimates have shown that there has been an increase in life expectancy of 3 months each year since the middle of the 19th century (Oeppen & Vaupel, 2002) that is likely to continue, raising the possibility that, in the not so distant future, a significant number of humans will live beyond 100 years.

Therefore, the conviction that Gompertz curves reflect an intrinsic biological principle of ageing, as was thought (Sas *et al.*, 2012), is losing strength. Instead, a recent survey on a large number of species has shown that mortality curves are more diverse than expected (Jones *et al.*, 2014).

1.2.2 Susceptibility to disease and mortality

Deaths graphically depicted in Gompertz curves for humans result from all causes of mortality, and the acceleration of mortality evidenced along ageing corresponds to the increased incidence of age-related diseases (Finch, 2007). Certainly, there is a clear age-related disease burden on older individuals more than 80 years old, compared with those 20–50 years old (Carnes *et al.*, 2003; Horiuchi *et al.*, 2003), although the incidences of particular conditions may show different patterns according to the period of life considered; for example, cardiovascular disorders are present in both groups but show higher incidence in the older group (Horiuchi *et al.*, 2003).

Older individuals, in contrast to younger one, are subjected to this enhanced disease burden because their organism becomes frail and vulnerable. Frailty is generally considered to be the consequence of functional capacity (reserve) involution, sufficient to bring body systems close to clinical manifestations (Campbell & Buchner, 1997; Fried *et al.*, 2004; Partridge *et al.*, 2012). Therefore, while the fragile individual does not exhibit overt clinical disease, he is at increased risk of doing so if subjected to internal or external stresses. This intuitive point of view is hard to assess quantitatively, in contrast to the straightforward verification of lifespan. In fact, it is more complex to determine how frail or functionally involuted an individual is because frailty extends to multiple systems simultaneously, and shows variable magnitude and severity. In addition, over time, such evaluation has received less attention and fewer resources compared with the study of clinical signs and symptoms because it is socially more acceptable to allocate research funds to obvious disease than to an unclear functional involution. Another difficulty is the choice of assessment method. It may focus on essential musculoskeletal, respiratory, nutritional and cognitive abilities (Campbell & Buchner, 1997) or may be a rather complex formula to include audiometry parameters, visual data, memory and brain magnetic resonance data, among others (Hochschild, 1990; Diehr *et al.*, 2013; Newman *et al.*, 2008; Sanders *et al.*, 2012a, b). For this reason too, it is most desirable to undertake an active search for the most appropriate parameters for prediction of ageing consequences, including disability and death. Despite the uncertainties, the general view that physical and mental performance declines along time is supported by a number of studies. It is apparent by the seventh decade and continues at a rate that, depending on the studied parameters, appears to be greater for physical decline than mental (Diehr *et al.*, 2013; Parker *et al.*, 2008).

The established age-related functional loss may be well recognized, but its starting point is unclear. For a demographer, examination of the Gompertz–Makeham curves shows that functional loss starts when mortality accelerates (Gavrilov & Gavrilova, 2006), but for a physiologist, to verify that point would require a longitudinal examination of a considerable number of volunteers to identify involution parameters that follow different patterns, according to the specific body systems. For example, muscle capacity peak occurs at age 18 and the maximum inspiratory capacity at age 20, whereas creativity or auditory discrimination might peak before the age of 10 (Cutler & Mattson, 2006). Nevertheless, it might be found that the efficiency of a particular system is only a part of the whole body functionality; for example, muscles and lungs may reach their functional peak around age 20, but the best times for marathon runners were reported for 25–30-year-old althletes (Fries, 1980), indicating that, beyond lung and muscle capacity, peak fitness requires additional abilities such as self-discipline.

1.2.3 Age-related and age-dependent diseases

Ageing is not a disease, but a disease susceptibility condition. Diseases, manifested as a set of abnormal signs and symptoms, may have external causes such as infectious, or infectious-like agents (virus, bacteria, parasites, prions) or physical and chemical hazards such as radiation or environmental toxins, or inappropriate nutritional habits; they may have internal causes, including hereditary and congenital ones, or late acquired abnormalities, such as tissue deposition of inorganic or organic material (e.g. stones or lipids of atheroma lesions) and progressive cell or tissue loss. External causes can strike any age and disappear shortly after the cause ceases. Yet when internal causes are considered, except for most monogenic genetic disorders, the effect tends to remain more or less indolent albeit progressive, which is associated with ageing phenotype characteristics.

Among age-associated disorders, a distinction between age-dependent and age-related diseases has been proposed (Brody & Schneider, 1986). The etiopathogenesis of the former is connected to ageing and its morbidity, and mortality increases with it as well, making ageing a major risk factor for disorder progression and severity. Characteristic degenerative diseases such as osteoporosis, Alzheimer and Parkinson diseases, type 2 diabetes and cardiovascular diseases caused by atherosclerosis belong to that group. The second group, age-related diseases, has a temporal relation with age but no relation in terms of increase in incidence; it includes multiple sclerosis, amyotrophic lateral sclerosis and gout.

Cancer appears to fit less well in this categorization. Its incidence increases until the sixth decade, where it occupies the first place, and declines at a more advanced age (Horiuchi *et al.*, 2003). Interestingly, in an incidence analysis of the 20 most common cancers in men and women, an increase was shown up to 80 years and a decline thereafter (Harding *et al.*, 2008). As almost all cancers follow this pattern, they unveil the suggestion that very old age prevents cancer by some quirky biological process.

Age-dependent diseases, owing to their progressive course and causes, are those that best fit into the involution process. It is noteworthy that their course involves the accumulation of abnormal biomolecules, which is considered to be a fundamental cause of ageing (Kirkwood, 2005). They also pose a semantic difficulty because along the course of their establishment, the difference between ageing and disease is difficult to distinguish until clinical symptoms appear. However, even in their absence, ageing should not be considered suitable as a cause of death. Although individuals with exceptional longevity may die before a specific diagnosis is established, autopsies reveal large numbers of lesions and evidence previous disorders, of which cardiovascular disease is most prevalent (Blumenthal, 2002; Roberts, 1998; Berzlanovich *et al.*, 2005). Indeed, the relation between ageing and disease will remain a most complex one to deal with and, while some well-known biogerontologists would favor a distinction (Hayflick, 2000), others do not find it necessary (Masoro, 2006; Holliday, 2004).

There is a common belief that enhanced longevity will result in additional disease and disability, but it may not be necessarily so; some data even suggest otherwise. In fact, because of the wider availability of medical resources in developed countries and the refinement of diagnostic procedures, more diseases are reported but they are also more adequately treated, thus postponing mortality and related disability to a later age. Interestingly, although the proportion of independent individuals may decline progressively along time, independence for common activities is still considerable at older ages (Lowsky *et al.*, 2014), including nonagenarians and centenarians (Christensen *et al.*, 2009). Moreover, in the evaluation of health conditions of super-centenarians, overt diseases or morbidity were not found in a number of them until a short time before their death (Andersen *et al.*, 2012).

This late-age decrement in morbidity and the deceleration of mortality rate previously discussed are not sufficiently consistent to extrapolate to the whole population, in part because the population assessed is very much selected – they are the last survivors of a large cohort of people. However, surprisingly, the data suggest that the limits of human longevity may expand and there is potential for very old people to have reasonable healthy lives. As this is a result of a favorable biology of the organism, it means that there are mechanisms that are amenable to study, and probably, modulation in order to ameliorate old-age disability. Such exciting biological issues are also challenging as they will require the involvement of the whole of society owing to their vast implications for health, education, social insurance and employment.

1.3 Fundamental causes

The susceptibility of organisms to fatal disorders follows the functional involution of cells and tissues, itself a consequense of random, cumulative molecular dysfunction and error-making (Kirkwood & Austad, 2000; Hayflick, 2004; Holliday, 2004; Terman, 2006; López-Ótin *et al.*, 2013). Despite the variety of maintenance and repair systems in cells, survival is also an opportunity to make more errors that result in the accumulation of more by-products (Hayflick, 2000; Kirkwood, 2005; Baraibar & Friguet, 2013). Thus, as these are a consequence of life itself, their mechanistic roots, that is, the causes of ageing, should lie in the essential processes of cell functioning.

The most fundamental one is, perhaps, the extraction of free energy from food and its processing into usable compounds, which is necessary to fuel exceptionally complex activities, such as cell division, or ordinary daily work, such as transmembrane solute gradient maintenance or constitutive protein synthesis. The most important energetic compound so obtained, adenosine triphosphate (ATP), is mainly synthesized in the mitochondria. Using an ingenious set of chemical reactions, the reducing power of electrons released during food oxidation is buffered by their delivery onto successive electron carriers until the final reduction of molecular oxygen; while doing so, the process generates a proton gradient that is then used to synthesize ATP.

As the system is not entirely efficient, some electrons escape the carriers and, instead of fully reducing the molecular oxygen to water, they partially reduce it into superoxide anion $O_2^{\bullet-}$, one of the reactive oxygen species (ROS). The amount of electrons that are lost in this way may depend on the specific cell type (Turrens, 2003) and the lifespan of species under consideration (Barja & Herrero, 1998). Yet it is estimated that 1–2% of the oxygen that diffuses into the mitochondria is reduced to superoxide anion (Turrens, 2003), which, in the mitochondrial matrix, attains 5- to 10-fold higher concentration compared with the cytosol or nucleus (Cadenas & Davies, 2000). Superoxide dismutases, either the copper–zinc (CuZnSOD) or the manganese (MnSOD) isoforms, rapidly convert superoxide anion into hydrogen peroxide (H_2O_2), which, although not a radical, is still an oxidant. It is able to diffuse across membranes and, when doing so, may cause molecular harm, either directly or upon its conversion into the highly reactive hydroxyl radical ($HO^{\bullet}$).

In the endoplasmic reticulum (ERet), prostaglandins, steroid hormones, drugs and xenobiotics are oxidized by cytochrome P450-catalyzed reactions (Zangar *et al.*, 2004) and additional contributors provide minor amounts of oxidizing species (Curtis *et al.*, 2012; Förstermann & Sessa, 2012).

ROS promote an oxidative burden on cells. When not buffered by anti-oxidants, whatever their origin, they impose an oxidative stress on most biomolecules that deranges their functioning. As a consequence, should the process continue, not only will these molecules become unable to exert their effects, but they also tend to accumulate in the cells and tissues of organisms over time (Bokov *et al.*, 2004). The possibility that this continued process might underlie ageing was theorized by Denham Harman in 1956 as the free radical theory of ageing (Harman, 1956), later refined by scientific achievements, as the discovery of SOD and the further involvement of mitochondria in ROS generation and targeting for oxidative damage, and renamed as the mitochondrial free radical theory of ageing (MFRTA) (Harman, 1972; Beckman & Ames, 1998). Since then, the further involvement of mitochondria in ageing has been extensively investigated (Gomez-Cabrera *et al.*, 2012; Bratic & Larsson, 2013).

Although the general theory and the MFRTA have been questioned over time (Perez *et al.*, 2009; Yang & Hekimi, 2010), the latter is supported by age-associated observations: (a) mitochondrial ROS production increases with age owing to organelle function decline; (b) the accumulation of mitochondrial DNA mutations during ageing impairs respiratory chain function; and (c) mitochondrial ROS-scavenging enzyme activity declines with age, which in turn results in further ROS increase and oxidative biomolecular damage (Castro *et al.*, 2012b). In addition, microinjection of aged mitochondria into young fibroblasts results in their rapid acquisition of aged properties (Corbisier & Remacle, 1990), and the rate of ROS production by short-lived species of mitochondria is higher than that by long-lived species (Perez-Campo *et al.*, 1998), further supporting the view that the ROS produced by mitochondria are involved in the ageing process.

1.4 Experimental approach to human ageing

1.4.1 Ageing models in dividing cells: Replicative senescence and telomere involvement

Normal somatic cells have long been utilized by researchers to study cellular senescence and have proved to be a useful *in vitro* model to unravel complex molecular mechanisms and pathways likely to underly the human ageing process. Senescent cell phenotypes reported to date have employed dividing cells *in vitro* as the preferred systems.

Replicative senescence (RS) was first described in 1961 by Hayflick and Moorhead, when they observed that normal human diploid fibroblasts in culture had a limited replicative potential and became irreversibly arrested even in the presence of mitogens (Hayflick & Moorhead, 1961). Such functional loss and distinctive features of RS were envisaged to be a manifestation of cellular ageing. Senescent cells also experience dramatic morphological alterations when compared with young proliferating cells, including the increase in cell surface area and volume (Greenberg *et al.*, 1977), the loss of typical small spindle-fusiform shape and the acquisition of large, flat, morphology, owing to changes in cytoskeleton protein expression (Nishio *et al.*, 2001).

Depending on the cell type, senescent cells can be kept quiescent in culture from weeks to years, although their organelles may change. Lysosomes increase in number and size (Lipetz & Cristofalo, 1972) and accumulate granules of lipofuscin (Brunk & Terman, 2002a). Also, partly reflecting the increase in lysosomal mass, senescent cells exhibit an increased activity of senescence associated β-galactosidase (SA β-gal) (Dimri *et al.*, 1995), a lysosomal enzyme extensively utilized as cellular senescence biomarker. In mitochondria, despite the increase in mass (Lee *et al.*, 2002), the respiratory chain function deteriorates (Boffoli *et al.*, 1994), the DNA acquires mutations (Mecocci *et al.*, 1993) and mitochondria accumulate oxidatively damaged proteins (Ahmed *et al.*, 2010). In the nucleus, chromatin condensation increase is the most conspicuous change, while electron-dense regions, the senescence-associated heterochromatin foci, are formed throughout the nucleoplasm of interphase nuclei. These regions relate to transcriptionally suppressed E2F-responsive genes (Narita *et al.*, 2003), which contribute to cell cycle progression inhibition.

When compared with young cells, RS cells exhibit an altered gene expression profile that is cell type dependent (Shelton *et al.*, 1999). Such genes are involved in diverse processes such as cell cycle regulation, immune response and inflammation, cytoskeleton, stress response and metabolism (Zhang *et al.*, 2003; Ly *et al.*, 2000; Yoon *et al.*, 2004). Typically, when compared with young proliferating cells, RS fibroblasts overexpress senescence-associated genes such as apolipoprotein J (ApoJ), fibronectin, osteonectin, transforming growth factor β-1 (TGFβ1) and insulin growth factor binding protein 3 (IGFBP3) (Debacq-Chainiaux *et al.*, 2008). In addition, just before the cells lose their replicative ability and become senescent, the cyclin dependent kinase inhibitor (CDKI) p21 overexpresses to return to normal as cells enter RS. At this stage, CDKI p16 increases significantly and becomes the major inhibitor for cyclin-dependent kinases (CDK) 4 and 6, maintaining the cells in an irreversible growth arrest in G1 phase (Alcorta *et al.*, 1996; Pignolo *et al.*, 1998). At the protein level, when compared with early passage fibroblasts, RS cells also exhibit a differential expression of several proteins that are components of the cytoskeleton, or implicated in key cellular functions, such as β-actin, tubulin β chain, vimentin, anexin I/VI and α-enolase (Trougakos *et al.*, 2006).

Resistance to apoptosis is another typical characteristic of RS cells, albeit dependent on the cell type and the pro-apoptotic signal. For example, senescent endothelial cells do not resist ceramide-induced apoptosis but RS fibroblasts do (Hampel *et al.*, 2004); RS fibroblasts resist growth factor deprivation- and oxidative stress-induced apoptosis but not Fas-mediated apoptosis (Chen *et al.*, 2000a; Tepper *et al.*, 2000). To explain the resistance to apoptosis, various reports implicated the upregulation of genes encoding survivin (Al-Khalaf & Aboussekhra, 2013), cellular myeloblastosys protein (c-myb; Lee *et al.*, 2010), major vault protein (Ryu *et al.*, 2008) and B cell-lymphoma 2 (bcl-2; Ryu *et al.*, 2007). More recently, epigenetic mechanisms involving locus-specific histone modifications, regulating *bcl-2:bax* (bcl-2 associated X protein) gene expression in senescent fibroblasts, were proposed to contribute to the apoptosis-resistant phenotype (Sanders *et al.*, 2013).

The number of doublings at which an entire cell population in a given culture reaches RS is fairly reproducible, suggesting the existence of a kind of cell division-counting mechanism. Currently, there is evidence in favor of telomere shortening as cells age in culture (Harley *et al.*, 1990). Telomeres are the natural nonblunted ends of chromosomes that consist of repetitive sequences (TTAGGG in humans) and specialized proteins, essential for maintaining genomic stability (Blackburn, 1991). Conventional DNA polymerases are unable to replicate completely the terminal ends of linear DNA molecules owing to the inherent RNA priming mechanism of DNA replication (Olovnikov, 1973). Instead, telomerase, a specialized DNA polymerase, is capable of synthesizing *de novo* TTAGGG repeats and adding them to human chromosome ends to compensate for telomeric DNA losses (Blackburn, 1992). As most normal somatic cells do not express telomerase, their telomeres shorten with each cell cycle. When telomere attrition is critical, it triggers a full senescence cell cycle inhibition response that limits the proliferative capacity of cultured cells. Actually, the ectopic expression of telomerase was sufficient to revert RS cells into a phenotypically youthful state (Bodnar *et al.*, 1998). Telomere attrition-induced cell cycle arrest may result from deletion of critical genes involved in cellular division located near telomeres (Allsopp, 1996) or from silencing of subtelomeric genes owing to heterochromatin shifting caused by telomere loss (Wright & Shay, 1992). Whatever the basic cause, critical telomere shortening triggers a DNA damage response that induces the overexpression of p53 and p21 proteins that block CDK activity in G1 phase (Huang *et al.*, 1996; Saretzki *et al.*, 1999).

1.4.2 Stress-induced premature senescence

Premature senescence, or stress-induced premature senescence (SIPS), can be experimentally achieved in a short period of time by exposing dividing cells to subcytotoxic levels of stressors, such as H_2O_2 (Chen & Ames, 1994), *tert*-butyl hydroperoxide (tBHP; Dumont *et al.*, 2000), hyperoxia (Saretzki *et al.*, 1998), ultraviolet B radiation (Debacq-Chainlaux *et al.*, 2005) or copper sulfate ($CuSO_4$; Matos *et al.*, 2012), among others. Similarly to RS cells, SIPS cells are irreversibly arrested in G1 phase (Chen *et al.*, 1998; von Zglinicki *et al.*, 1995) and share structural and molecular features, serving therefore as an excellent model for the study of cellular senescence. The most frequently used SIPS model is obtained upon exposure of early-passage fibroblasts to a subcytotoxic dose of H_2O_2 for 2 hours (H_2O_2-SIPS). Three days afterwards, most cells cease proliferation, develop senescent-like morphology and exhibit increased SA β-gal activity and altered gene expression (Chen & Ames, 1994; Chen *et al.*, 1998). In H_2O_2-SIPS cells, senescence is modulated by specific molecular changes that involve retinoblastoma (Rb) protein, enhanced actin stress fibers and cystoskeleton reorganization (Chen *et al.*, 2000b). In tBHP- and H_2O_2-induced SIPS, cells overexpress p21 and p16 that inhibit cyclinD-CDK4/6 complexes and block Rb protein phosphorylation, preventing cells progressing from G1 to S phase. Similarly to RS fibroblasts, SIPS cells have low Rb protein phosphorylation (Chen *et al.*, 1998; Dumont *et al.*, 2000) and senescence-associated genes, such as p21, ApoJ, fibronectin, IGFBP3 or TGFβ1, are overexpressed in hyperoxia- (Saretzki *et al.*, 1998), tBHP-, H_2O_2- (Dumont *et al.*, 2000) and $CuSO_4$-SIPS (Matos *et al.*, 2012). Using the H_2O_2-SIPS model, it was shown that TGFβ1 overexpression is required for the induction of senescent morphogenesis, increased mRNA levels of the senescence-associated genes fibronectin, ApoJ and osteonectin, and increased activity of SA β-gal (Frippiat *et al.*, 2001).

The involvement of telomere shortening in the establishment of SIPS is not clear. Several studies have demonstrated that, in hyperoxia- or H_2O_2-SIPS cells, telomeres shorten faster than in young fibroblasts (von Zglinicki *et al.*, 1995; Duan *et al.*, 2005), but others failed to show it (Chen *et al.*, 2001), suggesting that SIPS can be attained without telomere shortening. These conflicting observations may result from variation in the oxidative stress intensity and the type of targeted biomolecule. Whatever the particular conditions may be, oxidative stress indeed affects telomere attrition as cell culture supplementation with anti-oxidants results in decline of telomere erosion (von Zglinicki, 2000; Furumoto *et al.*, 1998) and enhanced expression of anti-oxidant enzymes such as glutathione peroxidase and CuZnSOD (Serra *et al.*, 2000). In this setting, telomeres are likely to act as oxidative stress sensors and, when the condition leads to single-strand DNA damage accumulation in telomeres, cell proliferation inhibition signals are conveyed through p53 and p21 overexpression (Saretzki *et al.*, 1999).

1.4.3 Ageing in organs and tissues

An important question in this issue regards the value of RS cells in living organisms and how much they contribute to the functional involution related to ageing. This is an unsettled matter mostly because a large number of tissues do not have a substantial amount of proliferating cells and those that have tend to produce cells that, instead of accumulating, are normally discarded from the organism or recycled.

In tissues from aged humans, the presence of somatic cells with traits of senescence has only rarely been reported. The major limitation to detecting senescent cells in living aged tissues is that a specific marker that would exclusively or unequivocally identify senescent cells does not exist. The most widely used marker, the senescence associated β-galactosidase histochemical (Dimri *et al.*, 1995; Itahana *et al.*, 2007, 2013), has nevertheless been questioned because under some conditions, it also identifies nonsenescent cells (Cristofalo, 2005; Yang & Hu, 2005).

More recent markers of senescence have been categorized as genes involved in the establishment and maintenance of senescent states (upregulated p16 or p21), markers of genotoxic stress (telomere-associated foci, TAF) and distinctive heterochromatin clusters (senescence-associated heterochromatin foci). Employing these biomarkers, it was reported that the number of senescent cells in various living tissues from humans, primates and rodents increases with age, in frequencies varying from less than 1% to around 15%, depending on the species and tissues (Dimri *et al.*, 1995; Pendergrass *et al.*, 1999; Paradis *et al.*, 2001; Ding *et al.*, 2001; Herbig *et al.*, 2006; Jeyapalan *et al.*, 2007; Wang *et al.*, 2009; Kreiling *et al.*, 2011; Hewitt *et al.*, 2012).

The concept underlying senescence is consolidating in a cluster of markers collectively designated as senescent-associated secretory phenotype, SASP (Hewitt *et al.*, 2012; Kuilman & Peeper, 2009). The concept implies that, although irreversibly arrested, senescent cells *in vivo* remain metabolically active as they secrete pro-inflammatory cytokines, chemokines, growth factors and proteases with profound effects on the surrounding microenvironment. SASP can exert four different types of actions: they act in an autocrine fashion, further fostering senescence development within the secreting cell (Wajapeyee *et al.*, 2008); they promote tumorigenesis on surrounding premalignant or transformed cells (Coppe *et al.*, 2008); they regulate immune clearance of senescent cells (Kang *et al.*,

2011); and they induce senescence in normal surrounding cells (Acosta *et al.*, 2013). Such changes in the tissue microenvironment would be expected to affect tissue homeostasis and function, and lead to tissue degeneration and organ dysfunction. The relation between *in vivo* ageing and cellular senescence in tissues was demonstrated using a mouse model where the removal of senescent cells was able to prevent or delay tissue dysfunction and extend lifespan (Baker *et al.*, 2011).

1.4.4 Lipofuscin deposition following organelle dysfunction and damage accumulation

In postmitotic cells, deposition of lipofuscin, often called the "age pigment", has long been considered a major cellular sign of ageing. Lipofuscin refers to the age-related brownish hue that is noticed in bright tissues on a simple macroscopic inspection.

Owing to the distinct color and natural autofluorescence, by absorbing light between 320 and 480 nm and emitting at 460–630 nm (Katz *et al.*, 1988), lipofuscin is easily detectable in the cytoplasm in nonstained tissue sections; moreover, it may be demonstrated by histochemistry, using techniques such as Sudan black for lipid or periodic acid–Schiff for carbohydrate staining (Dayan *et al.*, 1988). In ultrastructural observations, lipofuscin appears as intracytoplasmic, membrane bound granules, exhibiting an heterogeneous content that includes lipid-like material together with dense irregular features, sometimes with filamentous shape, that contain protein (Almeida *et al.*, 1998). In fact, lipofuscin is composed of oxidized proteins (30–70%), lipids (20–50%) and, in a lesser amount, carbohydrates and transition metals (Fe, Cu, Zn and Mn; Benavides *et al.*, 2002; Double *et al.*, 2008), which is evidence of the role of oxidation in its genesis and ability to oxidize even further.

Lipofuscin formation has been proposed to fall within a mitochondrial–lysosomal axis theory of ageing (Brunk & Terman, 2002b). In time, mitochondria from aged postmitotic cells produce less ATP and become particularly affected in their function owing to continued production of ROS. On the electron microscope, they enlarge, swell, lose cristae and, sometimes, show complete destruction of their inner membranes and the formation of amorphous electron-dense material (Terman *et al.*, 2003). In a normal situation, such dysfunctional organelles are conveyed to the lysosomes where they are destroyed. In addition, this process, named macroautophagy (discussed in Chapter 2), endows cells with the ability to recycle their own deteriorated biological material, which may include insoluble protein aggregates and deranged organelles such as mitochondria; autophagy also prevents their accumulation and therefore promotes cell economy when nutritional environmental conditions are hostile.

However, in ageing and experimental oxidative environments, lipofuscin granule accumulation in lysosomes is progressive; in time, lysosomes increase in number and size but also decrease in their degradative capacity (Terman *et al.*, 1999), thus leading to inefficient degradation of damaged mitochondria. The continuous mitochondrial generation of ROS and the accumulation of lipofuscin-bound redox-active iron result in enhanced harmful effects as H_2O_2 is converted to the highly reactive hydroxyl radical via the Fenton reaction; this event perpetuates oxidative stress and explains, at least in part, lipofuscin cytotoxicity (Hohn *et al.*, 2010). Its age-related accumulation has been of major interest in the nervous system (Shantha *et al.*, 1969), but has been shown in a diversity of tissues and species as well (Terman & Brunk, 1998).

The ERet is another cell compartment whose components are also affected by age. In addition to being the major intracellular Ca^{2+} store, the ER is the site for synthesis, processing, folding and posttranslational modifications of all lysosomal, cell membrane integral and secretory proteins. Several conditions, such as redox changes and calcium disturbance, are able to disrupt ERet homeostasis and originate ERet stress (discussed in Chapter 2), characterized by the accumulation of unfolded/misfolded proteins and the activation of the unfolded protein response, whose main goal is to restore ERet normal functioning. The efficiency of such a response is diminished with age, owing to impairment of the chaperoning system that verifies protein quality (Macario & Conway de Macario, 2002). Moreover, ERet resident chaperones, whose activity is crucial for an efficient unfolded protein response, are progressively oxidized with age, further contributing to their functional decline (Nuss *et al.*, 2008).

Proteins from the cytosol are also prone to oxidizing and having their function disturbed. Actually, while proteins in general are the main targets for ROS-mediated damage, cytosolic proteins appear to be particularly sensitive. In fact, actin, tubulin, vimentin, proteasome proteins, chaperones and ribosomal proteins, either isolated or in whole organisms, become markedly oxidized in ageing and in experimental conditions (Levine & Stadtman, 2001; Castro *et al.*, 2012a, 2013; Baraibar & Friguet, 2013; David *et al.*, 2010). The result is misfolding, functional impairment, irreversible carbonylation and the establishment of crosslinks.

To prevent the accumulation of damaged proteins, that is, to maintain proteostasis, cells use the proteasome as the first and most important nonlysosomal mechanism for protein turnover (Jung *et al.*, 2009). It is a complex catalytic structure that assembles as a 20S catalytic core, independent of ATP and ubiquitin tagging, or a 26S form that combines the 20S core and a 19S regulatory cap involved in ubiquitinated substrate recognition (Jung *et al.*, 2009). The 20S proteasome form is the main site for oxidized protein degradation, largely because of its relative resistance to oxidative stress (Reinheckel *et al.*, 1998). For 26S proteasome action, the ubiquitin system must first be activated. In succession, three enzymes activate the substrates with ubiquitin molecules (E1 ubiquitin activating enzyme), transfer and transport them (E2 ubiquitin conjugating enzyme), and finally deliver them to the proteasome (E3 ubiquitin ligase).

When oxidative conditions intensify, or when cells attain RS, the proteasome function declines (Davies & Shringarpure, 2006) and protein crosslinks increase, form aggregates and become insoluble. The process ultimately leads to lipofuscin formation and accumulation within lysosomes (Jung *et al.*, 2007). These damaging events are especially dramatic in postmitotic cells since they are not able to dilute this material by cell division.

1.4.5 Damage consequences: Dysfunctional organelles and cell functional decline. Cell loss

Damaged macromolecules and organelles are usually eliminated through proteosomal or lysosomal degradation systems in order to ensure the maintenance of cellular functions. However, during ageing, both systems are affected and their degradative activity declines significantly, resulting in the accumulation of altered proteins and defective organelles in aged cells.

The oxidatively modified structures that accumulate with age in postmitotic cells are functionally inefficient and, therefore, are frequently considered as biological "garbage" or "waste" material. Defective mitochondria and aggregated oxidized proteins are the most common forms of extra-lysosomal "garbage", while lipofuscin represents the intra-lysosomal one.

Accumulation of such materials is harmful because of the occupation of cytoplasm, interference with biological processes and likely toxic effects. In addition, lipofuscin-loaded cells exhibit diminished autophagic activity (Terman *et al.*, 1999) since most lysosomal enzymes are directed to lipofuscin-loaded lysosomes in futile attempts to degrade the indigestible pigment. In such a scenario, the recycling of defective mitochondria is inhibited, further increasing their accumulation. On the other hand, enhanced ROS generation at these dysfunctional organelles accelerates lipofuscin deposition, which again inhibits mitochondria turnover and further promotes ROS production through intralysosomal iron-catalyzed reactions. These cyclical events exhaust clearance mechanisms, leading to continuous age-related accumulation of intracellular "garbage", profound dysfunction and the death of postmitotic cells (Brunk & Terman, 2002b).

1.5 Involving genes in organism ageing and longevity

Although the ageing process appears to be intrinsically random, one may question whether and to what extent the genes contribute to ageing. Their impact may be simply recognized as "Yes, they do impact" because virtually every aspect of life maintenance implies the activity of gene expression products. Moreover, the appearance of by-products and their clearance or accumulation depend on the transcriptional activity as well. Yet, how they intervene or what is the relative contribution of any gene is much more difficult to answer.

The extreme complexity of life, and ageing, are illustrative of the multifactorial dimension of the genetic contribution to ageing. Moreover, as ageing is not a disease, much less a monogenic disease, genes cannot be taken as causing ageing in the sense that there is not one gene that may be held responsible for the ageing process. Otherwise, a mutation in this gene might lead to organism ageing retardation and extended longevity. Should it have a favorable trait, natural selection would provide its survival over the previous wild-type condition and the earth would be plentiful of very long-lived species.

1.5.1 Longevous humans

In contrast to other organism's models, whose relatively short lifespans are easily surveyed in the laboratory (e.g. the *Caenorhabditis elegans*, the *Drosophila melanogaster* or even the *Mus musculus*), the extensive lifespan of humans poses an immediate difficulty. To circumvent this, researchers have looked for genes, or combinations of genes, that may have been favorable for enhanced human longevity.

A strategy to tackle the problem has been to employ whole, or nearly whole, cohorts of humans, a reason why it has only recently become possible to conveniently examine a cohort whose members were born early in the 20th century. One benefit of such a study is the inclusion of centenarians and nonagerians who are likely to have genes or gene combinations that favor long life. In addition, the cohort may help to identify monozygotic twins who, because they sidestep natural genetic variation, are highly valued in approaching genetic vs environmental determinants.

In cohorts of Scandinavian twins it was estimated that the overall contribution of heritability to the age at death is 20–30% (Murabito *et al.*, 2012), being slightly higher for females compared with males (Herskind *et al.*, 1996) and, in any case, higher when compared with nontwin controls. An interesting finding is that the influence of genetics has a small impact until the sixth decade but increases thereafter (Hjelmborg *et al.*, 2006; Willcox *et al.*, 2006), thus converging with the results of centenarians. These may thus be seen as humans harboring the genetic complements of successful ageing. In addition, their siblings were found to have several-fold greater possibility of reaching 100 years, in contrast to nonsiblings (Perls *et al.*, 2002), thus favoring an intrafamiliar clustering for exceptional longevity (Perls *et al.*, 2000). Surprisingly, centenarian offspring may have enhanced mortality while they are children but, at old age, they exhibit lower mortality rates for all or specific causes of death, such as coronary heart disease and cancer (Terry *et al.*, 2004). A lower prevalence of cardiovascular diseases, a major cause of death at any adult age, is also noticed in centenarian offspring (Terry *et al.*, 2003). In general, the contribution of heredity to lifespan should be considered modest, compared with the contribution to other phenotypes such as Alzheimer disease or age at menarche or menopause (Murabito *et al.*, 2012), suggesting that the conditions underlying lifespan are more heterogeneous compared with the higher homogeneity of a neurological or a reproductive phenotype.

Regarding genetic involvement in longevity, genome-wide association studies have identified apolipoprotein E (*APOE*) gene polymorphisms as the most consistently related to longevity (Christensen *et al.*, 2009; Beekman *et al.*, 2013). *APOE2* allele was associated with enhanced longevity, whereas the *APOE4* allele was found at very low proportions in centenarians (Gerdes *et al.*, 2000) and was associated with enhanced mortality caused by atheromatous cardiovascular disorders and Alzheimer disease (Schachter *et al.*, 1994; Corder *et al.*, 1993). The APOE protein is a lipoprotein and cholesterol transporter between tissues; its APOE4 isoform has a better interaction with the cognate receptor (Mahley & Rall, 2000), resulting in a higher propensity for cholesterol to be taken up by targeted tissues. Except for the rare *E2/E2* homozygosity, the E2 isoform is more often related to reduced circulating total and low-density lipoprotein (LDL) cholesterol, whereas E4 results in the opposite (Mahley & Rall, 2000). In parallel with these observations, centenarian Ashkenazi Jew offspring exhibited higher high-density lipoprotein cholesterol, and males had lower LDL levels, compared with controls (Barzilai *et al.*, 2001).

Another gene found in association with long-lived individuals and replicated more than once is Forkhead box O 3A, *FOXO3A* (Willcox *et al.*, 2008; Flachsbart *et al.*, 2009). This gene encodes a transcription factor regulated mainly in the setting of insulin and the insulin-like growth factor 1 (IGF-1) signaling pathway discussed later.

Apart from evidence related to *APOE* alleles and *FOXO3A*, other studies in the field have reported associations with ageing, although less consistent, for other genes and telomere length (Brooks-Wilson, 2013; Wheeler & Kim, 2011). Telomere length as inversely correlated with the risk of death from specific diseases has been examined in the last decade, producing conflicting results (Christensen *et al.*, 2009); more recently, it was found to correlate with disease burden in general rather than with a single disorder (Sanders *et al.*, 2012b).

It is interesting that nearly all of the genes found to associate with longevity have some involvement in lipid metabolism or nutrient uptake and use by cells, which relates them to cell enrichment with lipids. Unsurprisingly, unfavorable serum patterns of lipoproteins, unfavorable *APOE* allele combinations and excess circulating insulin are associated with enhanced risk of atheromatous disease, a major cause of death in human adults.

1.5.2 Experimental approaches

The use of cells and tissues in the study of ageing has produced relevant knowledge and insights into the diversity of ageing patterns and their likely causes. Additional information, perhaps more relevant, may be obtained when the appraisal extends to whole organisms under experimental conditions. The laboratory is not the real world but allows the study of organisms under controlled conditions, which is quite suitable when the purpose is to determine their lifespans and record the causes of death. Appropriate accommodation may be very expensive though, which limits the type of organisms used. Among the species employed, the tiny nematode *C. elegans* has been most fruitful because of the simplicity of its husbandry, in-depth knowledge of its biology, the variety of strains and its mere 3 week life cycle. While the mouse is the easiest-to-use mammal, only a very restricted number of laboratories have access to nonhuman primates.

Animal strains with spontaneous mutations associated with enhanced longevity have been selected over time, but what deeply changed the field was the application of recombinant DNA technology. Such procedures, largely employed in *C. elegans*, showed how the inactivation or the overexpression of a single gene would result in substantial longevity change, drawing further attention to the role of genes. Surprisingly, such role did not unveil any cryptic or unprecedented process. Rather, ageing turned out to be centered on metabolism and its regulation, showing that, no matter how much complex any biological process is, it might be simplified to the use of food to survive.

In 1988, a strain of *C. elegans* with a 60% additional increment in longevity owing to a mutation in the *age-1* gene was described (Friedman & Johnson, 1988), but only some years later its product, the phosphatidylinositol-3-kinase (PI3K), was identified (Morris *et al.*, 1996). This kinase activates a discrete step in the intracellular insulin and IGF-1 signaling pathway, part of an endocrine axis with major reference points at the pituitary and the liver. Apart from being evolutionarily conserved in a variety of organisms, this axis is now recognized as having an extraordinary involvement in ageing and longevity (Fontana *et al.*, 2010).

Elucidation of the *age-1* gene product-specific role was probably the first precise mechanistic step that directly involved metabolism in ageing. However, more than 50 years previously, it had been recognized that reducing the laboratory diet to a defined amount, that is, employing energy restriction (ER), resulted in enhanced rodent longevity.

Thorough study in the 1970s and 1980s unveiled many other benefits, including reduction in chronic disorders and cancer incidence, and anti-inflammatory and anti-infectious preventive effects; in ER animals there is an enhanced but moderate cortisol/corticosterone secretion, reduced thyroid hormones and insulin resistance, increased degradation and decreased accumulation of oxidized proteins, enhanced proteasome activity and heat shock protein 90 (further reading is recommended in Speakman & Mitchell, 2011 and in Chapter 2). ER effects are thus global and detectable in virtually every body system. Owing to their interplay, some effects may not just be a consequence of the restriction *per se*, but secondary to changes that ER elicits in other systems; this is likely to be the case for endocrine systems where such interplay is larger. ER became thus a scientifically robust, nongenetically engineered model of longevity enhancement with health improvement for a wide variety of species that probably includes primates (Colman *et al.*, 2009; Mattison *et al.*, 2012).

During the search for the fine molecular mechanisms governing longevity extension, ER highlighted the major involvement of molecular regulators of metabolism: the insulin/IGF-1 axis, the adenosine monophosphate kinase sensing of intracellular ATP, the sirtuin signaling and target of rapamycin signaling pathways. Emphasis will now be given to insulin/IGF-1 axis; other mechanisms, while receiving some attention in the following sections, are more comprehensively discussed in Chapters 2 and 3.

1.5.2.1 The insulin/IGF-1 axis

In mammals, the pathway centered on the growth hormone (GH)/IGF-1 axis, may be tracked to the hypothalamic pulsatile secretion of growth hormone-releasing hormone (GHRH). In the anterior pituitary, GHRH binds to its cognate receptor (GHRHR) at the surface of somatotrophs and promotes GH synthesis and secretion to the blood. Upon interacting with its receptor on liver cells, GH activates a transductive pathway, which results in IGF-1 synthesis and release into the circulation. At the surface of target cells, IGF-1 binds to the IGF-1 receptor (IGF-1R), a member of the insulin/IGF-1R family, and starts another transductive pathway.

IGF-1R is present in a variety of cells, including fat, muscle and liver cells and therefore possesses a wide distribution in the body. Upon its synthesis as a single-chain propeptide, the receptor is processed into a mature heterodimer having one α and one β subunit covalently linked by a disulfide bond (Ullrich *et al.*, 1986). At the plasma membrane, it interacts with a similar heterodimer and acquires the functional heterotetramer structure composed of two α and two β chains incorporating the ligand binding and tyrosine kinase domains respectively; IGF-1R and insulin receptor heterodimers may assemble as hybrid heterotetramers with similar ability to bind ligands and trigger the intracellular signaling pathway (Pollak, 2012). Rodents bearing mutations affecting different levels of the IGF-1 secretion axis live longer than controls and are considerably smaller. They have provided relevant information on some mechanisms affecting ageing and longevity and insights on how to modulate them.

Mice with spontaneous homozygous GHRHR mutations, known as *Ghrhr*$^-$/*Ghrhr*$^-$ (or *lit/lit* mice owing to their small size) have an abnormal N-terminal, extracellular domain, resulting in an inability to interact with the ligand and, consequently, to synthesize GH; therefore, mice have low levels of circulating GH and IGF-1, are about half the size of wild-type strains and, when they are fed with a low-fat diet, the increase in mean and maximum lifespan extends their longevity by 25% (Godfrey *et al.*, 1993; Flurkey *et al.*, 2001).

Autosomal recessive isolated growth hormone deficiencies in humans owing to GHRHR mutations constitute about 10% of the total number of cases. As expected, most patients exhibit short stature, but their growth is proportional, intelligence is not affected and fertility is largely conserved (Mullis, 2010).

At a lower level of the IGF-1/GH axis stand the Ames and the Snell dwarf strains that result from spontaneous recessive mutations in the homeobox protein prophet of PIT1 (*Prop1*) and the pituitary-specific positive transcription factor 1 (*Pit1*) genes, respectively. During pituitary development, *Prop1* gene expression appears in anterior pituitary cells and becomes upregulated. The encoded protein, Prop1, forms homodimers that target specific gene regulatory sites, including *Pit1* gene, whose increasing activation parallels subsequent downregulation of *Prop1*. *Pit1* gene expression is necessary for the local differentiation of a variety of peptide-producing cells such as the thyrotrophs, lactotrophs and the somatotrophs (de Moraes *et al.*, 2012). Compared with controls, *Pit1* and *Prop1* mutants are about 50% smaller, their weights reduce to 30% and some tissues have increased activity of catalase and CuZnSOD isoform (Bartke, 2011; Flurkey *et al.*, 2001). Mice are usually infertile and their longevities are extended by 50% in males, and even more in females, compared with controls; moreover, mean and maximum lifespans are enhanced in Snell (Flurkey *et al.*, 2002) and in Ames strains (Brown-Borg *et al.*, 1996). The features of these animals are thought to be due to primary deficiency of GH secretion and consequent lack of IGF-1 secretion stimulation. However, they have additional deficiencies in TSH and prolactin, which contribute to the final phenotype.

Abnormalities at this level of IGF-1 axis were previously described in humans (Pfäffle & Klammt, 2011) who show a variable degree of hypopituitarism, with emphasis on short stature, affecting children and adolescents, but including additional hormonal deficiencies.

Other strains with deficient IGF-1 secretion are the result of selective gene inactivation. These comprise the homozygous GH receptor knockout strain (GHRKO, also known as GHR/GHBP knockout) that bears the inactive GHR and the GHR binding protein resulting from GHR extracellular domain proteolytic cleavage. The hallmark of the condition is enhanced resistance to GH and very low levels of circulating IGF-1, insulin and glucose (Bonkowski *et al.*, 2009). Mice have ~50% reduced size but increased average and maximum lifespan by a similar figure and the change also appears to delay ageing, as evidenced by the late appearance of age-associated diseases (Bartke, 2005).

Those mice, also known as Laron dwarfs, have a human counterpart in the Laron syndrome (Laron, 2004) that shows marked dwarfism, enhanced GH resistance and very low IGF-1 blood levels. It is not clear whether these patients live longer because they tend to die from external causes; however, except for cardiovascular diseases, whose mortality is similar to that of controls, Laron syndrome patients appear to be protected from age-associated diseases such as cancer and diabetes (Guevara-Aguirre *et al.*, 2011). Similarly to Ames/Snell dwarves, the Laron mice also lack the effects of GH. While in the former it is because of a developmental defect limiting strongly its synthesis, in the latter it is because the synthesis is conserved but the means to put it into action, the receptor, is not operational.

Mice with *IGF-1* gene knockout, which would minimize some of the confounding effects observed in the above-mentioned strains, have a poor outcome because shortly after birth many individuals die from respiratory impairment; moreover, the survivors show structural and functional abnormalities in various organs, including the gonad, which makes them infertile (Liu *et al.*, 2000). IGF-1R homozygous null mutants are also not viable; the heterozygous strain has elevated circulating IGF-1 levels, but as they lack a fully functional receptor, the gain in longevity is small, 16–33% depending on sex (Holzenberger *et al.*, 2003). They do not develop dwarfism, they have similar glucose and insulin levels, are fertile and appear to cope well with oxidative stressful conditions. In *C. elegans*, the ortolog of the insulin/IGF-1R is the *daf-2* gene (dauer formation or *daf* strains) that when mutated results in doubling of the organism lifespan (Kenyon *et al.*, 1993); in arthropods and yeasts, similar signaling cascades employing high-homology molecules have been found, whose mutation also results in prolonged longevity (Fontana *et al.*, 2010).

The likelihood that similar genetic variations might exist in humans prompted a search for IGF-1R gene variants that might be favorable to enhanced longevity. Such a search by sequencing IGF-1R genes of centenarians led to the identification of missense variants that, although rare in the population, appear enriched in centenarians (Tazearslan *et al.*, 2012).

1.5.2.2 IGF-1 signaling into FOXO proteins

Interestingly, IGF-1 involvement in longevity, rather than relying on its signaling pathway activation, is manifested when it is downregulated, as occurs during ER, for example. Upon IGF-1/IGF-1R interaction, receptor conformation is altered, which induces trans-phosphorylation in tyrosine residues of its intracellular domains (Fig. 1.1).

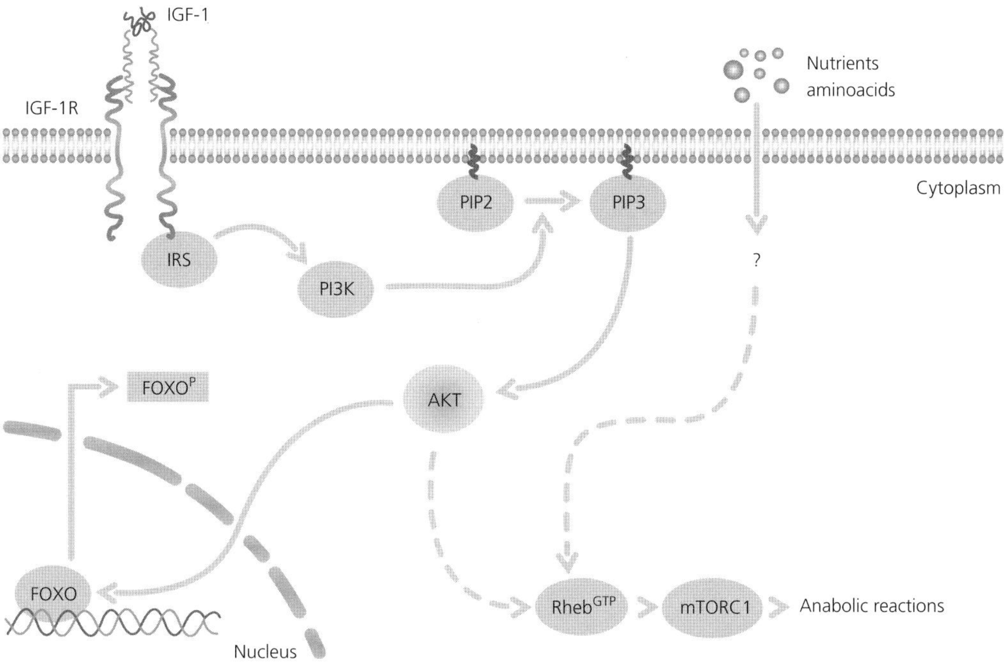

Figure 1.1 IGF-1R pathway activation. Upon interaction of insulin-like growth factor and cognate receptor (IGF-1/IGF-1R), receptor catalytic properties are activated. Insulin receptor substrate (IRS) isoforms then bind the receptor and recruit phosphatidylinositol-3-kinase (PI3K), which promotes phosphatidylinositol (3,4,5)-triphosphate (PIP3) synthesis and AKT activation. AKT then phosphorylates forkhead transcription factor (FOXO) proteins, which cease their transcription modulatory effect and leave the nucleus. AKT action also keeps the small GTPase Rheb in its GTP bound form, which keeps the mechanistic target of rapamycin complex 1 (mTORC1) active to promote its anabolism-favorable effect.

This change enables receptor catalytic activity, insulin receptor substrates isoforms binding and membrane-bound PI3K recruitment. PI3K then promotes AKT activation that targets distinct molecules such as the FOXO family of transcription factors (and daf-16, the single FOXO ortholog in nematodes).

In mammals, the FOXO group of proteins, part of a large family of forkhead transcription factors, is composed of four members (FOXO1, 3A, 4 and 6) that are expressed in specific tissues. When phosphorylated by AKT, FOXO proteins become deactivated and leave the nucleus to the cytoplasm, where they remain inactive. When dephosphorylated, FOXO proteins bind regulatory factors or undergo post-transcriptional modifications, regain activity and return to the nucleus, where they promote the transcription of genes that modulate a diversity of biological processes as follows.

FOXO proteins show a major participation in proteostasis maintenance (Webb & Brunet, 2014), thus indicating that the process is activated when IGF-1 signaling is turned off. They may act by direct upregulation of E3 ubiquitin ligase that attaches ubiquitinylated protein to the proteasome, or by directly regulating proteasome components. In addition, FOXO proteins foster macroautophagy by binding to promoters of relevant genes as light chain 3 β (*Lc3b*) or autophagy-related gene 12 (*Atg12)*, whose products are required for autophagosome formation (Webb & Brunet, 2014). Another mechanism is via the upregulation of glutamine synthetase; the increase in intracellular glutamine levels is accompanied by an inhibitory effect upon mTORC1, referred to later, resulting in additional autophagy promotion and survival (van der Vos *et al.*, 2012).

FOXO proteins, in addition, promote the upregulation of catalase, MnSOD and the growth arrest and DNA damage45 (Gadd45) protein (Manolagas & Almeida, 2007; Vurusaner *et al.*, 2012). While MnSOD, a characteristic mitochondrial enzyme, converts superoxide anion into H_2O_2, catalase breaks it into oxygen and water, and Gadd45 is fundamental for DNA repair following mutagenic damage.

Therefore, by activating different mechanisms, FOXO proteins prevent the harmful effects of oxidation, repair DNA damage and provide for proteostasis, by destroying abnormal proteins either at the proteasome or upon autophagy promotion. As a whole, this action mitigates the errors made when biochemical pathways are in progress, supports cell survival and extends longevity.

It is not surprising that, having such abilities, FOXO3A gene has been found to be associated with long-lived individuals in more than one study, providing further evidence that ageing, the progressive functional impairment that leads to death, is the result of cumulative molecular dysfunction and errors that evolve in the course of fundamental biological processes.

1.5.2.3 Other pathways

The mechanistic (originally, mammalian) target of rapamycin, mTOR, is a member of the phosphoinositide-3-kinase-related protein kinases family, which includes PI3K. In mammals, the enzyme is a component of two different protein complexes, the mTORC1 and the mTORC2 (Guertin & Sabatini, 2007).

Growth factors, such as IGF-1, amino acids and stressful conditions, such as hypoxia, all may activate mTORC1. Upon insulin or IGF-1 interaction with their receptors, a pathway signals to AKT activation in a process similar to FOXO activation. AKT then targets tuberin, a component of a GTPase activating protein, rendering it inactive; consequently, tuberin substrates such as Rheb (Ras homolog enriched in brain), a small GTPase protein, are kept at the GTP-bound, active form. In this situation, Rheb-GTP is able to exert its strong and essential role of promoting mTORC1 kinase activity (Cai *et al.*, 2006).

The activation of mTOR results in essential life maintenance biological processes such as protein synthesis, which includes RNA transcription, ribosome assembly and mRNA translation. In fact, mTORC1's main substrates are eIF-4E binding protein 1 (4E-BP1) and the S6 kinase 1 (S6K1). The 4E-BP1 protein is usually bound to the eukaryotic protein synthesis initiation factor 4E (eIF4E), which renders it unable to continue to perform mRNA activation and protein synthesis initiation; in anabolic conditions, mTORC1 phosphorylates 4E-BP1 protein, which dissociates from the eIF4E, which then associates with eIF4G and makes it ready to enter protein synthesis. Activation of S6K1 by mTORC1 results in phosphorylation of small ribosome subunit S6 and other substrates such as RNA polymerase I, essential for ribosomal RNA generation and protein production (Wullschleger *et al.*, 2006).

In addition, mTORC1 has an important involvement in autophagy, directly related to the intracellular and environmental metabolic conditions. When they are good, mTORC1 targets proteins such as Atg13, unc-51-like kinase 1 (ULK1) and ULK2, renders them inactive and blocks autophagosome formation (Rubinsztein *et al.*, 2011); in unfavorable nutritional conditions, mTORC1 is downregulated and the effect is reversed. Moreover, mTORC1 senses the intracellular energy level and redirects biological processes accordingly. When the AMP/ATP ratio increases, indicating a reduced energy content (Hardie & Hawley, 2001), AMP kinase is activated in order to enhance intracellular ATP level; this metabolic change results in mTORC1 signaling depression and a shift into an energy-sparing condition that includes protein synthesis downregulation and macromolecule catabolism to obtain usable energy.

Therefore, mTORC1 is very sensitive to the cell nutritional environment and is at the center of a successful biological process that appeared long ago in the evolutionary scale and persisted from yeast to mammals in a conserved fashion (Sabatini *et al.*, 1994). When the environment is one of abundance, it is signaled into the cell and recognized by an, as yet unknown, sensor molecule that triggers a transductive pathway resulting in cell growth; in unfavorable conditions such as nutrient shortage, mTORC1 expression is depressed, which stalls the anabolic effect and raises the inhibitory barrier to autophagy, that is, it sequesters cytoplasm portions in a membrane, digests them and recycles the contents (discussed in Chapter 2). In view of wide variation in the nutritional environment, these regulatory properties are very useful for survival because, in particular, when shortage is prolonged, as in ER, the change into an energy-sparing mode and the use of autophagy elicit an extension of longevity.

Much of the knowledge in this setting comes from the use of the mTORC1-specific and strong inhibitor rapamycin. The effect, observed in cells, is likely to take place in whole organisms and various species. In fact, there is substantial evidence that rapamycin administration to mice results in extension of their life, including an association with better health standards (Harrison *et al.*, 2009; Wilkinson *et al.*, 2012; Zhang *et al.*, 2014). These observations have highlighted the regulation of mTORC1 as a promising way to tackle human ageing.

1.6 Conclusions and prospects

> What matters to Mrs Jane Doe to be like a goldsmith shopfront: silver forehead, golden hair, emerald eyes, nacred face, rubi mouth, pearled teeth or crystal neck? Indeed, if she is inattentive somewhat, in time her old age hour will come ... Because silver tarnishes, gold dims, emeralds dull, the nacred darkens, rubis bleach, pearls lose luster, crystal cracks, and all changes, not just the shape but the substance too.
>
> *(In "Apólogos dialogais", Francisco Manuel de Mello, Portuguese writer, 1608–66.)*

Looking at all the scientific advances made so far, ageing, progressive time-related reduced functional ability remains intriguing. Ageing is a biological process and, as such, is amenable to analysis employing techniques suitable to the study of other biological processes of organisms such as cell signaling or the cell cycle. A major difference, however, is that, instead of being one event in a life, ageing is much more the event of life, after the developmental program is concluded. This point considerably changes the usual scientific strategies.

From one perspective, ageing emerged as a biological novelty because the process is rarely seen in the wild. Even for humans, although some have reached old age in the past, the possibility that a large number of them will see themselves ageing, is recent. What has changed is the ability to overcome external causes of longevity limitation such as bad sanitary conditions, including appropriate housing and nutrition, and infectious agents that once caused major human mortality. In the 14th century, in just a few years, the Black Death killed about 50% of Europeans; nowadays the agent *Yersinia pestis* still causes a serious, albeit treatable, infection. In this setting of public health, courageous decisions and the progress as a whole have resulted in amazing improvements, as evidenced by the increase of life expectancy: in Sweden for example, it rose from 45 years in 1840 to 84 years in 2012.

In a time of many questions being asked, and many being answered too, there remains the ever puzzling question of why we age. Regrettably, a final answer is not known yet.

We are convinced, though, that as ageing is the event of life, explanations for ageing should be sought in the essence of life-in-action. In our view, such essence is centered on the ingenious, sequential electron transport at the respiratory chain and, because the transport process is imperfect, on the simultaneous production of harmful by-products as oxygen free radicals. The hypothesis that these compounds cause ageing is quite attractive because of the mechanistic explanation provided; yet strangely, the hypothesis will never achieve final proof in the sense that it would not be possible to prove the reverse, that is, that a cell or tissue system will not age when free radical production is prevented – an experimental absurd, taking into account life as we know it.

Sound research favors the view that continuous, untoward metabolic errors, taking place throughout life, underlie the decline of the functional ability. Their permanent presence makes tissues and organisms become frail and susceptible to disease, which at a certain time will terminate the organism's life. That is, ageing is a risk factor for disease and disease is a risk factor for death.

Cancer and atheromatous cardiovascular diseases are the most common causes of death in older individuals and have been the subject of concern all over the world. Cancer is a kind of new event in the biology of cells that acquire new properties such as immortality. For the detection of these cells in individuals, screening programs and causal agent avoidance have been devised and implemented over time; the treatment is cell removal, which may be successful enough to achieve a cure or may be unsuccessful and terminate the organism's life. Cell from degenerative, age-dependent disorders are different. Instead of acquiring new vital properties, as cancer cells do, many of them exhibit the deposition of damaged molecules that break their functioning and may cause their death. As the selective disposal of accumulated products is unlikely, the treatment anticipated to be most effective will be old cell replenishment or replacement with new cells.

How do we address these matters hoping to ameliorate human ageing? As a biological issue, the first approach is experimental, although it is faced with an important difficulty, which is the choice of the model to employ. Cells are useful to analyze metabolic pathways but it is uncertain how much the *in vitro* ageing cell model reflects *in vivo* conditions. Therefore, animal studies are necessary and, despite the plasticity one may find in looking at different tissues, ageing concerns the whole organism and is a product of interdependence. The use of mammals is the most logical decision, but it faces husbandry challenges that other organisms such as flies and worms do not; in turn these are evolutionarily distant from humans.

As a societal issue, another action is to increase the public awareness of degenerative diseases and foster education concerning healthy lifestyles. It is interesting that the only experimental way to mitigate disease and enhance longevity in nongenetically engineered animals is by restricting the amount of daily energy ingestion. The conclusions are robust in rodents and may apply to nonhuman primates. Limited experience with human subjects who have decided to adhere to such a harsh dietary regime has produced results that appear comparable to those in small mammals. However, caution should be taken when comparing or extrapolating data obtained in evolutionarily distant species.

Public awareness is frequently distorted by attractive announcements of cures or treatments for ageing. In fact, there is no such thing – it should be remembered that ageing is not a disease, but a disease-prone condition. Therefore, a permanent educational effort is advisable to emphasize the benefits of improving the health of humans, in contrast to unreal expectations of extending their lifespan. Much as healthy ageing is the consensual aim for the gerontology scientist to investigate, it ought to be the purpose of the common man to seek.

Abstaining from environmental hazards and pursuing a lifestyle without excess in ingested food and sedentary habits is a good decision in view of epidemiologic data. It is also useful to have a favorable set of genes and, among them, those that regulate metabolism.

Exciting news is constantly arriving, reporting ways to modulate the profound cell mechanisms that control nutrient sensing, uptake and utilization. The *in vivo* application of some molecules in rodents provides evidence for benefits in terms of healthier and longer lifespan. There is hope that the same benefits may not reveal unwanted side effects when used in humans for the purpose of ameliorating health and postponing the establishment of disorders.

Acknowledgment

We thank Sérgio Evangelista, Laboratório de Iconografia, Faculdade de Medicina da Universidade do Porto, for art work.

References

Acosta, J. C., A. Banito, T. Wuestefeld, A. Georgilis, P. Janich, J. P. Morton, D. Athineos, T. W. Kang, F. Lasitschka, M. Andrulis, G. Pascual, K. J. Morris, S. Khan, H. Jin, G. Dharmalingam, A. P. Snijders, T. Carroll, D. Capper, C. Pritchard, G. J. Inman, T. Longerich, O. J. Sansom, S. A. Benitah, L. Zender, and J. Gil. 2013. A complex secretory program orchestrated by the inflammasome controls paracrine senescence. *Nat. Cell Biol.* 15:978–990.

Ahmed, E. K., A. Rogowska-Wrzesinska, P. Roepstorff, A. L. Bulteau, and B. Friguet. 2010. Protein modification and replicative senescence of WI-38 human embryonic fibroblasts. *Aging Cell* 9:252–272.

Alcorta, D. A., Y. Xiong, D. Phelps, G. Hannon, D. Beach, and J. C. Barrett. 1996. Involvement of the cyclin-dependent kinase inhibitor p16 (INK4a) in replicative senescence of normal human fibroblasts. *Proc. Natl Acad. Sci. USA* 93:13742–13747.

Al-Khalaf, H. H. and A. Aboussekhra. 2013. Survivin expression increases during aging and enhances the resistance of aged human fibroblasts to genotoxic stress. *Age (Dordr.)* 35:549–562.

Allsopp, R. C. 1996. Models of initiation of replicative senescence by loss of telomeric DNA. *Exp. Gerontol.* 31:235–243.

Almeida, H., M. C. Magalhães, and M. M. Magalhães. 1998. Age-related changes in the inner zone of the adrenal cortex of the rat – a morphologic and biochemical study. *Mech. Ageing Dev.* 105:1–18.

Andersen, S. L., P. Sebastiani, D. A. Dworkis, L. Feldman, and T. T. Perls. 2012. Health span approximates life span among many supercentenarians: compression of morbidity at the approximate limit of life span. *J. Gerontol. A. Biol. Sci. Med. Sci.* 67:395–405.

Baker, D. J., T. Wijshake, T. Tchkonia, N. K. Lebrasseur, B. G. Childs, B. Van De Sluis, J. L. Kirkland, and J. M. Van Deursen. 2011. Clearance of p16Ink4a-positive senescent cells delays ageing-associated disorders. *Nature* 479:232–236.

Baraibar, M. A. and B. Friguet. 2013. Oxidative proteome modifications target specific cellular pathways during oxidative stress, cellular senescence and aging. *Exp. Gerontol.* 48:620–625.

Barja, G. and A. Herrero. 1998. Localization at complex I and mechanism of the higher free radical production of brain nonsynaptic mitochondria in the short-lived rat than in the longevous pigeon. *J. Bioenerg. Biomembr.* 30:235–243.

Bartke, A. 2005. Minireview: role of the growth hormone/insulin-like growth factor system in mammalian aging. *Endocrinology* 146:3718–3723.

Bartke, A. 2011. Growth hormone, insulin and aging: the benefits of endocrine defects. *Exp. Gerontol.* 46:108–111.

Barzilai, N., I. Gabriely, M. Gabriely, N. Iankowitz, and J. D. Sorkin. 2001. Offspring of centenarians have a favorable lipid profile. *J. Am. Geriatr. Soc.* 49:76–79.

Beckman, K. B. and B. N. Ames. 1998. The free radical theory of aging matures. *Physiol. Rev.* 78:547–581.

Beekman, M., H. Blanche, M. Perola, A. Hervonen, V. Bezrukov, E. Sikora, F. Flachsbart, L. Christiansen, A. J. De Craen, T. B. Kirkwood, I. M. Rea, M. Poulain, J. M. Robine, S. Valensin, M. A. Stazi, G. Passarino, L. Deiana, E. S. Gonos, L. Paternoster, T. I. Sorensen, Q. Tan, Q. Helmer, E. B. Van Den Akker, J. Deelen, F. Martella, H. J. Cordell, K. L. Ayers, J. W. Vaupel, O. Tornwall, T. E. Johnson, S. Schreiber, M. Lathrop, A. Skytthe, R. G. Westendorp, K. Christensen, J. Gampe, A. Nebel, J. J. Houwing-Duistermaat, P. E. Slagboom, C. Franceschi, and GEHA Consortium. 2013. Genome-wide linkage analysis for human longevity: Genetics of Healthy Aging Study. *Aging Cell* 12:184–193.

Benavides, S. H., A. J. Monserrat, S. Farina and E. A. Porta. 2002. Sequential histochemical studies of neuronal lipofuscin in human cerebral cortex from the first to the ninth decade of life. *Arch. Gerontol. Geriatr.* 34:219–231.

Berzlanovich, A. M., W. Keil, T. Waldhoer, E. Sim, P. Fasching, and B. Fazeny-Dorner. 2005. Do centenarians die healthy? An autopsy study. *J. Gerontol. A. Biol. Sci. Med. Sci.* 60:862–865.

Blackburn, E. H. 1991. Structure and function of telomeres. *Nature* 350:569–573.

Blackburn, E. H. 1992. Telomerases. *Annu. Rev. Biochem.* 61:113–129.

Blumenthal, H. T. 2002. The autopsy in gerontological research: a retrospective. *J. Gerontol. A. Biol. Sci. Med. Sci.* 57:M433–437.

Bodnar, A. G., M. Ouellette, M. Frolkis, S. E. Holt, C. P. Chiu, G. B. Morin, C. B. Harley, J. W. Shay, S. Lichtsteiner, and W. E. Wright. 1998. Extension of life-span by introduction of telomerase into normal human cells. *Science* 279:349–352.

Boffoli, D., S. C. Scacco, R. Vergari, G. Solarino, G. Santacroce, and S. Papa. 1994. Decline with age of the respiratory chain activity in human skeletal muscle. *Biochim. Biophys. Acta* 1226:73–82.

Bokov, A., A. Chaudhuri, and A. Richardson. 2004. The role of oxidative damage and stress in aging. *Mech. Ageing Dev.* 125:811–826.

Bonkowski, M. S., F. P. Dominici, O. Arum, J. S. Rocha, K. A. Al Regaiey, R. Westbrook, A. Spong, J. Panici, M. M. Masternak, J. J. Kopchick, and A. Bartke. 2009. Disruption of growth hormone receptor prevents calorie restriction from improving insulin action and longevity. *PLoS One* 4:e4567.

Bratic, A. and N. G. Larsson. 2013. The role of mitochondria in aging. *J. Clin. Invest.* 123:951–957.

Brody, J. A. and E. L. Schneider. 1986. Diseases and disorders of aging: an hypothesis. *J. Chronic Dis.* 39:871–876.

Brooks-Wilson, A. R. 2013. Genetics of healthy aging and longevity. *Hum. Genet.* 132:1323–1338.

Brown-Borg, H. M., K. E. Borg, C. J. Meliska, and A. Bartke. 1996. Dwarf mice and the ageing process. *Nature* 384:33.

Brunk, U. T. and A. Terman. 2002a. Lipofuscin: mechanisms of age-related accumulation and influence on cell function. *Free Radic. Biol. Med.* 33:611–619.

Brunk, U. T. and A. Terman. 2002b. The mitochondrial–lysosomal axis theory of aging: accumulation of damaged mitochondria as a result of imperfect autophagocytosis. *Eur. J. Biochem.* 269:1996–2002.

Cadenas, E. and K. J. Davies. 2000. Mitochondrial free radical generation, oxidative stress, and aging. *Free Radic. Biol. Med.* 29:222–230.

Cai, S. L., A. R. Tee, J. D. Short, J. M. Bergeron, J. Kim, J. Shen, R. Guo, C. L. Johnson, K. Kiguchi, and C. L. Walker. 2006. Activity of TSC2 is inhibited by AKT-mediated phosphorylation and membrane partitioning. *J. Cell Biol.* 173:279–289.

Campbell, A. J. and D. M. Buchner. 1997. Unstable disability and the fluctuations of frailty. *Age Ageing* 26:315–318.

Carnes, B. A., S. J. Olshansky, and D. Grahn. 2003. Biological evidence for limits to the duration of life. *Biogerontology* 4:31–45.

Castro, J. P., C. Ott, T. Jung, T. Grune, and H. Almeida. 2012a. Carbonylation of the cytoskeletal protein actin leads to aggregate formation. *Free Radic. Biol. Med.* 53:916–925.

Castro, J. P., T. Jung, T. Grune, and H. Almeida. 2013. Actin carbonylation: from cell dysfunction to organism disorder. *J. Proteomics* 92:171–180.

Castro, R. M., E. Suarez, E. Kraiselburd, A. Isidro, J. Paz, L. Ferder, and S. Ayala-Torres. 2012b. Aging increases mitochondrial DNA damage and oxidative stress in liver of rhesus monkeys. *Exp. Gerontol.* 47:29–37.

Chen, Q. and B. N. Ames. 1994. Senescence-like growth arrest induced by hydrogen-peroxide in human-diploid fibroblast F65 cells. *Proc. Natl Acad. Sci. USA* 91:4130–4134.

Chen, Q. M., J. C. Bartholomew, J. Campisi, M. Acosta, J. D. Reagan, and B. N. Ames. 1998. Molecular analysis of H_2O_2-induced senescent-like growth arrest in normal human fibroblasts: p53 and Rb control G1 arrest but not cell replication. *Biochem. J.* 332:43–50.

Chen, Q. M., J. Liu, and J. B. Merrett. 2000a. Apoptosis or senescence-like growth arrest: influence of cell-cycle position, p53, p21 and bax in H2O2 response of normal human fibroblasts. *Biochem. J.* 347:543–551.

Chen, Q. M., V. C. Tu, J. Catania, M. Burton, O. Toussaint, and T. Dilley. 2000b. Involvement of Rb family proteins, focal adhesion proteins and protein synthesis in senescent morphogenesis induced by hydrogen peroxide. *J. Cell Sci.* 113:4087–4097.

Chen, Q. M., K. R. Prowse, V. C. Tu, S. Purdom, and M. H. Linskens. 2001. Uncoupling the senescent phenotype from telomere shortening in hydrogen peroxide-treated fibroblasts. *Exp. Cell Res.* 265:294–303.

Christensen, K., G. Doblhammer, R. Rau, and J. W. Vaupel. 2009. Ageing populations: the challenges ahead. *Lancet* 374:1196–1208.

Colman, R. J., R. M. Anderson, S. C. Johnson, E. K. Kastman, K. J. Kosmatka, T. M. Beasley, D. B. Allison, C. Cruzen, H. A. Simmons, J. W. Kemnitz, and R. Weindruch. 2009. Caloric restriction delays disease onset and mortality in rhesus monkeys. *Science* 325:201–204.

Comfort, A. 1956. The biology of ageing. *Lancet* 271:772–778.

Coppe, J. P., C. K. Patil, F. Rodier, Y. Sun, D. P. Munoz, J. Goldstein, P. S. Nelson, P. Y. Desprez, and J. Campisi. 2008. Senescence-associated secretory phenotypes reveal cell-nonautonomous functions of oncogenic RAS and the p53 tumor suppressor. *PLoS Biol.* 6:2853–2868.

Corbisier, P. and J. Remacle. 1990. Involvement of mitochondria in cell degeneration. *Eur. J. Cell Biol.* 51:173–182.

Corder, E. H., A. M. Saunders, W. J. Strittmatter, D. E. Schmechel, P. C. Gaskell, G. W. Small, A. D. Roses, J. L. Haines, and M. A. Pericak-Vance. 1993. Gene dose of apolipoprotein E type 4 allele and the risk of Alzheimer's disease in late onset families. *Science* 261:921–923.

Cristofalo, V. J. 2005. SA beta Gal staining: biomarker or delusion. *Exp. Gerontol.* 40:836–838.

Curtis, J. M., W. S. Hahn, E. K. Long, J. S. Burrill, E. A. Arriaga, and D. A. Bernlohr. 2012. Protein carbonylation and metabolic control systems. *Trends Endocrinol. Metab.* 23.399–406.

Cutler, R. G. and M. P. Mattson. 2006. The adversities of aging. *Ageing Res. Rev.* 5:221–238.

David, D. C., N. Ollikainen, J. C. Trinidad, M. P. Cary, A. L. Burlingame, and C. Kenyon. 2010. Widespread protein aggregation as an inherent part of aging in *C. elegans*. *PLoS Biol.* 8:e1000450.

Davies, K. J. and R. Shringarpure. 2006. Preferential degradation of oxidized proteins by the 20S proteasome may be inhibited in aging and in inflammatory neuromuscular diseases. *Neurology* 66:S93–96.

Dayan, D., I. Abrahami, A. Buchner, M. Gorsky, and N. Chimovitz. 1988. Lipid pigment (lipofuscin) in human perioral muscles with aging. *Experimental Gerontology* 23:97–102.

Debacq-Chainlaux, F., C. Borlon, T. Pascal, V. Royer, F. Eliaers, N. Ninane, G. Carrard, B. Friguet, F. De Longueville, S. Boffe, J. Remacle, and O. Toussaint. 2005. Repeated exposure of human skin fibroblasts to UVB at subcytotoxic level triggers premature senescence through the TGF-beta 1 signaling pathway. *J. Cell Sci.* 118:743–758.

Debacq-Chainiaux, F., T. Pascal, E. Boilan, C. Bastin, E. Bauwens, and O. Toussaint. 2008. Screening of senescence-associated genes with specific DNA array reveals the role of IGFBP-3 in premature senescence of human diploid fibroblasts. *Free Radic. Biol. Med.* 44:1817–1832.

De Moraes, D. C., M. Vaisman, F. L. Conceicao, and T. M. Ortiga-Carvalho. 2012. Pituitary development: a complex, temporal regulated process dependent on specific transcriptional factors. *J. Endocrinol.* 215:239–245.

Diehr, P. H., S. M. Thielke, A. B. Newman, C. Hirsch, and R. Tracy. 2013. Decline in health for older adults: five-year change in 13 key measures of standardized health. *J. Gerontol. A. Biol. Sci. Med. Sci.* 68:1059–1067.

Dimri, G. P., X. H. Lee, G. Basile, M. Acosta, C. Scott, C. Roskelley, E. E. Medrano, M. Linskens, I. Rubelj, O. Pereirasmith, M. Peacocke, and J. Campisi. 1995. A biomarker that identifies senescent human-cells in culture and in aging skin in-vivo. *Proc. Natl Acad. Sci. U.S.A* 92:9363–9367.

Ding, G., N. Franki, A. A. Kapasi, K. Reddy, N. Gibbons, and P. C. Singhal. 2001. Tubular cell senescence and expression of TGF-beta1 and p21(WAF1/CIP1) in tubulointerstitial fibrosis of aging rats. *Exp. Mol. Pathol.* 70:43–53.

Double, K. L., V. N. Dedov, H. Fedorow, E. Kettle, G. M. Halliday, B. Garner, and U. T. Brunk. 2008. The comparative biology of neuromelanin and lipofuscin in the human brain. *Cell. Mol. Life Sci.* 65:1669–1682.

Duan, J., Z. Zhang, and T. Tong. 2005. Irreversible cellular senescence induced by prolonged exposure to H2O2 involves DNA-damage-and-repair genes and telomere shortening. *Int. J. Biochem. Cell Biol.* 37:1407–1420.

Dumont, P., M. Burton, Q. M. Chen, E. S. Gonos, C. Frippiat, J. B. Mazarati, F. Eliaers, J. Remacle, and O. Toussaint. 2000. Induction of replicative senescence biomarkers by sublethal oxidative stresses in normal human fibroblast. *Free Radic. Biol. Med.* 28:361–373.

Finch, C. E. 2007. *The Biology of Human Longevity – Inflammation, Nutrition, and Aging in the Evolution of Lifespans.* Burlington, MA: Academic Press.

Flachsbart, F., A. Caliebe, R. Kleindorp, H. Blanche, H. Von Eller-Eberstein, S. Nikolaus, S. Schreiber, and A. Nebel. 2009. Association of FOXO3A variation with human longevity confirmed in German centenarians. *Proc. Natl Acad. Sci. USA* 106:2700–2705.

Flurkey, K., J. Papaconstantinou, R. A. Miller, and D. E. Harrison. 2001. Lifespan extension and delayed immune and collagen aging in mutant mice with defects in growth hormone production. *Proc. Natl Acad. Sci. USA* 98:6736–6741.

Flurkey, K., J. Papaconstantinou, and D. E. Harrison. 2002. The Snell dwarf mutation Pit1(dw) can increase life span in mice. *Mech. Ageing Dev.* 123:121–130.

Fontana, L., L. Partridge, and V. D. Longo. 2010. Extending healthy life span – from yeast to humans. *Science* 328:321–326.

Förstermann, U. and W. C. Sessa. 2012. Nitric oxide synthases: regulation and function. *Eur. Heart J.* 33:829–837, 837a–837d.

Fried, L. P., L. Ferrucci, J. Darer, J. D. Williamson, and G. Anderson. 2004. Untangling the concepts of disability, frailty, and comorbidity: implications for improved targeting and care. *J. Gerontol. A. Biol. Sci. Med. Sci.* 59:255–263.

Friedman, D. B. and T. E. Johnson. 1988. A mutation in the age-1 gene in *Caenorhabditis elegans* lengthens life and reduces hermaphrodite fertility. *Genetics* 118:75–86.

Fries, J. F. 1980. Aging, natural death, and the compression of morbidity. *New Engl. J. Med.* 303:130–135.

Frippiat, C., Q. M. Chen, S. Zdanov, J. P. Magalhães, J. Remacle, and O. Toussaint. 2001. Subcytotoxic H2O2 stress triggers a release of transforming growth factor-beta 1, which induces biomarkers of cellular senescence of human diploid fibroblasts. *J. Biol. Chem.* 276:2531–2537.

Furumoto, K., E. Inoue, N. Nagao, E. Hiyama, and N. Miwa. 1998. Age-dependent telomere shortening is slowed down by enrichment of intracellular vitamin C via suppression of oxidative stress. *Life Sci.* 63:935–948.

Gavrilov, L. A. and N. S. Gavrilova. 2006. Reliability theory of aging and longevity. *In:* E. J. Masoroand and S. N. Austad (eds) *Handbook of the Biology of Aging*, 6th edn. Burlington, MA: Academic Press.

Gerdes, L. U., B. Jeune, K. A. Ranberg, H. Nybo, and J. W. Vaupel. 2000. Estimation of apolipoprotein E genotype-specific relative mortality risks from the distribution of genotypes in centenarians and middle-aged men: apolipoprotein E gene is a "frailty gene," not a "longevity gene". *Genet. Epidemiol.* 19:202–210.

Godfrey, P., J. O. Rahal, W. G. Beamer, N. G. Copeland, N. A. Jenkins, and K. E. Mayo. 1993. GHRH receptor of little mice contains a missense mutation in the extracellular domain that disrupts receptor function. *Nat. Genet.* 4:227–232.

Gomez-Cabrera, M. C., F. Sanchis-Gomar, R. Garcia-Valles, H. Pareja-Galeano, J. Gambini, C. Borras, and J. Vina. 2012. Mitochondria as sources and targets of damage in cellular aging. *Clin. Chem. Lab. Med.* 50:1287–1295.

Greenberg, S. B., G. L. Grove, and V. J. Cristofalo. 1977. Cell size in aging monolayer cultures. *In Vitro* 13:297–300.

Guertin, D. A. and D. M. Sabatini. 2007. Defining the role of mTOR in cancer. *Cancer Cell* 12:9–22.

Guevara-Aguirre, J., P. Balasubramanian, M. Guevara-Aguirre, M. Wei, F. Madia, C. W. Cheng, D. Hwang, A. Martin-Montalvo, J. Saavedra, S. Ingles, R. De Cabo, P. Cohen, and V. D. Longo. 2011. Growth hormone receptor deficiency is associated with a major reduction in pro-aging signaling, cancer, and diabetes in humans. *Sci. Transl. Med.* 3:70ra13.

Hampel, B., F. Malisan, H. Niederegger, R. Testi, and P. Jansen-Durr. 2004. Differential regulation of apoptotic cell death in senescent human cells. *Exp. Gerontol.* 39:1713–1721.

Hardie, D. G. and S. A. Hawley. 2001. AMP-activated protein kinase: the energy charge hypothesis revisited. *Bioessays* 23:1112–1119.

Harding, C., F. Pompei, E. E. Lee, and R. Wilson. 2008. Cancer suppression at old age. *Cancer Res.* 68:4465–4478.

Harley, C. B., A. B. Futcher, and C. W. Greider. 1990. Telomeres shorten during ageing of human fibroblasts. *Nature* 345:458–460.

Harman, D. 1956. Aging: a theory based on free radical and radiation chemistry. *J. Gerontol.* 11:298–300.

Harman, D. 1972. The biologic clock: the mitochondria? *J. Am. Geriatr. Soc.* 20:145–147.

Harrison, D. E., R. Strong, Z. D. Sharp, J. F. Nelson, C. M. Astle, K. Flurkey, N. L. Nadon, J. E. Wilkinson, K. Frenkel, C. S. Carter, M. Pahor, M. A. Javors, E. Fernandez, and R. A. Miller. 2009. Rapamycin fed late in life extends lifespan in genetically heterogeneous mice. *Nature* 460:392–395.

Hayflick, L. 2000. The future of ageing. *Nature* 408:267–269.

Hayflick, L. 2004. The not-so-close relationship between biological aging and age-associated pathologies in humans. *J. Gerontol. A. Biol. Sci. Med. Sci.* 59:B547–550, discussion 551–543.

Hayflick, L. and P. S. Moorhead. 1961. Serial cultivation of human diploid cell strains. *Exp. Cell Res.* 25:585–621.

Herbig, U., M. Ferreira, L. Condel, D. Carey, and J. M. Sedivy. 2006. Cellular senescence in aging primates. *Science* 311:1257.

Herskind, A. M., M. Mcgue, T. I. Sorensen, and B. Harvald. 1996. Sex and age specific assessment of genetic and environmental influences on body mass index in twins. *Int. J. Obes. Relat. Metab. Disord.* 20:106–113.

Hewitt, G., D. Jurk, F. D. Marques, C. Correia-Melo, T. Hardy, A. Gackowska, R. Anderson, M. Taschuk, J. Mann, and J. F. Passos. 2012. Telomeres are favoured targets of a persistent DNA damage response in ageing and stress-induced senescence. *Nat. Commun.* 3:708.

Hjelmborg, J., I. Iachine, A. Skytthe, J. W. Vaupel, M. Mcgue, M. Koskenvuo, J. Kaprio, N. L. Pedersen, and K. Christensen. 2006. Genetic influence on human lifespan and longevity. *Hum. Genet.* 119:312–321.

Hochschild, R. 1990. Can an index of aging be constructed for evaluating treatments to retard aging rates? A 2,462-person study. *J. Gerontol.* 45:B187–214.

Hohn, A., T. Jung, S. Grimm, and T. Grune. 2010. Lipofuscin-bound iron is a major intracellular source of oxidants: role in senescent cells. *Free Radic. Biol. Med.* 48:1100–1108.

Holliday, R. 2004. The close relationship between biological aging and age-associated pathologies in humans. *J. Gerontol. A. Biol. Sci. Med. Sci.* 59:B543–546.

Holliday, R. 2006. Aging is no longer an unsolved problem in biology. *Ann. N. Y. Acad. Sci.* 1067:1–9.

Holzenberger, M., J. Dupont, B. Ducos, P. Leneuve, A. Geloen, P. C. Even, P. Cervera, and Y. Le Bouc. 2003. IGF-1 receptor regulates lifespan and resistance to oxidative stress in mice. *Nature* 421:182–187.

Horiuchi, S., C. E. Finch, F. Mesle, and J. Vallin. 2003. Differential patterns of age-related mortality increase in middle age and old age. *J. Gerontol. A. Biol. Sci. Med. Sci.* 58:495–507.

Huang, L. C., K. C. Clarkin, and G. M. Wahl. 1996. Sensitivity and selectivity of the DNA damage sensor responsible for activating p53-dependent G1 arrest. *Proc. Natl Acad. Sci. USA* 93:4827–4832.

Itahana, K., J. Campisi, and G. P. Dimri. 2007. Methods to detect biomarkers of cellular senescence: the senescence-associated beta-galactosidase assay. *Methods Mol. Biol.* 371:21–31.

Itahana, K., Y. Itahana, and G. P. Dimri. 2013. Colorimetric detection of senescence-associated beta galactosidase. *Methods Mol. Biol.* 965:143–156.

Jeyapalan, J. C., M. Ferreira, J. M. Sedivy, and U. Herbig. 2007. Accumulation of senescent cells in mitotic tissue of aging primates. *Mech. Ageing Dev.* 128:36–44.

Jones, O. R., A. Scheuerlein, R. Salguero-Gomez, C. G. Camarda, R. Schaible, B. B. Casper, J. P. Dahlgren, J. Ehrlen, M. B. Garcia, E. S. Menges, P. F. Quintana-Ascencio, H. Caswell, A. Baudisch, and J. W. Vaupel. 2014. Diversity of ageing across the tree of life. *Nature* 505:169–173.

Jung, T., N. Bader, and T. Grune. 2007. Lipofuscin: formation, distribution, and metabolic consequences. *Ann. NY Acad. Sci.* 1119:97–111.

Jung, T., B. Catalgol, and T. Grune. 2009. The proteasomal system. *Mol. Aspects Med.* 30:191–296.

Kang, T. W., T. Yevsa, N. Woller, L. Hoenicke, T. Wuestefeld, D. Dauch, A. Hohmeyer, M. Gereke, R. Rudalska, A. Potapova, M. Iken, M. Vucur, S. Weiss, M. Heikenwalder, S. Khan, J. Gil, D. Bruder, M. Manns, P. Schirmacher, F. Tacke, M. Ott, T. Luedde, T. Longerich, S. Kubicka, and L. Zender. 2011. Senescence surveillance of pre-malignant hepatocytes limits liver cancer development. *Nature* 479:547–551.

Katz, M. L., G. E. Eldred, A. N. Siakotos, and N. Koppang. 1988. Characterization of disease-specific brain fluorophores in ceroid-lipofuscinosis. *Am. J. Med. Genet. Suppl.* 5:253–264.

Kenyon, C., J. Chang, E. Gensch, A. Rudner, and R. Tabtiang. 1993. A *C. elegans* mutant that lives twice as long as wild type. *Nature* 366:461–464.

Kirkwood, T. 1999. *Time of Our Lives: The Science of Human Aging*. Oxford: Oxford University Press.

Kirkwood, T. B. 2005. Understanding the odd science of aging. *Cell* 120:437–447.

Kirkwood, T. B. and S. N. Austad. 2000. Why do we age? *Nature* 408:233–238.

Kreiling, J. A., M. Tamamori-Adachi, A. N. Sexton, J. C. Jeyapalan, U. Munoz-Najar, A. L. Peterson, J. Manivannan, E. S. Rogers, N. A. Pchelintsev, P. D. Adams, and J. M. Sedivy. 2011. Age-associated increase in heterochromatic marks in murine and primate tissues. *Aging Cell* 10:292–304.

Kuilman, T. and D. S. Peeper. 2009. Senescence-messaging secretome: SMS-ing cellular stress. *Nat. Rev. Cancer* 9:81–94.

Laron, Z. 2004. Laron syndrome (primary growth hormone resistance or insensitivity): the personal experience 1958–2003. *J. Clin. Endocrinol. Metab.* 89:1031–1044.

Lee, H. C., P. H. Yin, C. W. Chi, and Y. H. Wei. 2002. Increase in mitochondrial mass in human fibroblasts under oxidative stress and during replicative cell senescence. *J. Biomed. Sci.* 9:517–526.

Lee, Y. H., N. H. Lee, G. Bhattarai, P. H. Hwang, T. I. Kim, E. C. Jhee, and H. K. Yi. 2010. c-myb has a character of oxidative stress resistance in aged human diploid fibroblasts: regulates SAPK/JNK and Hsp60 pathway consequently. *Biogerontology* 11:267–274.

Levine, R. L. and E. R. Stadtman. 2001. Oxidative modification of proteins during aging. *Exp. Gerontol.* 36:1495–1502.

Lipetz, J. and V. J. Cristofalo. 1972. Ultrastructural changes accompanying the aging of human diploid cells in culture. *J. Ultrastruct. Res.* 39:43–56.

Liu, J. L., S. Yakar, and D. Leroith. 2000. Conditional knockout of mouse insulin-like growth factor-1 gene using the Cre/loxP system. *Proc. Soc. Exp. Biol. Med.* 223:344–351.

López-Ótin, C., M. A. Blasco, L. Partridge, M. Serrano, and G. Kroemer. 2013. The hallmarks of aging. *Cell* 153:1194–1217.

Lowsky, D. J., S. J. Olshansky, J. Bhattacharya, and D. P. Goldman. 2014. Heterogeneity in healthy aging. *J. Gerontol. A. Biol. Sci. Med. Sci.* 69:640–649.

Ly, D. H., D. J. Lockhart, R. A. Lerner, and P. G. Schultz. 2000. Mitotic misregulation and human aging. *Science* 287:2486–2492.

Macario, A. J. and E. Conway De Macario. 2002. Sick chaperones and ageing: a perspective. *Ageing Res. Rev.* 1:295–311.

Macieira-Coelho, A. 2003. *Biology of aging*. Springer-Verlag, Berlin, Heidelberg.

Mahley, R. W. and S. C. Rall, Jr. 2000. Apolipoprotein E: far more than a lipid transport protein. *Annu. Rev. Genomics Hum. Genet.* 1:507–537.

Manolagas, S. C. and M. Almeida. 2007. Gone with the Wnts: beta-catenin, T-cell factor, forkhead box O, and oxidative stress in age-dependent diseases of bone, lipid, and glucose metabolism. *Mol. Endocrinol.* 21:2605–2614.

Masoro, E. J. 2006. Are age-associated diseases an integral part of aging? *In:* E. J. Masoroand and S. N. Austad (eds) *Handbook of the Biology of Aging*, 6th edn. Burlington, MA: Academic Press.

Matos, L., A. Gouveia, and H. Almeida. 2012. Copper ability to induce premature senescence in human fibroblasts. *Age (Dordr.)* 34:783–794.

Mattison, J. A., G. S. Roth, T. M. Beasley, E. M. Tilmont, A. M. Handy, R. L. Herbert, D. L. Longo, D. B. Allison, J. E. Young, M. Bryant, D. Barnard, W. F. Ward, W. Qi, D. K. Ingram, and R. De Cabo. 2012. Impact of caloric restriction on health and survival in rhesus monkeys from the NIA study. *Nature* 489:318–321.

Mecocci, P., U. Macgarvey, A. E. Kaufman, D. Koontz, J. M. Shoffner, D. C. Wallace, and M. F. Beal. 1993. Oxidative damage to mitochondrial DNA shows marked age-dependent increases in human brain. *Ann. Neurol.* 34:609–616.

Medawar, P. B. 1952. *An Unsolved Problem of Biology: An Inaugural Lecture Delivered at University College, London, 6 December, 1951*. London: H.K. Lewis.

Melo, F. M. 1998. *Os Relógios Falantes incluída em Apólogos Dialogais*, Braga-Coimbra, Angelus Novus. (In portuguese).

Morris, J. Z., H. A. Tissenbaum, and G. Ruvkun. 1996. A phosphatidylinositol-3-OH kinase family member regulating longevity and diapause in *Caenorhabditis elegans*. *Nature* 382:536–539.

Mullis, P. E. 2010. Genetics of isolated growth hormone deficiency. *J. Clin. Res. Pediatr. Endocrinol.* 2:52–62.

Murabito, J. M., R. Yuan, and K. L. Lunetta. 2012. The search for longevity and healthy aging genes: insights from epidemiological studies and samples of long-lived individuals. *J. Gerontol. A. Biol. Sci. Med. Sci.* 67:470–479.

Narita, M., S. Nũnez, E. Heard, A. W. Lin, S. A. Hearn, D. L. Spector, G. J. Hannon, and S. W. Lowe. 2003. Rb-mediated heterochromatin formation and silencing of E2F target genes during cellular senescence. *Cell* 113:703–716.

Newman, A. B., R. M. Boudreau, B. L. Naydeck, L. F. Fried, and T. B. Harris. 2008. A physiologic index of comorbidity: relationship to mortality and disability. *J. Gerontol. A. Biol. Sci. Med. Sci.* 63:603–609.

Nishio, K., A. Inoue, S. Qiao, H. Kondo, and A. Mimura. 2001. Senescence and cytoskeleton: overproduction of vimentin induces senescent-like morphology in human fibroblasts. *Histochem. Cell Biol.* 116:321–327.

Nuss, J. E., K. B. Choksi, J. H. Deford, and J. Papaconstantinou. 2008. Decreased enzyme activities of chaperones PDI and BiP in aged mouse livers. *Biochem. Biophys. Res. Commun.*365:355–361.

Oeppen, J. and J. W. Vaupel. 2002. Demography. Broken limits to life expectancy. *Science* 296:1029–1031.

Olovnikov, A. M. 1973. A theory of marginotomy. The incomplete copying of template margin in enzymic synthesis of polynucleotides and biological significance of the phenomenon. *J. Theor. Biol.* 41:181–190.

Olshansky, S. J. 2010. The law of mortality revisited: interspecies comparisons of mortality. *J. Comp. Pathol.* 142 Suppl 1:S4–9.

Paradis, V., N. Youssef, D. Dargere, N. Ba, F. Bonvoust, J. Deschatrette, and P. Bedossa. 2001. Replicative senescence in normal liver, chronic hepatitis C, and hepatocellular carcinomas. *Hum. Pathol.* 32:327–332.

Parker, M., P. Schön, M. Lagergren, and M. Thorslund. 2008. Functional ability in the elderly Swedish population from 1980 to 2005. *Eur. J. Ageing* 5:299–309.

Partridge, J. S., D. Harari, and J. K. Dhesi. 2012. Frailty in the older surgical patient: a review. *Age Ageing* 41:142–147.

Pendergrass, W. R., M. A. Lane, N. L. Bodkin, B. C. Hansen, D. K. Ingram, G. S. Roth, L. Yi, H. Bin, and N. S. Wolf. 1999. Cellular proliferation potential during aging and caloric restriction in rhesus monkeys (*Macaca mulatta*). *J. Cell. Physiol.* 180:123–130.

Perez, V. I., A. Bokov, H. Van Remmen, J. Mele, Q. Ran, Y. Ikeno, and A. Richardson. 2009. Is the oxidative stress theory of aging dead? *Biochim. Biophys. Acta* 1790:1005–1014.

Perez-Campo, R., M. Lopez-Torres, S. Cadenas, C. Rojas, and G. Barja. 1998. The rate of free radical production as a determinant of the rate of aging: evidence from the comparative approach. *J. Comp. Physiol. B* 168:149–158.

Perls, T., M. Shea-Drinkwater, J. Bowen-Flynn, S. B. Ridge, S. Kang, E. Joyce, M. Daly, S. J. Brewster, L. Kunkel, and A. A. Puca. 2000. Exceptional familial clustering for extreme longevity in humans. *J. Am. Geriatr. Soc.* 48:1483–1485.

Perls, T. T., J. Wilmoth, R. Levenson, M. Drinkwater, M. Cohen, H. Bogan, E. Joyce, S. Brewster, L. Kunkel, and A. Puca. 2002. Life-long sustained mortality advantage of siblings of centenarians. *Proc. Natl Acad. Sci. USA* 99:8442–8447.

Pfäffle, R. and J. Klammt. 2011. Pituitary transcription factors in the aetiology of combined pituitary hormone deficiency. *Best Pract. Res. Clin. Endocrinol. Metab.* 25:43–60.

Pignolo, R. J., B. G. Martin, J. H. Horton, A. N. Kalbach, and V. J. Cristofalo. 1998. The pathway of cell senescence: WI-38 cells arrest in late G1 and are unable to traverse the cell cycle from a true G0 state. *Exp. Gerontol.* 33:67–80.

Pollak, M. 2012. The insulin receptor/insulin-like growth factor receptor family as a therapeutic target in oncology. *Clin. Cancer Res.* 18:40–50.

Rau, R., E. Soroko, D. Jasilionis and, J. W. Vaupel. 2008. Continued reductions in mortality at advanced ages. *Populat. Dev. Rev.* 34:747–768.

Reinheckel, T., N. Sitte, O. Ullrich, U. Kuckelkorn, K. J. Davies, and T. Grune. 1998. Comparative resistance of the 20S and 26S proteasome to oxidative stress. *Biochem. J.* 335:637–642.

Roberts, W. C. 1998. The heart at necropsy in centenarians. *Am. J. Cardiol.* 81:1224–1225.

Rubinsztein, D. C., G. Marino, and G. Kroemer. 2011. Autophagy and aging. *Cell* 146:682–695.

Ryu, S. J., Y. S. Oh, and S. C. Park. 2007. Failure of stress-induced downregulation of Bcl-2 contributes to apoptosis resistance in senescent human diploid fibroblasts. *Cell Death Differ.* 14:1020–1028.

Ryu, S. J., H. J. An, Y. S. Oh, H. R. Choi, M. K. Ha, and S. C. Park. 2008. On the role of major vault protein in the resistance of senescent human diploid fibroblasts to apoptosis. *Cell Death Differ.* 15:1673–1680.

Sabatini, D. M., H. Erdjument-Bromage, M. Lui, P. Tempst, and S. H. Snyder. 1994. RAFT1: a mammalian protein that binds to FKBP12 in a rapamycin-dependent fashion and is homologous to yeast TORs. *Cell* 78:35–43.

Sanders, J. L., R. M. Boudreau, B. W. Penninx, E. M. Simonsick, S. B. Kritchevsky, S. Satterfield, T. B. Harris, D. C. Bauer, A. B. Newman, and Health ABC Study. 2012a. Association of a modified physiologic index with mortality and incident disability: the Health, Aging, and Body Composition study. *J. Gerontol. A. Biol. Sci. Med. Sci.* 67:1439–1446.

Sanders, J. L., A. L. Fitzpatrick, R. M. Boudreau, A. M. Arnold, A. Aviv, M. Kimura, L. F. Fried, T. B. Harris, and A. B. Newman. 2012b. Leukocyte telomere length is associated with noninvasively measured age-related disease: the Cardiovascular Health Study. *J. Gerontol. A. Biol. Sci. Med. Sci.* 67:409–416.

Sanders, Y. Y., H. Liu, X. Zhang, L. Hecker, K. Bernard, L. Desai, G. Liu, and V. J. Thannickal. 2013. Histone modifications in senescence-associated resistance to apoptosis by oxidative stress. *Redox Biol.* 1:8–16.

Saretzki, G., J. Feng, T. Von Zglinicki, and B. Villeponteau. 1998. Similar gene expression pattern in senescent and hyperoxic-treated fibroblasts. *J. Gerontol. A. Biol. Sci. Med. Sci.* 53:B438–442.

Saretzki, G., N. Sitte, U. Merkel, R. E. Wurm, and T. Von Zglinicki. 1999. Telomere shortening triggers a p53-dependent cell cycle arrest via accumulation of G-rich single stranded DNA fragments. *Oncogene* 18:5148–5158.

Sas, A. A., H. Snieder, and J. Korf. 2012. Gompertz' survivorship law as an intrinsic principle of aging. *Med. Hypotheses* 78:659–663.

Schachter, F., L. Faure-Delanef, F. Guenot, H. Rouger, P. Froguel, L. Lesueur-Ginot, and D. Cohen. 1994. Genetic associations with human longevity at the APOE and ACE loci. *Nat. Genet.* 6:29–32.

Serra, V., T. Grune, N. Sitte, G. Saretzki, and T. Von Zglinicki. 2000. Telomere length as a marker of oxidative stress in primary human fibroblast cultures. *Ann. NY Acad. Sci.* 908:327–330.

Shantha, T. R., S. L. Manocha, and G. H. Bourne 1969. Morphology and cytology of neurons. *In:* G. H. Bourne (ed.) *The Structure and Function of Nervous Tissue. Vol. II.* New York: Academic Press.

Shelton, D. N., E. Chang, P. S. Whittier, D. Choi, and W. D. Funk. 1999. Microarray analysis of replicative senescence. *Curr. Biol.* 9:939–945.

Speakman, J. R. and S. E. Mitchell. 2011. Caloric restriction. *Mol. Aspects Med.* 32:159–221.

Tazearslan, C., M. Cho, and Y. Suh. 2012. Discovery of functional gene variants associated with human longevity: opportunities and challenges. *J. Gerontol. A. Biol. Sci. Med. Sci.* 67:376–383.

Tepper, C. G., M. F. Seldin, and M. Mudryj. 2000. Fas-mediated apoptosis of proliferating, transiently growth-arrested, and senescent normal human fibroblasts. *Exp. Cell Res.* 260:9–19.

Terman, A. 2006. Catabolic insufficiency and aging. *Ann. NY Acad. Sci.* 1067:27–36.

Terman, A. and U. T. Brunk. 1998. Lipofuscin: mechanisms of formation and increase with age. *APMIS* 106:265–276.

Terman, A., H. Dalen, and U. T. Brunk. 1999. Ceroid/lipofuscin-loaded human fibroblasts show decreased survival time and diminished autophagocytosis during amino acid starvation. *Exp. Gerontol.* 34:943–957.

Terman, A., H. Dalen, J. W. Eaton, J. Neuzil, and U. T. Brunk. 2003. Mitochondrial recycling and aging of cardiac myocytes: the role of autophagocytosis. *Exp. Gerontol.* 38:863–876.

Terry, D. F., M. Wilcox, M. A. Mccormick, E. Lawler, and T. T. Perls. 2003. Cardiovascular advantages among the offspring of centenarians. *J. Gerontol. A. Biol. Sci. Med. Sci.* 58:M425–431.

Terry, D. F., M. A. Wilcox, M. A. Mccormick, J. Y. Pennington, E. A. Schoenhofen, S. L. Andersen, and T. T. Perls. 2004. Lower all-cause, cardiovascular, and cancer mortality in centenarians' offspring. *J. Am. Geriatr. Soc.* 52:2074–2076.

Trougakos, I. P., A. Saridaki, G. Panayotou, and E. S. Gonos. 2006. Identification of differentially expressed proteins in senescent human embryonic fibroblasts. *Mech. Ageing Dev.* 127:88–92.

Turrens, J. F. 2003. Mitochondrial formation of reactive oxygen species. *J. Physiol.* 552:335–344.

Ullrich, A., A. Gray, A. W. Tam, T. Yang-Feng, M. Tsubokawa, C. Collins, W. Henzel, T. Le Bon, S. Kathuria, E. Chen, and Et Al. 1986. Insulin-like growth factor I receptor primary structure: comparison with insulin receptor suggests structural determinants that define functional specificity. *EMBO J.* 5:2503–2512.

Van Der Vos, K. E., P. Eliasson, T. Proikas-Cezanne, S. J. Vervoort, R. Van Boxtel, M. Putker, I. J. Van Zutphen, M. Mauthe, S. Zellmer, C. Pals, L. P. Verhagen, M. J. Groot Koerkamp, A. K. Braat, T. B. Dansen, F. C. Holstege, R. Gebhardt, B. M. Burgering, and P. J. Coffer. 2012. Modulation of glutamine metabolism by the PI(3)K-PKB-FOXO network regulates autophagy. *Nat. Cell Biol.* 14:829–837.

Vaupel, J. W. 2010. Biodemography of human ageing. *Nature* 464:536–542.

Vaupel, J. W., J. R. Carey, K. Christensen, T. E. Johnson, A. I. Yashin, N. V. Holm, I. A. Iachine, V. Kannisto, A. A. Khazaeli, P. Liedo, V. D. Longo, Y. Zeng, K. G. Manton, and J. W. Curtsinger. 1998. Biodemographic trajectories of longevity. *Science* 280:855–860.

Von Zglinicki, T. 2000. Role of oxidative stress in telomere length regulation and replicative senescence. *Ann. NY Acad. Sci.* 908:99–110.

Von Zglinicki, T., G. Saretzki, W. Docke, and C. Lotze. 1995. Mild hyperoxia shortens telomeres and inhibits proliferation of fibroblasts – a model for senescence. *Exp. Cell Res.* 220:186–193.

Vurusaner, B., G. Poli, and H. Basaga. 2012. Tumor suppressor genes and ROS: complex networks of interactions. *Free Radic. Biol. Med.* 52:7–18.

Wajapeyee, N., R. W. Serra, X. Zhu, M. Mahalingam, and M. R. Green. 2008. Oncogenic BRAF induces senescence and apoptosis through pathways mediated by the secreted protein IGFBP7. *Cell* 132:363–374.

Wang, C., D. Jurk, M. Maddick, G. Nelson, C. Martin-Ruiz, and T. Von Zglinicki. 2009. DNA damage response and cellular senescence in tissues of aging mice. *Aging Cell* 8:311–323.

Webb, A. E. and A. Brunet. 2014. FOXO transcription factors: key regulators of cellular quality control. *Trends Biochem. Sci.* 39:159–169.

Wheeler, H. E. and S. K. Kim. 2011. Genetics and genomics of human ageing. *Philos. Trans. R. Soc. Lond. B: Biol. Sci.* 366:43–50.

Wilkinson, J. E., L. Burmeister, S. V. Brooks, C. C. Chan, S. Friedline, D. E. Harrison, J. F. Hejtmancik, N. Nadon, R. Strong, L. K. Wood, M. A. Woodward, and R. A. Miller. 2012. Rapamycin slows aging in mice. *Aging Cell* 11:675–682.

Willcox, B. J., D. C. Willcox, Q. He, J. D. Curb, and M. Suzuki. 2006. Siblings of Okinawan centenarians share lifelong mortality advantages. *J. Gerontol. A. Biol. Sci. Med. Sci.* 61:345–354.

Willcox, B. J., T. A. Donlon, Q. He, R. Chen, J. S. Grove, K. Yano, K. H. Masaki, D. C. Willcox, B. Rodriguez, and J. D. Curb. 2008. FOXO3A genotype is strongly associated with human longevity. *Proc. Natl Acad. Sci. USA* 105:13987–13992.

Wright, W. E. and J. W. Shay. 1992. The two-stage mechanism controlling cellular senescence and immortalization. *Exp. Gerontol.* 27:383–389.

Wullschleger, S., R. Loewith, and M. N. Hall. 2006. TOR signaling in growth and metabolism. *Cell* 124:471–484.

Yang, N. C. and M. L. Hu. 2005. The limitations and validities of senescence associated-beta-galactosidase activity as an aging marker for human foreskin fibroblast Hs68 cells. *Exp. Gerontol.* 40:813–819.

Yang, W. and S. Hekimi. 2010. A mitochondrial superoxide signal triggers increased longevity in *Caenorhabditis elegans*. *PLoS Biol.* 8:e1000556.

Yoon, I. K., H. K. Kim, Y. K. Kim, I. H. Song, W. Kim, S. Kim, S. H. Baek, J. H. Kim, and J. R. Kim. 2004. Exploration of replicative senescence-associated genes in human dermal fibroblasts by cDNA microarray technology. *Exp. Gerontol.* 39:1369–1378.

Zangar, R. C., D. R. Davydov, and S. Verma. 2004. Mechanisms that regulate production of reactive oxygen species by cytochrome P450. *Toxicol. Appl. Pharm.* 199:316–331.

Zhang, H., K. H. Pan, and S. N. Cohen. 2003. Senescence-specific gene expression fingerprints reveal cell-type-dependent physical clustering of up-regulated chromosomal loci. *Proc. Natl Acad. Sci. USA* 100:3251–3256.

Zhang, Y., A. Bokov, J. Gelfond, V. Soto, Y. Ikeno, G. Hubbard, V. Diaz, L. Sloane, K. Maslin, S. Treaster, S. Rendon, H. Van Remmen, W. Ward, M. Javors, A. Richardson, S. N. Austad, and K. Fischer. 2014. Rapamycin extends life and health in C57BL/6 mice. *J. Gerontol. A. Biol. Sci. Med. Sci.* 69:119–130.

CHAPTER 2

To eat or not to eat – Anti-ageing effects of energy restriction

Delminda Neves,[1] Maria João Martins,[2] Emanuel dos Passos[2,3] and Inês Tomada[1]

[1] *Department of Experimental Biology, Faculty of Medicine, and Institute for Molecular and Cell Biology, University of Porto, Porto, Portugal*

[2] *Department of Biochemistry, Faculty of Medicine, and Instituto de Investigação e Inovação em Saúde, University of Porto, Porto, Portugal*

[3] *CIAFEL – Research Centre in Physical Activity, Health and Leisure, Faculty of Sport, University of Porto, Porto, Portugal*

Part 1

2.1 Energy restriction as more than a weight-loss strategy

For at least 500 years, restricting intake of food has been regarded as beneficial to health, and conversely, it has been believed that overconsumption promotes disease and ultimately early death (Speakman & Mitchell, 2011). Energy restriction (ER), often called caloric restriction, refers to feeding protocols that employ the reduction of energy intake while maintaining essential nutrient requirements. Experimental mammalian models of ER involve a reduction in energy intake that normally varies from 25 to 40% of the *ad libitum* diet through the lifespan of the animal. However, when this kind of protocol is used, not only the amount of energy is reduced but also the levels of macro- and micronutrients to a similar extent. Thus, it is often necessary to normalize the levels of the micronutrients to the recommended daily intake levels. Primarily, diet patterns that involve ER result in a decrease in body weight (BW), disproportionately contributed to by white adipose tissue (WAT), thus causing a percentage increment in lean body mass (LBM), without reducing the energy expenditure *per unit* of body mass (McCarter & Palmer, 1992) nor significantly or persistently modifying oxygen-free radical production (Pamplona *et al.*, 2002). This diet pattern results in an increase in lifespan in organisms from yeast to primates (Colman *et al.*, 2009), accounting for an extension of maximum lifespan of 30–40% in rodents (McCay *et al.*, 1935; Weindruch *et al.*, 1986) or even nearly doubling the lifespan in mice when combined whith favorable mutations (Ikeno *et al.*, 2013). Moreover, ER reduces the incidence and the rate of progression of most age-associated diseases. The extension of lifespan and the reduction of the incidence of diseases are secondary to the biological adaptations that occur in response to prolonged ER, including metabolic, hormonal, biochemical and gene expression modifications. The overall physiological processes of aged rodents maintained in a long-term ER regimen are more like those found in the young, compared with animals fed *ad libitum* (Masoro,

Anti-Ageing Nutrients: Evidence-Based Prevention of Age-Associated Diseases, First Edition. Edited by Delminda Neves.

2002). Experiments carried out in other species such as dogs, cows and nonhuman primates corroborate previous findings in rodents. In addition, observations in humans support the hypothesis that ER induces physiological modifications equivalent to those found in other mammals. Thus, owing to its vast effects on organisms, one should consider ER to be much more than a weight-loss strategy.

2.2 Restriction of energy vs restriction of nutrients

Most of the ER protocols consist of the reduction of the amount of food available, after quantification of *ad libitum* consumption on an individual basis. Restriction is further calculated and, if necessary, adjusted during the experiment considering that nutritional needs, and consequently *ad libitum* intake, are not constant throughout the lifespan. In these protocols food portions are provided individually and daily. However, not only how much food is ingested but also when it is ingested may influence which downstream pathways are activated. Hence, other protocols of food restriction were developed in the 1990s that consist of providing food *ad libitum* to a restricted group intermittently with periods of fasting. These protocols often consist of feeding every other day (also called alternate day fasting). If the fasting days do not alternate, the protocol is generally called intermittent fasting or intermittent feeding. These feeding protocols do not consist of a severe restriction in the total amount of energy provided from food (Speakman & Mitchell, 2011). Interestingly, they present beneficial effects to health and longevity (Goodrick *et al.*, 1990), particularly in the prevention of cardiovascular disease (CVD) and neurodegeneration (Anson *et al.*, 2005; Mattson & Wan, 2005), in part because intermittent feeding regimens trigger similar biological pathways to ER (increase in autophagy and mitochondrial respiratory efficiency, discussed later). Nonetheless, intermittent feeding apparently acts in a genotype-dependent fashion, considering the absence of beneficial effects in growth hormone (GH) receptor-knockout mice compared with wild-type counterparts, and the unexpected induction of diabetes and obesity and the worsening of atherosclerosis observed in low-density lipoprotein (LDL)-receptor-knockout mice (Westbrook *et al.*, 2014; Dorighello *et al.*, 2013).

The reduction of certain macronutrients intake without reduction of overall energy provided from diet could also exert a favorable influence on the health, and probably on the lifespan, of mammals resembling that provoked by ER. In fact, it was reported that reducing the protein content of the diet by 40% for 7 weeks in rats decreased mitochondrial production of reactive oxygen species (ROS), without changes in mitochondrial oxygen consumption, and reduced oxidative damage of nuclear and mitochondrial DNA in the liver (Sanz *et al.*, 2004). These results suggest that part of the decrease in ageing rate induced by ER could be due to the corresponding decrease in protein intake. Supporting that, several studies have reported that protein restriction itself increases the maximum lifespan in rodents (reviewed in Pamplona & Barja, 2006). Moreover, ER does not reduce concentrations of insulin-like growth factor 1 (IGF-1), strongly associated with an increase in lifespan in mammals (Yuan *et al.*, 2009) (discussed in Chapter 1), in humans, unlike in rodents, unless protein intake is also reduced (Fontana *et al.*, 2008). Restriction of other macronutrients such as lipids or carbohydrates does not exert similar effects (Sanz *et al.*, 2006a, b).

The individual restriction of specific amino acids demonstrated that restriction of methionine, and to a lesser extent tryptophan, by reducing 80% of the baseline methionine intake and substituting it with glutamate, induced a significant positive effect on lifespan in rats and mice independently of global energy intake (Orentreich *et al.*, 1993; Sun *et al.*, 2009; Ooka *et al.*, 1988). In addition, methionine restriction, at levels similar to those observed in 40% protein restriction, mimics the effects of this treatment, namely it decreases mitochondrial ROS production, the concentration of complexes I and III, oxidative damage of DNA and proteins, glycoxidation or lipoxidation, fatty acid unsaturation and apoptosis-inducing factor (Pamplona & Barja, 2006; Caro *et al.*, 2008). The positive effects of 80% methionine restriction were also evident in aged rats that presented reduced BW and visceral adiposity when compared with age-matched *ad libitum*-fed controls, concomitantly with decreases in glucose, insulin, leptin and IGF-1, and increases in adiponectin plasma levels. Furthermore, methionine restriction blunts the age-related increase in cholesterol and triglyceride levels (Malloy *et al.*, 2006). In fact, methionine restriction mirrors the changes that occur under ER, suggesting that it may play a contributory role in the effects of this diet pattern. Methionine-restricted diet reduces the incidence of tumors and improves survival in experimental animals exposed to carcinogens, which is in agreement with the fact that many cancer cells exhibit dependence on methionine to survive and proliferate (reviewed in Cavuoto & Fenech, 2012).

2.2.1 Experimental models of energy restriction

In 1935, McCay reported for the first time that 40% ER from the age of weaning increases maximal longevity in rats. Since then many other studies have shown that ER slows ageing in yeast, flies, worms, mice and rats, and extends average and maximal lifespan in mice, cows and dogs (Weindruch, 1992; Pinney *et al.*, 1972; Kealy *et al.*, 2002). Despite there being a broad conservation of pathways concerned with the control of lifespan among species, considerable differences exist as well (Speakman & Mitchell, 2011). Thus, this chapter is focused on data described in mammals (mice and rats, and also nonhuman primates and human trials). The main outcomes of ER in mammals are summarized in Table 2.1.

Most of the studies concerning the effects of ER in mammals have been carried out in small rodents, and unexpectedly, the effect observed for this diet pattern varies among species and strains in both mice and rats (reviewed in Merry, 2005). In fact, it has been demonstrated that ER increases lifespan in a range of outbred, inbred, obese, mutant, knockout and transgenic strains of rodents. However, while in rats ER further decreases the age-specific mortality rate and retards the rate of ageing, the same outcome is not evident in mice, only a delay in ageing rather than a reduction in the rate of ageing being observed (Merry, 2005). Despite ER being normally beneficial, responses to this diet pattern can vary in rodents, particularly when animals are subjected to different levels of restriction (Speakman & Mitchell, 2011). Broadly, in mice, an increase in longevity proportional to the severity of dietary restriction is observed, to a maximum of 65% restriction (Weindruch *et al.*, 1986). However, this finding does not agree with observations in inbred strains of mice, which exhibited both increase and decrease in mean lifespan when subjected to 40% ER (Liao *et al.*, 2010). One potential explanation formulated by Speakman & Mitchell (2011) is that all rodent strains respond positively to ER, but the level of restriction at which their responses

Table 2.1 Main outcomes on energy-restricted individuals.

Species/study	Age at baseline	ER regimen	Main outcomes on energy-restricted individuals
Mouse (Weindruch *et al.*, 1986)	21–28 days	25–65% restriction from *ad libitum*-ingested amount	↑ Mean and maximum lifespan ↑ Longevity proportional to the severity of ER ↓ Tumor incidence
Mouse (Dhahbi *et al.*, 2004)	19 months	40% restriction from *ad libitum*-ingested amount	↑ Mean time to death ↑ Mean and maximum lifespan ↓ Tumor incidence Modification in gene expression profile
Mouse (Donato *et al.*, 2013)	14–16 weeks	40% restriction from *ad libitum*-ingested amount	↓ Body weight ↓ Total body fat mass ↑ Total daily activity ↓ Systolic and diastolic blood pressure ↓ Triglycerides levels in blood Prevention of age-related stiffening of large elastic arteries ↓ Oxidative stress Preservation of endothelial and vascular function ↑ Arterial activity of Sirt1 ↓ mTOR activation
Mouse (Vera *et al.*, 2013)	3 months	40% restriction from *ad libitum*-ingested amount	↓ Body weight ↓ Total body fat mass ↑ Glucose tolerance ↑ Maintenance and/or elongation telomeres
Mouse (Han *et al.*, 2012)	4 months	40% restriction from *ad libitum*-ingested amount	↓ Body weight ↓ Total body fat mass ↓ Left ventricular mass Preservation of cardiac contractile function ↑ Cardiomyocyte function ↑ Insulin sensitivity ↑ Phosphorylation of AMPK ↓ mTOR activation ↑ Myocardial autophagy
Rat (Jiang *et al.*, 2005)	4 months	40% restriction from *ad libitum*-ingested amount	↓ Body weight Prevention of kidney interstitial fibrosis ↓ Extracellular matrix accumulation in kidney Prevention of age-associated renal disease
Mouse (Someya *et al.*, 2010)	2 months	25% restriction from *ad libitum*-ingested amount	↓ Body weight Prevention of age-related hearing loss ↓ Serum triglycerides levels ↓ Serum insulin fasting levels ↓ Oxidative damage in multiple tissues
Mouse (Mouton *et al.*, 2009)	17–18 months	40% restriction from *ad libitum*-ingested amount	↓ Body weight ↓ Formation of amyloid plaques in brain
Rat (Tomada *et al.*, 2013b)	2 months	25% restriction from *ad libitum*-ingested amount	↓ Body weight ↓ Adiposity ↓ Serum insulin fasting levels ↑ Adiponectin Reversal of age-related connective tissue deposition in *corpus cavernosum*

Continued

Table 2.1 Continued

Dog (Kealy *et al.*, 2002)	2 months	25% restriction from *ad libitum*-ingested amount	↑ Mean lifespan ↓ Body weight ↓ Total body fat mass Delay of onset of age-associated diseases ↓ Serum triglycerides levels ↓ Serum triiodothyronine levels ↓ Serum glucose and insulin fasting levels
Lemur *Microcebus murinus* (Dal-Pan *et al.*, 2011a, b; Marchal *et al.*, 2012, 2013)	38 months	30% restriction from *ad libitum*-ingested amount	↓ Body weight ↓ Daily energy expenditure ↑ Insulin sensitivity ↑ Cognitive performance
Rhesus macaques, *Macaca mulatta* (Colman *et al.*, 2009)	7 or 14 years	30% restriction from *ad libitum*-ingested amount	↓ Age-related deaths ↓ Total body fat mass ↓ In decline in muscle mass Metabolic improvement ↓ Neoplasia incidence ↓ Cardiovascular disease Delay of onset of age-associated diseases ↓ Age-associated brain atrophy ↑ Survival Younger outward appearance
Rhesus macaques, *Macaca mulatta* (Mattison *et al.*, 2003, 2012; Messaoudi *et al.*, 2006)	1–17 years	22–24% after a period of 30% restriction from *ad libitum*-ingested amount	↓ Body weight ↓ Total body fat mass ↓ Trunk fat mass Delay in skeletal development ↓ Bone mineral content Delay in reproductive maturation ↓ Glucose and insulin fasting levels Amelioration of plasma lipids ↓ Body temperature ↓ Decline of DHEA levels ↓ Decline of melatonin levels ↓ Incidence of chronic diseases ↓ Oxidative stress (plasma-free isoprostane) Delay of senescence of the immune system
Human/ nonrandomized study with members of the Caloric Restriction Society (Cangemi *et al.*, 2010; Fontana *et al.*, 2004, 2008; Meyer *et al.*, 2006; Mercken *et al.*, 2013)		Self-imposed diet of 1112–1958 kcal/day	↓ Body weight ↓ Total body fat mass ↓ Glucose and insulin fasting levels Amelioration of plasma lipids ↓ C-reactive protein levels in blood ↓ Levels of TNF-α and TGF-β in blood ↓ Systolic and diastolic blood pressure ↓ Carotid artery intima–media thickness ↓ 17 β-estradiol and testosterone levels ↓ Levels of serum triiodothyronine Younger transcriptional profile in skeletal muscle Inhibition of IGF-1/insulin pathway in skeletal muscle
CALERIE Phase I, Tufts University (Das *et al.*, 2007; Meydani *et al.*, 2011)	24–42 years	30% restriction (recommended) from *ad libitum*-ingested amount for 12 months	↓ Body weight Amelioration of plasma lipids ↓ Insulin fasting levels ↑ Plasma glutathione peroxidase activity ↓ Plasma protein carbonyl levels

Continued

Table 2.1 Continued

CALERIE Phase I, Pennington Biomedical Research Center (Civitarese *et al.*, 2007; Heilbronn *et al.*, 2006; Larson-Meyer *et al.*, 2006; Lefevre *et al.*, 2009; Redman *et al.*, 2007)	25–50 years	25% restriction from *ad libitum*-ingested amount for 6 months	↓ Body weight ↓ Total body fat mass ↓ Visceral and subcutaneous fat mass ↓ Fat cell size and intrahepatic fat ↓ Insulin fasting levels ↑ Insulin sensitivity Amelioration of plasma lipids Improvement in cardiovascular health ↓ Body temperature ↓ Daily energy expenditure ↓ DNA damage ↑ Muscular expression of genes involved in mitochondrial function ↑ Muscle mitochondrial biogenesis
CALERIE Phase I Washington University (Hofer *et al.*, 2008; Racette *et al.*, 2006; Weiss *et al.*, 2006)	50–60 years	20% restriction from *ad libitum*-ingested amount for 12 months	↓ Body weight ↓ Total body fat mass ↓ Visceral and subcutaneous fat mass ↓ Blood insulin fasting levels ↓ Leptin ↑ Insulin sensitivity ↓ DNA and RNA oxidation levels in white blood cells
CALERIE Phase II	25–50 years	25% restriction from *ad libitum*-ingested amount for 2 years	No published data

AMPK, AMP-activated protein kinase; CALERIE, Comprehensive Assessment of Long-term Effects of Reducing Intake of Energy; DHEA, dehydroepiandrosterone; ER, energy restriction; IGF-1, insulin-like growth factor 1; mTOR, mechanistic target of rapamycin; Sirt1, sirtuin 1; TGF, transforming growth factor; TNF, tumor necrosis factor.

switch from life extension to life shortening differs between strains. Supporting this assumption, no adverse effect was observed for 20% ER from *ad libitum* consumption, which resulted in lifespan enhancement for all of the rodent strains tested. Higher levels of ER cause different responses among strains in terms of lifespan extension. The protective effects of ER reported in rodents are due to multiple mechanisms that include reduction of the incidence of tumors (Weindruch *et al.*, 1986; Dhahbi *et al.*, 2004), changes in body composition with reduction of adipose tissue, decrease in triglycerides in blood, prevention of stiffening of large elastic arteries, decrease in oxidative stress, preservation of endothelial and vascular functions, increase in arterial activity of sirtuin 1 (Sirt1) and decrease in mechanistic target of rapamycin (mTOR) activation (Donato *et al.*, 2013), improvement in myocardial and cardiomyocyte contractile function and autophagy (Han *et al.*, 2012), prevention of kidney interstitial fibrosis and age-associated kidney disease (Jiang *et al.*, 2005), prevention of age-associated cochlear cell death and hearing loss (Someya *et al.*, 2010), mitigation of neurological damage arising from ageing, mostly by reduction in amyloid deposition (Mouton *et al.*, 2009), amelioration of metabolic syndrome and reversal of age-related connective tissue deposition in *corpus cavernosum* (Tomada *et al.*, 2013b).

Many other studies not mentioned in this chapter have been carried out, and globally have contributed to knowledge concerning the effects of ER in small rodents. On the other hand, studies in nonhuman primates are scarce, but equally very important for the study of the ER effects in humans.

A study known as RESTRIKAL used 42 small primates, *Microcebus murinus*, which have a median survival time of 5.7 years and a maximum survival time of 12 years in captivity, divided into three groups, including one subjected to long-term ER. Starting at 38 months, these animals experienced a 30% ER relative to the amount of food supplied to the *ad libitum*-fed controls (Dal-Pan *et al.*, 2011a), which resulted in decrease in BW and daily energy expenditure, an increase in insulin sensitivity, the prevention of age-related DNA and RNA oxidative damage and an enhancement of cognitive performance, suggesting that ER has beneficial effects on brain function, even in adults (Dal-Pan *et al.*, 2011a, b; Marchal *et al.*, 2012, 2013). Interestingly, equivalent results to those found in ER-treated lemurs were observed in animals treated with 200 mg/kg/day of resveratrol, an ER mimetic discussed later.

There are two active randomized studies in nonhuman long-lived primates rhesus monkeys, *Macaca mulatta*, that started approximately two decades ago, testing the effects of long-term ER on longevity and disease, one at the University of Wiscosin–Madison and the other at the National Institute on Ageing (NIA) (Colman *et al.*, 2009; Mattison *et al.*, 2003, 2012). These studies extended ER findings beyond the laboratory rodents to a long-lived primate (rhesus monkeys, average lifespan in captivity 27 years, with the maximum reported lifespan being 40 years). The main outcomes of these paralleled studies are summarized in Table 2.1. Both studies demonstrated beneficial effects of 20–30% ER throughout life on rhesus monkeys. Restricted animals presented reduced BW mainly through decreased trunk fat mass, lower age-associated decline in muscle mass, metabolic improvement and lower incidence of chronic and age-associated diseases, including neoplasia, CVD, arthritis, diverticulosis and diabetes. In both studies, age-associated diseases were detected in control monkeys at an earlier age than in ER monkeys, but in the NIA study the difference did not achieve statistical difference. Surprisingly, concerning the survival outcomes, the findings obtained by the NIA group contrast with those observed by its counterpart in the University of Wiscosin–Madison, since the former did not observe improvement in this parameter (Mattison *et al.*, 2012), while the latter demonstrated improved survival and a significant decrease in the number of age-associated deaths (Colman *et al.*, 2009). These discrepancies could be justified by differences in experimental design and in diet composition, since the diet used in the NIA study had a natural ingredient base, containing flavonoids and fats from plant and fish origins, in contrast to that used in Colman *et al.*'s study, which was purified, with fat mainly derived from corn oil and supplemented with minerals and vitamins as separate components. Actually, an important difference in these studies concerns the supplementation of minerals and vitamins, taking into account that, in the NIA but not in the University of Wiscosin–Madison study, the same diet was used in ER and control groups, which led to an over-supplementation of control monkeys. In addition, these control animals were subjected to a 10% ER relative to *ad libitum*, which could contribute to the mitigation of differences between ER-treated animals and controls. Despite these recognized differences that in part justify the outcomes of the experiments, Mattison *et al.* (2012) suggested a separation of ER effects in health, morbility and mortality in primates.

Interestingly, many of the metabolic and hormonal adaptations typical of the ER-treated rodents did not occur in the ER-treated monkeys.

2.2.2 Observational studies and the first human trial of energy restriction: CALERIE study

How ER affects the human body and extends longevity in healthy individuals remains an unanswered question, particularly because the supporting data are mostly derived from the implementation of dietary reduction to induce weight loss among overweight or obese persons. Nevertheless, some healthy persons have adopted a self-restricted lifestyle for long periods and formed the Calorie Restriction Society in the USA in 1994, in 2002 renamed the Calorie Restriction Society International and classified as a nonprofit organization (www.calorierestriction.org). Members of this organization who practice ER in a voluntary regimen and design their diets so as to consume a balance of foods that supply greater than 100% of the Recommended Daily Intake for all of the essential nutrients, while minimizing energy content (1112–1958 kcal/day), have been studied; valuable data concerning the beneficial effects of ER were obtained, in particular improvements in cardiovascular and hormonal profile, glucose control and body composition (Cangemi *et al.*, 2010; Fontana *et al.*, 2004, 2008). However, this does not constitute a randomized controlled trial, which makes it difficult to strictly associate the observed health status with an ER regimen. Equivalent limitations were found in the analysis of the Okinawan centenarians, whose extreme longevity is apparently related to their long-term low-energy diet (83% of the Japanese average total energy intake as reported by Kagawa, 1978). Currently, the dietary pattern of the younger generation of Okinawans is suffering from Westernization, characterized by an increase in fat, meat and bread consumption. The traditional diet of Okinawans ca. 1950 was rich in vegetables, which represented 69% of total energy on average, in particular sweet potatoes, and low in sugars, grains (rice and wheat) and proteins of animal origin (fish, meat, eggs and dairy products), which jointly supplied less than 4% of total diet energy. Total energy provided by proteins in the diet of Okinawan centenarians did not exceed 9% (Willcox *et al.*, 2007). Despite the mortality registries in this cohort not having been carefully studied, which impedes the establishment of a clear connection between dietary pattern and causes of death, evidence suggests that death rates from heart and vascular diseases as well as cancer were markedly lower than those observed in the overall Japanese population. Supporting the idea that ER delays ageing features, the levels of the biomarkers of ageing dehydroepiandrosterone (DHEA), which decreases over time, measured in a cohort of 54 septuagenarians in Okinawa were significantly higher than in nonrestricted age-matched American individuals, the differences being higher among women than men from the two studied groups (Willcox *et al.*, 2006, 2007). However, despite the percentage of very old people being higher in Okinawa than elsewhere, the oldest people are not older than the oldest people in other parts of the world, which means that ER in Okinawans increases the average but not the maximum longevity (Holloszy & Fontana, 2007). These findings contrast with observations in ER rodents that present increased average and maximum longevities compared with *ad libitum*-fed counterparts.

In fact, studying the effect of ER on longevity in humans is not feasible, since the average life time expectancy is close to 80 years for the population in developed countries and these kinds of studies are challenging to conduct. Thus, surrogate measures, such as signals of biological adaptation, changes in risk factors for age-associated diseases or physiological variables that deteriorate progressively with ageing are used to evaluate ER impact in human ageing.

In an attempt to elucidate whether long-term ER interferes with human health in a similar fashion to that observed in small mammals and nonhuman primates, the first randomized human trial of ER effects in nonobese, healthy individuals, named CALERIE (Comprehensive Assessment of Long-term Effects of Reducing Intake of Energy), was initiated by the NIA and developed at three research centers (Tufts University, Pennington Biomedical Research Center and Washington University), coordinated by Duke University. CALERIE Phase 1 has already been completed; interventions lasted 6 months to 1 year and involved various ER protocols and age groups, integrated in three pilot studies (Das *et al.*, 2007; Heilbronn *et al.*, 2006; Racette *et al.*, 2006; Weiss *et al.*, 2006): (a) individuals aged 24–42 years were subjected to a 30% reduction in energy consumption for 12 months (Tufts University); (b) individuals aged 25–50 years were treated for 6 months with 25% ER (Pennington Biomedical Research Center); and (c) 50–60-year-old individuals were subjected to 20% energy reduction for 12 months (Washington University). All trials started with healthy but overweight subjects, and ER groups were compared with age-matched healthy individuals on typical American diets during the same period (control group). In line with results obtained in the experimental models, ER for 6 months to 1 year led to reductions in BW, lean mass, subcutaneous and visceral fat and circulating insulin, and improved lipid profile (Das *et al.*, 2007; Heilbronn *et al.*, 2006; Lefevre *et al.*, 2009; Redman *et al.*, 2007; Racette *et al.*, 2006; Weiss *et al.*, 2006). In addition, it was demonstrated that 6 months of 25% ER decreases average fat cell size, intrahepatic fat deposition and DNA damage, and increases the expression of genes involved in mitochondrial biogenesis and efficiency, such as endothelial nitric oxide synthase (eNOS), peroxisome proliferator-activated receptor gamma coactivator 1 alpha (PPARGC-1α or PGC-1α) and Sirt1, as demonstrated in skeletal muscle harvested by biopsy (Civitarese *et al.*, 2007; Heilbronn *et al.*, 2006; Larson-Meyer *et al.*, 2006). One year of 20% ER decreases DNA and RNA oxidation levels in white blood cells, putatively by decreasing systemic oxidative stress (Hofer *et al.*, 2008). In line with these findings, 30% ER for 1 year increases glutathione peroxidase (GPx) activity and decreases protein carbonyl levels in plasma (Meydani *et al.*, 2011).

Conversely to the CALERIE Phase I trial, the ongoing Phase II harmonized protocols enrolled 218 healthy voluntary participants (2% from the first screening step, since selection of participants able to maintain adherence to a 2 year ER program constituted a great challenge) with body mass index (BMI) between 22 and 28 kg/m^2 who are being subjected to a 25% ER pattern over 2 years (Rochon *et al.*, 2011). The main goal of the CALERIE Phase II study is to test the hypothesis that 2 years of sustained ER in healthy nonobese individuals results in the same beneficial effects as observed in other animals subjected to similar levels of ER, such as reduction in resting metabolic rate (RMR), core body temperature, serum triiodothyronine levels, serum tumor necrosis factor (TNF)-α levels and oxidative damage. Changes in body composition, immune system modulation, hormonal profile, plasma lipids, growth factors, inflammatory cytokines and C-reactive protein (CRP) concentrations, and modulation of gene expression in skeletal muscle and adipose tissues, as well as cognitive function and affective and physical status were also evaluated. Biological samples (plasma, biopsy samples, circulating cells and urine) were stored in a repository for further studies (Rochon *et al.*, 2011). The findings from this multicenter study will be published in the near future.

Despite the fact that we only have preliminary evidence based on surrogate measures of how ER might impact on human longevity, most available data indicate that ER exerts similar adaptive responses in humans as in experimental models and prevents the development of age-associated diseases; however it remains to be shown whether ER will extend lifespan in humans. It would be desirable to have a longer-term follow-up comprising a period longer than 2 years allotted to CALERIE, and also to perform a long-term observational study on participants after they complete the 2-year intervention. Even though the influence of ER patterns is predominantly positive to the health of the individuals, we cannot disregard hunger, which is a common plaint in individuals who adhere to ER and is not alleviated with the continuation of treatment, causing major discomfort and hindering lifelong compliance with this dietary pattern.

2.3 Effects of energy restriction on organisms

Epidemiological and experimental data indicate that diet plays a central role in the avoidance of many age-associated chronic diseases, and in the biology of ageing itself (Rizza *et al.*, 2014). In particular, ER is a recognized simple method for inducing a highly reproducible extension of lifespan in certain species, along with delaying age-related physiological changes and the onset of diseases (Xiang & He, 2011).

The first known report concerning the effects of food restriction in animals dates from 1917. Osborne *et al.* (1917) showed that restricting the food intake of rats had a positive impact on their lifespan and reproductive performance in later life. These findings were corroborated by the study of McCay *et al.* (1935) that demonstrated a dramatic extension in lifespan in rats subjected to 40% ER from the age of weaning. Following these earlier studies in rodents, subsequent data have consistently shown that ER slows ageing and prolongs maximum lifespan in many other species, from yeasts to vertebrates (Speakman & Mitchell, 2011). These animals not only live longer and are healthier, but at any time they are physiologically younger than *ad libitum*-fed animals (Masoro, 2005). Broadly, a 10–50% reduction in energy intake below the usual *ad libitum* intake causes a proportionate increase in maximum lifespan, whereas ER exceeding 50% typically causes undernutrition and increases mortality (Rizza *et al.*, 2014).

Interestingly, in the last century, the shortage of food during World War II was associated with a fall in mortality from CVD (Fontana *et al.*, 2004), reinforcing the beneficial effects of ER on human cardiovascular health. Indeed, despite the lack of validated biomarkers of ageing and the difficulty of conducting randomized, diet-controlled, long-term survival studies in humans, epidemiologic data show that ER positively affects many factors involved in the pathogenesis of ageing and life expectancy in humans (Omodei & Fontana, 2011). However, the causal association between ER and longevity has not been definitively proven, nor is the optimal energy intake for life prolongation known. Notwithstanding, the available data suggest that, in humans, ER with an adequate nutrient intake is as beneficial as it is in animal models (Anton & Leeuwenburgh, 2013). Below, the main effects of ER on organism physiology are discussed, thus explaining how this nutritional pattern intervenes in late-life quality by lessening the chronic disease burden that strongly contributes to mortality in the elderly (Willcox *et al.*, 2007).

2.3.1 Increased longevity and health of energy-restricted organisms

Rodents provide an extremely valuable and flexible animal model to determine the effects of ER, and for a long time were the only mammals in which ER had clearly been shown to increase both average and maximal lifespan, and to decelerate age-dependent physiological and structural changes in multiple organs and tissues (Omodei & Fontana, 2011). However, as mentioned earlier, recent findings from nonhuman primate studies suggest that prolonged ER presents equivalent effects to those found in rodents (Anton & Leeuwenburgh, 2013).

In addition to its effects on longevity, the extent of lifespan independent of the biological ageing process, ER increases healthspan by preventing or delaying the occurrence of a wide range of chronic diseases. Nevertheless, there are some controversies concerning the best age to start ER. Pugh *et al.* (1999) reported that initiating ER later in life significantly extends lifespan in rodents, although the effect is significantly lower compared with that observed when ER starts at weaning. On the other hand, Dhahbi *et al.* (2004) demonstrated that in rodents ER initiated at adulthood (12–19 months of age) is as effective as ER begun early in life in decelerating mortality rate, extending remaining lifespan and modifying gene expression profile.

Studies performed in rhesus monkeys corroborate evidence from rodent models of ER, showing that a reduction of daily energy intake of 30% leads to an increase in maximum lifespan compared with control animals (Colman & Anderson, 2011). A younger outward appearance has been also observed after 20 years of decreased energy intake (Colman *et al.*, 2009). In addition, rhesus monkeys subjected to ER showed decreased age-associated pathologies. These primates presented increased insulin sensitivity, reduced adiposity and oxidative damage, and improved cardiovascular profile, reinforcing the effect of ER on reduction of age-associated pathologies and therefore extension of lifespan (Colman *et al.*, 2009; Colman & Anderson, 2011; Pan *et al.*, 2012; Roth & Polotsky, 2012).

The incidence of a wide range of age-associated chronic diseases in humans, such as chronic nephropathies, cardiomyopathies, atherosclerotic lesions, diabetes mellitus (DM), hypertension and autoimmune and respiratory diseases, can be avoided or prevented by ER (Chung *et al.*, 2013). Studies conducted in humans, including the CALERIE trial, have noted favorable ER-dependent changes in biomarkers related to cardiovascular and glucoregulatory function, which probably relate to longevity (Trepanowski *et al.*, 2011). There are many evidences indicating that long-term self-imposed ER (3–15 years) results in several metabolic adaptations that reduce the risk of developing CVD and cancer, and opposes the expected age-associated alterations in myocardial stiffness and autonomic function, while improving recovery of cardiac function following ischemia (Fontana *et al.*, 2004; Lefevre *et al.*, 2009; Rizza *et al.*, 2014). For instance, both left ventricular diastolic function and heart rate variability indexes, two markers of cardiovascular ageing, are significantly improved by ER, and resemble those of individuals 20 years younger on a typical Western diet (Meyer *et al.*, 2006; Stein *et al.*, 2012). Reduced arterial stiffness and improved endothelial dysfunction of the arteries were observed in ER individuals (Meyer *et al.*, 2006; Stein *et al.*, 2012). Similarly, ER also slows down the transcriptional changes associated with ageing in skeletal muscle, causing it to resemble that of much younger individuals (Mercken *et al.*, 2013). In line with this, long-term ER in rodents prevents age-associated hypertrophy and apoptosis of cardiomyocytes (Dhahbi *et al.*, 2006), and reduces perivascular collagen deposition in myocardium (Dhahbi *et al.*, 2006; Tomada *et al.*, 2013b).

On the basis of a range of cardiovascular risk factors, long-term self-imposed ER (for an average of 6 years) has been associated with a protective effect against atherosclerosis (consolidated by a 40% reduction in carotid artery intima-media thickness), reduction in hypertension (showing consistently lower levels of both systolic and diastolic blood pressures), inflammation (recording a significant reduction in inflammatory markers such as plasma levels of CRP, TNF-α and interleukin-6, IL-6), plasma levels of triglycerides, and total and LDL-cholesterol, and an increase in the plasma level of high-density lipoprotein (HDL)-cholesterol (Fontana *et al.*, 2004).

Undoubtedly, ER is protective against becoming overweight/obese, but also against the development of type 2 DM. In fact, ER clearly improves glucoregulatory function, reducing fasting glycemia and insulinemia, and increasing insulin sensitivity (Fontana *et al.*, 2010a; Golubović *et al.*, 2013). Furthermore, markers of oxidative stress, such as hydrogen peroxide, protein carbonyls and nitrotyrosine, are significantly reduced in the serum of obese individuals upon an ER regimen (Dandona *et al.*, 2001; Trepanowski *et al.*, 2011).

The ER regimen was also proven to prevent age-associated decline in psychomotor and spatial memory tasks, and the loss of dendritic spines, necessary for learning in animal models, resulting in the promotion of brain plasticity and ability to self-repair (Mattson, 2000). It was observed that ER decreases neurodegeneration and β-amyloid deposition in the brain and enhances neurogenesis in animal models of Alzheimer disease, Parkinson disease, Huntington disease and stroke (Omodei & Fontana, 2011).

ER has been shown to inhibit spontaneous, chemically induced and radiation-induced tumors in several murine models of cancer (Longo & Fontana, 2010). For instance, a 15–53% reduction in energy relative to *ad libitum* ingestion caused a proportionate linear 20–62% reduction in malignant tumor incidence in rodents. Also in monkeys, young-onset 30% ER completely prevented cancer, while adult-onset 30% ER reduced cancer incidence by 50% compared with controls (Colman *et al.*, 2009; Mattison *et al.*, 2012). Whether ER reduces cancer incidence in humans is unknown, but data from studies of long-term ER suggest that the metabolic and physiological responses to ER in humans are equivalent to those in rodents and monkeys (Fontana *et al.*, 2010a).

The mechanisms behind ER-mediated beneficial effects on cancer observed in rodents and nonhuman primates are thought to involve the metabolic adaptations to ER itself, including: (a) decreased production of growth factors and anabolic hormones; (b) decreased ROS production and upregulation of the endogenous anti-oxidant systems, which decrease oxidative stress and free radical-induced DNA damage; (c) decreased plasma concentrations of inflammatory cytokines and increased circulating anti-inflammatory molecules, such as corticosteroids, ghrelin and adiponectin; and (d) protection against age-associated deterioration in immunosurveillance. In addition, ER simultaneously affects multiple processes that are involved in the pathogenesis of cancer, including DNA repair processes, autophagy and the removal of damaged cells through apoptosis, and protection against the damaging effects of a wide range of toxic and genotoxic compounds (Longo & Fontana, 2010). Recently, it was demonstrated, in rectal tissue biopsies obtained from obese patients, that ER may contribute to the prevention of telomere shortening, an initiating event in cancer that may cause genome instability (O'Callaghan *et al.*, 2009). This finding may be of crucial importance not only in the pathogenesis of cancer, but also in the whole biology of ageing.

Nonetheless, the effects of ER on cancer are not homogeneous. The age at which ER is initiated, the severity of ER and the strain/genetic background of the animals determine the magnitude of cancer prevention or delay. Furthermore, some cancers show a greater response to ER than others, and a small proportion of tumors, unfortunately, seems to be resistant to the effects of ER (Longo & Fontana, 2010).

In mammals, ER induces primary changes in the neuroendocrine system and decreases the nicotinamide adenine dinucleotide $(NAD)^+$ to NADH conversion rate. The primary result of this change is a reduced secretion of GH and insulin. Low GH, in turn, decreases the levels of IGF-1 produced in the liver (Dabhade & Kotwal, 2013). In mice, mutations in the homeobox protein prophet of PIT-1 (Prop-1) or pituitary-specific positive transcription factor 1 (Pit-1) genes, which cause severe deficiency in secretion of GH and IGF-1, extend lifespan by 25–65% and cause dwarfism (McKee *et al.*, 2010). In fact, the deficiency of those hormones appears to mediate the effects of Prop-1 and Pit-1 mutations on longevity, since mice that cannot release GH in response to GH-releasing hormone also live longer. Moreover, both dwarf mice with high plasma GH, but a 90% lower IGF-1 (GHR/BP null mice), and heterozygous female IGF-1 receptor knockout mice not only live longer than wild-type controls (Holzenberger *et al.*, 2003) but also present lower incidence and delayed occurrence of tumors (particularly spontaneous tumors), increased insulin sensitivity and a reduction in age-dependent cognitive impairment (Vergara *et al.*, 2004; Ikeno *et al.*, 2009). Furthermore, although GH- and IGF-1-deficient dwarf mice become obese at middle age (Berryman *et al.*, 2004), when these animals are subjected to ER, they no longer become obese and can live up to 100% longer than wild-type and *ad libitum*-fed mice, suggesting that ER activates additional mechanisms independent of the GH/IGF-1 axis repression (Bartke *et al.*, 2008). In contrast, mice overexpressing the GH receptor have very high concentrations of IGF-1, larger body size, shorter lifespan and an increased incidence of cancer and kidney and neurodegenerative diseases (Bartke *et al.*, 2002). Interestingly, low IGF-1 signals and reduced cancer incidence are simultaneously observed in ER mice, a mechanism that might be partly explained by their increased resistance to oxidative damage. However, while ER decreases serum IGF-1 concentration by 30–40% in rodents, equivalent effects have not been observed in healthy humans unless protein intake is also reduced (Fontana *et al.*, 2008).

The activation of the transcription factor nuclear factor-erythroid 2 p45-related factor 2 (Nrf2), which increases the transcription and activity of a variety of anti-oxidative and carcinogen-detoxification enzymes, might be important in mediating the anticancer effects of ER. This is supported by experiments performed in Nrf2-deficient mice, in which the antitumorigenesis effects of ER were significantly impaired (Pearson *et al.*, 2008a). Notwithstanding, more studies are needed to elucidate the exact molecular mechanisms that underlie the beneficial effects of ER in preventing cancer by avoiding accumulation of DNA damage or by potentiating the regression of pre-neoplastic lesions. How ER can block cancer before it becomes invasive or metastatic should also be investigated and clarified.

In brief, ER extends the maximal lifespan of several species, which is maximized when the magnitude of ER is expanded to the highest possible value and duration without inducing undernutrition (Trepanowski *et al.*, 2011; Roth & Polotsky, 2012). In accordance with studies of Meyer *et al.* (2006), when optimal nutritional choices, such as those that are advocated by the Mediterranean diet (discussed in Chapter 11), are coupled to ER, an increase in life expectancy in humans is made possible. Regardeless of the benefits described earlier, it should be emphasized that severe ER can have harmful consequences at an organic level and can negatively affect general health. Excessive restriction of energy intake has been associated with impaired wound healing, anemia, muscle wasting, neurologic deficits, lower extremity edema, weakness, dizziness, lethargy, irritability and depression. Furthermore, it can result in impaired regulation of body temperature (BT) and cell-mediated immunity, dry and atrophic skin, thin and sparse hair, suppressed cell production in the bone marrow, decreased cardiac muscle mass, hypotension, bradycardia, amenorrhea and osteoporosis (Soare *et al.*, 2014).

2.3.2 Body composition, temperature and resting metabolic rate

One of the most overt effects of ER is the change in body composition. This diet pattern leads to loss of fat mass, particularly visceral white adipose tissue (vWAT), which is causally linked to the lifespan-enhancing effects of ER. Indeed, surgical excision of rat vWAT not only improves their insulin sensitivity (Barzilai *et al.*, 2000), but also allows them to live longer than *ad libitum*-fed controls (although not as long as animals on 40% ER; Muzumdar *et al.*, 2008). Data from studies conducted in rodent models suggest that the effects of ER on maximum lifespan are mediated by ER itself and are not simply a result of leanness induced by such restriction. Supporting that, it was found that maximum lifespan did not increase in male rats that maintained a low body fat mass (BFM) by performing regular exercise on running wheels, but increased in sedentary paired-weight male rats that were food restricted (Holloszy *et al.*, 1985; Craig *et al.*, 1987). Moreover, maximum lifespan was higher in ER genetically obese (ob/ob) mice than in a*d libitum*-fed, genetically normal, lean mice, even though BFM in the ER ob/ob mouse was more than twice as high as in genetically normal and lean mice (Harrison *et al.*, 1984).

Endocrine regulation is largely responsible for many changes in body composition. GH is one of the most important hormones, regulating growth, body composition and bone strength. However, as mentioned earlier, GH-deficient and GH receptor-deficient mice live substantially longer than wild-type counterparts, while mice overexpressing GH receptor have a larger body size but shorter lifespan (Bartke *et al.*, 2002). In humans, although GH and/or IGF-1 deficiency promotes obesity and hyperlipidemia, and the treatment of GH-deficient individuals with GH causes a beneficial effect on body composition and dyslipidemia, the replenishment of GH increases intima media thickness and the number of atherosclerotic carotid plaques, indicating that the obesity associated with GH or GH receptor deficiency may not be detrimental (Oliveira *et al.*, 2007).

Recently, Kim *et al.* (2009) aimed to determine the effect of ageing and ER (40% less than age-matched *ad libitum*-fed male Fisher 344 rats) on adipogenesis in WAT. The authors verified that the expression of the two key regulatory mediators of the adipogenesis process (peroxisome proliferator-activated receptor-γ, PPARγ, and sterol regulatory element-binding protein, SREBP-1) was significantly increased in WAT from aged-ER animals compared with *ad libitum*-fed counterparts. This observation suggests that ER can mitigate the decreased expression and activity of transcription factors related to adipogenesis in WAT during the ageing process. In this study, it was also observed that modulation of lipid accumulation by ER through increased carnitine palmitolytransferase-1 (CPT-1) activity is important to the anti-ageing action of ER and to its ability to attenuate age-associated metabolic diseases (Kim *et al.*, 2009).

A decline in LBM and bone mass density (osteopenia and osteoporosis) tends to occur as people age, as well as a rise in BFM and its redistribution (Gomez-Cabello *et al.*, 2012;

Bazzocchi *et al.*, 2013). Nevertheless, these changes in body composition cannot be blamed entirely on the ageing process *per se*, but instead on the increasingly sedentary behavior of individuals as they grow older. Reduced physical activity leads to loss of muscle and, as a direct consequence, body metabolic rate (BMR) falls. A lower BMR implies that older people need to eat less energy to maintain the same BW. Regardless of BW, the changes in BFM distribution are definitively considered one of the major age-related physiological modifications that might underlie a wide range of negative health effects (Wang *et al.*, 2008a).

Skeletal muscle mass and strength decrease (sarcopenia) and associated decrease in LBM have been associated with increased mortality (Cesari *et al.*, 2009). Interestingly, in rhesus monkeys ER prevents or delays this age-related loss of muscle function and mass (Colman *et al.*, 2009; McKiernan *et al.*, 2010), but unfortunately, in humans, the ER regimen does not appear to retard the age-related loss of LBM (Weiss *et al.*, 2007).

Although there are conflicting data concerning ER effects on bone mineral mass in humans (Santarpia *et al.*, 2013), it is interesting to note that ER in rhesus monkeys does not alter bone mineral metabolism measured by biochemical markers of bone turnover, such as serum levels of osteocalcin, parathyroid hormone and 25(OH)vitamin D (Lane *et al.*, 2001; Colman *et al.*, 2012); however, these nonhuman primates present lower total body bone mineral density in comparison to controls, which is not associated with increased bone fractures (Mattison *et al.*, 2003; Colman *et al.*, 2012). Hence, it is believed that the lowest bone mass in ER animals reflects the smaller body size of rhesus monkeys and not a pathological osteopenic condition (Colman *et al.*, 2012).

ER is correlated with a marked lowering of energy metabolism (Redman *et al.*, 2009). At the whole-animal level, it is clear that, to reach energy balance, animals under ER must experience a reduction in their total rate of energy expenditure equivalent to the level of restriction. Since the effect of ER on lifespan is directly related to the percentage restriction, then the total utilization of energy is similar in animals under different levels of restriction, however for different lifespans. This belief agrees with one of the most attractive theories put foward to explain how ER increases lifespan, the *rate of living theory* (Hulbert *et al.*, 2007), which states that a decrease in the BMR (rate of living) lowers the flow of energy, with a consequent decrease in ROS production and oxidative damage to living tissues (Sanz *et al.*, 2006c).

Direct measurements of RMR in mice under 20% ER have demonstrated a reduction in this parameter that apparently contributes about 24% to the overall energy savings (Hambly & Speakman, 2005). Furthermore, considering that the effect of ER on total expenditure of energy is negative, animals tend to become physically smaller to increase the efficiency of the use of energy. For example, an animal under 30% ER, to attain energy balance, may reduce the size of all of its organs by 30%. Alternatively, it may decrease its organs by only 20% and save the additional 10% energy by depressing cellular energy use, or it might reduce the size of its organs by 40%, allowing it to increase expenditure at the tissue level by 10% (Speakman & Mitchell, 2011).

However, the concept that ER modulates lifespan by decreasing the BMR, with the accrual of macromolecule damage over time, has been replaced during the last decade by the concept that ER influences the activity of several signaling pathways that regulate energy metabolism. The most widely studied of these are the sirtuins, particularly Sirt1, PGC-1α, AMP-activated protein kinase (AMPK), IGF-1 and mTOR protein kinase signaling (Testa *et al.*, 2014), further discussed later.

The reduction of hormones that regulate cellular metabolism and thermogenesis, such as thyroid hormones and cathecolamines, constitutes an adaptation mechanism that has been hypothesized to play an important role in mediating the anti-ageing and life-extending effects of ER (Fontana & Klein, 2007). Indeed, ER is associated with decreased circulating triiodothyronine (T3) levels and sympathetic nervous system activity, causing a decrease in BT in rodents and in nonhuman primates and in the whole-body resting energy expenditure (Weindruch *et al.*, 1979; Cheney *et al.*, 1983; Lane *et al.*, 1996; Blanc *et al.*, 2003; Ferguson *et al.*, 2007; Carrillo & Flouris, 2011). This drop in BT is similar to that observed in hibernation, which leads to the consideration that ER and hibernation states may be co-adaptive responses (Walford & Spindler, 1997). Studies performed in the Ames dwarf mouse (Hunter *et al.*, 1999) and the GH receptor/binding protein knockout mouse (Hauck *et al.*, 2001) demonstrate that both present low BT, supporting the role of lower BT in extended lifespan and in the prevention of tumor development. On the other hand, when wild-type mice are housed at thermoneutral conditions, the effect of ER on BT is reduced, and there is a corresponding reduction in the effect of ER on lifespan and cancer prevention (Koizumi *et al.*, 1996). Also interesting is the fact that *ad libitum*-fed transgenic mice overexpressing the uncoupling protein 2 (UCP2) in hypocretin neurons (Hcrt-UCP2 mice) have a lower BT and a 16% greater life expectancy than wild-type animals, regardless of total energy intake (Conti *et al.*, 2006). Notwithstanding, it should be emphasized that there are marked differences in the BT response to ER among mouse strains, as shown in a comparison of 28 different strains on 30% ER for 4 months (Rikke *et al.*, 2003). Many strains had a BT that was lower (excluding periods of torpor) by 1–2 °C, but in others the reductions were more profound and averaged 3–5 °C. In humans, long-term ER is also associated with significant reductions in BT regardless of BFM (Soare *et al.*, 2011). This ER-mediated adaptation seems to contribute to lifespan extension, as demonstrated in the Baltimore Longitudinal Study of Aging, in which men with a lower BT lived significantly longer (Roth *et al.*, 2002).

2.3.3 Metabolism and insulin sensitivity

Ageing is associated with changes in glucose metabolism, which may lead to the development of a variety of health problems, particularly type 2 DM and CVD. However, epidemiological and experimental studies have shown that type 2 DM and CVD are neither caused by ageing *per se*, nor inevitable consequences of age. Rather, changes in glucose metabolism render the body more vulnerable to the development of those diseases. Age-related loss of LBM, decreased β-cell proliferation and dysregulation of insulin signaling result in insulin resistance and glucose intolerance, conditions that promote the development of DM (Taguchi & White, 2008).

Chronic ER improves insulin sensitivity and significantly reduces fasting glycemia, fasting insulinemia and serum fructosamine concentration, a marker of nonenzymatic glycation of serum proteins (Fontana *et al.*, 2010a; Golubović *et al.*, 2013). The accumulation of advanced glycation end-products (AGE) is also reduced by ER, which is particularly important in CVD prevention, since AGE interaction with their specific receptors results in activation of signal transduction mechanisms, including oxidative stress, modification in extracellular matrix features, release of inflammatory and chemotactic cytokines and growth factors, and increased expression of adhesion molecules (Fontana, 2009).

Recent evidence suggests that decreased insulin signaling, and not enhanced insulin sensitivity, may be implicated in the delayed ageing phenotype of some of the animal models of increased longevity. In fact, long-lived mouse strains such as fat-specific insulin-receptor knockout (which lack the insulin receptor expression in the adipose tissue), brain insulin receptor substrate-2 null, insulin receptor substrate-1 null and Klotho gene overexpressing animals present reduced insulin signaling and/or mild lifelong insulin resistance (Kurosu *et al.*, 2005; Taguchi *et al.*, 2007; Selman *et al.*, 2008). Interestingly, long-term severe ER is associated with impaired glucose tolerance in some individuals, presumably owing to decreased insulin-mediated glucose disposal, associated with lower circulating levels of IGF-1, total testosterone and T3, which are also typical adaptations to ER in rodents (Fontana *et al.*, 2010a). Thus, it seems plausible that severe ER decreases signaling through the insulin pathway in some tissues and that this may play a role in downregulation of the expression of pro-ageing genes by reducing AKT/protein kinase B (PKB) while increasing the activity of the transcription factors of the forkhead box O (FOXO) family (Salih & Brunet, 2008; Kenyon, 2010). In fact, two decades ago, Kenyon *et al.* (1993) published the first paper indicating that the inhibition of the insulin/IGF-1/FOXO pathway dramatically extends lifespan in worms. Since then, accumulating data have shown that this pathway is evolutionarily conserved and that dietary and genetic manipulations of the insulin/IGF-1/FOXO pathway promote health and extend lifespan in rodents (Kennedy *et al.*, 2007; Piper & Bartke, 2008) and in humans (van Heemst *et al.*, 2005; Suh *et al.*, 2008). In addition, a downregulation of the insulin/IGF-1/FOXO pathway, both at transcriptional and post-transcriptional levels, is observed in humans on long-term 30% ER (Mercken *et al.*, 2013).

2.3.4 Immune system and inflammatory modulation

Chronic inflammation plays a central role in the pathogenesis of several age-associated chronic diseases (e.g. atherosclerosis, cancer, arthritis, dementia and osteoporosis) and in the ageing process itself (Fontana, 2009). While excessive energy intake and adiposity, in particular visceral adiposity, cause a state of low-grade chronic inflammation, reflected by increased levels of circulating IL-1β, IL-6, IL-8, IL-18, TNF-α, monocyte chemoattractant protein-1 (MCP-1), fibrinogen and CRP, ER reduces systemic inflammation, which constitutes one of its interventions in the retardation of ageing and the prevention/delay of chronic diseases (Fontana & Klein, 2007; Chung *et al.*, 2013). Supporting this, several studies on animals have consistently shown that chronic ER results in low levels of circulating inflammatory adipocytokines, low blood lymphocyte levels, reduced production of inflammatory cytokines by the white blood cells and serum cortisol levels in the high normal range. In this setting, it is important to note that the ER-induced lower inflammatory state does not occur passively from an absence of inflammatory stimuli, but instead depends on coordinated actions of specific metabolic, hormonal and gene expression products that actively repress responses to potential inflammatory stimuli (Fontana, 2009). In fact, ER enhances the ability to cope with intense inflammatory stimuli, and protects against age-associated deterioration of immune function, including reduced immune response capability, thymic involution and shifts in leukocyte and lymphocyte subsets (Fontana, 2009). Data from self-imposed ER and from short-term ER intervention studies have shown that ER in humans also results in a reduction of systemic pro-inflammatory cytokines, chemokines and cell-surface adhesion molecules, and increased anti-inflammatory cytokines (Racette *et al.*, 2006; Weiss *et al.*, 2006; Fontana *et al.*, 2007; Chung *et al.*, 2013). For instance, middle-aged humans on ER have very low levels of chronic inflammation, as reflected in remarkably low levels of CRP (0.3 mg/L compared with values in the 1.5–2.0 mg/L range in healthy controls) and TNF-α (50% lower than controls; Fontana *et al.*, 2004, 2006; Meyer *et al.*, 2006).

Moreover, BW loss induced by ER reduces macrophage activation and its infiltration in the adipose tissue, which leads to noticeable improvements in insulin sensitivity and a better circulating adipokine profile (Xydakis *et al.*, 2004). The reduction in systemic inflammation and oxidative stress that results from ER is associated with increased eNOS levels and activity, resulting in greater nitric oxide (NO) bioavailability and reduction in arterial stiffness (Csiszar *et al.*, 2009; Zanetti *et al.*, 2010; Samaras *et al.*, 2013).

ER also exerts its anti-inflammatory effects through increased endogenous corticosteroid production. Chronic ER rodents have significantly higher daily mean plasma free corticosterone concentration than *ad libitum*-fed animals throughout their lifespan, apparently without increased hypothalamic–pituitary activity, since plasma adrenocorticotropic hormone (ACTH) concentrations are lower in the former than in *ad libitum* fed counterparts (Han *et al.*, 2001). It is important to underline that the rise in corticosteroid levels has inhibitory effects on inflammatory gene expression, and also a role in autoimmune diseases prevention (Rhen & Cidlowski, 2005).

Increased immune system response caused by ER may involve the elevation of circulating ghrelin, an orexigenic hormone secreted by the stomach, concomitantly with reduction in leptin levels, which intervention in the neuroendocrine axes is discussed later (Speakman & Mitchell, 2011). Ghrelin infusion is known to partially reverse age-related thymic involution, while inhibiting the production of pro-inflammatoiry cytokines in T-cells (Dixit, 2008).

A suggested mechanism underpinning the positive effects of ER on immune function is the reduction in ROS production that may damage T-lymphocytes, impeding their ability to combat tumor cells. However, since ROS are an integral component of the response to pathogens, lowered capacity to generate ROS may then lead to negative impacts on the immune system in ER animals with respect to their capacity to resist infections (Speakman & Mitchell, 2011). In fact, even though ER has been shown to delay the age-dependent decline in certain immune functions, and reduces the morbidity of autoimmune diseases (Trepanowski *et al.*, 2011), severe ER may increase susceptibility to infections by bacteria, virus and worms (Kristan, 2008). In addition, ER can impair wound healing, as shown in skin wounds in long-term ER mice compared with *ad libitum*-fed mice, the healing process being greatly accelerated by a short period of *ad libitum* feeding before the wound is inflicted (Reed *et al.*, 1996).

2.3.5 Neuroendocrine axes and adipokines

The molecular mechanisms by which ER regulates the neuroendocrine system remain obscure. Nevertheless, the effects of ER may be explained from an evolutionary perspective; organisms have developed neuroendocrine signals and metabolic response systems to maximize survival during periods of food shortage. When organisms encounter a period of food scarcity, they suspend growth and reproduction, and induce the production of defense molecules, like glucocorticoid hormones and heat shock proteins. For instance, increased glucocorticoid hormone levels in response to ER are critical for mobilizing energy reserves and immune responses (Berner & Stern, 2004).

ER modulates the secretion of adipose tissue-derived peptides, generally adipokines (the main functions of which are summarized in Table 2.2), such as adiponectin, a peptide

Table 2.2 Summary of main biological and molecular properties of adipokines.

Adipokine	Effects of ER vs obesity on circulating levels	Benefic biological and molecular properties
Adiponectin (Ouchi *et al*., 2001, 2003; Xydakis *et al*., 2004; Zhu *et al*., 2004; Otabe *et al*., 2007; Shinmura *et al*., 2007, 2008; Jung *et al*., 2008; Niemann *et al*., 2008; Fontana *et al*., 2010a; Polyzos *et al*., 2010; Qiao *et al*., 2011; Mattu & Randeva, 2013; Tomada *et al*., 2013b, 2014; Vielma *et al*., 2013)	Plasma levels inversely related to adipose tissue accretion; reflects adverse fat distribution and adipose tissue dysfunction ↑ ER ↓ Obesity	↓ Hypertension ↓ Myocardial infarction ↓ Coronary heart disease (in diabetics) ↓ Myocardial hypertrophy ↑ Vasodilatation ↓ Coronary artery disease ↑ Angiogenesis ↓ Insulin resistance (↓ serum glucose; ↓ insulin levels) ↑ Insulin sensitivity ↓ Atherosclerosis ↓ Vascular adhesion molecules expression ↓ Transformation of macrophages into foam cells ↓ Systemic inflammation ↓ TNF-α-induced NF-κB activation ↓ Apoptosis of endothelial cells ↓ Proliferation of vascular smooth muscle cells ↓ Liver inflammation and fibrosis
Leptin (Vidal *et al*., 1996; Fantuzzi & Faggioni, 2000; Yamagishi *et al*., 2001; Lee *et al*., 2004; Sierra-Johnson *et al*., 2007; Wannamethee *et al*., 2007; Leal & Mafra, 2013; Mattu & Randeva, 2013; Santarpia *et al*., 2013)	Plasma levels directly related with obesity severity ↓ ER ↑ Obesity	*Low levels* ↓ Orexigenic and ↑ anorexigenic peptide synthesis in the hypothalamus, thereby reducing appetite ↓ Gonadal, growth hormone and thyroidal axes ↑ Glucocorticoid system *High levels* ↑ Hypertension (↑ mean arterial blood pressure) ↑ Heart rate ↑ Myocardial infarction and stroke ↑ Coronary artery disease ↑ Vasodilation (in coronary artery disease) ↑ Insulin resistance ↑ Hemostasis imbalance ↑ Inflammation ↑ Atherosclerosis ↑ Hypertrophy in cardiomyocytes ↓ Cardiac lipotoxicity
Resistin (Azuma *et al*., 2003; Silha *et al*., 2003; Verma *et al*., 2003; Rajala *et al*., 2004; Bokarewa *et al*., 2005; Kusminski *et al*., 2005; Sato *et al*., 2005; Fontana *et al*., 2010a; Edwards *et al*., 2011; Mattu & Randeva, 2013; Yu *et al*., 2013)	Increased in obesity; predictive marker of cardiovascular disease risk ↓ ER ↑ Obesity	↑ Insulin resistance ↑ Dyslipidemia ↑ Systemic inflammation ↑ Levels in myocardial infarction ↑ Atherosclerosis ↑ Endothelial dysfunction ↑ Expression of VCAM-1 and ICAM-1 ↓ Sirtuin1

Continued

Table 2.2 Continued

Visfatin (Ognjanovic & Bryant-Greenwood, 2002; Smith *et al.*, 2006; Dahl *et al.*, 2007; Takebayashi *et al.*, 2007; Busso *et al.*, 2008; de Luis *et al.*, 2008; Kovacikova *et al.*, 2008; Lim *et al.*, 2008; Bo *et al.*, 2009)	Circulating levels directly related to abdominal fat mass ↓ ER ↑ Obesity	Regulation of glucose homeostasis ↓ Vascular smooth muscle apoptosis ↓ Cardiac contractibility ↑ HDL ↑ Endothelial dysfunction ↓ Infarct size ↑ Expression of pro-inflammatory cytokines (IL-1β, IL-6 and TNF-α) ↑ Expression of VCAM-1 and ICAM-1, via oxidative stress-dependent NF-κB activation ↑ Plaque destabilization (patients with unstable carotid and coronary atherosclerosis)
Vaspin (Chang *et al.*, 2010; Auguet *et al.*, 2011; Phalitakul *et al.*, 2011; Bluher, 2012)	Circulating levels directly related to body fat mass accretion ↓ ER ↑ Obesity	↑ Activity of anti-orexigenic factors ↓ TNF-α-induced expression of ICAM-1 Prevents ROS generation and subsequent activation of NF-κB Improves glucose metabolism (at low levels)
Omentin (Yang *et al.*, 2006b; de Souza Batista *et al.*, 2007; Yamawaki *et al.*, 2010; Auguet *et al.*, 2011; Moreno-Navarrete *et al.*, 2011; Shibata *et al.*, 2012; Zhong *et al.*, 2012)	Circulating levels inversely related with visceral fat mass ↑ ER ↓ Obesity	↓ Endothelial dysfunction ↑ Insulin-induced glucose uptake ↓ Inflammation ↓ TNF-α-induced expression of adhesion molecules in endothelial cells via NF-κB inhibition activation
Apelin (Boucher *et al.*, 2005; Kuba *et al.*, 2007; Weir *et al.*, 2009; Yue *et al.*, 2010; Krist *et al.*, 2013)	Serum levels increase in obesity ↓ ER ↑ Obesity	*Positive inotrope* ↓ Atrial fibrillation ↓ Levels in ischemic cardiomyopathy ↑ Levels in hypoxia ↑ Vasodilatation Anti-inflammatory Anti-atherogenic Improves glucose metabolism
Chemerin (Goralski *et al.*, 2007; Sell *et al.*, 2009, 2010; Chakaroun *et al.*, 2012; Roman *et al.*, 2012)	Directly associated with cardiometabolic risk factors ↓ ER ↑ Obesity	↓ Insulin sensitivity ↑ Subclinical inflammation Adipogenesis regulation

ER, energy restriction; HDL, high-density-lipoprotein cholesterol; ICAM-1, intercellular adhesion molecule-1; IL, interleukin; NF-κB, nuclear factor kappa-light-chain enhancer of activated B cells; ROS, reactive oxygen species; Sirt1, Sirtuin 1; TNF, tumor necrosis factor; VCAM-1, vascular cell adhesion molecule-1.

with recognized anti-inflammatory, anti-atherogenic, anti-diabetic and cardioprotective properties (Qiao *et al.*, 2011; Mattu & Randeva, 2013; Vielma *et al.*, 2013). The circulating levels of adiponectin are inversely associated with WAT accretion, and might be an important mechanistic component of the action of ER, as its serum levels markedly increase upon ER in rodents (Zhu *et al.*, 2004; Shinmura *et al.*, 2007, 2008; Niemann *et al.*, 2008; Tomada *et al.*, 2013b, 2014) and humans (Xydakis *et al.*, 2004; Jung *et al.*,

2008; Fontana *et al.*, 2010a). In line with this, some authors suggest that BW loss owing to ER appears to be the most effective intervention to increase adiponectin gene expression (Qiao *et al.*, 2011). Conversely, the consumption of diets rich in saturated fatty acids significantly reduces adiponectin gene expression and circulating levels in rodents (Flachs *et al.*, 2006; Bueno *et al.*, 2008; Ribot *et al.*, 2008; Tomada *et al.*, 2013b). Adiponectin-deficient mice show a marked insulin resistance (Kadowaki *et al.*, 2006), whereas overexpression of adiponectin in transgenic mice prevents several abnormalities induced by this diet, in particular elevated serum glucose and insulin levels (Otabe *et al.*, 2007).

Adiponectin has several positive effects on endothelial health and whole-body metabolism. It improves insulin sensitivity through activation of AMPK in liver and skeletal muscle, reduces the hepatic expression of enzymes envolved in gluconeogenesis, and attenuates liver inflammation and fibrosis via activation of AMPK and PPARα pathways (Polyzos *et al.*, 2010). Moreover, adiponectin levels are inversely associated with adhesion molecule expression and the transformation of macrophages into foam cells (Ouchi *et al.*, 2001). Adiponectin also reduces the apoptosis of endothelial cells and inhibits the proliferation of vascular smooth cells (Ouchi *et al.*, 2003), which together with its anti-inflammatory effects contribute to the reduction of atherosclerotic risk. Studies *in vitro* have also shown that adiponectin can reduce the inflammatory response of endothelial cells through inhibition of TNF-α-induced nuclear factor kappa-light chain enhancer of activated B cell (NF-κB) activation (Ouchi *et al.*, 2000).

Concomitantly with the increase in adiponectin, ER reduces the circulating levels of leptin, an adipokine with multiple biological effects including the control of adipose tissue growth and the modulation of inflammation and autoimmune reactivity (Fantuzzi & Faggioni, 2000). Leptin is almost exclusively expressed and produced by differentiated adipocytes of WAT, subcutaneous WAT (sWAT) being its main source (Zha *et al.*, 2009). Its plasma concentrations and mRNA expression in adipose tissue are directly related to obesity severity (Considine *et al.*, 1996; Vidal *et al.*, 1996); hence, it may represent the best indicator of body composition characteristics and changes in overweight and obese individuals. Leptin controls adipose tissue growth through the central nervous system. In addition, leptin released from expanding adipocytes acts in GABA (γ-aminobutyric acid)-nergic neurons to reduce appetite and increase energy expenditure (Leal & Mafra, 2013) and inhibits the hypothalamic production of the robust orexigenic mediator neuropeptide Y (NPY) while stimulating the anorexigenic pro-opiomelanocortin (POMC). As a long-term food intake regulator, it signals nutritional status to several other physiological systems and modulates their function. That is, when plasma leptin levels decline following fasting or long-term ER, neuroendocrine changes (like the suppression of the gonadal, GH and thyroidal axes and the enhancement of the glucocorticoid system) are induced as adaptive responses to maximize organism survival (Shimokawa & Higami, 2001). Thus, it has a 2-fold regulatory role: when BW is stable, it favors BFM stores; conversely during BW loss, it contributes to energy balance regulation by increasing appetite and decreasing energy expenditure (Santarpia *et al.*, 2013). In this context, it is important to note that the hunger that affects animals under ER conditions is matched by the neuropeptide profile in the hypothalamus, such as elevated NPY and Agouti-regulated peptide (AgRP) levels in response to diminished leptin levels (Minor *et al.*, 2009). Furthermore, circulating ghrelin increases during ER-induced BW loss in obese rodents and humans (Speakman & Mitchell, 2011), suggesting that this hormone may contribute to the sustained appetite associated with ER. The increase in ghrelin blood levels is apparently favored by the reduced levels of circulating leptin observed in individuals under ER-dependent BFM loss conditions (Hambly *et al.*, 2012). In the general population, hyperleptinemia is associated with atherosclerosis, hypertension and metabolic syndrome (a cluster of cardiometabolic risk factors, such as insulin resistance/type 2 DM, hypertension, dyslipidemia and abdominal obesity; Mattu & Randeva, 2013). Leptin plays an important role in the early stages of atherosclerosis development by initiating leukocyte and macrophage recruitment to the endothelial wall, achieved by the induction of mitochondrial superoxide production and expression of MCP-1 in endothelial cells (Yamagishi *et al.*, 2001). Furthermore, increased leptin serum concentrations in humans are also associated with an increased risk of myocardial infarction and stroke, independently of obesity status and the presence of cardiovascular risk factors (Sierra-Johnson *et al.*, 2007). This may be explained in part by the fact that increased leptin levels *per se* lead to increased insulin resistance, hemostasis imbalance and vascular inflammation (Wannamethee *et al.*, 2007).

ER also modulates the serum concentrations of many other adipokines (evident after modest BW losses of 5–10% of the initial BW in overweight and obese individuals; Fontana, 2009). One such adipokine is resistin, circulating levels of which reduce as a result of BW loss induced by ER, exercise and/or bariatric surgery (Azuma *et al.*, 2003; Bokarewa *et al.*, 2005; Edwards *et al.*, 2011). Conversely, resistin over-expression is found in obesity, and is associated with insulin resistance and dyslipidemia (Silha *et al.*, 2003; Rajala *et al.*, 2004; Kusminski *et al.*, 2005; Sato *et al.*, 2005). It is a potent pro-inflammatory molecule (Bokarewa *et al.*, 2005; Fontana *et al.*, 2010a) that induces insulin resistance via increased expression of gluconeogenic enzymes and decreased activity of AMPK, as well as insulin receptor substrate-2 expression in liver (Sheng *et al.*, 2008). In addition, resistin injures endothelium through the induction of secretion of endothelin-1 by endothelial cells, and increased vascular cell adhesion molecule (VCAM)-1 and MCP-1 expression (Verma *et al.*, 2003). Recently, Yu *et al.* (2013) demonstrated that resistin is a negative regulator of Sirt1 expression in both human hepatoma cell line HepG2 and mouse hepatocytes, and that it might play an important role in the development of senescence-associated liver diseases.

Visceral WAT and macrophages of humans also produce visfatin, an adipokine involved in the control of glucose homeostasis by regulating pancreatic β-cell function through the NAD^+ biosynthetic pathway (Busso *et al.*, 2008). Although its circulating levels are not associated with insulin sensitivity, and similar concentrations have been shown in type 2 DM patients and normoglycemic subjects (Berndt *et al.*, 2005; Pagano *et al.*, 2006), visfatin is increased in abdominal obesity (Mattu & Randeva, 2013). Bo *et al.* (2009) reported that plasma visfatin concentrations increase by about 2.4 ng/mL per cm increase in waist circumference. However, the effect of BW loss in visfatin levels is uncertain, as both a decrease and an increase in circulating visfatin levels were reported in morbidly obese subjects after surgically induced BW loss (Haider *et al.*, 2006; Krzyzanowska *et al.*, 2006; Garcia-Fuentes *et al.*, 2007; Botella-Carretero *et al.*, 2008; Swarbrick *et al.*, 2008). Interestingly, several studies have shown that individuals following ER diets had reduced plasma visfatin levels as a function of BW loss (Kovacikova *et al.*, 2008; de Luis *et al.*, 2008). For instance, individualized dietary and exercise recommendations followed for 1 year by metabolic syndrome patients determined a small, but not statistically significant reduction in visfatin circulating values, whereas controls, who had worsened metabolic and inflammatory patterns, showed a significant increase in their adipokine levels. At 1 year, the between-group difference in visfatin was highly significant, and a significant positive correlation was found between high-sensitivity (hs)CRP and TNF-α and changes in serum visfatin concentrations (Bo *et al.*, 2009). On the other hand, Richard *et al.* (2013) showed that the BW reduction over a 20-week period in metabolic syndrome obese patients who consumed the Mediterranean diet (discussed in Chapter 11) had no significant impact on the reduction of plasma visfatin concentrations, even when patients reduced their usual energy intake by 500 kcal/day. Nevertheless, variations in this adipokine were significantly correlated with concurrent variations in inflammatory markers such as IL-6 and TNF-α (Richard *et al.*, 2013). Increasing evidence supports the participation of visfatin in inflammatory processes (partly through increased expression of VCAM-1 and intercellular adhesion molecule 1, ICAM-1, via oxidative stress-dependent NF-κB activation; Dahl *et al.*, 2007) as its plasma values are significantly increased in proinflammatory states such as rheumatoid arthritis, inflammatory bowel disease and polycystic ovary syndrome (Otero *et al.*, 2006; Tan *et al.*, 2006; Moschen *et al.*, 2007). An interesting crosstalk between inflammatory cytokines and visfatin may exist, since there is evidence showing that inflammatory cytokines induce visfatin synthesis, and visfatin *per se* stimulates their expression (Ognjanovic *et al.*, 2001; Ognjanovic & Bryant-Greenwood, 2002).

Visfatin appears to have a mixed role in CVD. Albeit visfatin has been positively correlated with HDL-cholesterol (Smith *et al.*, 2006) and reduction in cardiomyocyte death and myocardial infarct size (Lim *et al.*, 2008), high visfatin levels are also associated with endothelial dysfunction (Takebayashi *et al.*, 2007) and plaque destabilization in patients with unstable carotid and coronary atherosclerosis (Dahl *et al.*, 2007). Overall, it appears to contribute to CVD more than alleviate it.

Vaspin, a vWAT-derived serpin (serpin A12 according to the serpin nomenclature), was identified as a putative member of the serine protease inhibitor family that was originally found to be expressed in vWAT of Otsuka Long Evans Tokushima Fatty (OLETF) rats at the age when obesity and insulin plasma concentrations peak (Hida et al., 2005; Bluher, 2012). Vaspin expression was shown to decrease with worsening of diabetes and BW loss, whereas its serum levels could be normalized by insulin or pioglitazone treatment (Hida et al., 2005). Consistent with that, it was found that increased vaspin mRNA expression in human WAT was associated with obesity, insulin resistance and type 2 DM (Klöting et al., 2006). The exact mechanism of how vaspin secretion may be linked to deterioration of glucose metabolism and insulin sensitivity is not clear. However, it was postulated that this adipokine inhibits a protease that plays a role in the degradation of a hormone or molecule with direct or indirect glucose-lowering effects (Bluher, 2012). In addition to its sustained blood glucose-lowering effects, central vaspin administration also acutely reduces food intake (Klöting et al., 2011), supporting the hypothesis that vaspin is an adipokine that triggers anorectic pathways in the hypothalamus, where reduction of NPY and increase in POMC mRNA levels mediate feeding inhibition (Brunetti et al., 2011). Until now, the mechanism of how vaspin regulates feeding behaviour has been unclear, but it has been proposed that vaspin may also inhibit a protease that degrades an anti-orexigenic factor (Brunetti et al., 2011). It also inhibits TNF-α-induced expression of ICAM-1 by preventing ROS generation and subsequent activation of NF-κB (Phalitakul *et al.*, 2011). Curiously, BFM accretion is associated with increased vaspin expression and circulating levels, whereas modest BW loss decreases serum vaspin concentrations simultaneously with improvements in parameters relevant to insulin resistance (Chang *et al.*, 2010). These interesting findings indicate that vaspin may provide a compensatory response to antagonize the action of proteases that could be upregulated in states of insulin resistance (Auguet *et al.*, 2011).

Omentin is another adipokine strongly expressed in stromal vascular cells of vWAT. Its levels in blood are inversely related to obesity and suppressed by an increase in glycemia and insulinemia (de Souza Batista *et al.*, 2007; Auguet *et al.*, 2011). Omentin enhances the insulin-induced glucose uptake in human visceral and subcutaneous adipocytes through increased phosphorylation of AKT/PKB (Yang *et al.*, 2006b), and like vaspin, downregulates TNF-α-induced expression of adhesion molecules in endothelial cells via NF-κB inhibition. Thus, omentin may be of potential benefit owing to its anti-inflammatory ability to attenuate endothelial dysfunction and atherosclerosis (Zhong *et al.*, 2012). In fact, it was observed that pre-treatment with omentin in isolated rat aorta and mesenteric artery directly induced endothelium-dependent vasodilation, through increased endothelium-derived NO (Yamawaki *et al.*, 2010). Circulating omentin levels were recently considered a biomarker of metabolic disorders, since this parameter is negatively correlated with endothelial dysfunction (Moreno-Navarrete *et al.*, 2011) and, therefore, with several metabolic risk factors (Shibata *et al.*, 2012).

The adipokine apelin is widely expressed in rat and human tissues (including the heart, and large or small conduit vessels) and endothelial cells, and its serum levels increase in obese and insulin-resistant patients in an apparent attempt to compensate metabolic dysregulation (Boucher *et al.*, 2005; Krist *et al.*, 2013). It has been shown that apelin plays a role in the regulation of mechanisms so different as cardiovascular function, glucose homeostasis, food intake, cell proliferation and angiogenesis. Apelin-null mice have impaired insulin sensitivity, an effect that could be reversed by the administration of exogenous apelin (Yue *et al.*, 2010). The glucose-lowering effects of this adipokine seem to involve eNOS, AMPK and AKT, further suggesting that apelin also interferes in endothelial function. In addition, throughout ageing apelin-knockout mice develop progressive impairment of cardiac contractility associated with systolic dysfunction, demonstrating that apelin is crucial to maintaining cardiac contractility in pressure overload and ageing (Kuba *et al.*, 2007). Recently, Krist *et al.* (2013) demonstrated in obese and insulin-resistant patients that BW loss induced by ER, exercise and/or bariatric surgery led to significantly reduced apelin serum concentrations, which resulted in improved insulin sensitivity and subclinical inflammation. Taken together, these data reinforce the hypothesis that circulating apelin increases as a compensatory mechanism to improve insulin sensitivity, which in turn may lead to decreased apelin levels. Indeed, lower apelin serum concentrations in healthy lean individuals seem to be a consequence rather than a cause of insulin sensitivity (Krist *et al.*, 2013).

Chemerin is a recently described adipokine that has been related to adipogenesis regulation and adipocyte metabolism (Goralski *et al.*, 2007). Although the molecular mechanisms of its action are still controversial (Bondue *et al.*, 2011), its expression and circulating levels are positively related to the presence of metabolic syndrome features, such as increased blood pressure, hypertriglyceridemia and insulin resistance (Sell *et al.*, 2009; Roman *et al.*, 2012). While administration of chemerin exacerbates glucose intolerance in obese mice (Ernst *et al.*, 2010), in humans, BW loss induced by ER and/or bariatric surgery is associated with the reduction of circulating levels of chemerin, which in turn contributes to improved insulin sensitivity and subclinical inflammation (Sell *et al.*, 2010; Chakaroun *et al.*, 2012).

2.3.6 Growth factors and cytoprotective effects

Metabolic, hormonal and growth factor changes associated with increased food consumption, decreased physical activity and excessive adiposity affect the defense mechanisms, and cells under permissive conditions most probably undergo malignant transformation (Longo & Fontana, 2010). Conversely, ER is a potent and reproducible physiological intervention for protecting mammals against cancer, as it reduces the levels of several anabolic hormones, growth factors and inflammatory cytokines, decreases oxidative stress and cell proliferation, enhances autophagy and promotes DNA repair processes (Fontana & Klein, 2007). ER induces mild cellular stress, in response to which the cell takes adaptive measures by synthesizing many cytoprotective proteins, including neurotrophic factors such as brain-derived neurotrophic factor, protein chaperones such as heat-shock proteins, transcription factors such as Nrf2, and mitochondrial uncoupling proteins, which crosstalk in triggering resistance to oxidative and metabolic insults (Sykiotis *et al.*, 2011; Mattson *et al.*, 2003; Hayes & Dinkova-Kostova, 2014). The main ER-induced cytoprotective molecular mechanisms are discussed in the following sections.

2.4 Cellular and molecular effects of energy restriction

The anti-ageing effects of ER on most animal species are highly conserved, and reflect the widespread cellular and molecular mechanisms that mediate these beneficial effects. Actually, multiple molecular mechanisms have been proposed to mediate the effects of ER on cells, including promotion of the maintenance of chromatin integrity (Vaquero & Reinberg, 2009) and gene inactivation, which results from a selective heterochromatinization of large parts of the genome, which might include many genes. The sirtuins actively participate in this process, owing to their NAD^+-dependent deacetylase activity in histones, promoting condensation of chromatin. In addition, ER leads to a decreased exposure of DNA to ROS, ensuing its decreased production in ER conditions, partly owing to an increase in the efficiency of both mitochondrial electron transport and oxidative phosphorylation, and in anti-oxidant defenses (Xia *et al.*, 1995). DNA oxidative damage, including mitochondrial DNA, is indeed prevented (Lanza *et al.*, 2012), as well as the onset of replicative senescence phenotype and the shortening of telomeres (von Zglinicki, 2002). The latter process is dependent on telomerase activity that apparently is better preserved in animals under ER (Vera *et al.*, 2013). It has also been demonstrated that ER increases DNA repair mechanisms, avoiding the accumulation of altered nuclear DNA (Heydari *et al.*, 2007). In effect, ER has been shown to increase most DNA repair mechanisms, including base excision repair (Cabelof *et al.*, 2003), nucleotide excision repair (Guo *et al.*, 1998), mismatch repair (Tsao *et al.*, 2002) and double-strand nonhomologous end joining (Lee *et al.*, 2011b).

Intimately linked with ER is the modulation of specific signaling pathways such as those that involve insulin/IGF-1 and mTOR that keenly interfere with the activation of cellular autophagy. These mechanisms are discussed later.

Concerning cell organization, ER, owing to the decrease in oxidative processes, leads to reduction of cellular accumulation of damaged proteins, mainly owing to carbonylation, glycation and crosslinking reactions. The accumulation of dolichol in cell membranes is also retarded in ER-treated animals, which confers protection of the physiological properties and the signal transduction ability of membranes (Parentini *et al.*, 2005).

2.4.1 Modulation of gene expression

Over the last two decades, genes controlling nutrient sensors and metabolic functions have been demonstrated to influence ageing mechanisms and longevity in a long list of species including the yeast *Saccharomyces cerevisiae*, the fruit fly *Drosophila melanogaster* and murine models. Although ER constitutes a nongenetic manipulation, most of the effects that result from this dietary pattern stem from modulation of gene expression. In fact, ER induces major changes in gene expression patterns, an effect that is not due to an overall alteration in the general transcriptional apparatus of the cell, but conversely results from a selected modulation of gene expression that globally influences physiological features of different cells in a common pattern (Han & Hickey, 2005). Globally, the genes targeted by ER can be classified in different groups that, despite the tissue-specificity of responses, usually belong to the families of metabolic pathways, stress response, DNA damage repair, regulation of the structure of chromatin, detoxification and mitochondria-related processes (Vaquero & Reinberg, 2009).

Among the nutrient-sensing pathways involved in the longevity response to ER are mTOR, sirtuins, AMPK, insulin/IGF-1 signaling and transcription factor Nrf2, as discussed later. In mice, an inverse correlation between IGF-1 levels and lifespan was observed in inbred strains (Yuan *et al.*, 2009), as well as in small dogs, which live longer than larger ones because they possess a single allele of the IGF-1 gene (Sutter *et al.*, 2007). In line with those findings, it was recognized that mutations known to impair IGF-1 receptor signaling relate to increased longevity in humans (Kojima *et al.*, 2004; Suh *et al.*, 2008). However, most of the transcriptional programs induced by ER in aged mice seem to be independent of alteration in IGF-1 levels (Barger *et al.*, 2008), since an increase in longevity that strongly resembles that induced by ER was observed in mice after inhibition of mTOR signaling, an effect that was not further increased by ER (Harrison *et al.*, 2009). One of the main effects of mTOR inhibition is the upregulation of autophagy, as discussed later. However, this outcome seems to be indirectly regulated and dependent on the expression of genes affected by PHA-4 (which specifically determines pharyngeal fate *in Caenorhabditis elegans* cells) and forkhead box A transcription factors, as demonstrated in *C. elegans* (Hansen *et al.*, 2008). Concerning AMPK and sirtuins, overexpression is strongly associated with ER-dependent lifespan expansion in mammals. Their crosstalk in cells is presented in the next point.

Prolla postulated that the global gene expression profile of each tissue can be used to evaluate its biological age, because such profiles correlate preferentially with biological as opposed to chronological age (cited by Lee *et al.*, 1999). In effect, 25% ER prevents 90% of age-related changes in gene expression, as demonstrated in DNA microarrays of the heart of 30-month-old mice, with more than half of these modifications presenting a significant variation (Barger *et al.*, 2008). Differences observed in the skeletal muscle and brain of the same animals are not so marked; only 19–26% of the genes had modified expression in ER rats compared with their age-matched controls. Interestingly, 9 years of ER treatment in rhesus monkeys did not reverse the upregulation of transcripts involved in inflammation and oxidative stress induced by ageing in the quadriceps muscle, and inversely, this nutrional pattern increased the expression of cytoskeletal protein-encoding genes and repressed genes involved in mitochondrial function, suggesting that the impact of ER in transcriptional modulation in primates is probably smaller than in shorter-lived organisms (Kayo *et al.*, 2001). Concerning the hippocampus of the rat, ER presents the opposite effects to age in the regulation of genes related to oxidative phosphorylation, response to oxidative stress, mitochondrial function, deubiquitinating pathways and antigen presentation, showing, however, a differential pattern among regions of the hippocampus (Zeier *et al.*, 2011). In fact, transcriptional activity adjusts differentially in tissues to age, animal species and ER pattern too (reviewed in Park & Prolla, 2005; Fu *et al.*, 2006; Han & Hickey, 2005). Among the genes that consistently vary in the various analyzed tissues, those that intervene in chromatin remodeling and histone expression and define the transcriptional and epigenetic states, present a marked impact in ER-treated rats, consistent with promotion of the preservation of genome stability in these conditions and therefore retarding some aspects of the ageing processes in the long-term (Barger *et al.*, 2008).

Interestingly, NF-κB has been suggested to be an intermediate activator of age-related transcriptional changes in both mouse and human tissues (Adler *et al.*, 2007); its blockade reversed global gene expression in the skin of aged mice to a gene expression pattern equivalent to that observed in young mice.

So far, knowledge of how ER modulates gene expression in humans is at an early stage, as is that of genetic variants that contribute to exceptional longevity (Ferrario *et al.*, 2012). However, increased prevalence of variants of genes Ca^{2+}/calmodulin-dependent protein kinase-4, ataxin-1, doublecortin and Ca^{2+}/calmodulin-dependent protein kinase-like-1 was verified in a cohort of 410 individuals of exceptional longevity enrolled in the Southern Italian Centenarian Study (Malovini *et al.*, 2011), and also gene FOXO3A in a cohort of 213 Japanese American men who lived for at least 95 years (Willcox *et al.*, 2008). The most convincing correlation was found between increased longevity and reduction of apolipoprotein E4 allele, which strongly decreases the prevalence of CVD and Alzheimer disease (Schächter *et al.*, 1994). Moreover, longitudinal analysis demonstrated an association between increased longevity in humans and genetic variation in the TERC locus of the telomerase gene that codifies the RNA component of this enzyme, and in the genes that codify Mn-superoxide dismutase and GPx1. For these genes encoding proteins protecting against ROS, a synergistic effect was observed for specific polymorphisms (Soerensen *et al.*, 2009, 2012). Other gene variants were also reported to be associated with human longevity; however, studies across populations failed to demonstrate consistent replication of results.

A very recent study analyzed the transcriptional profile within skeletal muscle of members of the Calorie Restriction Society who had practiced 30% ER for long periods (4–20 years), comparatively with younger and age-paired individuals fed a typical Western diet (Mercken *et al.*, 2013). In line with observations in the rodent, the authors demonstrated that restricted individuals presented a younger gene expression profile, independent of genetic and geographical characteristics of the human cohort, showing a consistent and uniform reprogramming of molecular pathways that shifted cellular metabolism from growth to maintenance and repair activities. These changes included a downregulation of phosphoinositide-3-kinase (PI3K) and AKT/PKB transcripts, a decrease in cyclin D2, a master-regulator of cell cycle progression, and an increase in superoxide dismutase 2, DNA damage-binding 1, a molecular repair factor, and molecules involved in macroautophagic mechanisms expressed downstream to FOXO, as well as Sirt2, Sirt4, Sirt5, AMPKβ and γ and PGC-1α transcripts (Mercken *et al.*, 2013). This evidence indicates that humans share with other species transcriptional responses to ER that are typically associated with improved health and longevity.

However, the shift in gene expression by ER is not universal; a large fraction of genes that change with age are not altered by ER, and conversely, a large number of genes that do not change with age are altered by ER. In addition, several other mechanisms are conjugated in the ER-dependent extension of lifespan in mammals, namely genetic background and environmental influences.

2.4.2 Molecular mechanisms of sirtuins

Mammalian sirtuins (Sirt1–7) belong to a family of seven enzyme orthologs of the silent information regulator 2 (Sir2) of the yeast. The sirtuins belong to the class III of NAD^+-dependent deacetylases (Landry *et al.*, 2000) and present deacetylase and ADP-ribosylase activies that are mechanistically similar; in both reactions a NAD^+ is cleaved. More than a dozen nonhistone deacetylation substrates are known for sirtuins (reviewed in Haigis & Guarente, 2006). Mammalian sirtuins present a highly conserved NAD^+-dependent catalytic domain (North & Verdin, 2004), but could intervene in different pathways, affect a broad range of cellular functions and present different cellular locations (Table 2.3). Moreover, expression of sirtuins is tissue specific (Michishita *et al.*, 2005).

In the yeast, Sir2 extends replicative lifespan, silences genes by histone deacetylation, enables DNA repair and suppresses the formation of extrachromosomal rDNA circles. In the worm *C. elegans* and in the fruit fly *D. melanogaster*, the presence of orthologs of Sir2 also increases longevity, mediating the ER lifespan-extending pathway (Tissenbaum & Guarente, 2001; Rogina & Helfand, 2004). This evidence strongly links sirtuins to ER and longevity. In mammals, so far, no role in lifespan regulation has been determined for any sirtuin; however, it is recognized that ER conditions induce expression of Sirt1 (Cohen *et al.*, 2004) in several tissues of the mouse, such as the cortex and hippocampus of the brain, skeletal muscle and adipose tissues, and also the *corpus cavernosum* of the rat, but repress Sirt1 expression in the liver, the cerebellum and the midbrain (Chen *et al.*, 2008a,b; Tomada *et al.*, 2014).

2.4.2.1 Sirtuin 1

Sirt1 localizes in both the nucleus and the cytoplasm (Michishita *et al.*, 2005; Tomada *et al.*, 2013a, 2014), and is known to regulate many physiological processes. First, regulation of gene expression: Sirt1 deacetylates histones (H1, H3 and H4), promoting the formation of heterochromatin and the repression of gene expression (Vaquero *et al.*, 2004). It induces post-translational modification of transcription factors, such as hypoxia inducible factor (HIF)-1α and HIF-2α, which apparently compete for Sirt1 binding, inhibiting the downstream response to hypoxia (Lim *et al.*, 2010), the FOXO family, which regulates response to oxidative stress (Brunet *et al.*, 2004; Alcendor *et al.*, 2007), and p53, which controls cell survival and senescence (Luo *et al.*, 2001). In addition, Sirt1 interacts in the nucleus with PPARα, which activates genes encoding fatty acid oxidation enzymes, and PGC-1α (Purushotham *et al.*, 2009) and deacetylates NF-κB, which suppress its ability to activate pro-inflammatory transcriptional targets, and even promotes cell apoptosis in stressfull conditions (Yeung *at al.*, 2004). Sirt1, whose deacetylase activity is circadian, is required for high-magnitude circadian transcription of several core CLOCK (circadian locomotor output cycles kaput) genes. It is also physically associated with CLOCK protein and regulates the acetylation state of its targets (Asher *et al.*, 2008; Nakahata *et al.*, 2008). This evidence suggests a possible connection between circadian rhythm and lifespan.

Table 2.3 Main characteristics of mammalian sirtuins.

Sirtuin	Activity	Targets	Subcellular localization	Variation of its expression	Main biological functions
Sirt1	Protein deacetylase	H4K16, H3K9, H1 HIF-1α, HIF-2α FOXO1 FOXO3 PGC-1α p53 NF-κB Cytoplasmic acetyl–CoA synthetase	Cytoplasmic Nuclear	↓ Hypoxia ↑ ER ↓ Ageing	Regulation of gene expression Control of cell cycle Improvement of DNA repair Control of cell survival Metabolism (gluconeogenesis, lipolysis and insulin secretion control) Vascular protection Promotion of endothelial function Attenuation of inflammatory response Promotes autophagy
Sirt2	Protein deacetylase	H4K16 α-Tubulin FOXO1	Cytoplasmic Nuclear	↑ ER	Cell cycle control Modulation of oxidative stress Promotion of lipolysis Adipocyte differentiation and proliferation
Sirt3	Protein deacetylase	H4K16 Ku-70 Isocitrate dehydrogenase 2 FOXO3 Manganese superoxide dismutase Ornithine transcarbamoylase Mitochondrial acetyl–CoA synthetase	Mitochondrial Cytoplasmic Nuclear	↑ ER	Cell stress and death protection Improvement of thermogenesis Improvement of mitochondrial function Control of fatty acid oxidation Metabolism control Regulation of urea cycle Regulation of AMPK activation Tumor suppressor
Sirt4	ADP-ribosyltransferase	Glutamate dehydrogenase	Mitochondrial	↓ ER	Control of cell survival during fasting Control of insulin secretion Metabolism control
Sirt5	Protein deacetylase	Carbamoyl phosphate synthetase 1 Cytochrome c	Mitochondrial	↓ ER	Regulation of urea cycle
Sirt6	ADP-ribosyltransferase Protein deacetylase	H3K9, H3K56 NF-κB	Nuclear	↑ ER ↑ Ageing	Base excision DNA repair Attenuates inflammatory response
Sirt7	Protein deacetylase	p53	Nucleolar		Ribossomal DNA transcriptional regulation Control of cell of survival and proliferation

AMPK, AMP-activated protein kinase; ER, Energy restriction; FOXO, transcription factors of the forkhead family; HIF, hypoxia inducible factor; H1, histone H1; H3K9, histone H3 acetylated at lysine 9; H4K16, histone H4 acetylated at lysine 16; H3K56, histone H3 acetylated at lysine 56; NF-κB, nuclear factor kappa-light chain enhancer of activated B cells; PGC, peroxisome proliferator-activated receptor gamma coactivator; Sirt, sirtuin.

Second, Sirt1 regulates control of the cell cycle and cell proliferation: Sirt1 deacetylates and dowregulates p53, which inhibits apoptosis and could extend the longevity of cells (Luo *et al.*, 2001). Other studies have demonstrated antiproliferative effects for Sirt1 during cancer development, as in breast cancer 1 gene (BRCA1) mutant cell lines where Sirt1 represses survivin expression after histone deacetylation (Wang *et al.*, 2008b). Thus, the role of Sirt1 as a potential tumor suppressor remains controversial.

Third, Sirt1 regulates the maintenance of genomic stability, promoting DNA repair in stressful conditions (Oberdoerffer *et al.*, 2008; Wang *et al.*, 2008c).

Fourth, Sirt1 regulates neuron survival: Sirt1 is recruited to local DNA double-strand breaks and cooperates in their repair through the nonhomologous end-joining pathway in postmitotic neurons, contributing thus to maintaining genomic stability, promoting neuron survival and avoiding neurodegeneration (Dobbin *et al.*, 2013; Donmez *et al.*, 2012; Kim *et al.*, 2007).

Fifth, Sirt1 regulates blood vessel growth and endothelial function, stimulating angiogenesis and targeting eNOS for deacetylation, increasing its activity (Guarani & Potente, 2010; Mattagajasingh *et al.*, 2007). It thus prevents endothelial dysfunction, premature senescence of the endothelial cells and also oxidative stress-induced damage of the heart (Alcendor *et al.*, 2007).

Sixth, Sirt1 regulates gluconeogenesis, by deacetylation and activation of the transcription factor PGC-1α, which activate genes involved in gluconeogenesis during prolonged fasting, and also FOXO1, the ability of which to promote expression of genes involved in gluconeogenesis under oxidative stress conditions after Sirt1-mediated deacetylation has been demonstrated (Rodgers *et al.*, 2005; Frescas *et al.*, 2005).

Seventh, Sirt1 regulates lipolysis, repressing the key regulator of metabolism, PPARγ, and mobilizing fat from adipocytes (Picard *et al.*, 2004). Interestingly, its coactivator PGC-1α can itself stimulate Sirt1 expression after interaction with Sirt1 gene promoter, as demonstrated by the fact that its disruption strongly inhibits Sirt1 expression in vascular cells, leading to a senescence phenotype (Xiong *et al.*, 2013).

Eighth, Sirt1 regulates insulin secretion, positively regulating insulin secretion by pancreatic β-cells in response to glucose (Moynihan *et al.*, 2005). In addition, Sirt1 represses transcription of the gene that codifies UCP-2 in the mitochondria, leading to more efficient energy generation. This mechanism is, however, attenuated in animals under food deprivation, which modifies the insulin responsiveness of β-cells (Bordone *et al.*, 2006). Moreover, Sirt1 apparently promotes the survival of pancreatic β-cells under acute metabolic stress through FOXO1 deacetylation (Kitamura and Kitamura, 2007).

Finally, Sirt1 regulates autophagy, positively regulating macroautophagy (Lee *et al.*, 2008), as discussed later. All of these mechanisms are affected during ageing and are modulated by ER (Moynihan *et al.*, 2005; Haigis & Guarente, 2006).

It was also reported that Sirt1 deacetylates cytoplasmic enzyme acetyl–CoA synthetase (Hallows *et al.*, 2006), which favors the synthesis of fatty acids and cholesterol, but the expression of this enzyme is repressed by fasting (Sone *et al.*, 2002). Furthermore, Sirt1 overexpression in transgenic mice demonstrates its protective effects against diabetes, liver steatosis, bone loss and inflammatory diseases, in a similar pattern to that observed in ER animal models (Bordone *et al.*, 2006). The whole expression of Sirt1 in tissues presents an age-dependent pattern that could vary among tissues. However, Sirt1 activity tends to decrease with ageing in liver, heart, kidney and lung of the rat owing to the decreased bioavailability of NAD^+ (Braidy *et al.*, 2011). An equivalent variation of

Sirt1 activity and NAD+ levels was also observed in skin collected from male, but not female, patients (Massudi *et al.*, 2012). The NAD+ dependence of sirtuins strongly links its activity to the metabolic state of the cell, creating thus an intricate connection between acetylation/deacetylation, energetic state and gene expression (Finkel *et al.*, 2009).

2.4.2.2 Sirtuin 6

Sirtuin 6 is also a nuclear protein (Michishita *et al.*, 2005) upregulated by ER (Kanfi *et al.*, 2008), although some controversy exists concerning regulation of its expression under this dietary pattern (Kawakami *et al.*, 2012). Further, to present a robust ADP–phosphoribosyl transferase activity (Liszt *et al.*, 2005), this enzyme is also involved in the deacetylation of histones (Michishita *et al.*, 2008; Gil *et al.*, 2013) and base excision repair. However, lack of Sirt6 apparently does not interfere with the other DNA repair mechanisms. Sirt6 knockout mice present a premature ageing phenotype (Mostoslavsky *et al.*, 2006). On the other hand, Sirt6 overexpression leads to metabolic features such as low levels of circulating IGF-1 and glucose that regulate lifespan in the male mice (Kanfi *et al.*, 2012). Interestingly, Sirt6 expression is upregulated in the skeletal muscle of the aged rats (Koltai *et al.*, 2010).

2.4.2.3 Sirtuin 7

Sirtuin 7 is a nucleolar enzyme that fails to deacetylate histone H4 acetylated at lysine 16 (H4K16), a known target to other mammalian sirtuins (Michishita *et al.*, 2005), but not p53, supported by demonstration of elevated levels of acetylated p53 found in Sirt7 knockout mice (Vakhrusheva *et al.*, 2008a). Sirt7 expression is higher in tissues with a high proliferation rate where it is involved in the regulation of the expression of rRNA genes, being a component of the RNA polymerase I transcriptional machinery and also an activator of its own transcription (Ford *et al.*, 2006). In particular, Sirt7 is involved in the survival of cardiomyocytes under stress conditions (Vakhrusheva *et al.*, 2008a), further exerts an antiproliferative role that may improve tissue integrity in aged animals (Vakhrusheva *et al.*, 2008b), and represses hypoxia-inducible factors expression, as recently reported (Hubbi *et al.*, 2013). Taken together, these findings suggest that Sirt7 activity could exert an antitumorigenic action. In fact, knockout animals for Sirt7 gene presented a decreased lifespan, but deaths were attributed to a premature-ageing-like phenotype, and not to increased incidence of tumors (Vakhrusheva *et al.*, 2008a). So far, no nutrient dependency of Sirt7 expression has been demonstrated.

2.4.2.4 Sirtuin 3

Conversely, Sirt3 has been demonstrated to be upregulated under fasting or ER conditions in adipose and skeletal tissue, but not in cardiac muscle, of mice (Shi *et al.*, 2005; Palacios *et al.*, 2009). Actually, Sirt3 activates mitochondrial acetyl–CoA synthetase by deacetylation (Schwer *et al.*, 2006), regulating the entry of carbons from acetate into central metabolism, which ensures full incorporation of dietary or ketone-derived acetate under energy limitation conditions (Haigis & Guarente, 2006). It was initially thought that Sirt3 location was restricted to the mitochondria (Michishita *et al.*, 2005), since cleavage of the signal sequence is necessary for enzymatic activity (Schwer *et al.*, 2002), but recent evidence shows that it also exists in the nucleus and the cytoplasm (Scher *et al.*, 2007). Sirt3 possess a strong deacetylase activity, and as well as intervening in AMPK activation (discussed later) (Palacios *et al.*, 2009), it interferes in mitochondrial function by upregulating expression of the genes that codify uncoupling protein 1 (UCP1) and PGC1-α, reducing free radical levels and improving thermogenesis regulation (Shi *et al.*, 2005). Moreover, Sirt3 leads to the reduction of oxidative damage through upregulation of the mitochondrial glutathione anti-oxidant defense system (which prevents age-related hearing loss in mice; Someya *et al.*, 2010), Mn-superoxide dismutase (which is also deacetylated in response to ER; Qiu *et al.*, 2010) and catalase (which protects against cardiac hypertrophy; Sundaresan *et al.*, 2008, 2009). Recent evidence, reviewed by Guarente (2011), indicates Sirt3 as an important tumor suppressor in human cancers, which agrees with the fact that it is the only sirtuin that is linked to longevity in humans (Bellizzi *et al.*, 2005).

2.4.2.5 Sirtuins 4 and 5

Similarly to Sirt3, Sirt4 and Sirt5 are mitochondrial (Michishita *et al.*, 2005), and together they regulate several mitochondrial enzymes, such as glutamate dehydrogenase, which is crucial for metabolic adaptation to ER (Haigis *et al.*, 2006), and also enzymes of the urea cycle, which play an important role in the ammonia detoxification during fasting (Nakagawa *et al.*, 2009; Hallows *et al.*, 2011). Sirt3- and Sirt4-coordinated actions are also responsible for maintaining NAD^+ levels in mitochondria, thus dictating cell survival during starvation (Yang *et al.*, 2007). Sirt4 interacts with insulin-degrading enzyme, and apparently dowregulates pancreatic insulin secretion (Ahuja *et al.*, 2007). Interestingly, ER leads to the dowregulation of Sirt4 activity, inducing a decrease in amino acid-stimulated insulin secretion and ADP-ribosylation of glutamate dehydrogenase (Haigis & Guarente, 2006). On the other hand, Sirt5 was found to deacetylate cytochrome c, and apparently intervenes in the regulation of this protein in respiration and apoptosis (Gertz & Steegborn, 2010).

2.4.2.6 Sirtuin 2

Sirtuin 2 is mainly detected in the cytoplasm (Michishita *et al.*, 2005), where it colocalizes with the microtubule network, targeting α-tubulin for deacetylation (North *et al.*, 2003). This enzyme is upregulated during mitosis, being subsequently degraded, which suggests a role for Sirt2 in cell cycle regulation (Dryden *et al.*, 2003). Sirt2 colocalizes with chromatin during the G_2/M transition (Vaquero *et al.*, 2006), thus being able to deacetylate H4K16, also a substrate to Sirt1. Taking these findings into account, and also the low levels of Sirt2 observed in several cancer lines, this protein has been proposed to be a tumor suppressor (North & Verdin, 2004). In addition, Sirt2 modulates oxidative stress (Wang *et al.*, 2007), promotes lipolysis and inhibits adipocyte differentiation and proliferation in ER conditions (Wang & Tong, 2009).

Interestingly, novel evidence suggests that the mammalian sirtuins crosstalk inside the cells and cooperate in the molecular responses to ER. In accordance with this, levels of Sirt6, Sirt2, Sirt1 and Sirt3 increase in ER conditions, and Sirt1 itself activates expression of Sirt3 (Bell & Guarente, 2011). In addition, Sirt1 and Sirt6 both repress NF-κB activity and ensuing age-related transcriptional changes and inflammatory effects (Kawahara *et al.*, 2009), and Sirt7, Sirt1, Sirt3, which share deacetylations targets such as FOXO3, crosstalk in the protection of cardiac hypertrophy. On the other hand, Sirt1 and Sirt4 seem to oppose their regulatory functions in insulin secretion in response to glucose and amino acids (Haigis *et al.*, 2006), as well as Sirt1 and Sirt2 interventions concerning neurodegenerative diseases, in particular in Parkinson disease (reviewed in Donmez & Outeiro, 2013).

2.4.3 AMPK

AMPK is a heterotrimeric enzyme composed of a catalytic α subunit and two regulatory β and γ subunits, allosterically activated by AMP, which makes it a crucial sensor of the energy status of the cell. In fact, it is activated when AMP/ATP or ADP/ATP ratios increase, which develop under ER conditions, hypoxia or increased ATP consumption (Hardie, 2011), and also by phosphorylation by upstream kinases. ER is thus considered an activator of AMPK activity, especially when implemented throughout life (Edwards *et al.*, 2010; Han *et al.*, 2012), despite no differences being found in its activity in vital organs such as heart, skeletal muscle and liver of young mice under ER for 4 months, and a decrease being observed in the liver of ER-treated 6-month-old rats compared with controls (Gonzalez *et al.*, 2004; To *et al.*, 2007). On the other hand, it has recently been demonstrated that the AMPK signaling pathway is indispensible for energy regulation and myocardial adaptation in mice subjected to ER, and that these effects are absent in AMPKα2 knockout littermates (Chen *et al.*, 2013). In fact, AMPK plays an important role in cellular energy homeostasis and at the whole-body level too (Hardie *et al.*, 2012). In addition, AMPK constitutes a well-known target to inhibit cell growth and proliferation, which apparently mediates its tumor-suppressor effects.

Interestingly, AMPK activity can be upregulated by plant-derived compounds, including resveratrol, epigallocatechin gallate (EGCG) and capsaicin, which share a mitochondrial-inhibiting function (Hardie, 2011); AMPK activation to pharmacological or physiological stimuli being less responsive in aged rodents than in young animals (Reznick *et al.*, 2007). Once activated by mitochondrial inhibition, AMPK upregulates catabolic pathways that generate ATP, both in the short-term, by increased glycolysis and fatty acid oxidation, and in a long-term pattern, by activation of mitochondrial function (Cantó & Auwerx, 2010). Concomitantly, AMPK represses ATP-consuming pathways, such as the syntheses of proteins, glucose, glycogen and lipids. One of the main AMPK repressed pathways under ER is that of mTOR, which indeed inhibits protein synthesis.

AMPK modulates the expression of genes that codify catabolic or anabolic enzymes, through phosphorylation of a wide variety of transcription factors or coregulators (Hardie, 2011). In particular, AMPK activates by phosphorylation several members of the FOXO family of transcription factors (Greer *et al.*, 2007), which appear to protect cells from stressors and promote the longevity of organisms (Kenyon, 2010), and also upregulates PGC-1α, which activates mitochondrial biogenesis (Zong *et al.*, 2002). Moreover, AMPK is strictly linked to the modulation of the activity of Sirt1 (Suchankova *et al.*, 2009), in part through the control of bioavailability of its substrate NAD^+ (Cantó *et al.*, 2009). In line with this finding, Sirt1 contributes to the activation of PGC-1α, catalyzing its deacetylation (Rodgers *et al.*, 2005). AMPK-mediated PGC1-α phosphorylation at Thr_{177} and Ser_{538} (Cantó *et al.*, 2009), enables its complete activation. In fact, AMPK and Sirt1 activities strongly cooperate in the pathways triggered by ER, in particular in aged individuals (Cantó & Auwerx, 2011).

2.4.4 Oxidative stress and metabolic reprogramming

Energy and/or nutrient restriction-induced increase in mitochondrial respiration (possibly associated with augmented mitochondrial biogenesis) and fatty acid oxidation (mice under ER oxidize 4 times more fat than *ad libitum*-fed counterparts; Speakman & Mitchell, 2011), linked to a decrease in carbohydrate oxidation, momentarily leads to a mild increase in reactive species levels, which contributes to explain the beneficial effects of different dietary restriction regimens through the activation of the transcription factor Nrf2 (Vincent *et al.*, 2009; Sykiotis *et al.*, 2011; Hine & Mitchell, 2012; Testa *et al.*, 2014). In addition to those mechanisms, energy and/or nutrient restriction mimetics including resveratrol and curcumin, potentially induce a small and transient increase in oxidative stress by activating phase I oxidases, and then activate Nrf2 (Kluth *et al.*, 2007; Sykiotis *et al.*, 2011; Hine & Mitchell, 2012; Cardozo *et al.*, 2013; Hayes & Dinkova-Ksotova, 2014; Csiszár *et al.*, 2014).

Nrf2 target genes can be organized in two extensive groups: genes ubiquitously needed vs genes specifically needed by particular tissues (Kitteringham *et al.*, 2010; Sykiotis *et al.*, 2011). Nrf2 activation leads to the induction and/or repression of genes from Phase I to III detoxification and anti-oxidant responses, including NADPH-generating enzymes (first group), and of genes involved in metabolism (second group), among others. The molecular response to Nrf2 is indeed mostly associated with an effector role in longevity signaling accompanying energy and/or nutrient restriction regimens or mimetics (Kwak *et al.*, 2003; Kitteringham *et al.*, 2010; Sykiotis *et al.*, 2011; Hine & Mitchell, 2012; Seo & Lee 2013; Wan Hasan *et al.*, 2014; Hayes & Dinkova-Ksotova, 2014).

Concerning metabolic pathways, the effects of Nrf2 are vast considering that it leads to inhibition of pyruvate kinase (preventing the glycolytic flux) and increases glucose-6-phosphate and 6-phosphogluconate dehydrogenases, transaldolase and transketolase gene expression, overall promoting flux through the pentose phosphate pathway, allowing increased provision of NADPH, erythrose-4-phosphate and ribose-5-phosphate for reductive synthesis and/or nucleotides, nucleic acids, amino acids and phospholipids synthesis. Adding to these effects, Nrf2 promotes *de novo* purine synthesis by stimulating methylenetetrahydrofolate dehydrogenase and phosphoribosyl pyrophosphate amidotransferase gene expression (reviewed in Hayes & Dinkova-Ksotova, 2014). Nrf2 exerts a negative regulation of hepatic fatty acid synthesis/desaturation and cholesterol synthesis by downregulating ATP-citrate lyase, acetyl-CoA carboxylases 1 and 2, fatty acid synthase, stearoyl CoA desaturase 1, fatty acid elongases, 3-hydroxy-3-methylglutaryl coenzyme A synthase and reductase, and SREBP-1c and SERBP-2 gene expression (Tanaka *et al.*, 2008; Shin *et al.*, 2009; Kitteringham *et al.*, 2010; Sykiotis *et al.*, 2011; Hayes & Dinkova-Ksotova, 2014). The increase in fatty acid oxidation is promoted after decreasing malonyl-CoA levels, following the decrease of acetyl-CoA carboxylases and stearoyl CoA desaturase 1 gene expression, and increasing CD36 gene expression (this latter gene is also Nrf2-induced), all contributing to increased fatty acid transport/import into mitochondria (Shin *et al.*, 2009; Zhang *et al.*, 2013; Hayes & Dinkova-Ksotova, 2014). Conversely, impairment of Nrf2 action is associated with an increase in hepatic free fatty acid levels as well as with fatty liver and steatohepatitis development (Tanaka *et al.*, 2008; Chowdhry *et al.*, 2010; Sugimoto *et al.*, 2010; Sykiotis *et al.*, 2011; Wang *et al.*, 2013; Hayes & Dinkova-Ksotova, 2014). Nrf2 also modulates lipid metabolism in adipose tissue, although contradictory results have been reported for the role of Nrf2 in adipocyte differentiation and obesity, probably owing to differences in experimental protocols (Sykiotis *et al.*, 2011; Seo & Lee 2013). Depolarization of mitochondria and impairment of oxidative phosphorylation, resulting in the decline of ATP levels, occur after Nrf2 impairment, while Nrf2 activation improves these parameters (Holmström *et al.*, 2013).

Nrf2 controls intermediary metabolism in several and interconnected ways, ensuring a prime role in metabolic reprograming during ER and stress (reviewed in Hayes & Dinkova-Ksotova, 2014).

2.4.5 Autophagy and mTOR signaling

Autophagy is an evolutionary conserved process that involves the degradation of own-cell components through a lysosomal pathway. Eukaryotic cells present several autophagic mechanisms that differ in the conditions that trigger activation and the type of molecules/structures degraded too. There are three main types of autophagy. The first is microautophagy, which occurs when cytoplasmic components are, prior to degradation, involved by direct invagination or protusion of the lysosomal or endosomal membrane, and is the least studied form of autophagy (Sahu *et al.*, 2011). The second type is chaperone-mediated autophagy (CMA), which is only present in higher organisms and is the mostly selective mechanism of lysosomal degradation of proteins. CMA does not require the formation of intermediate vesicles and is selective for a restricted group of cytosolic proteins that possess a specific motif biochemically related to the pentapeptide KFERQ, recognized by the proper chaperone heat shock protein 70 (hsp70) and respective co-chaperones. Further, the substrate protein is targeted to the lysosome-associated receptor protein type 2A, translocated to the lysosomal matrix and ultimately degraded by proteases (Massey *et al.*, 2004). Knowledge of regulation of microautophagy and CMA in relation to ageing is currently limited. However, it has been shown not only that CMA decreases with ageing owing to the decrease in CMA-substrate traffic to lysosomes, but also that CMA decrease could be induced by nutritional factors or oxidative stress (Massey *et al.*, 2004; Cuervo *et al.*, 2005). The third type of autophagy is macroautophagy, an evolutionary conserved intracellular process activated by stressors, and quantitatively the most important form of autophagy, responsible for enzymatic degradation of organelles or damaged cellular components such as proteins, lipids, sugars and nucleic acids, resulting in the formation of precursors of macromolecules that can be reused inside the cell in multiple functions. In this process, entire regions of the cytosol are involved by membranes that seal in vesicles named autophagosomes that fuse with lysosomes of the cell for the degradation of the sequestered cellular components. In addition to be inducible in response to stress signals, new evidence demonstrates that macroautophagy also intervenes in the maintenance of cellular homeostasis (Nakai *et al.*, 2007), through the removal of damaged components and replacement with newly formed molecules. This housekeeping mechanism is particularly relevant in ageing cells, since damaged proteins that could not be degraded in the main ubiquitin–proteasome system, which is exclusively targeted to unfolded proteins and decreases in activity during ageing, accumulate in cells and form toxic aggregates (Li & Li, 2011). In fact, accumulation of ubiquitinated proteins is a common age-related feature (Pan *et al.*, 1993; Scrofano *et al.*, 1998). Furthermore, the proteasome is unable to degrade molecules other than proteins, such as oxidized nucleic acids, lipids or damaged organelles that also form during ageing, which implies that lysosomal intervention in the cellular homeostasis has increased importance in senescent cells. In opposition to the increased degradation demands, the ability of the lysosomes to digest intracellular components and to fuse and degrade the autophagic structures (Terman *et al.*, 2007) tends to decrease with ageing, partly owing to the accumulation of undigested materials inside lysosomes, namely lipofuscin (discussed in Chapter 1; Ward, 2002). Thus, autophagy failure presents deleterious consequences for the maintenance of long-lived postmitotic cells, such as neurons, cardiomyocytes and skeletal muscle fibers (Cuervo *et al.*, 2005), where intracellular accumulation of material extra- and intralysossomally is frequently observed, namely aggregated indigestible proteins, aggresomes, in the cytosol, accumulation of lipofuscin in the lysosomes, and enlarged mitochondria presenting desintegration of cristae, a condition that is often associated with increased production of ROS (Sohal & Sohal, 1991). Interestingly, ROS are themselves activators of autophagy, which is particularly important in the degradation of damaged mithochondria (Scherz-Shouval & Elazar, 2011), nonfunctional peroxisomes (Kim & Klionsky, 2000; Donati, 2006) and plasma membranes with high dolichol content (Marino *et al.*, 1998). In fact, the concerted degradation of these cellular structures greatly increases the whole cell function. Mitochondria are specifically degraded by a very selective form of macroautophagy, named mitophagy, that only targets damaged mitochondria (Lemasters, 2005).

Although macroautophagy was initially thought to be a widespread nonspecific degradation process, new evidence shows that additional macroautophagy pathways exist that are strictly regulated and that substrate elimination occurs in a very selective manner (Kraft *et al.*, 2010). Moreover, it was recently demonstrated that a member of B cell-lymphoma 2 (Bcl2)-associated athanogen (BAG) family of proteins, BAG3, functions as an important chaperone in addressing aggregated proteins to macroautophagy, since it is able to form large multichaperone complexes. In fact, BAG3-mediated degradation of proteins seems to be highly increased in the aged cells (Gamerdinger *et al.*, 2009). Furthermore, BAG3 was demonstrated to be involved in the active transport of protein substrates inside the cell, along the microtubules toward the nucleus (Behl, 2011).

Nutrients are the main exogenous modulators of autophagy, which is not surprising because it could be considered a mechanism of cell survival during starvation. In line with this, autophagy requires the expression of multiple genes essential to longevity increase in organisms as varied as *S. cerevisiae, D. melanogaster, C. elegans,* and mammals. ER increases the inducible forms of autophagy: (a) CMA, through an increase in the number of lysosomes presenting the luminal chaperone, constitutively expressed protein of the heat shock family of 70 kDa (hsc70) necessary to CMA-substrate translocation (Massey *et al.*, 2004), but as age progresses, the levels of this protein significantly decrease (Cuervo & Dice, 2000); and (b) macroautophagy (Gelino & Hansen, 2012), to levels equivalent to those observed in young animals (Donati *et al.*, 2001), although its activation is mainly regulated in mammals by levels of amino acids and hormones, including glucagon and insulin, with stimulatory and inhibitory effects, respectively. In fact, autophagy is essential for maintaining an adequate pool of amino acids for gluconeogenesis and the synthesis of proteins (Yoshimori, 2004). Interestingly, the activation of autophagy in response to low levels of amino acids following overnight fasting, or to high glucagon levels, tends to decrease in older rodents (Del Roso *et al.*, 2003; Bergamini *et al.*, 1993). ER has been demonstrated to prevent the age-dependent decrease in the *in vivo* induction of macroautophagy (Del Roso *et al.*, 2003), avoiding the accumulation of altered mitochondria (Yen & Klionsky, 2008), peroxisomes and dolichol-modified membranes in older cells (Donati, 2006), which is associated with an increased lifespan (Cavallini *et al.*, 2001).

Macroautophagy is a multistep process that involves a rearrangement of subcellular membranes to sequester cytoplasm and organelles for fusing with lysosomes where the degradation reactions take place. In brief, a double membrane, called an isolation membrane, the exact origin of which remains uncertain but which is apparently synthesized *de novo*, encompasses a portion of the cytoplasm and closes, forming an autophagosome. Autophagosomes can fuse either with endosomes or lysosomes in cells, resulting in autolysosome formation where the hydrolytic enzymes from the lysosome degrade the components in an acidic medium (Hannigan & Gorski, 2009). It is largely accepted that macroautophagy develops through the following steps: induction, vesicle nucleation and expansion, lysosome targeting, lysosome docking and autophagosome–lysosome fusion, vesicle breakdown and recycling (Klionsky & Emr, 2000). Several autophagy-related genes (ATG) are upregulated during the specific steps and the overall process of macroautophagy. Most of the 30 ATG genes described in the yeast, where the autophagic pathways were primarily elucidated (Suzuki & Ohsumi, 2007), present a conserved equivalent in mammals.

Interestingly, macroautophagy is regulated by the same conserved factors that regulate metabolism and ageing. In fact, it is suppressed in the presence of amino acids, such as leucine and tyrosine, by activation of mTOR complex 1 (Kanazawa *et al.*, 2004), in an AKT/PKB kinase-dependent pathway. Thus, it is possible to modify the macroautophagy rate according to the proteins ingested. The same is in part true for carbohydrates and lipids, since both are able to indirectly modulate macroautophagy through their effects on insulin levels (Hannigan & Gorski, 2009). While carbohydrates increase insulin levels, lead to activation of mTOR and suppress autophagy, lipids exert the opposite effect. Other dietary components can modulate the cellular autophagy. It has been demonstrated *in vitro* that caffeine present in coffee and tea, polyphenols such as curcumin, genistein and resveratrol (discussed later), and vitamins C, D, E and K2 favor autophagy. On the other hand, quercetin apparently inhibits autophagic processes (reviewed in Hannigan & Gorski, 2009). We should, however, take into account that the evidence needs further clarification with regard to the effects of nutrients after ingestion by entire organisms, since compounds could be differently metabolized in the gastrointestinal tract and reach organs to variable degrees. Nutrient interference in the whole foodstuffs could also occur, affecting bioavailability and biological activity. Thus, most aspects of nutritional intervention in cellular autophagy mechanisms remain to be elucidated, and so far only fasting seems to be a straight autophagy-promoting strategy for whole organisms.

Inhibition of mTOR in mammalian cells ensuing starvation results in dephosphorylation of the orthologs of the yeast autophagy genes, *Atg*1, *Atg*11 and *Atg*13, that together with *Atg*17, form the initiation complex unc-51 like kinase 1(ULK1)/*Atg*1 (Kawamata *et al.*, 2008; Fig. 2.1). This complex is also actively regulated by the nutrient sensor regulator of autophagy AMPK, although in the opposite direction to mTOR (Kim *et al.*, 2011b). Interestingly, Sirt1 deficiency results in mTOR signaling activation, and consequently repression of autophagic processes (Ghosh *et al.*, 2010). Further formation of the autophagosome in mammalian cells requires activity of the class III, PI3K vacuolar protein sorting (Vps)34 that integrates the autophagy-regulating complex (PI3K complex), together with Beclin1/Atg6, Atg14/Barker and p150/Vps15 (Ravikumar *et al.*, 2010). The vesicle expansion step involves the recruitment of proteins of the ATG family, mammalian Atg9 for membrane increment provided by other organelles (Young *et al.*, 2006) and, for formation of the autophagosome, ATG12 and ATG5, which engages ATG16 for recruitment of microtubule-associated protein light chain 3 (MAP-LC3) or protein light chain 3 (LC-3/ATG8) that is further conjugated to phosphatidylethanolamine (PE). LC-3PE binds to the engulfment membrane that cycles in the autophagosome formation and remains bound until fusion to the lysosome (Rajawat *et al.*, 2009), functioning thus as a cellular marker of autophagy. The autophagosomes are formed randomly in the mammalian cell cytoplasm and move along microtubules (Ravikumar *et al.*, 2010) in

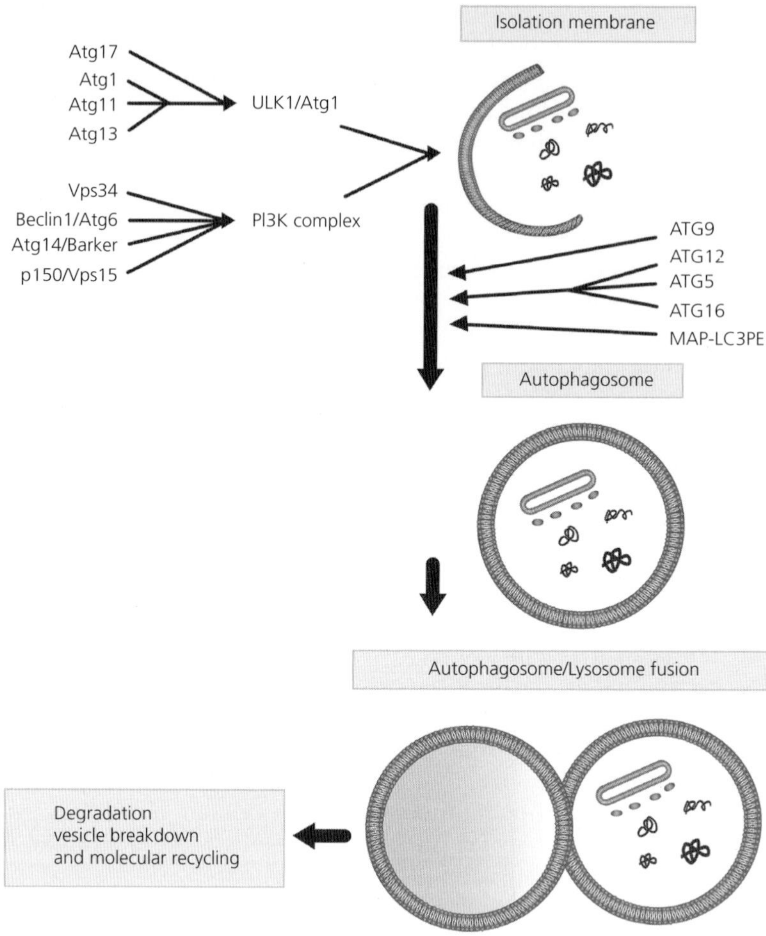

Figure 2.1 Summary of the main molecular pathways intervening in macroautophagy multistep degradation process. Atg/ATG, Autophagy-related genes; MAP-LC3PE, microtubule-associated protein light chain 3 phosphatidylethanolamine; PI3K, phosphatidylinositol 3-kinase; ULK1, unc-51 like kinase 1;Vps, vacuolar protein sorting.

the sense of the centrosome. In effect, LC-3 associated with Golgi-associated ATPase enhancer of 16 kDa (GATE-16) and γ-aminobutyric acid type A receptor-associated protein (GABARAP) interacts with the initiation complex ULK1 for vesicle expansion, maturation and intracellular trafficking (Okazaki *et al.*, 2000). The machinery necessary for the process of vesicle fusion includes the soluble *N*-ethylmaleimide-sensitive factor activating protein receptor (SNARE) proteins and the class C Vps/homotypic fusion and protein sorting (HOPS) complex (Nair *et al.*, 2011).

Macroautophagy can be activated pharmacologically by treatment with antilipolytic agents, especially when associated with fasting, or with the antibiotic rapamycin, which inhibits the mTOR pathway (Donati, 2006). In fact, reduced mTOR activity activates autophagy, which has been shown to influence the ageing process and extend lifespan in many organisms. Interestingly, the life-extending effects of Sirt1 activators are lost in autophagy-deficient *C. elegans* mutant, which strongly suggests that ER- and Sirt1-dependent effects on the extension of longevity are mediated by the activation of autophagy (Morselli *et al.*, 2010). In mammals, Sirt1 has been demonstrated to positively regulate autophagy, in part through upregulation of the expression of autophagy-related genes (Lee *et al.*, 2008), and also through the activation of transcription factors linked to the autophagic processes, such as FOXO1 which moves to the nucleus after Sirt1-mediated deacetylation (Hariharan *et al.*, 2010). An additional member of FOXO family, target of Sirt1-deacetylation (Brunet *et al.*, 2004), FOXO3, also intervenes in autophagy, apparently by promoting PI3K–AKT1-dependent phosphorylation and translocation of FOXO1 from the nucleus to the cytoplasm, resulting in an increase in FOXO1-induced autophagy (Zhou *et al.*, 2012). FOXO1 presents a dual function in autophagy regulation, intervening both in transcription and as mediator of the process in the cytoplasm. In addition, considering that Sirt1 intervenes in NAD^+-dependent direct deacetylation of the proteins Atg5, Atg7 and Atg8 (Lee *et al.*, 2008), acetylation/deacetylation seems to constitute an important post-translational modification in the mechanism of autophagosome formation (Rajawat *et al.*, 2009).

Impairment of autophagy, mainly through the loss of activity of ATG genes, is associated with neurodegenerative diseases that result from the accumulation of aggregated proteins. In fact, it was demonstrated in murine models of Parkinson and Huntington diseases that induction of autophagy by mTOR-dependent mechanisms ameliorated the symptoms of these diseases (Ravikumar *et al.*, 2004; Berger *et al.*, 2006). On the other hand, the role of autophagy in cancer progress remains far from being clarified. Autophagy apparently interferes in a specific fashion with the survival or suppression of each tumor cell population; it either increases cell survival under conditions of limited oxygen and nutrients or favors removal of damaged or mutated proteins and organelles (reviewed in Gelino & Hansen, 2012; Sato *et al.*, 2007).

2.5 Energy restriction mimetics

Despite the fact that controlled trials of long-term ER in humans remain limited, its benefits in added years of healthy life are evident. However, this nutritional pattern is hard to maintain owing to hunger, cold and diminished libido that assist mammals to cope with these conditions (Speakman & Mitchell, 2011). The need to elucidate the molecular pathways and cellular modifications that are associated with ER has prompted the scientists to develop strategies to mimic the effects of food restriction. These strategies include a group of drugs, named "ER mimetics" that intervene in the major pathways affected by ER with the intention of obtaining its benefits while avoiding the undesirable side effects of this nutritional regimen. In fact, the ideal ER mimetic should produce metabolic, hormonal and physiological effects similar to those of ER without reducing the food intake and provide beneficial effects on mortality and age-associated diseases (Ingram *et al.*, 2006). According to the interventional mechanism, the ER mimetics can be classified into four groups: (a) drugs that stimulate sirtuin activity; (b) drugs that intervene in the IGF-1/insulin signaling pathway; (c) drugs that inhibit mTOR signaling; and (d) other interventions, including antilipolytic effects. The main biological and molecular interventions of ER mimetics are summarized in Table 2.4.

Table 2.4 Summary of ER mimetics molecular interventions.

Compound	Class of ER mimetic	Main biological and molecular effects
Resveratrol	Sirtuin activity stimulator	↑ AMPK ↑ Sirt1 gene expression Shift in transcriptional profile of mice that overlaps ER effect ↑ Mitochondrial biogenesis ↑ Autophagy ↑ Longevity in high-fat diet fed mice ↓ Inflammation in mice and human ↑ Vascular function in mice and human ↑ Motor coordination in mice ↓ Cataract formation in mice Improvement of metabolic profile in mice and human ↓ Intrahepatic lipid deposition in human
Metformin	Antidiabetic drugs	↑ Lifespan in mice ↑ Healthspan in mice ↓ Glucose levels in blood ↑ Cardiovascular protection ↓ AGE formation ↑ AMPK ↓ Levels of insulin and IGF-1 in blood ↑ Autophagy ↓ mTOR
Pioglitazone		↑ AMPK ↑ Sensibility to insulin ↓ AGE formation ↑ Telomerase ↓ Stress-induced endothelial cells apoptosis
Rapamycine	Inhibitor of mTOR	↑ Autophagy
Spermidine	Polyamines	↓ Histone acetyltransferases activity ↑ Autophagy ↓ Oxidative stress
Acipimox	Antilipolytic drugs	↓ Free fatty acids and glucose levels in blood ↑ Glucagon/insulin ratio ↑ Autophagy
3,5-Dimethylpyrazole		↓ Membrane dolychol accumulation

AGE, advanced glycation end-products; AMPK, AMP-activated protein kinase; ER, energy resctriction; IGF-1, insulin-like growth factor 1; mTOR, mechanistic target of rapamycin; Sirt1, sirtuin 1.

2.5.1 Sirtuin activity stimulators

Sirtuin activity stimulators were the first class of drugs proposed to mimic the molecular effects of ER (Wood *et al.*, 2004). Some described activators of Sirt1 are naturally present in food, such as omega-3 and omega-9 fatty acids, and the polyphenolic compounds butein, piceatannol, fisetin, quercetin and resveratrol (Xue *et al.*, 2012; Lim *et al.*, 2013; Wood *et al.*, 2004). The most studied Sirt1 activator is resveratrol, a stilbene polyphenol (3,5,4′-trihydroxystilbene), the anti-obesity effects of which are described later. Although resveratrol's role was originally thought to be restricted to direct enhancent of deacetylase activity of Sirt1, some evidence supports the hypothesis that activation of Sirt1 by resveratrol could be primarily mediated by activation of AMPK, which acts as a primer sensor of NAD^+ levels, leading to its increase when low, which then results in Sirt1 activation (Hu *et al.*, 2011; Park *et al.*, 2012). In addition, resveratrol also induces Sirt1 mRNA transcription in a dose-dependent fashion, as demonstrated in retinal stem cells (Peng *et al.*, 2010), and activates Nfr2 (Sykiotis *et al.*, 2011; Csiszár *et al.*, 2014). Resveratrol treatment was shown to delay mortality in high-fat-diet-treated mice (Baur *et al.*, 2006), but apparently not in normal rodent-chow-treated animals (Strong *et al.*, 2013; Pearson *et al.*, 2008b; Miller *et al.*, 2011). ER leads to an adjustment of the transcriptional profile that overlaps with that observed in the heart, skeletal muscle and brain of resveratrol-treated mice, which interestingly diverges from that observed in the same tissues when aged (Pearson *et al.*, 2008b; Baur *et al.*, 2006; Barger *et al.*, 2008). In fact, resveratrol, through dietary supplementation, is as effective as ER in opposing the majority of age-related transcription alterations in the ageing heart (Barger *et al.*, 2008). In addition, resveratrol-fed elderly mice presented an amelioration of age-associated features, such as those that affect inflammatory state, endothelial function, vascular elasticity, motor coordination, cataract formation (Pearson *et al.*, 2008b) and metabolic profile, including insulin sensitivity and mitochondria biogenesis (Baur *et al.*, 2006).

Resveratrol is present at low levels and shows low bioavailability in foodstuffs, and indeed novel sirtuin activators, including reformulated versions of resveratrol and also structurally unrelated molecules, have been developed (Villalba & Alcaín, 2012), so far with limited applicability as a mimetic of beneficial ER effects. Nutraceutical formulations containing high-doses of resveratrol were demonstrated to reproduce the gene expression profile of ER, enhance mitochondria biogenesis and improve metabolic and inflammatory pathways in mice fed a high-calorie diet (Smith *et al.*, 2009), and also to produce beneficial effects in healthy and hypertensive obese men, ameliorating circulating glucose and lipids levels, inflammation markers, endothelium-dependent vasodilatation and decreasing intra-hepatic lipid deposition (Timmers *et al.*, 2011; Wong *et al.*, 2011, 2013). Concerning other compounds with recognized sirtuin-activator ability, several synthetic products (Milne *et al.*, 2007) have been tested in murine models and have been shown to induce similar effects to those observed in resveratrol treatments (reviewed in Villalba & Alcaín, 2012).

Interestingly, some everyday medication has been demonstrated in *in vitro* studies to modulate Sirt1 expression; in particular, L-thyroxin, insulin and sodium nitroprusside were shown to present upregulatory effects (Engel & Mahlknecht, 2008). In addition, it was recently reported that one of the pleiotropic vascular-protecting effects of statins encompasses the Sirt1 activation ability (Ota *et al.*, 2010). Despite the promising effects of sirtuin activators, to date, none has been shown to increase the lifespan of mice fed a normal diet.

2.5.2 Antidiabetic drugs

Several studies in the mouse suggest that treatment with biguanides that are widely used as antidiabetic drugs increase the mean and the maximum lifespan, and strongly decrease the incidence of spontaneous tumors (reviewed in Speakman & Mitchell, 2011). Among others, metformin, which currently is the oral biguanide most frequently prescribed to hyperglycemic patients, was recently demonstrated to improve healthspan and lifespan in mice (Martin-Montalvo *et al.*, 2013). In addition, it was reported that metformin is more effective than insulin in reducing all-cause mortality and diabetes-related endpoints in diabetic patients, providing cardiovascular protection independently of its hypoglycemic effects (Kirpichnikov *et al.*, 2002). Metformin inhibits hepatic glucose production and increases sensitivity to insulin while reducing glucotoxicity in type 2 DM (Wiernsperger & Bailey, 1999), and is the best studied biguanide in the context of mimicking ER effects. By reducing glucose in blood, metformin decreases the formation of AGE, a hallmark of cells and tissues in the elderly, and reduces oxidative and nitrosative stress as shown in type 2 DM patients (Chakraborty *et al.*, 2011). In non-diabetics, metformin therapy also elicits beneficial effects, inducing the reduction of plasma levels of insulin and of free IGF-1 (Fruehwald-Schultes *et al.*, 2002). Moreover, it has been demonstrated that metformin, in an indirect manner via an increase in AMP/ATP and ADP/ATP ratios, activates AMPK (Zhou *et al.*, 2001), and also autophagy, presenting protective effects as demonstrated in the heart of type 1 DM mice (Xie *et al.*, 2011). Metformin has also recently been reported to inhibit mTOR (Kalender *et al.*, 2010), thereby suggesting a potential overlap in the signaling pathways induced by both metformin and rapamycin (discussed later). Concerning mitochondria, namely the complex I activity, the effect of metformin remains far from being clarified, owing to recently reported evidence of its ability to increase mitochondrial activity in cultured muscular cells (Vytla & Ochs, 2013), conversely to its classically considered repressive action (Owen *et al.*, 2000).

Pioglitazone is a member of the family of thiazolidin–dione compounds used in the treatment of diabetes, and similarly to metformin, sensitizes peripheral tissues to insulin and activates AMPK (Coletta *et al.*, 2009). As an inhibitor of glycation, pioglitazone reduces AGE formation in tissues (Rahbar *et al.*, 2000) and is thus considered an anti-ageing drug, at least in *D. melanogaster* (Jafari *et al.*, 2007). In addition, pioglitazone activates aortic telomerase and prevents stress-induced endothelial apoptosis in mice and human cultured cells (Werner *et al.*, 2011). It was also demonstrated that mRNA levels of Sirt1 were increased in nondiabetic subjects treated with pioglitazone, combined with ephedrine and caffeine (Bogacka *et al.*, 2007), supporting the existence of additional crosstalk between pathways activated by pioglitazone that mimic ER-induced protection.

2.5.3 Rapamycine

Rapamycine and other drugs that inhibit the mTOR pathway could be used as ER mimetics, particularly because they are able to increase longevity in mice, even when treatment is initiated later in life (Harrison *et al.*, 2009; Miller *et al.*, 2011). Interestingly, it was recently reported that mTOR signaling in human cell lines and mouse tissues may be negatively regulated by Sirt1 (Ghosh *et al.*, 2010). The inhibition of mTOR strongly activates autophagy in cells, and this could be the main intervention in the ER-like effects that it produces. Interestingly, autophagy seems to be a common pathway of several (if not all) life-prolonging measures (Madeo *et al.*, 2010). Other classes of compounds, discussed later, also intervene in the upregulation of autophagy, and indeed present beneficial effects.

2.5.4 Polyamines

Spermidine is a polyamine, cellular levels of which decrease with ageing, which could also be considered an ER mimetic owing to its ability to induce autophagy and to increase longevity (Eisenberg *et al.*, 2009). In fact, spermidine exogenous supply triggers epigenetic deacetylation of histone H3 through inhibition of histone acetyltransferases, apparently through a mechanism independent but complementary to that activated by Sirt1. The altered acetylation status of the chromatin leads to significant upregulation of various autophagy-related transcripts, promoting autophagy in yeast, flies, worms and human cells. It also mitigates oxidative stress and suppresses necrosis in ageing yeast and potently inhibits the increase in oxidative stress in elderly mice.

2.5.5 Antilipolytic drugs

Antilipolytic drugs, such as 3,5-dimethylpyrazole or Acipimox, inhibit lipolysis, which causes a sudden decline in free fatty acids and glucose and an increase in glucagon/insulin ratio in blood, a decrease in liver membrane dolichol accumulation and the promotion of autophagy (Bergamini *et al.*, 1993; Donati *et al.*, 2004). In addition to the effects on insulin and glucagon secretion, treatment with antilipolytic drugs may influence the secretion of other hormones, such as glucocorticoids (Bergamini *et al.*, 1993) and GH (Peino *et al.*, 1996). This class of medicinal products is able to promote and intensify the anti-ageing effects of ER (Bergamini *et al.*, 2003), even when administered once a week. On the other hand, Acipimox does not affect autophagy and biomarkers of ageing if given to rats fed *ad libitum* (Donati *et al.*, 2004).

Part 2

2.6 Obesity and ageing

Obesity, defined as excessive body fat accumulation, is a heterogeneous disorder with a final common pathway in which energy intake chronically exceeds energy expenditure. The energy imbalance and, therefore, the body fat accretion frequently begin in childhood. Considering that obesity acquired in this period of life tends to persist into adulthood, obesity prevention should begin in early life (Kelishadi, 2007). Preventing overweight is highly preferable to initiating BW loss treatment after weight gain occurs, because the failure rate in achieving and maintaining BW loss is very high.

Obesity rates have increased worldwide in recent years, with the condition now being referred to as an epidemic, or even pandemic, affecting almost every country and age group. Overweight is a frequent cause of disability and serious diseases, with significant impact on the global incidence of CVD, type 2 DM, hypertension, dyslipidemia, nonalcoholic fatty liver disease (NAFLD), cancer, infertility and pregnancy complications, among many other conditions, including psychological issues (Longo & Fontana, 2010; Stevens *et al.*, 2012; Soare *et al.*, 2014). More recently, it has become evident that hyperglycemia and disturbed glycoregulation by modifications of the insulin receptor-mediated cell reactions, in addition to being related to type 2 DM development, can also contribute to cognitive decline and to age-associated dementias, such as Alzheimer disease (Robert, 2010).

In fact, data from large population studies suggest that lifestyle factors, such as sedentary lifestyle and excessive dietary intake, contribute to obesity, which may be responsible for up to 70% of chronic diseases and to reduced longevity (Eyre *et al.*, 2004). Considering that the number of aged people is increasing worldwide, the number of aged obese also follows this tendency.

As previously described, adipose tissue has been recognized as an active endocrine organ that secretes a large number of bioactive polypeptides, that is, adipokines. Adipokines act centrally to regulate appetite and energy expenditure, and peripherally affect insulin sensitivity, oxidative capacity and lipid uptake. The adipokine profile changes in response to the amount and condition of adipose tissue and, in obesity, the imbalanced release of these molecules leads to metabolic disturbances that play a central role in the development of additional diseases. Obesity constitutes thus a particularly deleterious condition in the elderly and strongly contributes to the onset and progression of age-associated diseases and, ultimately, to decreased lifespan (Fontana *et al.*, 2010b; Leal & Mafra, 2013).

2.6.1 Obesity as a premature death inducer

Obesity is clearly associated with increased morbidity and mortality, and therefore with a higher risk of premature death (Patel & Abate, 2013). In clinical practice, obesity has commonly been assessed by expressing BW as a function of height, the most frequently used index being the BMI. Numerous studies have shown that there is a J-shaped relationship between the BMI and morbidity/mortality risk. Thus a very low BMI is associated with increased mortality, even after correction for the presence of eventual underlying morbid conditions. On the other side of the spectrum, there is a progressive increase in the risk of comorbidities associated with an increase in BMI (Tchernof & Després, 2013). Notwithstanding the linear relationship between BMI and metabolic disturbances leading to CVD, this index does not take into account the heterogeneity of regional BFM deposition (Després *et al.*, 2001).

Extensive scientific evidence supports the association of greater BFM, especially if centrally distributed, with a higher risk of CVD, including coronary heart disease, heart failure and sudden death (Fox *et al.*, 2007). There is consensus that insulin resistance is the key underlying pathophysiologic process for the development of many of the obesity-associated comorbidities (Patel & Abate, 2013). However, obesity and adiposity seem to interfere in disease onset in a more complex fashion, since obese men without other metabolic or cardiovascular risk factors are at increased risk for cardiovascular events and death compared with nonobese individuals also without risk factors (Kuk & Ardern, 2009; Arnlov *et al.*, 2010), and on the other hand, subjects who have a BMI within normal range but have high adiposity present a higher prevalence of cardiometabolic dysregulation, metabolic syndrome and cardiovascular risk factors (Romero-Corral *et al.*, 2010). The classification of these metabolically dysfunctional obese individuals correlates with the presence of crown-like structures, which are histological features characterized by the accumulation of macrophages around dead adipocytes in inflamed adipose tissue (Murano *et al.*, 2008). Since a key function of macrophages is to remove apoptotic cells in an immunologically silent manner to prevent the release of noxious substances, it is reasonable to speculate that the presence of crown-like structures in adipose tissue reflects a pro-inflammatory state that is, in part, due to an impairment of the macrophage-mediated phagocytic process (Ouchi *et al.*, 2011).

Insulin resistance and related metabolic abnormalities may be due to differential distribution of adipose tissue and/or adipose tissue dysfunction (Patel & Abate, 2013). Although the underlying mechanisms are not fully known, visceral adiposity is more closely associated with obesity-related pathology than peripheral subcutaneous fat, even if localized in the abdominal region. It is important to note that, whereas peripheral sWAT tends to decrease with age, vWAT does not seem to be affected (Cartwright *et al.*, 2007). This is particularly important since many investigators have reported that vWAT is a major contributor to metabolic risk, whereas sWAT may have a protective role (McLaughlin *et al.*, 2011). sWAT located in the gluteofemoral region is particularly protective, even when present in large cells (Manolopoulos *et al.*, 2010).

In fact, adipocytes in sWAT easily differentiate and expand to store large amounts of triacylglycerol. This storage capacity serves to limit vWAT mass and ectopic lipid deposition in the liver, the heart and muscle, which is associated with obesity-induced insulin resistance (Wang *et al.*, 2008a; Kursawe *et al.*, 2013).

The importance of BFM distribution has been extensively studied. There is compelling evidence that adipose compartments differ in their endocrine activity and paracrine secretion profiles, with different impacts on glucose homeostasis, and thus the accompanying metabolic risk and morbidity (Hammar & Östgren, 2013). Broadly, a truncal distribution of BFM owing to vWAT accumulation is more closely connected with increased death rates for CVD, but also with cancer at multiple sites (Hammar & Östgren, 2013). Furthermore, perivascular fat depots may trigger local vascular inflammation and remodeling. In agreement with this, it was demonstrated that periaortic fat is independently associated with the prevalence of peripheral artery disease (Fox *et al.*, 2010), and greater pericardial fat correlates positively with the presence of coronary calcification (Rosito *et al.*, 2008; Liu *et al.*, 2010).

Regardless of the relevance of BFM distribution, several lines of experimental evidence suggest that the cellular characteristics of fat depots, including adipocyte size, macrophage accumulation, arteriolar dysfunction, angiogenesis and cellular hypoxia, are related to a greater cardiometabolic risk, independently of the absolute volume of adipose tissue in any given depot (Pasarica *et al.*, 2009; Gealekman *et al.*, 2011; Farb *et al.*, 2012; Rosenquist *et al.*, 2013; Lafontan, 2014). Adipocyte volume is a determinant of the cell's functionality, with larger adipocytes predicting more adverse cardiometabolic risk. In fact, fat depots with higher lipid content and lipolytic activity can increase systemic free fatty acids, which leads to increased lipid synthesis, gluconeogenesis and muscle and hepatic insulin resistance, resulting in hyperlipidemia, glucose intolerance, hypertension and ultimately atherosclerosis (Koutsari & Jensen, 2006; Lafontan, 2014). Fat cell size is inversely associated with insulin sensitivity, and the presence of large adipocytes in abdominal sWAT is considered an indicator of decreased adipogenic potential and can be the trigger for increased macrophage infiltration and inflammatory process activation (Lundgren *et al.*, 2007). Indeed, subcutaneous abdominal adipocyte hypertrophy is considered to be an independent risk factor for developing type 2 DM, regardless of BMI, adiposity and BFM distribution (Weyer *et al.*, 2000).

The existence of a deficit in the vascular NO bioavailability – endothelial dysfunction – is the first stage in the transition from normal vascular function to vasodilation disability, inflammation, atherogenesis and ultimately overt atherosclerosis. In fact, NO bioavailability is inversely related to the progression of vascular disease (Sandoo *et al.*, 2010). Accordingly, endothelial dysfunction is an early indicator of atherosclerotic damage and a high-quality prognostic marker of future cardiac events (Akcakoyun *et al.*, 2008). Endothelial dysfunction in aged individuals vasculature has been consistently described in rodents, nonhuman primates and humans (Ungvari *et al.*, 2010; Lind *et al.*, 2011; Seals *et al.*, 2011). This evidence demonstrates that ageing is an independent and unmodifiable factor associated with endothelial dysfunction even in the absence of obesity-related morbilities (Rodriguez-Mañas *et al.*, 2009), conditions that *per se* impair endothelium-dependent vasodilation. In fact, obesity is a chief contributor to endothelial dysfunction in the elderly, and conversely, ER is a simple strategy that results in improvement in endothelial function in aged animals (Nisoli *et al.*, 2005; Ungvari *et al.*, 2008; Csiszar *et al.*, 2009; Kondo *et al.*, 2009), including humans (Sasaki *et al.*, 2002; Raitakari *et al.*, 2004; Meyer *et al.*, 2006; Pierce *et al.*, 2008). ER confers vasoprotection in ageing and in pathological conditions that promote accelerated vascular ageing, such as oxidative stress and inflammation (Feige *et al.*, 2008; Ungvari *et al.*, 2008; Csiszar *et al.*, 2009; Ketonen *et al.*, 2010; Rippe *et al.*, 2010).

Obesity also interferes in endothelial function through regulation of circulating vascular growth factors levels. Adipose tissue is well vascularized and is regarded as a key source of these regulatory molecules (Rehman *et al.*, 2003; Bell *et al.*, 2006; Cao, 2007). Accordingly, obese individuals have higher serum levels of vascular endothelial growth factor (VEGF), hepatocyte growth factor and soluble tyrosine kinase with immunoglobulin-like and EGF-like domains (Tie)-2, whereas data regarding angiopoietin 2 are conflicting (Rehman *et al.*, 2003; Silha *et al.*, 2005; Bell *et al.*, 2006; Lieb *et al.*, 2009, 2010; Loebig *et al.*, 2010; Kaess *et al.*, 2012). Evidence indicates that adipogenesis and angiogenesis (new blood vessel formation) are temporal and spatially related (Tang *et al.*, 2008; Rutkowski *et al.*, 2009), with growth of newer vessels occurring in parallel with adipocyte hyperplasia. Indeed, adipocyte-secreted adipokines with pro-angiogenic activity, such as VEGF, placental growth factor, leptin and apelin, as well as antiangiogenic factors such as thrombospondin and endostatin, are a central requisite for adipose tissue expansion

(Nishimura *et al.*, 2007; Lafontan, 2014). However, as well as local effects, these adipokines may influence other vascular beds, and induce pathogenic neovascularization, such as that observed in the atherosclerotic plaque. Indeed, the levels of the aforementioned angiogenic factors secreted by adipose tissue are elevated in serum of obese patients, and ultimately intervene in the pathogenesis of CVD and cancer (Silha *et al.*, 2005; Rehman *et al.*, 2003). As angiogenesis is required for adipose tissue expansion, inhibitors of angiogenesis may inhibit adipose tissue expansion, and hence reverse obesity in genetic and diet-induced rodent models of obesity (Cao, 2010). The heterogeneity and scarcity of studies in humans, particularly in those who are elderly, which is associated with impaired angiogenesis, limit straightforward conclusions. Nevertheless, the most promising studies and anti-obesity nutrients presenting anti-angiogenic effects are discussed later.

2.6.2 Adipose tissue and metabolic dysregulation

Numerous studies have elucidated the intervention of adipose tissue and adipocyte dysfunction in the pathophysiology of insulin resistance and other obesity-related diseases, considering the strong association between high BFM and dysfunctional metabolism (Lafontan, 2014).

Adipose tissue consists of a variety of cells other than adipocytes, such as vascular cells, fibroblasts, macrophages stromal cells and monocytes, and its accretion, through adipocyte hypertrophy and hyperplasia, could lead to regions of hypoxia and increased cellular oxidative stress or endoplasmic reticulum (ERet) stress, discussed later (Lafontan, 2014). Hypoxia effects in adipose tissue deserve special attention, as they are thought to be involved in the induction of fibrosis and stimulation of local inflammatory responses (Halberg *et al.*, 2009). The activation of the transcription factor HIF-1α in visceral adipocytes from mice is critical for the progression of obesity-associated pathologies such as glucose intolerance, insulin resistance and cardiomyopathy (Krishnan *et al.*, 2012). Likewise, other adipose tissue-secreted molecules related to inflammation or metabolic disturbances are also hypoxia-induced, such as macrophage migration inhibitory factor, matrix metalloproteinase (MMP)-2 and MMP-9, IL-6, TNF-α, MCP-1, plasminogen activator inhibitor-1 (PAI-1), VEGF and leptin. In support of this idea, adipose tissue-specific genetic repression of endogenous HIF-1α activity, or treatment with an inhibitor (PX-478), resulted in the improvement of adipose tissue metabolic dysfunction and reduction of macrophage infiltration in mice (Jiang *et al.*, 2011; Leal & Mafra, 2013; Sun *et al.*, 2013). Thus, inhibition of HIF-1α activity in adipose tissue may be a promising strategy to improve obesity and insulin resistance.

The main role of WAT is triglyceride storage and fatty acid release over periods of starvation; however, adipocytes are not simple depots (Leal & Mafra, 2013). Instead, WAT is a dynamic endocrine organ that secretes several molecules, such as adipokines and pro-inflammatory cytokines (Leal & Mafra, 2013; Vielma *et al.*, 2013). As individuals accumulate fat and their adipocytes enlarge, adipose tissue undergoes molecular and cellular alterations, macrophages accumulate and inflammation ensues (Cancello *et al.*, 2005). Infiltrated and activated macrophages in adipose tissue are responsible for most pro-inflammatory cytokine production, in particular IL-6 and TNF-α, and also repress the production of anti-inflammatory and insulin-sensitizing adipokines, such as adiponectin (Ouchi *et al.*, 2011). This state of inflammation interferes with insulin signaling, not only locally, but also establishing global insulin resistance (Lafontan, 2014). Moreover, enhanced fibrotic processes in adipose tissue, in response to inflammation, can worsen inflammation in a vicious circle that leads toward irreversibility.

Although ageing *per se* has been reported to affect mechanisms involved in the development of insulin resistance (Einstein *et al.*, 2010), adipose tissue accretion apparently possesses a prevalent effect. Supporting this assumption, ER could be a useful tool to avoid and/or ameliorate insulin resistance because it mitigates inflammation (Esposito *et al.*, 2003). In contrast, it was reported that the removal of large amounts of subcutaneous abdominal fat by liposuction improves neither inflammation nor other cardiometabolic risk factors (Klein *et al.*, 2004).

Recently, many studies have shown that muscle triglyceride accumulation is an important causative factor for the progression of metabolic disorders (van Herpen & Schrauwen-Hinderling, 2008). In fact, enhanced intramyocellular lipid content is indicative of an oversaturation of the lipid storage capacity in WAT, thereby creating a spillover phenomenon that may also affect other organs. This ectopic accumulation of lipids in cells other than adipocytes promotes a number of lipotoxic insults in those cells, thereby leading to (or worsening) insulin resistance and the inflammatory state (Unger *et al.*, 2010). In this setting, ER exhibits an exceptionally broad protective effect against age-related changes in lipid metabolism, including adiposity and TG levels. Although it is recognized that ER clearly reduces the age-related increase in adiposity, the precise mechanisms of ER concerning the relation between adipogenesis and ectopic lipid accumulation are not fully known (van Herpen & Schrauwen-Hinderling, 2008).

2.6.2.1 Adipose tissue and disruption of endocrine secretion of adipokines

One of the aspects recently recognized to be associated with increased adiposity is the induction of neuroendocrine effects, including sympathetic nervous and angiotensin system activation, and alteration of adipokine secretion (Fontana, 2009).

Dysregulated production/secretion of adipokines by hypertrophied adipocytes is strongly associated with obesity-related disturbances. In fact, these cells hypersecrete pro-inflammatory and pro-diabetic adipokines while decreasing production of adipokines affording protection against inflammation and diabetes. For instance, in larger adipocytes leptin production is markedly increased (Guo *et al.*, 2004), but the synthesis of adiponectin and apelin, two adipokines with beneficial effects on insulin sensitivity and vascular function, is impaired (Lafontan, 2014).

In obesity, increased adipose mass in the presence of hyperleptinemia indicates resistance to endogenous leptin, although paradoxically, hyperleptinemia by itself causes leptin resistance by increasing the expression of proteins that block its signaling. One such protein is the muscle suppressor of cytokine signaling-3 (SOCS-3), overexpression of which not only inhibits insulin signaling but also leads to suppression of leptin-regulated genes involved in fatty acid oxidation and mitochondrial function, contributing to ectopic accumulation of lipids and to insulin resistance (Yang *et al.*, 2012; Jorgensen *et al.*, 2013). Furthermore, since hyperleptinemia induces macrophage activation, increasing levels of TNF-α, ROS and inducible NO synthase-derived NO potentially present deleterious effects on the cardiovascular system (Leal & Mafra, 2013).

2.6.3 Mitochondrial dysfunction

Ageing and obesity are two strong contributors to mitochondrial dysfunction, the former being involved in insufficiency of mitochondrial quality control and turnover mechanisms (such as attenuated autophagy). Adaptation to an excess nutrient

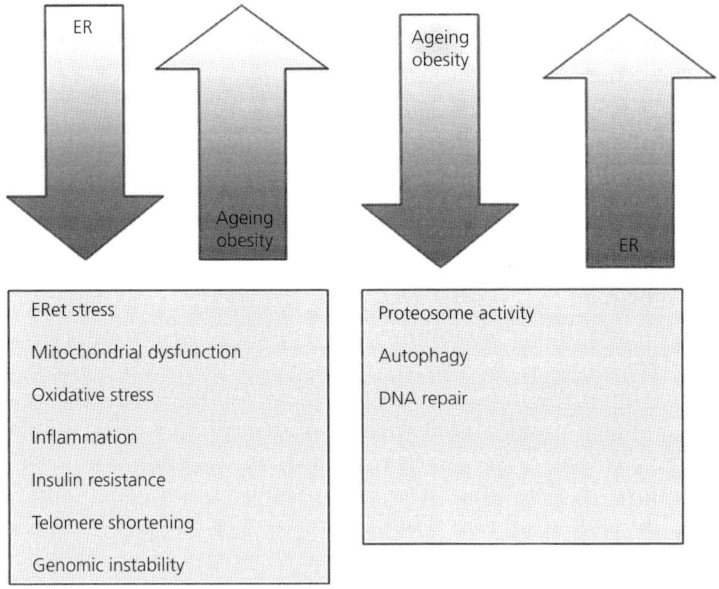

Figure 2.2 Resume of the main cellular functions inversely affected by ageing/obesity and ER. ER, energy restriction; ERet, endoplasmic reticulum.

environment interferes with mitochondrial function in a magnitude that reflects the duration to which the organism has been exposed to overnutrition (reviewed in Liesa & Shirihai, 2013). Conversely, ER counteracts these effects. The main cellular functions inversely affected by ageing/obesity and ER are summarized in Fig. 2.2. In a very interesting and recent study, Schmeisser *et al.* showed that, regarding lifespan, mitochondrial complex I inhibition exerts an effect similar to ER, but independently of FOXO, AMPK or sirtuins signaling (Schmeisser *et al.*, 2013). Complex I inhibition-induced longevity extension is dependent on p38 MAPK and Nrf2 activation, resulting from a momentary increase in mitochondrial ROS production (Schmeisser *et al.*, 2013). The outcomes of Nrf2 activation on oxidative stress defenses and metabolic control can be found in Section 2.4.4.

2.6.4 Endoplasmic reticulum stress

As a complex process characterized by an inexorable progressive loss of function and homeostasis, ageing is associated with a decrease in the cellular capacity to respond to several forms of stress that might contribute to an impaired functionality of the cells, tissues and organs (Hussain & Ramaiah, 2007; Inagi, 2009; Wu *et al.*, 2010), even in the absence of pathological conditions (Wu *et al.*, 2010). In addition to increased levels of oxidative damage and mitochondria-dependent mechanisms of apoptosis (Stadtman, 2001; Rabek *et al.*, 2003), some studies have recently suggested that impaired functionality of the ERet may also play an important role in the ageing process (Stadtman, 2001; Ikeyama *et al.*, 2003; Rabek *et al.*, 2003; Hussain & Ramaiah, 2007; Pfaffenbach & Lee, 2011). Moreover, strong evidence demonstrates that obesity contributes to the age-related decline of the cellular response to ERet stress.

2.6.4.1 Endoplasmic reticulum stress-induced unfolded protein response

ERet is a large membrane-enclosed-sensing cellular stress compartment, in which nascent membrane and secretory proteins are synthesized and folded into the final three-dimensional structures as well as a site where steroids, cholesterol and other lipids are synthesized (Schroder & Kaufman, 2005; Ron & Walter, 2007; Kitamura, 2008; Zhang & Kaufman, 2008). The ERet lumen is characterized by an oxidative environment and high calcium levels (and plays a role in calcium storage and homeostasis). In fact, protein folding is an oxidative process that generates ROS as by-products (Zhang & Kaufman, 2008).

ERet is the central regulator of protein folding, quality control, trafficking and targeting, and its ability to adapt and manage adverse conditions appears thus to be of paramount importance for the cell. Nowadays, it is well known that several physiological, such as ageing, and also pathological conditions may decrease the ERet protein-folding, quality control and trafficking machinery, leading to a cellular perturbation termed *ERet stress*, which is characterized by the accumulation of unfolded and/or misfolded proteins in the ERet (Kaufman, 2002; Ozcan *et al.*, 2004; Schroder & Kaufman, 2005; Ron & Walter, 2007; Hetz *et al.*, 2011; Hetz, 2012). In response to the accumulation of unfolded and/or misfolded proteins, the ERet orchestrate a coordinated adaptive response collectively known as the *unfolded protein response* (UPR) in order to cope with stressful conditions (Kitamura, 2008; Back & Kaufman, 2012; Hetz, 2012). The UPR results from the activation of three distinct signal transduction pathways mediated by the protein kinase-activated by double-strand RNA (PKR)-like ERet kinase (PERK), the inositol requiring enzyme 1 (IRE1) and the activating transcription factor (ATF)-6 (Kaufman, 2002; Ron, 2002; Ron & Walter, 2007; Malhi & Kaufman, 2011). Under conditions of ERet homeostasis, these three UPR transmembrane sensors are inactive through binding of the glucose related protein 78/immunoglobulin heavy chain-binding protein (GRP78/BiP) (Hotamisligil, 2010). However, under ERet stress conditions, when the protein load in the ERet overcomes the ERet folding and/or quality control capability, leading to the accumulation of unfolded and/or misfolded proteins in the ERet lumen, BiP is released from the UPR sensors resulting in their activation. Then, activation of PERK, ATF-6 and IRE1 triggers complex downstream signaling pathways (Ron & Walter, 2007). The activation of PERK leads to eukaryotic initiation factor (eIF)2α phosphorylation and, consequently, global attenuation of protein synthesis and subsequent reduction of the ERet workload (Hotamisligil, 2010). Alternatively, activation of the PERK-eIF2α pathway induces the translation of the ATF-4 gene as well as of the genes involved in the ERet redox control, such as Nrf2 (Cullinan *et al.*, 2003; Cullinan & Diehl, 2004, 2006). When detached from BiP, ATF-6 transits to the Golgi apparatus where it is activated by site-1 and site-2 proteases. Then, activated ATF-6 translocates to the nucleus where it triggers the activation of several UPR effectors (including chaperones and signal transducers) involved in protein folding, processing and degradation (Hotamisligil, 2010; Hetz *et al.*, 2011). Additionally, activated IRE1 catalyzes the removal of a small intron from the mRNA encoding the X-box binding protein-1 (XBP1), through an alternative mechanism of splicing of the XBP1. Spliced XBP1, alone or in conjugation with ATF-6, induces the expression of chaperones and proteins involved in ERet biogenesis, phospholipids synthesis and ERet-associated degradation (Hotamisligil, 2010; Lee *et al.*, 2011a).

The main purpose of this complex and coordinated activation of the UPR is to mitigate the ERet stress by attenuating general protein translation, increasing misfolded or unfolded protein degradation and increasing the expression of chaperones that assist the protein folding process in the ERet lumen (Ron & Walter, 2007; Rutkowski & Kaufman, 2007; Hotamisligil, 2010; Fu *et al.*, 2012). Therefore, the first phase of the UPR activation is generally regarded as a pro-survival mechanism, which provides a "*window of opportunity*" for cells to readjust the ERet environment in order to cope with stress (Kitamura, 2008). Nevertheless, if the adaptive response fails to mitigate the ERet stress and homeostasis is not restored, cell functioning is compromised and apoptotic-signaling pathways may be triggered, which leads to cell death (Oslowski & Urano, 2010; Fonseca *et al.*, 2011; Fu *et al.*, 2012; Hetz, 2012).

2.6.4.2 Ageing-induced modification in unfolded protein response

The ageing process is characterized by accumulation of misfolded and modified proteins and by harmful protein aggregates (Salminen & Kaarniranta, 2010), clearly suggesting reduced ERet functionality (Fig. 2.3). In fact, increasing evidence associates alterations in

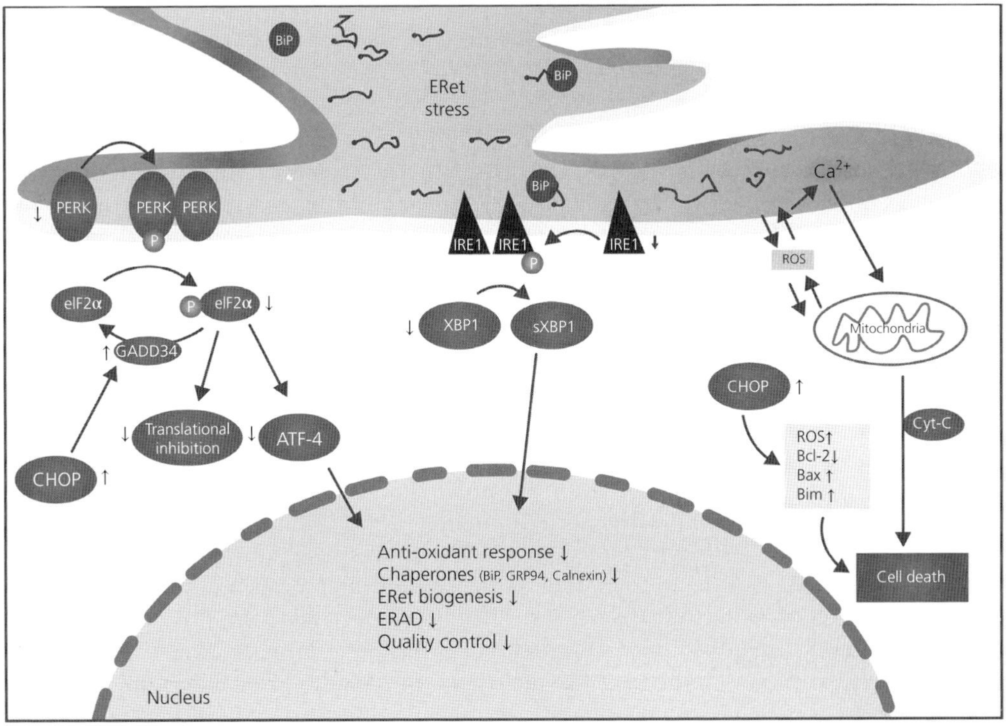

Figure 2.3 Endoplasmic reticulum stress in the ageing process. ATF-4, activating transcription factor-4; Bax, Bcl-2-associated X protein; Bim, Bcl-2 interacting mediator of cell death; Bcl-2, anti-apoptotic protein; BiP, immunoglobulin heavy chain-binding protein; Ca^{2+}, calcium ion; CHOP, C/EBP homologous protein; Cyt-c, cytochrome C; eIF2α, eukaryotic initiation factor 2α; ERAD, endoplasmic reticulum-associated protein degradation; ERet, endoplasmic reticulum; GADD34, growth arrest and DNA damage-inducible protein 34; GRP94, glucose-regulated protein 94; IRE1-inositol requiring enzyme 1; PERK, protein kinase-activated by double-strand RNA (PKR)-like-endoplasmic reticulum kinase; ROS, reactive oxygen species; sXBP1, spliced X-box binding protein 1; XBP1, X-box binding protein 1.

the ERet morphology and decline in the expression of ERet chaperones and transducers with ageing (Salminen & Kaarniranta, 2010). Taken together, these modifications affect protein-processing efficiency (Rabek *et al.*, 2003; Kourtis & Tavernarakis, 2011) and consequently create an unstable ERet environment unable to sustain cellular homeostasis (Kourtis & Tavernarakis, 2011), resulting in ERet misfolded protein accumulation.

Indeed, it is likely that "*misfolded protein syndromes*" of aged tissues might be primarily caused by the failure of the ERet chaperone and transducer machinery (Rabek *et al.*, 2003; Salminen & Kaarniranta, 2010). Accordingly, several studies demonstrate that the efficiency of the ERet stress–UPR system declines during the ageing process (Naidoo, 2009a, 2009b). Considering that in normal physiological conditions ERet quality control efficiency avoids accumulation of protein aggregates (Brown & Naidoo, 2012), it is plausible to hypothesize that accumulation of unfolded and/or misfolded proteins during the ageing process could be a result of compromised protein quality control in the ERet. Additionally, age-related accumulation of misfolded proteins might be a result of an impaired cleansing system owing to the decline in the proteasomal degradation and autophagic processes, thus reinforcing the idea that the functionality of the protein quality control system is compromised (Salminen & Kaarniranta, 2010; Brown & Naidoo, 2012).

The decrease in the efficiency of the ERet functionality can be explained, at least in part, by a reduction in ERet resident chaperones (such as BiP, GRP94 and calnexin), lower activity of protein disulfide isomerase (PDI; catalyzes protein disulfide bond formation and isomerization) and increased carbonylation of ERet proteins (Rabek *et al.*, 2003; Nuss *et al.*, 2008; Salminen & Kaarniranta, 2010). Accompanying these alterations, eIF2α phosphorylation level, which is responsible for shutting down protein translation, and ATF-4 and XBP1 expression are clearly reduced in the ageing process (Paz Gavilan *et al.*, 2006; Hussain & Ramaiah, 2007), which might result from the reduced expression of the upstream ERet stress signal transducers PERK and IRE1 (Paz Gavilan *et al.*, 2006).

Nevertheless, there is solid evidence demonstrating that ageing is accompanied by a shift in the balance between the protective adaptive response and cell death signaling. In fact, complementary to the ERet stress, which reduces the capacity to restore cellular homeostasis, the expression of growth arrest and DNA damage-inducible protein 34 (GADD34) and C/EBP homologous protein (CHOP; the major ERet stress-related apoptosis inducer) is enhanced in the ageing context (Ikeyama *et al.*, 2003; Li & Holbrook, 2004; Paz Gavilan *et al.*, 2006; Hussain & Ramaiah, 2007; Naidoo *et al.*, 2008), thereby suggesting that ageing cells are more susceptible to ERet stress-induced apoptosis. CHOP appears to mediate cell death signaling using two different mechanisms: it increases expression of ERet oxidoreductase 1α, which transfers electrons from PDI during protein disulfide-bound formation to molecular oxygen, thus generating hydrogen peroxide as a by-product; and, simultaneously, it decreases the levels of anti-apoptotic protein Bcl-2 and enhances levels of pro-apoptotic proteins Bcl-2 associated X protein (Bax) and Bcl-2 interacting mediator of cell death (Bim). Additionally, the ERet stress-induced ROS production may cause calcium leak from the ERet, leading to mitochondrial calcium accumulation, which, in turn, promotes mitochondrial depolarization and exacerbates ROS production further amplifying ERet stress and mitochondrial dysfunction (Kaufman *et al.*, 2010; Zhang, 2010). On the other hand, CHOP antagonizes the inhibition of protein translation imposed by the PERK-eIF2α pathway through the increase in GADD34 expression (Marciniak *et al.*, 2004; Oyadomari & Mori, 2004; Szegezdi *et al.*, 2009).

GADD34 dephosphorylates eIF2α, contributing to cell recovery from protein translation shut-down imposed by eIF2α phosphorylation (Novoa *et al.*, 2001). Under unmitigated ERet stress conditions, increase in newly synthesized protein results in additional protein load augmenting the ERet stress, in a vicious circle.

Therefore, over time, it is plausible that unmitigated ERet stress probably plays an important role in some age-associated pathologies. In fact, ERet stress has been shown to be increased in type 2 DM, Alzheimer disease, Parkinson disease, NAFLD and chronic renal disease and CVD (Naidoo *et al.*, 2008; Inagi, 2009; Wu *et al.*, 2010; Brown & Naidoo, 2012). It appears that, in all of these disorders, proteins or fragments of proteins are modified from their natural soluble forms to insoluble fibrils forms, which accumulate owing to the decreased efficiency of the proteosomal degradation system, causing organ dysfunction (Naidoo *et al.*, 2008; Brown & Naidoo, 2012).

2.6.4.3 Obesity-induced endoplasmic reticulum stress

Obesity imposes significant metabolic challenge and disturbance, where an additional demand on the cellular synthetic and degradation machinery occurs in tissues, such as the liver, adipose tissue and pancreas, and results in the loss of homeostasis on tissues, organs and organisms (Hotamisligil, 2010).

Numerous factors, such as increased oxidative stress, mitochondrial dysfunction and chronic low-grade inflammation, underlie tissue damage in an obese environment (Ogihara *et al.*, 2004; Anderson *et al.*, 2009; Barazzoni *et al.*, 2012; Rector *et al.*, 2013). Additionally, obesity promotes ERet stress, which is relevant in the propagation of obesity-induced metabolic disturbance (Fig. 2.4; Ozcan *et al.*, 2004; de Ferranti & Mozaffarian, 2008; Engin & Hotamisligil, 2010). Indeed, ERet stress plays a major role in the activation and amplification of inflammatory signaling and insulin resistance in response to obesity (Zhang *et al.*, 2006; Zhang & Kaufman, 2008; Hotamisligil, 2010; Gregor & Hotamisligil, 2011; Malhi & Kaufman, 2011; Lee *et al.*, 2012; Miani *et al.*, 2012) and sustained ERet stress has been described in humans and rodent models of obesity and/or NAFLD (Puri *et al.*, 2008; Cnop *et al.*, 2012; Zhang *et al.*, 2014).

IRE1 and PERK pathways present an important function in the interconnection of ERet stress with the inflammatory signaling pathway (Urano *et al.*, 2000; Hu *et al.*, 2006; Zhang & Kaufman, 2008; Solinas & Karin, 2010). IRE1 activates not only IκB kinase, which phosphorylates NF-κB inhibitor (IκB) and leads to its degradation followed by NF-κB activation, but also the c-jun N-terminal kinase (JNK), increasing pro-inflammatory cytokine expression (Urano *et al.*, 2000; Hu *et al.*, 2006; Zhang & Kaufman, 2008). Furthermore, PERK-eIF2α-mediated suppression of protein translation leads to decreased expression of IκB, resulting in NF-κB activation with production of pro-inflammatory mediators (Deng *et al.*, 2004; Zhang & Kaufman, 2008). Conversely, IL-1β, TNFα and interferon gamma, which are increased in the context of obesity and relate to pancreatic β-cells dysfunction, are able to induce ERet stress, mainly through downregulation of the sarco/ERet pump Ca^{2+}ATPase (SERCA)2b (and therefore depletion of Ca^{2+} from the ERet) and eventual decrease in the expression of several ERet chaperones, such as BiP and GRP94 (Cardozo *et al.*, 2005; Gregor & Hotamisligil, 2007; Akerfeldt *et al.*, 2008). ERet stress and inflammatory signaling pathways are also interconnected through intercellular ROS generation (Zhang, 2010; Gregor & Hotamisligil, 2011). Consequently, alterations in the redox status (and/or ROS generation) could affect ERet homeostais and protein folding (Malhotra & Kaufman, 2007), with increased oxidative stress representing

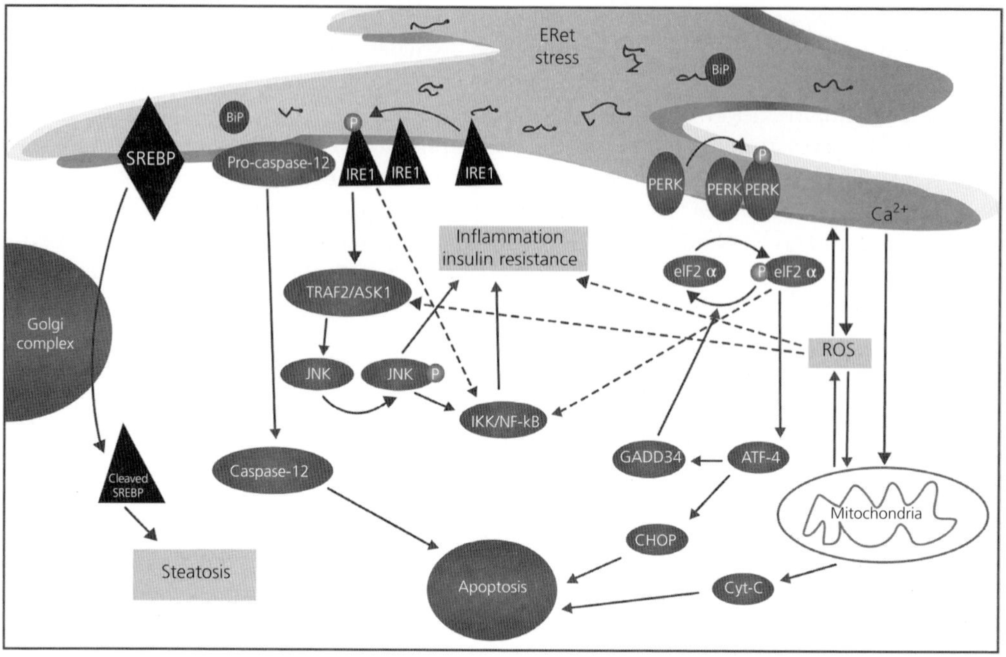

Figure 2.4 Endoplasmic reticulum stress in obesity. ATF-4, activating transcription factor-4; BiP, immunoglobulin heavy chain-binding protein; Ca^{2+}, calcium ion; CHOP-C/EBP, homologous protein; Cyt-c, cytochrome c; eIF2α, eukaryotic initiation factor 2α; ERet, endoplasmic reticulum; GADD34, growth arrest and DNA damage-inducible protein 34; IKK/NF-κB, IκB kinase/nuclear factor kappa-light chain enhancer of activated B cells; IRE1, inositol-requiring enzyme 1; PERK, protein kinase-activated by double-strand RNA (PKR)-like-endoplasmic reticulum kinase; JNK, c-jun N-terminal kinase; ROS, reactive oxygen species; SREBP-sterol regulatory element-binding protein; TRAF2/ASK1, TNF receptor-associated factor 2/apoptosis signal regulating kinase 1.

another mechanism bridging obesity to ERet stress (Gregor & Hotamisligil, 2007). Accordingly, in an opposite approach, it was demonstrated that ERet stress in the liver could be reduced/normalized through anti-inflammatory and anti-oxidant therapies, which resulted in the blockage of steatosis and insulin resistance (Shi *et al.*, 2013) and improved protein folding and secretion (Malhotra *et al.*, 2008), respectively. Therefore, in the context of obesity, ERet stress can amplify the inflammatory signaling but inflammation can also induce ERet stress (Cardozo *et al.*, 2005; Gregor & Hotamisligil, 2007; Akerfeldt *et al.*, 2008; Miani *et al.*, 2012), thereby resulting in a vicious circle. Consequently, this mutual amplification between ERet stress and inflammatory signaling might render cells less able to recover from injury, which can be even aggravated in the ageing setting.

Several downstream effectors of the UPR appear to be involved in the disruption of the insulin signaling cascade, with the activation of IRE1 and/or PERK pathways involved in the process (Ozcan *et al.*, 2004; Eizirik *et al.*, 2008; Zhang & Kaufman, 2008). The precise mechanisms by which obesity-induced ERet stress impairs insulin signaling and metabolic control are complex and occur at different levels of the insulin signaling pathway (Fu *et al.*, 2012). Obesity has been associated with increased JNK activation in the liver and adipose tissue (Hirosumi *et al.*, 2002; Eizirik *et al.*, 2008; Hotamisligil, 2008; Boura-Halfon & Zick, 2009), a via also activated by ERet stress that has been critically implicated in the development and progression of insulin resistance through inhibitory serine phosphorylation of insulin receptor substrates 1 and 2 (Hirosumi *et al.*, 2002; Solinas & Karin, 2010; Malhi & Kaufman, 2011; Cnop *et al.*, 2012; Ozcan & Tabas, 2012). In order to compensate for the ongoing impaired insulin signaling, pancreatic β-cells increase insulin production, thus resulting in increased demand in β-cells for protein synthesis, folding and quality control and, consequently, in pancreatic ERet stress (Ozcan & Tabas, 2012).

Obesity-associated increase in hepatic lipid droplets accumulation can be explained by enhanced hepatic lipogenesis, enhanced fatty acid uptake and/or decreased hepatic lipoprotein secretion (Wang & Kaufman, 2012; Zámbó *et al.*, 2013). Nevertheless, nowadays it is well accepted that UPR pathway activation can play a major role in the regulation of lipogenesis and in the size and composition of lipid droplets, including regulation of cholesterol metabolism (Gregor & Hotamisligil, 2007; Collison *et al.*, 2009; Hotamisligil, 2010). The proteins of the SREBP family are involved in those processes. These proteins are codified by two genes in humans, SREBP1 and SREBP2, and are synthesized and located on the ERet membrane. The activation process of the SREBP proteins, which can be induced by the ERet stress, requires their translocation to the Golgi apparatus where they undergo successive cleavages by site-1 and site-2 proteases (similarly to the ATF-6 pathway activation), yielding the active transcription-regulatory forms SREBP-1a, SREBP-1c and mature SREBP-2, involved in cholesterol metabolism, lipid synthesis and/or storage (Kammoun *et al.*, 2009; Damiano *et al.*, 2010; Zhang *et al.*, 2011, 2012; Lee *et al.*, 2012; Lhoták *et al.*, 2012; Fang *et al.*, 2013; Xiao and Song, 2013). Alteration in ERet phospholipid composition (higher concentration of phosphatidylcholine compared with phosphatidylethanolamine, owing to stimulation of lipid synthesis), simultaneously with SREBP activation, observed in the obese liver, inhibits SERCA2b activity, disrupts calcium homeostasis and induces ERet stress (Fu *et al.*, 2011). Reinforcing the tight interconnection between ERet stress and NAFLD, hepatic overexpression of BiP or SERCA2b mitigates ERet stress and slows down hepatic lipogenesis, decreasing the risk for NAFLD onset (Ozcan *et al.*, 2006; Kammoun *et al.*, 2009; Fu *et al.*, 2011; Lee & Ozcan, 2014; Zhang *et al.*, 2014). Furthermore, the IRE1 pathway regulates the transcription of several genes involved in fatty acid/triacylglycerols/phospholipids synthesis, such as stearoyl-CoA desaturase-1, acetyl-CoA carboxylase 2 and diacylglycerol acyltransferase 2 (Hotamisligil, 2010). However, the relationship between ERet stress and lipid metabolism is bidirectional: activation of the UPR pathways can induce lipogenesis and altered lipid homeostasis while intracellular accumulation of (saturated) fatty acyl-CoA, aberrant lipid metabolism and alterations in the phospholipid composition of the ERet lead to ERet stress (Fu *et al.*, 2011; Basseri & Austin, 2012; Zámbó *et al.*, 2013), thus creating a vicious circle.

Obesity impairs autophagy, which also increases ERet stress and insulin resistance (Yang *et al.*, 2010). Autophagy is a homeostatic process of intracellular self-degradation of long-lived protein aggregates and damaged organelles (Kawakami *et al.*, 2009; Yang *et al.*, 2010; Decuypere *et al.*, 2011) and ERet stress-induced autophagy can be an adaptive mechanism to set out misfolded proteins that have escaped the ERet-associated proteosomal degradation and, thus, assist the ERet in restoring cellular homeostasis (Ogata *et al.*, 2006; Yang *et al.*, 2010). Since the ageing process is accompanied by decreased autophagy, we could postulate that obesity in the ageing context could reinforce the failure in the autophagic system, thus resulting in further ERet dysfunction, creating a vicious circle and, consequently, contributing to metabolic deterioration and exacerbating age-related cellular and tissue features.

2.6.5 Anti-obesity effects of natural compounds extracted from plants

A majority of older adults in the USA and Europe are overweight or obese. Beyond the ER dietary pattern, some natural compounds available in food, especially when plant-derived, have been described as factors that ameliorate obesity (Meydani & Hasan, 2010; Hurt & Wilson, 2012). Their effects could be due to multiple mechanisms, and their main advantage is their accessibility and apparent safety of their consumption. The most studied anti-obesity compounds present in food are discussed later and the main effects are summarized in Table 2.5.

2.6.5.1 Polyphenols

Polyphenols constitute a vast class of compounds that possess anti-oxidant capacities, and thus their consumption significantly inhibits oxidative stress, atherogenesis and atherosclerotic lesion development, which strongly protects various organs and in particular the cardiovascular system. Regular intake of polyphenols contributes to the delay or avoidance of age-associated diseases, as demonstrated in mice and humans. In addition, polyphenols directly intervene in the four main periods of the adipocyte life cycle: differentiation, proliferation, lipid accumulation and cell death. The main classes of polyphenols available in food with apparent anti-obesity effects are focused on later. However, since most of the clinical studies have been done on young adults, polyphenol supplement use in the elderly should be treated with caution.

2.6.5.1.1 Cathechins

Green tea prepared from the unfermented dried leaves of the plant *Camellia sinensis* (Theaceace) is one of the most popular beverages in the world, and has been extensively studied for its putative disease-preventive effects. It is a beverage rich in polyphenolic flavonoids, in particular catechins, such as epicatechin, catechin gallate, epicatechin gallate, gallocatechin, gallocatechin gallate, epigallocatechin and EGCG, which is the most abundant, and reportedly has anti-obesity and anti-adipogenic effects.

The molecular pathways of anti-adipogenic mechanisms of EGCG at the adipocyte level have recently been elucidated in cultured 3T3-L1 cells. It was demonstrated that EGCG dose-dependently inhibits, first, lipid droplet formation and differentiation into mature adipocytes (Chan *et al.*, 2011). The repression of adipocyte phenotype is partly due to the downregulation of the expression of PPARγ and CCAAT enhancer binding protein α (C/EBPα) (Furuyashiki *et al.*, 2004), adipogenic transcription factors involved in the expression of fatty acid binding protein (FABP) 4, a lipid-metabolizing enzyme involved in fat accumulation, and other lipid metabolizing enzymes. Concomitantly, EGCG upregulates β-catenin expression, and in particular favors its nuclear localization, demonstrating that EGCG-induced inhibition of adipogenesis is at least partially dependent on the Wingless and INT-1 (WNT)/β-catenin pathway (Lee *et al.*, 2013). Second, EGCG inhibits cellular proliferation, suppressing the clonal expansion of adipocytes via insulin signaling and stress-dependent MAPK/ERK (extracellular-signal-regulated kinase) and PI3K/AKT pathways, through inactivation of FOXO1 (Kim & Sakamoto, 2012). Third, it induces apoptosis of adipocytes (Lin *et al.*, 2005).

Over the past 10 years, there have been a number of studies in experimental animal models that support the anti-obesity effect of regular intake of catechins. In fact, it has been demonstrated that EGCG administration to both mice and rats avoids the BW

Table 2.5 Anti-obesity effects of natural compounds provided by food.

Compound	Class	Food source	Anti-obesity mechanisms
EGCG	Polyphenol	Tea	↓ Lipid droplet formation ↓ Adipocyte differentiation ↓ Clonal expansion of adipocytes ↑ Apoptosis of adipocytes ↓ High-fat diet induced weight gain in rodents ↓ Total percentage of body fat in rats ↓ Subcutaneous and mesenteric adipose tissue mass in rodents ↓ Fat deposition in liver in rodents ↓ Lipogenesis in rat liver ↑ Fecal excretion of fat and nitrogen rich-nutrients ↓ Cholesterol absorption on gastrointestinal tract ↓ Pancreatic lipases ↓ Angiogenesis ↑ Weight loss in metabolic syndrome elderly patients and obese individuals ↓ Appetite ↓ Leptin levels in the rodent blood
Curcumin		Turmeric	↓ Lipid accumulation in droplets ↓ Adipocyte differentiation ↓ Fatty acid synthase in adipocytes ↑ Apoptosis of adipocytes ↓ Angiogenesis ↓ Fat deposition in liver in high-fat-treated rodents ↓ Macrophage infiltration in adipose tissue and liver in high-fat-treated rodents ↑ Glycemic control in type 2 diabetes mellitus mice ↑ Adiponectin in rodents ↓ Hepatic activity of NF-κB in rodents
Resveratrol		Grapes Red wine Peanuts	↑ Adiponectin in cultured adipocytes ↓ mRNA expression of atherogenic adipokines ↓ Triacylglycerol content on adipocytes ↓ Adipocyte differentiation ↓ Adipocyte proliferation ↑ Apoptosis of adipocytes ↓ Angiogenesis Improves body weight in high-fat fed mice ↓ Subcutaneous, mesenteric and retroperitoneal adipose tissue mass in mice ↓ Ectopic fat deposition ↑ Energy expenditure in mice ↑ Satiety and resting metabolic rate in grey mouse lemurs during the winter body-weight-gain period ↓ Resting metabolic rate in humans ↑ Ectopic deposition of lipids on skeletal muscle of humans ↓ Ectopic deposition of lipids on the liver of humans
Quercetin		Capers Lovage Apples Onions Grapes	↓ Adipocyte differentiation ↑ Apoptosis of adipocytes ↓ Adipogenesis Transient ↑ energy expenditure in mice ↓ Liver steatosis ↓ High-fat-diet-induced weight gain in mice ↓ Visceral fat deposition in high-fat diet fed mice ↓ BMI, body weight and waist circumference in APOE3/3 individuals

Continued

Table 2.5 Continued

Daidzein		Soy	↓ Adipocyte differentiation ↓ High-fat-diet-induced weight gain in rats ↓ Fat deposition in liver of high-fat-diet-fed rats Regulates thermogenesis in brown adipose tissue
Genistein		Soy	↓ Adipocyte differentiation ↓ High-fat-diet-induced weight gain in mice ↓ High-fat-diet-induced fat accretion in mice ↓ Fat deposition in liver of high-fat diet fed rats ↓ Food intake, fat accumulation and adipocyte apoptosis in ovariectomized mice
Isoflavone extract		Soy	↓ Fatty acid synthase expression in liver of high-fat-fed ovariectomized rats ↓ Subcutaneous and retroperitoneal adipose tissue mass in rats ↑ Adiponectin in blood of obese postmenopausal women
Magnesium	Mineral		Improves insulin resistance in obese individuals ↓ Central obesity body fat percentage and BMI in aged type 2 diabetes mellitus patients

APOE, Apolipoprotein E; BMI, body mass index; EGCG, (–)epigallocatechin gallate; NF-κB, nuclear factor kappa-light chain enhancer of activated B cells.

increase induced by a high-fat diet (Wolfram *et al.*, 2005). In addition, others authors found a decrease in the mass of subcutaneous and epididymal adipose pads (Lee *et al.*, 2009) and in lipid deposition in liver (Bose *et al.*, 2008) of catechin-treated rodents. In line with this, Chen *et al.* (2009) demonstrated that long-term treatment with green or black tea reduces the magnitude of fat gain of rats on a 15% fat diet, while a low dose of EGCG, 1 mg/kg, decreases the percentage of fat mass without affecting BW. It was also found that tea consumption leads to the downregulation of genes related to adipocyte differentiation or extracellular triacylglycerol hydrolysis (PPARγ, C/EBP-β and lipoprotein lipase) in perirenal and epidydimal WAT (Chen *et al.*, 2009; Lee *et al.*, 2009), and increases the number of apoptotic adipocytes in visceral adipose tissue in the rat (Monteiro *et al.*, 2008). Moreover, short-term treatment with EGCG reduces the expression of fatty acid synthase and other genes involved in lipogenesis, in the liver of mice in the postprandial state, as well as increasing fecal energy excretion in the form of fat- and nitrogen-rich nutrients (Friedrich *et al.*, 2012), which could be partly justified by the inhibitory effect of EGCG on the activity of the pancreatic lipases (Wang *et al.*, 2006). However, we should take into account that other components of tea, such as saponins, also possess pancreatic lipase inhibitory effect, which could synergize with that of EGCG. There is evidence for the anti-obesity effects of saponins (reviewed in de la Garza *et al.*, 2011). EGCG has also been shown to decrease cholesterol absorption from the gastrointestinal tract (Wolfram *et al.*, 2005). Aditionally to produce effects in high-fat-treated rodents, it was also demonstrated that tea catechins modulate lipid metabolism in nonobese counterparts, reducing mesenteric and liver fat accretion (Ito *et al.*, 2008). In aged rats, it was shown that 6 months' consumption of green tea or catechin extract with low content of EGCG induces an apparent diminished atherosclerotic progression in cavernous tissue coupled to a decrease in the expression of VEGF and its main receptor VEGFR2, demonstrating a modulatory effect in tissue angiogenesis in the elderly (Neves *et al.*, 2008).

Concerning studies in humans, the effects of catechins in obesity control are far from being established. It was recently demonstrated that postmenopausal women receiving 300 mg daily of EGCG in caffeine-free green tea for 12 weeks coupled to an exercise program did not show significant differences in waist circumference, or in total or intra-abdominal adipose tissue (Hill *et al.*, 2007), which suggests that the anti-obesity effect of catechins decreases in the elderly. On the other hand, it was reported that the consumption of green tea for 2 months was effective in inducing weight loss, reducing the BMI and waist circumference of elderly patients with metabolic syndrome (Vieira *et al.*, 2012), and that consumption of extract of green tea with 208 mg of EGCG for 3 months by obese individuals aged 30–60 years significantly reduced BMI, waist circumference and blood lipids (Suliburska *et al.*, 2012), apparently by a mechanism independent of the increase in energy expenditure (Thielecke *et al.*, 2010). Nonetheless, others reported that green tea or catechins coupled to caffeine elicit an increase in energy expenditure, suggesting that they act synergistically in the short- and long-term (Bérubé-Parent *et al.*, 2005; Westerterp-Plantenga *et al.*, 2005). Whether catechins increase energy expenditure independently of caffeine or not remains to be elucidated. It was also demonstrated that ingestion for 8 weeks of green tea, or encapsulated extracts with equivalent levels of EGCG, resulted in a similar effect on BW variation in obese patients, leading to a lowered lipid peroxidation (Basu *et al.*, 2010), indicating that it could ameliorate the oxidative processes characteristic of the ageing phenotype. An additional contributor to the anti-obesity effects of catechins in humans, in line with observations in the rodents, could be the decreased absorption of nutrients in the gastrointestinal tract, particularly of carbohydrates and probably fat. In fact, several reports indicate that catechins reduce glucose absorption and that intake of cathechin-enriched oolong tea increases the fecal fat content by 50% when compared with periods of placebo intake by the same patients (Zhong *et al.*, 2006; Hsu *et al.*, 2006). However, the loss of energy in feces owing to tea intake could be partly due to protein malabsorption (Unno *et al.*, 2009), which in the elderly could be considered an undesirable effect. Moreover, green tea catechins such as EGCG may contribute to inhibition of the appetite. The satiating power of beverages containing both catechins and fiber is greatly increased and reduces the energy ingestion in other meals (Carter & Drewnowski, 2012), which could be an important trigger for control of over-ingestion of food and ensuing overweight. Supporting that, it was demonstrated that EGCG intraperitoneal injection to rats led not only to BW reduction, but also to a decrease in leptin levels and reduction of food intake compared with controls. Similar results were observed in lean and obese male Zucker rats (Kao *et al.*, 2000).

2.6.5.1.2 Curcumin

Curcumin is a naturally occurring polyphenol (dyferuloylmethane) found in the Indian spice turmeric, the ground rhizome of the perennial herb *Curcuma longa*, largely used as a spice and colorant and long been used in traditional Indian medicine because of its recognized beneficial effects. It has been recently recognized as an anti-ageing nutrient (Lima *et al.*, 2011; Shen *et al.*, 2013) despite the low bioavailability found in curcumin owing to its hydrophobic nature, which limits its activity. Curcumin dietary supplementation lowers oxidative stress and improves vascular dysfunction both in young and aged experimental rodent models (Fleenor *et al.*, 2013). It was demonstrated that curcumin exerts direct effects on WAT, inhibiting differentiation of pre-adipocytes by activation of

WNT/β-catenin signaling in a dose-dependent fashion (Ahn *et al.*, 2010), leading to reduction in oil red O-stained lipid droplets and downregulating the expression of the genes that codify PPARγ, C/EBNα and adipokines (Kim *et al.*, 2011a). It is also a potent inhibitor of fatty acid synthase in adipocytes and an inducer of apoptosis (Ejaz *et al.*, 2009; Zhao *et al.*, 2011), reducing the fat content and the number of adipocytes in adipose tissue. In addition, curcumin exerts an anti-angiogenic role in cultured endothelial cells and in murine adipose tissue by downregulating the expression of VEGF and VEGFR2 and reducing the microvessel density in WAT (Ejaz *et al.*, 2009). Angiogenesis repression seems to be partly responsible for the amelioration of BW observed in curcumin-treated mice. Moreover, curcumin treatment suppresses LDL receptor expression in cultured rat isolated hepatic stellate cells (Kang & Chen, 2009). It also reduces lipogenic gene expression in the liver, intrahepatic lipid content and macrophage infiltration in both WAT and liver of high-fat diet-treated mice (Shao *et al.*, 2012), apparently contributing to the avoidance of the hepatic fibrogenesis, common in obese individuals. In line with previous demonstration of the ability to control obesity, it was demonstrated that orally ingested curcumin reverses the main inflammatory and metabolic derangements associated with obesity and improves glycemic control in high-fat-diet-induced obesity and leptin-deficient ob/ob male C57BL/6J mice models of type 2 DM (Weisberg *et al.*, 2008). The authors found that curcumin-fed animals presented an increase in the production of adiponectin and a decrease in the hepatic activity of NF-κB.

Concerning human trials, it was reported that curcuminoid supplementation, 1 g/day for 30 days, in a randomized, double-blind, placebo-controlled, crossover trial that enrolled 30 participants, led to a significant reduction in serum triglycerides concentrations but did not have a significant influence on other lipid profile parameters, or BMI or total BFM (Mohammadi *et al.*, 2013). However, longer treatments or an increase in daily curmumin doses could induce weight loss, since no dose-limiting toxicity has been reported for curcumin. Phase I clinical trials indicated that oral doses as high as 15 g/day for 3 months are safe (Aggarwal & Sung, 2008). Curcumin has indeed been proposed as a putative nutraceutical for the treatment of metabolic syndrome owing to its conjugated beneficial effect on hypertension, obesity, endothelial dysfunction, insulin resistance and plasmatic lipids (reviewed in Sahebkar, 2013). Its relatively low cost, safety and proven efficacy make it advisable to include curcumin as part of the diet, not only as an anti-ageing but also as an anti-obesity factor. Interestingly, and despite the beneficial role of curcumin in obesity-related low-grade inflammation and impaired immune response, it does not superimpose the effect of ER (Wang *et al.*, 2013).

Some of the effects observed after curcumin treatment in obesity-induced adipose tissue inflammation are comparable to those found for recognized activators of Sirt1; however, no demonstration exists of direct activation of Sirt1 by curcumin (Bradford, 2013). Nevertheless, Weisberg *et al.* (2008) demonstrated a significant increase in Sirt1 expression after curcumin treatment in the adipose tissue of a murine model of obesity.

2.6.5.1.3 Resveratrol

Resveratrol is a well-studied polyphenolic compound naturally present in red grapes, red wine and peanuts and a recognized activator of Sirt1, as discussed earlier. Studies in cultured adipocytes have demonstrated that treatment with resveratrol strongly alters the expression profile of proteins (Rosenow *et al.*, 2012), reverses the secretion and mRNA expression of the atherogenic adipokines PAI-1 and IL-6, induced by TNF-α, and stimulates secretion of adiponectin (Ahn *et al.*, 2007). In addition, it promotes the fatty acid β-oxidation pathway in mitochondria and reduces triacylglycerol content (Mercader *et al.*, 2011). Similar results were also observed in human adipose tissue explants triggered *in vitro* with IL-1β for 24 h (Olholm *et al.*, 2010). Anti-adipogenic effects in 3T3-L1 adipocytes were observed for resveratrol-rich extracts of grape skin too (Zhang *et al.*, 2012). Interestingly, resveratrol seems to have effects in cultured adipocytes equivalent to those observed for curcumin: it inhibits adipogenic differentiation and proliferation, inducing cell cycle arrest in the early phase of adipogenesis (Fischer-Posovszky *et al.*, 2010; Kwon *et al.*, 2012), reduces fat accumulation (Gomez-Zorita *et al.*, 2013) and downregulates expression of PPARγ, C/EBPα, SREBP1 and fatty acid synthase mRNAs, as well as favoring adipocytes apoptosis (Rayalam *et al.*, 2008; Chen *et al.*, 2012). Moreover, resveratrol inhibited inflammatory and angiogenic response to hypoxia in human adipocytes removed from adipose tissue of nonoverweight women (Cullberg *et al.*, 2013).

Resveratrol also improves BW, as demonstrated in a cohort of male C57Bl/6J mice that were given a dose of 200 or 400 mg/kg/day of resveratrol concomitantly with either a standard chow or high-fat diet for 15 weeks (Lagouge *et al.*, 2006). An equivalent study in C57BL/6J mice demonstrated an additional effect of resveratrol treatment with 0.4% *trans*-resveratrol-supplemented high-fat diet for 9 weeks, which was a decrease in expression of inflammation and adipogenesis-related signaling molecules compared with high-fat-fed matched animals (Kim *et al.*, 2011c). Under control diet conditions, resveratrol-treated mice tended to gain less weight as compared with controls, presenting lower mass of epididymal, perirenal, mesenteric and retroperitoneal WAT. In fact, on a high-fat diet, rats treated with resveratrol, even at low dose, weighed almost the same as the controls (Lagouge *et al.*, 2006; Cho *et al.*, 2012), apparently owing to an increase in energy expenditure, since energy intake was unaffected in resveratrol-treated groups. Resveratrol effect is dose-dependent (Macarulla *et al.*, 2009) and seems to have a biphasic effect on energy expenditure (Baur, 2010); at low doses it caused a modest, but significant increase in the BW of mice, without any significant effect on food intake (Pearson *et al.*, 2008b). In contrast, in a study carried out in the primate grey mouse lemurs, *Microcebus murinus*, it was observed that 200 mg/kg/day of resveratrol reduced body-mass gain during the winter body-mass-gain period, by increasing satiety and RMR (Dal-Pan *et al.*, 2010). Resveratrol has consistently been found to ameliorate insulin resistance in obese animals, an effect that is related to a reduction in ectopic fat deposits in nonadipose tissues, particularly in the liver (Baur *et al.*, 2006).

To our knowledge, there has been no controlled study of resveratrol effects on BW for long-term treatments in humans. A recently conducted study in a cohort of 11 obese adults given 150 mg/day *trans*-resveratrol for 30 days demonstrated that the treatment partly mimetized the effects of ER, causing significant reductions in sleeping and RMR, which however do not agree with data from murine models. Concerning BW, no differences were noted between resveratrol- and placebo-treated groups, although ER causes metabolic adaptations partly through weight loss. An increased lipid deposition inside skeletal muscular cells was also observed after oil red O staining in biopsied tissues samples, coupled to a decrease in intrahepatic lipids assayed by proton magnetic resonance spectroscopy on a 3 T whole-body scanner in resveratrol-treated individuals (Timmers *et al.*, 2011). This study is partly corroborated by findings reported by Poulsen *et al.* (2013) that demonstrated no effect of resveratrol treatment for 4 weeks on oxidation rates of lipids, ectopic or visceral fat content, resting energy expenditure and inflammatory and metabolic biomarkers in obese men. In line with this, resveratrol 75 mg/day treatment for 12 weeks did not ameliorate either BW or metabolic profile in nonobese individuals (Yoshino *et al.*, 2012). Further studies with a higher number of participants, longer treatment periods and different dosages/formulations of resveratrol are necessary to certify the real potential of resveratrol in BW control and the effects of long-term supplementation. Nonetheless, it will take years to determine the efficacy of resveratrol for improving health and lowering the incidence of obesity and other age-associated diseases in the elderly population.

2.6.5.1.4 Quercetin

Quercetin is a major flavonol abundantly found in plant products, such as capers, lovage, apples, onions and grapes, and presents anti-adipogenic properties. Indeed, quercetin induces apoptosis of cultured 3T3-L1 pre-adipocytes, inhibiting Bcl-2 and activated caspase-3, Bax and Bcl-2 homologous antagonist/killer (Bak) proteins (Hsu & Yen, 2006), decreases the expression of C/EBPα, PPARγ and SREBP-1, thereby suppressing the differentiation of preadipocytes to adipocytes, and attenuates adipogenesis through the upregulation of the AMPK pathway (Ahn *et al.*, 2008).

It has been reported that mice fed 1.2% quercetin-supplemented high-fat diet for 8 weeks (lipids in diet increase the total bioavailability of quercetin, as demonstrated in an experimental model of pigs; Lesser *et al.*, 2004) showed transiently increased energy expenditure but persistently decreased circulating markers of inflammation. However, quercetin supplement did not affect the BW, nor the total adiposity as evaluated by nuclear magnetic resonance. Interestingly, a metabolic adaptation occurred relative to quercetin bioavailability in these animals, since a decrease in its circulating levels was observed between 3 and 8 weeks of treatment (Stewart *et al.*, 2008). The upregulated expression of caspase-3 found in quercetin-treated animals was shown to attenuate liver steatosis (Panchal *et al.*, 2012). In an additional study, it was demonstrated that supplementation of a high-fat Western diet with 0.025% quercetin for 9 weeks, or 0.05% for 20 weeks, decreased BW, visceral and hepatic fat deposition in mice, improved systemic parameters related to metabolic syndrom, and selectively regulated expression at the mRNA of genes involved in lipid metabolism in the liver in high-fat-treated animals (Jung *et al.*, 2013; Kobori *et al.*, 2011).

So far, some clinical trials have not demonstrated a clear anti-obesity effect of quercetin supplementation. In a double-blind, randomized, placebo-controlled study that enrolled 93 overweight subjects (25–65 years), who presented several polymorphisms of apolipoprotein E, quercetin-treated subjects received 150 mg/day, a dose that represents 15-fold the mean estimated daily intake, for 6 weeks (Egert *et al.*, 2010). All of the participants maintained their habitual diet and physical activity levels during the treatment. This study demonstrated that the apolipoprotein E genotype may be an important determinant of the responsiveness of serum lipids and blood pressure to daily quercetin treatment in human intervention studies, despite the absence of BW, waist circumference and body composition amelioration in treated individuals. In another study that used the same dose of quercetin but for 8 weeks, it was demonstrated that treatment moderately but significantly reduced BMI, BW and waist circumference in apolipoprotein E (APOE)3/3 but not in APOE4 subjects, reinforcing the importance of the genotype in the responsiveness to nutritional modulation (Pfeuffer *et al.*, 2013). The dose of quercetin employed in these studies does not modify resting energy expenditure, as evidenced in young normal-weight women (Egert *et al.*, 2011). A clinical trial in a heterogeneous group of 941 individuals, treated in a double-blind fashion with 500 or 1000 mg/day of quercetin for 12 weeks, was conducted by Knab *et al.* (2011), and failed to demonstrate differences in body mass or body composition between treated and placebo groups, either in normal-weight or in overweight and obese subjects.

2.6.5.1.5 Isoflavones

Emerging evidence suggests that supplementation or consumption of foods rich in isoflavones, such as daidzein, genistein and glycitein, found in soy and soy products, may have a beneficial effect on obesity in animals and humans. Similarly to other polyphenols whose effects have been described, soy isoflavones inhibit adipocyte differentiation by downregulation of PPARγ and C/EBPα genes (Harmon *et al.*, 2002; Shen *et al.*, 2006). In line with this, a dose-dependent inhibition of adipogenic differentiation of cultured human adipose tissue-derived pluripotent mesenchymal stem cells by daidzein and genistein was observed. However, different sets of mechanisms of the two isoflavones on adipogenesis are involved: while genistein exerts an anti-adipogenic effect through activation of WNT/β-catenin signaling, daidzein inhibits adipogenesis through stimulation of lipolysis (Kim *et al.*, 2010).

In rat experimental models, it was demonstrated that isoflavone-enriched chow treatment for 3 weeks decreased epididymal and retroperitoneal fat pad accretion in males (Manzoni *et al.*, 2005), and that supplementation of the soy minor isoflavone daidzein for 14 days, concomitantly with a high-fat diet, reduced weight gain and fat content of the liver. In addition, daidzein affected transcription factors and lipogenic enzymes, particularly stearoyl coenzyme A desaturase 1, and increased UCP1, an important enzyme for thermogenesis in brown adipose tissue (Crespillo *et al.*, 2011). In line with this, genistein treatment of high-fat-diet-treated mice reduced BW, fat accretion and hepatic lipid deposition (Yang *et al.*, 2006a; Lee *et al.*, 2006). However, it was also shown that genistein at low levels, equivalent to those present in Eastern and Western diets, presents an adipogenic effect in male mice, coupled to a significant increase in the epididymal and renal fat pads. This effect was not observed in males treated with pharmacological doses (200 mg/kg/day) of genistein or in females (Penza *et al.*, 2006). In ovariectomized mice, genistein further decreased fat accumulation, owing to reduction of food intake, and increased the apoptosis of mature adipocytes (Kim *et al.*, 2006). These results agree with findings obtained in high-fat-fed ovariectomized rats treated with isoflavone, which prevented obesity, in part by decreasing liver fatty acid synthase expression (Na *et al.*, 2008). These results are promising for the control of obesity in postmenopausal women. In fact, in a randomized prospective human cohort study in obese postmenopausal women, it was demonstrated that soy isoflavone extract treatment for 6 months significantly increased levels of blood adiponectin (Llaneza *et al.*, 2011), despite the absence of differences in BW and composition. However, in a recently conducted study in a cohort of 39 postmenopausal Caucasian and African American women, it was shown that ingestion of a soy protein plus isoflavone supplement significantly reduced subcutaneous and total abdominal fat in Caucasian, and total body fat in African, women (Christie *et al.*, 2010). Most of the clinical trials are conducted in postmenopausal women, considering the resemblance of isoflavones to endogenous estrogen. Isoflavones compete with 17β-estradiol for binding to the intranuclear estrogen receptors and exert estrogenic or antiestrogenic effects in the various tissues, and could be used as an alternative to hormone replacement therapy (reviewed in Bedell *et al.*, 2014). Moreover, evidence suggests that the benefits of isoflavones for blood lipids and obesity in humans increase when they are consumed in combination with soy protein (reviewed in Ørgaard & Jensen, 2008). In fact, some clinical studies showed that soy protein-based meals with high concentration of isoflavones not only decreased BW, fat mass and waist circumference, but also ameliorated the blood lipid profile (Allison *et al.*, 2003; Deibert *et al.*, 2004).

Other polyphenolic compounds, such as proanthocyanidines and anthocyanins, abundant in blueberries, have been shown to possess modulatory effects in adiposity and obesity. However, evidence in experimental models is scarce and this is far from being established, since effect of treatments with isolated polyphenols markedly differ from those induced by natural blueberry juice ingestion (Meydani & Hasan, 2010). So far, no clinical trial has been successfully conducted on proanthocyanidines and anthocyanin-based treatments.

2.6.6 Anti-obesity effects of minerals (magnesium)

Obesity is associated with an increased incidence of low magnesium intake and low serum magnesium levels. Low magnesium intakes and/or serum levels can be linked with other conditions that are also associated with obesity, such as glucose intolerance, metabolic syndrome, type 2 DM, inflammation, hypertension and atherosclerosis (some representing a chronic state; Champagne, 2008; Nielsen, 2010; Rosanoff *et al.*, 2012; Fuentes *et al.*, 2013; Kang, 2013; Kaur, 2014). Additionally, those metabolic and inflammatory pathological alterations also are associated with ageing (Barbagallo *et al.*, 2009) and a deficient magnesium status frequently occurs in elderly individuals (Gullestad *et al.*, 1994; Barbagallo *et al.*, 2009; Huang *et al.*, 2012; Rowe, 2012).

Magnesium deficiency was demonstrated to further impair the insulin signaling pathway in newly weaned male Wistar Hannover rats fed with a high-fat diet for 32 days, but, on the other hand, it did not modify values of body mass gain or adiposity index (Sales *et al.*, 2014). Nevertheless, maternal magnesium restriction in weanling Wistar/NIN rats increased the percentage of body fat and decreased LBM and fat-free mass as well as BW in 90- and 180-day- and 18-month-old offspring, pointing to the role of maternal magnesium status in short- and long-term variation of offspring adipose, muscle and bone mass (Venu *et al.*, 2005, 2008). Insulin secretion after a glucose challenge decreased in 180-day- and 18-month-old animals, indicating another irreversible effect of maternal magnesium restriction (Venu *et al.*, 2005, 2008). The increased percentage of body fat (and associated increase in central adiposity) observed in 18-month-old animals was most possibly due to increased fatty acid synthesis and transport (Venu *et al.*, 2008).

So far, no evidence exists demonstrating the influence of extracellular magnesium concentration on differentiation of 3T3-L1 pre-adipocytes exposed simultaneously to dexamethasone and insulin (Castiglioni *et al.*, 2013). On the other hand, the specific increase in intracellular free magnesium level induced by pioglitazone (as low as 300 nM) was observed in freshly isolated rat adipocytes, which could contribute to its beneficial effects on metabolism (Nadler & Scott, 1994).

Regarding human studies, Rodriguez-Morán and Guerrero-Romero (2004) reported that, in a group of 162 individuals, comprising a large range of BMI values (<25, ≥ 25 to <30

and ≥30 kg/m^2) and without inflammatory pathologies, diabetes or high blood pressure (mean age ~41 years), low serum magnesium levels were associated with high serum TNF-α levels in the obese-person subgroup. The study conducted by Evangelopoulos *et al.* (2008) agrees with these findings. It reported that serum magnesium levels were inversely correlated with serum high-sensitivity CRP values and the presence of metabolic syndrome in 117 overweight/obese adults (mean age ~66 years). Coherently, serum magnesium levels decreased with the increasing number of metabolic syndrome features (Evangelopoulos *et al.*, 2008). Interestingly, the importance of magnesium intake in human metabolic regulation seems to begin early in life, as shown by Celik *et al.* (2011), who demonstrated an association between low serum magnesium levels and insulin resistance development in 117 obese children and adolescents (vs 86 controls). Huerta *et al.* (2005) found that serum magnesium deficiency in 24 obese nondiabetic children and adolescents (aged 8–17 years; BMI ≥85th percentile for age and gender) vs 24 lean (BMI <85th percentile) controls (with correspondence for gender and puberty status) could result from low dietary mineral intake. Both dietary magnesium intake and fasting serum magnesium levels were negatively and positively correlated with fasting insulin and quantitative insulin sensitivity check index, respectively, pointing to a correlation with insulin resistance. Magnesium supplementation could be thus considered as a beneficial approach in the regulation of metabolic dysfunction and even in the control of obesity. In line with this, Cahill *et al.* (2013) hypothesized, after a large populational study (including 2295 healthy normal weight, overweight and obese individuals, mean age ~43 years), that overweight/obese persons are more likely to benefit from dietary magnesium intake. They found a negative relationship between insulin resistance markers (serum insulin, homeostatic model assessment-insulin resistance and homeostatic model assessment-β values) and dietary magnesium intake in the entire cohort. For homeostatic model assessment-insulin resistance, the association was more evident in overweight/obese persons (especially when corrected for percentage of body fat instead of BMI). In aged type 2 DM patients (age ≥65 years), a negative association between magnesium intake and central obesity, body fat percentage and BMI was also noted (Huang *et al.*, 2012).

Several mechanistic explanations have been given to account for the increased risk of metabolic and inflammatory impairment when a magnesium deficiency status occurs in an obesity environment (Busserolles *et al.*, 2003; Takaya *et al.*, 2004; Rayssiguier *et al.*, 2006; Nielsen, 2010; Pachikian *et al.*, 2010; Rosanoff *et al.*, 2012; Fuentes *et al.*, 2013; Fukuda & Ohno, 2014), highlighting the relevance of the results of Cahill *et al.* (2013), or in old ages (Barbagallo *et al.*, 2009). An interesting study conducted by Chacko *et al.* (2011) suggested that magnesium intervenes in the modulation of gene and protein profiles after demonstration that 4 weeks of magnesium supplementation in 14 healthy overweight/obese individuals (mean age ~44 years; BMI 26–32 kg/m^2) not only decreased fasting blood C-peptide and insulin concentrations but also altered gene expression in blood cells [with negative regulation of 36 genes (counting C1q and TNF-related protein 9 and pro-platelet basic protein, from metabolic and inflammatory pathways) and positive regulation of 24 genes (counting cation channels, with a prime role in magnesium homeostasis)] and urine proteomics (by varying numerous peptides and proteins levels). However, the full extension of the magnesium role in cell and organism metabolism remains to be elucidated.

Obesity is a complex problem, particularly in the elderly. Owing to the lack of clinical studies in this age group and the concomitant diseases that affect old people, the efficacy and safety of nutraceuticals or supplement use for weight loss have not been demonstrated in older adults. Thus, the strategies for weight loss should be carefully individualized, and the administration of nutritional supplements or nutraceuticals must be strictly monitorized for potential toxicity or undesirable effects.

2.7 Conclusion

The effect of ER on human lifespan remains an unsolved problem. However, more important than the increase in lifespan is the increase in healthspan, defined as the length of time prior to the onset of an age-associated disease, which currently constitutes an alternative measure of ageing. The prolonging of the healthy period for an individual may be of higher importance than the increase in the life expectancy. Concerning this aspect, all the evidence supports the hypothesis that implementation or mimicking the ER could significantly and positively affect the health and quality of life of elderly people. Nevertheless, additional studies are warranted to identify the precise ER-induced metabolic and molecular adaptations associated with healthy longevity, as well as the proper energy content, macronutrient and micronutrient composition of the diet, in order to fit the requirements of each individual based on age, sex, disease predisposition and genetic background.

Acknowledgment

The authors thank Sérgio Evangelista from Laboratório de Iconografia, Faculdade de Medicina da Universidade do Porto, for artwork for Figs 2.1, 2.3 and 2.4.

References

Adler, A. S., S. Sinha, T. L. Kawahara, J. Y. Zhang, E. Segal, and H. Y. Chang. 2007. Motif module map reveals enforcement of aging by continual NF-kappaB activity. *Genes Dev.* 21:3244–3257.

Aggarwal, B. B. and B. Sung. 2008. Pharmacological basis for the role of curcumin in chronic diseases: an age-old spice with modern targets. *Trends Pharmacol. Sci.* 30:85–94.

Ahn, J., H. Lee, S. Kim, and T. Ha. 2007. Resveratrol inhibits TNF-alpha-induced changes of adipokines in 3T3-L1 adipocytes. *Biochem. Biophys. Res. Commun.* 364:972–977.

Ahn, J., H. Lee, S. Kim, J. Park, and T. Ha. 2008. The anti-obesity effect of quercetin is mediated by the AMPK, and MAPK signaling pathways. *Biochem. Biophys. Res. Commun.* 373:545–549.

Ahn, J., H. Lee, S. Kim, and T. Ha. 2010. Curcumin-induced suppression of adipogenic differentiation is accompanied by activation of Wnt/beta-catenin signaling. *Am. J. Physiol. Cell. Physiol.* 298:C1510–C1516.

Ahuja, N., B. Schwer, S. Carobbio, D. Waltregny, B. J. North, V. Castronovo, P. Maechler, and E. Verdin. 2007. Regulation of insulin secretion by SIRT4, a mitochondrial ADP-ribosyltransferase. *J. Biol. Chem.* 282:33583–33592.

Akcakoyun, M., R. Kargin, A. C. Tanalp, S. Pala, O. Ozveren, M. Akcay, I. Barutcu, and C. Kirma. 2008. Predictive value of noninvasively determined endothelial dysfunction for long-term cardiovascular events and restenosis in patients undergoing coronary stent implantation: a prospective study. *Coron. Artery Dis.* 19:337–343.

Akerfeldt, M. C., J. Howes, J. Y. Chan, V. A. Stevens, N. Boubenna, H. M. McGuire, C. King, T. J. Biden, and D. R. Laybutt. 2008. Cytokine-induced beta-cell death is independent of endoplasmic reticulum stress signaling. *Diabetes* 57:3034–3044.

Alcendor, R. R., S. Gao, P. Zhai, D. Zablocki, E. Holle, X. Yu, B. Tian, T. Wagner, S. F. Vatner, and J. Sadoshima. 2007. Sirt1 regulates aging, and resistance to oxidative stress in the heart. *Circul. Res.* 100:1512–1521.

Allison, D. B., G. Gadbury, L. G. Schwartz, R. Murugesan, J. L. Kraker, S. Heshka, K. R Fontaine, and S. B. Heymsfield. 2003. A novel soy-based meal replacement formula for weight loss among obese individuals: a randomized controlled clinical trial. *Eur. J. Clin. Nutr.* 57:514–522.

Anderson, E. J., M. E. Lustig, K. E. Boyle, T. L. Woodlief, D. A. Kane, C. T. Lin, J. W. Price, 3rd, L. Kang, P. S. Rabinovitch, H. H. Szeto, J. A. Houmard, R. N. Cortright, D. H. Wasserman, and P. D. Neufer. 2009. Mitochondrial H2O2 emission, and cellular redox state link excess fat intake to insulin resistance in both rodents, and humans. *J. Clin. Invest.* 119:573–581.

Anson, R. M., B. Jones, and R. de Cabo. 2005. The diet restriction paradigm: a brief review of the effects of every-other-day feeding. *Age* 27:17–25.

Anton, S. and C. Leeuwenburgh. 2013. Fasting and caloric restriction? *Exp. Gerontol.* 48:1003–1005.

Arnlov, J., E. Ingelsson, J. Sundström, and L. Lind. 2010. Impact of body mass index and the metabolic syndrome on the risk of cardiovascular disease and death in middle-aged men. *Circulation* 121:230–236.

Asher, G., D. Gatfield, M. Stratmann, H. Reinke, C. Dibner, F. Kreppel, R Mostoslavsky, F. W. Alt, and U. Schibler. 2008. SIRT1 regulates circadian clock gene expression through PER2 deacetylation. *Cell* 134:317–328.

Auguet, T., Y. Quintero, D. Riesco, B. Morancho, X. Terra, A. Crescenti, M. Broch, C. Aguilar, M. Olona, J. A. Porras, M. Hernandez, F. Sabench, D. del Castillo, and C. Richart. 2011. New adipokines vaspin and omentin. Circulating levels and gene expression in adipose tissue from morbidly obese women. *BMC Med. Genet.* 12:60.

Azuma, K., F. Katsukawa, S. Oguchi, M. Murata, H. Yamazaki, A. Shimada, and T. Saruta. 2003. Correlation between serum resistin level and adiposity in obese individuals. *Obes. Res.* 11:997–1001.

Back, S. H. and R. J. Kaufman. 2012. Endoplasmic reticulum stress, and type 2 diabetes. *Annu. Rev. Biochem.* 81:767–793.

Barazzoni, R., M. Zanetti, G. Gortan Cappellari, A. Semolic, M. Boschelle, E. Codarin, A. Pirulli, L. Cattin, and G. Guarnieri. 2012. Fatty acids acutely enhance insulin-induced oxidative stress, and cause insulin resistance by increasing mitochondrial reactive oxygen species (ROS) generation, and nuclear factor-kappaB inhibitor (IkappaB)–nuclear factor-kappaB (NFkappaB) activation in rat muscle, in the absence of mitochondrial dysfunction. *Diabetologia* 55:773–782.

Barbagallo, M., M. Belvedere, and L. J. Dominguez. 2009. Magnesium homeostasis, and aging. *Magnes. Res.* 22:235–246.

Barger, J. L., T. Kayo, J. M. Vann, E. B. Arias, J. Wang, T. A. Hacker, Y. Wang, D. Raederstorff, J. D. Morrow, C. Leeuwenburgh, D. B. Allison, K. W. Saupe, G. D. Cartee, R. Weindruch, and T. A. Prolla. 2008. A low dose of dietary resveratrol partially mimics caloric restriction, and retards aging parameters in mice. *PLoS One* 3:e2264.

Bartke, A., V. Chandrashekar, B. Bailey, D. Zaczek, and D. Turyn. 2002. Consequences of growth hormone (GH) overexpression and GH resistance. *Neuropeptides* 36:201–208.

Bartke, A., M. Bonkowski, and M. Masternak. 2008. How diet interacts with longevity genes. *Hormones (Athens)* 7:17–23.

Barzilai, N., J. A. Cases, X. H. Ma, X. M. Yang, B. Q. Liu, and L. Rossetti. 2000. Decreased visceral fat entirely accounts for the effects of caloric restriction on insulin action in aging rats. *Diabetologia* 43:603.

Basseri, S. and R. C. Austin. 2012. Endoplasmic reticulum stress, and lipid metabolism: mechanisms, and therapeutic potential. *Biochem. Res. Int.* 2012:841362.

Basu, A., K. Sanchez, M. J. Leyva, M. Wu, N. M. Betts, C. E. Aston, and T. J. Lyons. 2010. Green tea supplementation affects body weight, lipids, and lipid peroxidation in obese subjects with metabolic syndrome. *J. Am. Coll. Nutr.* 29:31–40.

Baur, J. A. 2010. Biochemical effects of SIRT1 activators. *Biochim. Biophys. Acta* 1804:1626–1634.

Baur, J. A., K. J. Pearson, N. L. Price, H. A. Jamieson, C. Lerin, A. Kalra, V. V. Prabhu, J. S. Allard, G. Lopez-Lluch, K. Lewis, P. J. Pistell, S. Poosala, K. G. Becker, O. Boss, D. Gwinn, M. Wang, S. Ramaswamy, K. W. Fishbein, R. G. Spencer, E. G. Lakatta, D. Le Couteur, R. J. Shaw, P. Navas, P. Puigserver, D. K. Ingram, R. de Cabo, and D. A. Sinclair. 2006. Resveratrol improves health, and survival of mice on a high-calorie diet. *Nature* 444:337–342.

Bazzocchi, A., D. Diano, F. Ponti, A. Andreone, C. Sassi, U. Albisinni, G. Marchesini, and G. Battista. 2013. Health and ageing: a cross-sectional study of body composition. *Clin. Nutr.* 32:569–578.

Bedell, S., M. Nachtigall, and F. Naftolin. 2014. The pros, and cons of plant estrogens for menopause. *J. Steroid Biochem. Mol. Biol.* 139:225–236.

Behl, C. 2011. BAG3, and friends. Co-chaperones in selective autophagy during aging, and disease. *Autophagy* 7:795–798.

Bell, E. L. and L. Guarente. 2011. The sirt3 divining rod points to oxidative stress. *Mol. Cell* 42:561–568.

Bell, L. N., J. L. Ward, M. Degawa-Yamauchi, J. E. Bovenkerk, R. Jones, B. M. Cacucci, C. E. Gupta, C. Sheridan, K. Sheridan, S. S. Shankar, H. O. Steinberg, K. L. March, and R. V. Considine. 2006. Adipose tissue production of hepatocyte growth factor contributes to elevated serum HGF in obesity. *Am. J. Physiol. Endocrinol. Metab.* 291:E843–E848.

Bellizzi, D., G. Rose, P. Cavalcante, G. Covello, S. Dato, F. De Rango, V. Greco, M. Maggiolini, E. Feraco, V. Mari, C. Franceschi, G. Passarino, and G. De Benedictis. 2005. A novel VNTR enhancer within the SIRT3 gene, a human homologue of SIR2, is associated with survival at oldest ages. *Genomics* 85:258–263.

Bergamini, E., A. Del Roso, V. Fierabracci, Z. Gori, P. Masiello, M. Masini, and M. Pollera. 1993. A new method for the investigation of endocrine-regulated autophagy, and protein degradation in rat liver. *Exp. Mol. Pathol.* 59:13–26.

Bergamini E., G. Cavallini, A. Donati, and Z. Gori. 2003. The anti-ageing effects of caloric restriction may involve stimulation of macroautophagy, and lysosomal degradation, and can be intensified pharmacologically. *Biomed. Pharmacother.* 57:203–208.

Berger, Z., B. Ravikumar, F. M. Menzies, L. G. Oroz, B. R. Underwood, M. N. Pangalos, I. Schmitt, U. Wullner, B. O. Evert, C. J. O'Kane, and D. C. Rubinsztein. 2006. Rapamycin alleviates toxicity of different aggregate-prone proteins. *Hum. Mol. Genet.* 15:433–442.

Berner, Y. N. and F. Stern. 2004. Energy restriction controls aging through neuroendocrine signal transduction. *Ageing Res. Rev.* 3:189–198.

Berndt, J., N. Klöting, S. Kralisch, P. Kovacs, M. Fasshauer, M. R. Schön, M. Stumvoll, and M. Blüher. 2005. Plasma visfatin concentrations and fat depot-specific mRNA expression in humans. *Diabetes* 54:2911–2916.

Berryman, D. E., E. O. List, K. T. Coschigano, K. Behar, J. K. Kim, and J. J. Kopchick. 2004. Comparing adiposity profiles in three mouse models with altered GH signaling. *Growth Horm. IGF Res.* 14:309–318.

Bérubé-Parent, S., C. Pelletier, J. Doré, and A. Tremblay. 2005. Effects of encapsulated green tea, and Guarana extracts containing a mixture of epigallocatechin-3-gallate, and caffeine on 24 h energy expenditure, and fat oxidation in men. *Br. J. Nutr.* 94:432–436.

Blanc, S., D. Schoeller, J. Kemnitz, R. Weindruch, R. Colman, W. Newton, K. Wink, S. Baum, and J. Ramsey. 2003. Energy expenditure of rhesus monkeys subjected to 11 years of dietary restriction. *J. Clin. Endocrinol. Metab.* 88:16–23.

Bluher M. 2012. Vaspin in obesity and diabetes: pathophysiological and clinical significance. *Endocrine* 41:176–182.

Bo, S., G. Ciccone, I. Baldi, R. Gambino, C. Mandrile, M. Durazzo, L. Gentile, M. Cassader, P. Cavallo-Perin, and G. Pagano. 2009. Plasma visfatin concentrations after a lifestyle intervention were directly associated with inflammatory markers. *Nutr. Metab. Cardiovasc. Dis.* 19:423–430.

Bogacka, I., T. W. Gettys, L. de Jonge, T. Nguyen, J. M. Smith, H. Xie, F. Greenway, and S. R. Smith. 2007. The effect of beta-adrenergic, and peroxisome proliferator-activated receptor-gamma stimulation on target genes related to lipid metabolism in human subcutaneous adipose tissue. *Diabetes Care* 30:1179–1186.

Bokarewa, M., I. Nagaev, L. Dahlberg, U. Smith, and A. Tarkowski. 2005. Resistin, an adipokine with potent proinflammatory properties. *J. Immunol.* 174:5789–5795.

Bondue, B., V. Wittamer, and M. Parmentier. 2011. Chemerin and its receptors in leukocyte trafficking, inflammation and metabolism. *Cytokine Growth Factor Rev.* 22:331–338.

Bordone, L., M. C. Motta, F. Picard, A. Robinson, U. S. Jhala, J. Apfeld, T. McDonagh, M. Lemieux, M. McBurney, A. Szilvasi, E. J. Easlon, S. J. Lin, and L. Guarente. 2006. Sirt1 regulates insulin secretion by repressing UCP2 in pancreatic beta cells. *PLoS Biol.* 4:e31.

Bose, M., J. D. Lambert, J. Ju, K. R, Reuhl, S. A. Shapses, and C. S. Yang. 2008. The major green tea polyphenol, (−)-epigallocatechin-3-gallate, inhibits obesity, metabolic syndrome, and fatty liver disease in high-fat-fed mice. *J. Nutr.* 138. 1677–1683.

Botella-Carretero, J. I., M. Luque-Ramirez, F. Alvarez-Blasco, R. Peromingo, J. L. San Millan, and H. F. Escobar-Morreale. 2008. The increase in serum visfatin after bariatric surgery in morbidly obese women is modulated by weight loss, waist circumference, and presence or absence of diabetes before surgery. *Obes. Surg.* 18:1000–1006.

Boucher, J., B. Masri, D. Daviaud, S. Gesta, C. Guigné, A. Mazzucotelli, I. Castan-Laurell, I. Tack, B. Knibiehler, C. Carpéné, Y. Audigier, J. S. Saulnier-Blache, and P. Valet. 2005. Apelin, a newly identified adipokine up-regulated by insulin and obesity. *Endocrinology* 146:1764–1771.

Boura-Halfon, S. and Y. Zick. 2009. Phosphorylation of IRS proteins, insulin action, and insulin resistance. *Am. J. Physiol. Endocrinol. Metab.* 296:E581–591.

Bradford, P. G. 2013. Curcumin, and obesity. *Biofactors* 39:78–87.

Braidy, N., G. J. Guillemin, H. Mansour, T. Chan-Ling, A. Poljak, and R. Grant. 2011. Age related changes in NAD^+ metabolism oxidative stress, and Sirt1 activity in wistar rats. *PLoS One* 6:e19194.

Brown, M. K. and N. Naidoo. 2012. The endoplasmic reticulum stress response in aging, and age-related diseases. *Front Physiol* 3:263.

Brunet, A., L. B. Sweeney, J. F. Sturgill, K. F. Chua, P. L. Greer, Y. Lin, H. Tran, S. E. Ross, R. Mostoslavsky, H. Y. Cohen, L. S. Hu, H. L. Cheng, M. P. Jedrychowski, S. P. Gygi, D. A. Sinclair, F. W. Alt, and M. E. Greenberg. 2004. Stress-dependent regulation of FOXO transcription factors by the SIRT1 deacetylase. *Science* 303:2011–2015.

Brunetti, L., C. Di Nisio, L. Recinella, A. Chiavaroli, S. Leone, C. Ferrante, G. Orlando, and M. Vacca. 2011. Effects of vaspin, chemerin and omentin-1 on feeding behavior and hypothalamic peptide gene expression in the rat. *Peptides* 32:1866–1871.

Bueno, A. A., L. M. Oyama, C. de Oliveira, L. P. Pisani, E. B. Ribeiro, V. L. Silveira, and C. M. Oller do Nascimento. 2008. Effects of different fatty acids and dietary lipids on adiponectin gene expression in 3T3-L1 cells and C57BL/6J mice adipose tissue. *Pflugers Arch.* 455:701–709.

Busserolles, J., E. Gueux, E. Rock, A. Mazur, and Y. Rayssiguier. 2003. High fructose feeding of magnesium deficient rats is associated with increased plasma triglyceride concentration, and increased oxidative stress. *Magnes. Res.* 16:7–12.

Busso, N., M. Karababa, M. Nobile, A. Rolaz, F. Van Gool, M. Galli, O. Leo, A. So, and T. De Smedt. 2008. Pharmacological inhibition of nicotinamide phosphoribosyltransferase/visfatin enzymatic activity identifies a new inflammatory pathway linked to NAD. *PLoS One* 3:2267.

Cabelof, D. C., S. Yanamadala, J. J. Raffoul, Z. Guo, A. Soofi, and AR. Heydari. 2003. Caloric restriction promotes genomic stability by induction of base excision repair, and reversal of its age-related decline. *DNA Repair* 2:295–307.

Cahill, F., M. Shahidi, J. Shea, D. Wadden, W. Gulliver, E. Randell, S. Vasdev, and G. Sun. 2013. High dietary magnesium intake is associated with low insulin resistance in the Newfoundland population. *PLoS One* 8:e58278.

Cancello, R., C. Henegar, N. Viguerie, S. Taleb, C. Poitou, C. Rouault, M. Coupaye, V. Pelloux, D. Hugol, J. L. Bouillot, A. Bouloumie, G. Barbatelli, S. Cinti, P. A. Svensson, G. S. Barsh, J. D. Zucker, A. Basdevant, D. Langin, and K. Clement. 2005. Reduction of macrophage infiltration and chemoattractant gene expression changes in white adipose tissue of morbidly obese subjects after surgery induced weight loss. *Diabetes* 54:2277–2286.

Cangemi, R., A. J. Friedmann, J. O. Holloszy, and L. Fontana. 2010. Long-term effects of calorie restriction on serum sex-hormone concentrations in men. *Aging Cell* 9:236–242.

Cantó, C. and J. Auwerx. 2010. AMP-activated protein kinase, and its downstream transcriptional pathways. *Cell. Mol. Life Sci.* 67:3407–3423.

Cantó, C. and J. Auwerx. 2011. Calorie restriction: Is AMPK a key sensor, and effector? *Physiology* 26:214–224.

Cantó, C., Z. Gerhart-Hines, J. N. Feige, M. Lagouge, L. Noriega, J. C. Milne, P. J. Elliott, P. Puigserver, and J. Auwerx. 2009. AMPK regulates energy expenditure by modulating NAD^+ metabolism, and SIRT1 activity. *Nature* 458:1056–1060.

Cao, Y. 2007. Angiogenesis modulates adipogenesis and obesity. *J. Clin. Invest.* 117:2362–2368.

Cao, Y. 2010. Adipose tissue angiogenesis as a therapeutic target for obesity and metabolic diseases. *Nat. Rev. Drug Discov.* 9:107–115.

Cardozo, A. K., F. Ortis, J. Storling, Y. M. Feng, J. Rasschaert, M. Tonnesen, F. Van Eylen, T. Mandrup-Poulsen, A. Herchuelz, and D. L. Eizirik. 2005. Cytokines downregulate the sarcoendoplasmic reticulum pump Ca^{2+} ATPase 2b, and deplete endoplasmic reticulum Ca^{2+}, leading to induction of endoplasmic reticulum stress in pancreatic beta-cells. *Diabetes* 54:452–461.

Cardozo, L. F., L. M. Pedruzzi, P. Stenvinkel, M. B. Stockler-Pinto, J. B. Daleprane, M. Leite, Jr. and D. Mafra. 2013. Nutritional strategies to modulate inflammation and oxidative stress pathways via activation of the master antioxidant switch Nrf2. *Biochimie* 95:1525–1533.

Caro, P., J. Gómez, M. López-Torres, I. Sánchez, A. Naudí, M. Jove, R. Pamplona, and G. Barja. 2008. Forty percent, and eighty percent methionine restriction decrease mitochondrial ROS generation, and oxidative stress in rat liver. *Biogerontology* 9:183–196.

Carrillo, A. E. and A. D. Flouris. 2011. Caloric restriction and longevity: effects of reduced body temperature. *Ageing Res. Rev.* 10:153–162.

Carter, B. E. and A. Drewnowski. 2012. Beverages containing soluble fiber, caffeine, and green tea catechins suppress hunger, and lead to less energy consumption at the next meal. *Appetite* 59:755–761.

Cartwright, M. J., T. Tchkonia, and J. L. Kirkland. 2007. Aging in adipocytes: potential impact of inherent, depot-specific mechanisms. *Exp. Gerontol.* 42:463–471.

Castiglioni, S., M. Leidi, E. Carpanese, and J. A. Maier. 2013. Extracellular magnesium, and in vitro cell differentiation: different behaviour of different cells. *Magnes. Res.* 26:24–31.

Cavallini, G., A. Donati, Z. Gori, M. Pollera, and E. Bergamini. 2001. The protection of rat liver autophagic proteolysis from the age-related decline co-varies with the duration of anti-ageing food restriction. *Exp. Gerontol.* 36:497–506.

Cavuoto, P. and M. F. Fenech. 2012. A review of methionine dependency, and the role of methionine restriction in cancer growth control, and life-span extension. *Cancer Treat. Rev.* 38:726–736.

Celik, N., N. andiran, and A. E. Yilmaz. 2011. The relationship between serum magnesium levels with childhood obesity, and insulin resistance: a review of the literature. *J. Pediatr. Endocrinol. Metab.* 24:675–678.

Cesari, M., M. Pahor, F. Lauretani, V. Zamboni, S. Bandinelli, R. Bernabei, J. M. Guralnik, and L. Ferrucci. 2009. Skeletal muscle and mortality results from the InCHIANTI Study. *J. Gerontol.* 64:377–384.

Chacko, S. A., J. Sul, Y. Song, X. Li, J. LeBlanc, Y. You, A. Butch, and S. Liu. 2011. Magnesium supplementation, metabolic, and inflammatory markers, and global genomic, and proteomic profiling: a randomized, double-blind, controlled, crossover trial in overweight individuals. *Am. J. Clin. Nutr.* 93:463–473.

Chakaroun, R., M. Raschpichler, N. Kloting, A. Oberbach, G. Flehmig, M. Kern, M. R. Schön, E. Shang, T. Lohmann, M. Dreßler, M. Fasshauer, M. Stumvoll, and M. Blüher. 2012. Effects of weight loss and exercise on chemerin serum concentration and adipose tissue expression in human obesity. *Metabolism* 61:706–714.

Chakraborty, A., S. Chowdhury, and M. Bhattacharyya. 2011. Effect of metformin on oxidative stress, nitrosative stress, and inflammatory biomarkers in type 2 diabetes patients. *Diabetes Res. Clin. Pract.* 93:56–62.

Champagne, C. M. 2008. Magnesium in hypertension, cardiovascular disease, metabolic syndrome, and other conditions: a review. *Nutr. Clin. Pract.* 23:142–151.

Chan, C. Y., L. Wei, F. Castro-Muñozledo, and W. L. Koo. 2011. (−)-Epigallocatechin-3-gallate blocks 3T3-L1 adipose conversion by inhibition of cell proliferation, and suppression of adipose phenotype expression. *Life Sci.* 89:779–785.

Chang, H. M., H. J. Lee, H. S. Park, J. H. Kang, K. S. Kim, Y. S. Song, and Y. J. Jang. 2010. Effects of weight reduction on serum vaspin concentrations in obese subjects: modifications by insulin resistance. *Obesity* 18:2105–2110.

Chen, D., J. Bruno, E. Easlon, S. J. Lin, H. L. Cheng, F. W. Alt, and L. Guarente. 2008a. Tissue-specific regulation of SIRT1 by calorie restriction. *Genes Dev.* 22:1753–1757.

Chen, D., A. D. Steele, G. Hutter, J. Bruno, A. Govindarajan, E. Easlon, S. J. Lin, A. Aguzzi, S. Lindquist, and L. Guarente. 2008b. The role of calorie restriction, and SIRT1 in prion-mediated neurodegeneration. *Exp. Gerontol.* 43:1086–1093.

Chen, N., R. Bezzina, E. Hinch, P. A. Lewandowski, D. Cameron-Smith, M. L. Mathai, M. Jois, A. J. Sinclair, D. P. Begg, J. D. Wark, H. S. Weisinger, and R. S. Weisinger. 2009. Green tea, black tea, and epigallocatechin modify body composition, improve glucose tolerance, and differentially alter metabolic gene expression in rats fed a high-fat diet. *Nutr. Res.* 29:784–793.

Chen, S., X. Xiao, X. Feng, W. Li, N. Zhou, L. Zheng, Y. Sun, Z. Zhang, and W. Zhu. 2012. Resveratrol induces Sirt1-dependent apoptosis in 3T3-L1 preadipocytes by activating AMPK, and suppressing AKT activity, and survivin expression. *J. Nutr. Biochem.* 23:1100–1112.

Chen, K., S. Kobayashi, X. Xu, B. Viollet, and Q. Liang. 2013. AMP activated protein kinase is indispensable for myocardial adaptation to caloric restriction in mice. *PLoS One* 8:e59682.

Cheney, K. E., R. K. Liu, G. S. Smith, P. J. Meredith, M. R. Mickey, and R. L. Walford. 1983. The effect of dietary restriction of varying duration on survival, tumor patterns, immune function, and body-temperature in B10C3F1 female mice. *J. Gerontol.* 38:420–430.

Cho, S. J., U. J. Jung, and M. S. Choi. 2012. Differential effects of low-dose resveratrol on adiposity, and hepatic steatosis in diet-induced obese mice. *Br. J. Nutr.* 108:2166–2175.

Chowdhry, S., M. H. Nazmy, P. J. Meakin, A. T. Dinkova-Kostova, S. V. Walsh, T. Tsujita, J. F. Dillon, M. L. Ashford and J. D. Hayes. 2010. Loss of Nrf2 markedly exacerbates nonalcoholic steatohepatitis. *Free Radic. Biol. Med.* 48:357–371.

Christie, D. R., J. Grant, B. E. Darnell, V. R. Chapman, A. Gastaldelli, and C. K. Sites. 2010. Metabolic effects of soy supplementation in postmenopausal Caucasian, and African American women: a randomized, placebo-controlled trial. *Am. J. Obstet. Gynecol.* 203:153. e1–9.

Chung, K. W., D. H. Kim, M. H. Park, Y. J. Choi, N. D. Kim, J. Lee, B. P. Yu, and H. Y. Chung. 2013. Recent advances in calorie restriction research on aging. *Exp. Gerontol.* 48:1049–1053.

Civitarese, A. E., S. Carling, L. K. Heilbronn, M. H. Hulver, B. Ukropcova, W. A. Deutsch, S. R. Smith, E. Ravussin, and CALERIE Pennington Team. 2007. Calorie restriction increases muscle mitochondrial biogenesis in healthy humans. *PLoS Med.* 4:e76.

Cnop, M., F. Foufelle, and L. A. Velloso. 2012. Endoplasmic reticulum stress, obesity, and diabetes. *Trends Mol. Med.* 18:59–68.

Cohen, H. Y., C. Miller, K. J. Bitterman, N. R. Wall, B. Hekking, B. Kessler, K. T. Howitz, M. Gorospe, R. de Cabo, and D. A. Sinclair. 2004. Calorie restriction promotes mammalian cell survival by inducing the SIRT1 deacetylase. *Science* 305:390–392.

Coletta, D. K., A. Sriwijitkamol, E. Wajcberg, P. Tantiwong, M. Li, M. Prentki, M. Madiraju, C. P. Jenkinson, E. Cersosimo, N. Musi, and R. A. Defronzo. 2009. Pioglitazone stimulates AMP-activated protein kinase signalling, and increases the expression of genes involved in adiponectin signalling, mitochondrial function, and fat oxidation in human skeletal muscle in vivo: a randomised trial. *Diabetologia* 52:723–732.

Collison, K. S., S. M. Saleh, R. H. Bakheet, R. K. Al-Rabiah, A. L. Inglis, N. J. Makhoul, Z. M. Maqbool, M. Z. Zaidi, M. A. Al-Johi, and F. A. Al-Mohanna. 2009. Diabetes of the liver: the link between nonalcoholic fatty liver disease, and HFCS-55. *Obesity (Silver Spring)* 17:2003–2013.

Colman, R. J. and R. M. Anderson. 2011. Nonhuman primate calorie restriction. *Antioxid. Redox Signal.* 14:229–239.

Colman, R. J., R. M. Anderson, S. C. Johnson, E. K. Kastman, K. J. Kosmatka, T. M. Beasley, D. B. Allison, C. Cruzen, H. A. Simmons, J. W. Kemnitz, and R. Weindruch. 2009. Caloric restriction delays disease onset, and mortality in rhesus monkeys. *Science* 325:201–204.

Colman, R. J., T. M. Beasley, D. B. Allison, and R. Weindruch. 2012. Skeletal effects of long-term caloric restriction in rhesus monkeys. *Age (Dordr).* 34:1133–1143.

Considine, R. V., M. K. Sinha, M. L. Heiman, A. Kriauciunas, T. W. Stephens, M. R. Nyce, J. P. Ohannesian, C. C. Marco, L. J. McKee, T. L. Bauer, and J. F. Caro. 1996. Serum immunoreactive-leptin concentrations in normal-weight and obese humans. *New Engl. J. Med.* 334:292–295.

Conti, B., M. Sanchez-Alavez, R. Winsky-Sommerer, M. C. Morale, J. Lucero, S. Brownell, V. Fabre, S. Huitron-Resendiz, S. Henriksen, E. P. Zorrilla, L. de Lecea, and T. Bartfai. 2006. Transgenic mice with a reduced core body temperature have an increased life span. *Science* 314:825–828.

Craig, B. W., S. M. Garthwaite, and J. O. Holloszy. 1987. Adipocyte insulin resistance: effects of aging, obesity, exercise, and food restriction. *J. Appl. Physiol.* 62:95–100.

Crespillo, A., M. Alonso, M. Vida, F. J. Pavón, A. Serrano, P. Rivera, Y. Romero-Zerbo, P. Fernández-Llebrez, A. Martínez, V. Pérez-Valero, F. J. Bermúdez-Silva, J. Suárez, and F. R. de Fonseca. 2011. Reduction of body weight, liver steatosis, and expression of stearoyl-CoA desaturase 1 by the isoflavone daidzein in diet-induced obesity. *Br. J. Pharm.* 164:1899–1915.

Csiszar, A., N. Labinskyy, R. Jimenez, J. T. Pinto, P. Ballabh, G. Losonczy, K. J. Pearson, R. de Cabo, and Z. Ungvari. 2009. Anti-oxidative and anti-inflammatory vasoprotective effects of caloric restriction in aging: role of circulating factors and SIRT1. *Mech. Ageing Dev.* 130:518–527.

Csiszár, A., A. Csiszar, J. T. Pinto, T. Gautam, C. Kleusch, B. Hoffmann, Z. Tucsek, P. Toth, W. E. Sonntag, and Z. Ungvari. 2014. *Resveratrol encapsulated in novel fusogenic liposomes activates Nrf2 and attenuates oxidative stress in cerebromicrovascular endothelial cells from aged rats. J. Gerontol. A. Biol. Sci. Med. Sci.*, in press.

Cuervo, A. M. and J. F. Dice. 2000. Age-related decline in chaperone-mediated autophagy. *J. Biol. Chem.* 275:31505–31513.

Cuervo, A. M, E. Bergamini, U. T. Brunk, W. Dröge, M. Ffrench, and A. Terman. 2005. Autophagy, and aging. The importance of maintaining "clean" cells. *Autophagy* 1:131–140.

Cullberg, K. B., J. Olholm, S. K. Paulsen, C. B. Foldager, M. Lind, B. Richelsen, and S. B. Pedersen. 2013. Resveratrol has inhibitory effects on the hypoxia-induced inflammation, and angiogenesis in human adipose tissue in vitro. *Eur. J. Pharm. Sci.* 49:251–257.

Cullinan, S. B. and J. A. Diehl. 2004. PERK-dependent activation of Nrf2 contributes to redox homeostasis, and cell survival following endoplasmic reticulum stress. *J. Biol. Chem.* 279:20108–20117.

Cullinan, S. B. and J. A. Diehl. 2006. Coordination of ER, and oxidative stress signaling: the PERK/Nrf2 signaling pathway. *Int. J. Biochem. Cell Biol.* 38:317–332.

Cullinan, S. B., D. Zhang, M. Hannink, E. Arvisais, R. J. Kaufman, and J. A. Diehl. 2003. Nrf2 is a direct PERK substrate, and effector of PERK-dependent cell survival. *Mol. Cell. Biol.* 23:7198–7209.

Dabhade, P. and S. Kotwal. 2013. Tackling the aging process with bio-molecules: a possible role for caloric restriction, food-derived nutrients, vitamins, amino acids, peptides, and minerals. *J. Nutr. Gerontol. Geriatr.* 32:24–40.

Dahl, T. B., A. Yndestad, M. Skjelland, E. Oie, A. Dahl, A. Michelsen, J. K. Damas, S. H. Tunheim, T. Ueland, C. Smith, B. Bendz, S. Tonstad, L. Gullestad, S. S. Frøland, K. Krohg-Sørensen, D. Russell, P. Aukrust, and B. Halvorsen. 2007. Increased expression of visfatin in macrophages of human unstable carotid and coronary atherosclerosis: possible role in inflammation and plaque destabilization. *Circulation* 115:972–980.

Dal-Pan, A., S. Blanc, and F. Aujard. 2010. Resveratrol suppresses body mass gain in a seasonal non-human primate model of obesity. *BMC Physiol.* 10:11.

Dal-Pan, A., J. Terrien, F. Pifferi, R. Botalla, I. Hardy, J. Marchal, A. Zahariev, I. Chery, P. Zizzari, M. Perret, J. L. Picq, J. Epelbaum, S. Blanc, and F. Aujard. 2011a. Caloric restriction or resveratrol supplementation, and ageing in a non-human primate: first-year outcome of the RESTRIKAL study in Microcebus murinus. *Age* 33:15–31.

Dal-Pan, A., F. Pifferi, J. Marchal, J. L. Picq, F. Aujard, and RESTRIKAL Consortium. 2011b. Cognitive performances are selectively enhanced during chronic caloric restriction or resveratrol supplementation in a primate. *PLoS One* 6:e16581.

Damiano, F., S. Alemanno, G. V. Gnoni, and L. Siculella. 2010. Translational control of the sterol-regulatory transcription factor SREBP-1 mRNA in response to serum starvation or ER stress is mediated by an internal ribosome entry site. *Biochem. J.* 429:603–612.

Dandona, P., P. Mohanty, H. Ghanim, A. Aljada, R. Browne, W. Hamouda, A. Prabhala, A. Afzal, and R. Garg. 2001. The suppressive effect of dietary restriction and weight loss in the obese on the generation of reactive oxygen species by leukocytes, lipid peroxidation, and protein carbonylation. *J. Clin. Endocrinol. Metab.* 86:355–362.

Das, S. K., C. H. Gilhooly, J. K. Golden, A. G. Pittas, P. J. Fuss, R. A. Cheatham, S. Tyler, M. Tsay, M. A. McCrory, A. H. Lichtenstein, G. E. Dallal, C. Dutta, M. V. Bhapkar, J. P. Delany, E. Saltzman, and S. B. Roberts. 2007. Long-term effects of 2 energy-restricted diets differing in glycemic load on dietary adherence, body composition, and metabolism in CALERIE: a 1-y randomized controlled trial. *Am. J. Clin. Nutr.* 85:1023–1030.

Decuypere, J. P., G. Monaco, L. Missiaen, H. De Smedt, J. B. Parys, and G. Bultynck. 2011. IP(3) Receptors, Mitochondria, and Ca signaling: implications for aging. *J. Aging Res.* 920178.

de Ferranti, S. and D. Mozaffarian. 2008. The perfect storm: obesity, adipocyte dysfunction, and metabolic consequences. *Clin. Chem.* 54:945–955.

Deibert, P., D. König, A. Schmidt-Trucksaess, K. S. Zaenker, I. Frey, U. Landmann, and A. Berg. 2004. Weight loss without losing muscle mass in pre-obese, and obese subjects induced by a high-soy-protein diet. *Int. J. Obes. Relat. Metab. Disord.* 28:1349–1352.

de la Garza, A.L., F. I. Milagro, N. Boque, J. Campión, and J. A. Martínez. 2011. Natural inhibitors of pancreatic lipase as new players in obesity treatment. *Planta Med.* 77:773–785.

Del Roso, A., S. Vittorini, G. Cavallini, A. Donati, Z. Gori, M. Masini, M. Pollera, and E. Bergamini. 2003. Ageing-related changes in the in vivo function of rat liver macroautophagy, and proteolysis. *Exp. Gerontol.* 38:519–527.

de Luis, D. A., M. Gonzalez Sagrado, R. Conde, R. Aller, O. Izaola, and E. Romero. 2008. Effect of a hypocaloric diet on serum visfatin in obese non-diabetic patients. *Nutrition* 24:517–521.

Deng, J., P. D. Lu, Y. Zhang, D. Scheuner, R. J. Kaufman, N. Sonenberg, H. P. Harding, and D. Ron. 2004. Translational repression mediates activation of nuclear factor kappa B by phosphorylated translation initiation factor 2. *Mol. Cell. Biol.* 24:10161–10168.

De Souza Batista, C. M., R. Z. Yang, M. J. Lee, N. M. Glynn, D. Z. Yu, J. Pray, K. Ndubuizu, S. Patil, A. Schwartz, M. Kligman, S. K. Fried, D. W. Gong, A. R. Shuldiner, T. I. Pollin, and J. C. McLenithan. 2007. Omentin plasma levels and gene expression are decreased in obesity. *Diabetes* 56:1655–1661.

Després, J. P., I. Lemieux, and D. Prud'homme. 2001. Treatment of obesity: need to focus on high risk abdominally obese patients. *BMJ* 322:716–720.

Dhahbi, J. M., H. J. Kim, P. L. Mote, R. J. Beaver, and S. R. Spindler. 2004. Temporal linkage between the phenotypic, and genomic responses to caloric restriction. *Proc. Natl Acad. Sci. USA* 101:5524–5529.

Dhahbi, J. M., T. Tsuchiya, H. J. Kim, P. L. Mote, and S. R. Spindler. 2006. Gene expression and physiologic responses of the heart to the initiation and withdrawal of caloric restriction. *J. Gerontol. A. Biol. Sci. Med. Sci.* 61:218–231.

Dixit, V. D. 2008. Adipose-immune interactions during obesity and caloric restriction: reciprocal mechanisms regulating immunity and health span. *J. Leukoc. Biol.* 84:882–892.

Dobbin, M. M., R. Madabhushi, L. Pan, Y. Chen, D. Kim, J. Gao, B. Ahanonu, P. C. Pao, Y. Qiu, Y. Zhao, and L. H. Tsai. 2013. SIRT1 collaborates with ATM, and HDAC1 to maintain genomic stability in neurons. *Nat. Neurosci.* 16:1008–1015.

Donati, A. 2006. The involvement of macroautophagy in aging, and anti-aging interventions. *Mol. Aspects Med.* 27:455–470.

Donati, A., G. Cavallini, C. Paradiso, S. Vittorini, M. Pollera, Z. Gori, and E. Bergamini. 2001. Age-related changes in the autophagic proteolysis of rat isolated liver cells: effects of antiaging dietary restrictions. *J. Gerontol. A. Biol. Sci. Med. Sci.* 56:B375–B383.

Donati, A., G. Cavallini, C. Carresi, Z. Gori, I. Parentini, and E. Bergamini. 2004. Anti-aging effects of anti-lipolytic drugs. *Exp. Gerontol.* 39:1061–1067.

Donato, A. J., A. E. Walker, K. A. Magerko, R. C. Bramwell, A. D. Black, G. D. Henson, B. R. Lawson, L. A. Lesniewski, and D. R. Seals. 2013. Life-long caloric restriction reduces oxidative stress, and preserves nitric oxide bioavailability, and function in arteries of old mice. *Aging Cell* 12:772–783.

Donmez, G. and T. F. Outeiro. 2013. SIRT1, and SIRT2: emerging targets in neurodegeneration. *EMBO Mol. Med.* 5:344–352.

Donmez, G., A. Arun, C. Y. Chung, P. J. McLean, S. Lindquist, and L. Guarente. 2012. SIRT1 protects against α-synuclein aggregation by activating molecular chaperones. *J. Neurosci.* 32:124–132.

Dorighello, G. G., J. C. Rovani , C. J. Luhman, B. A. Paim, H. F. Raposo, A. E. Vercesi, and H. C. Oliveira. 2013. Food restriction by intermittent fasting induces diabetes, and obesity, and aggravates spontaneous atherosclerosis development in hypercholesterolaemic mice. *Br. J. Nutr.* 1:1–8.

Dryden, S. C., F. A. Nahhas, J. E. Nowak, A. S. Goustin, and M. A. Tainsky. 2003. Role for human SIRT2 NAD-dependent deacetylase activity in control of mitotic exit in the cell cycle. *Mol. Cell. Biol.* 23:3173–3185.

Edwards, A. G., A. J. Donato, L. A. Lesniewski, R. A. Gioscia, D. R. Seals, and R. L. Moore. 2010. Life-long caloric restriction elicits pronounced protection of the aged myocardium: a role for AMPK. *Mech. Ageing Dev.* 131:739–742.

Edwards, C., A. K. Hindle, S. Fu, and F. Brody. 2011. Downregulation of leptin and resistin expression in blood following bariatric surgery. *Surg. Endosc.* 25:1962–1968.

Egert, S., C. Boesch-Saadatmandi, S. Wolffram, G. Rimbach, and M. J. Müller. 2010. Serum lipid, and blood pressure responses to quercetin vary in overweight patients by apolipoprotein E genotype. *J. Nutr.* 140:278–284.

Egert, S., G. Rimbach, and M. J. Müller. 2011. No evidence for a thermic effect of the dietary flavonol quercetin: a pilot study in healthy normal-weight women. *Eur. J. Appl. Physiol.* 111:869–873.

Einstein, F. H., D. M. Huffman, S. Fishman, E. Jerschow, H. J. Heo, G. Atzmon, C. Schechter, N. Barzilai, and R. H. Muzumdar. 2010. Aging per se increases the susceptibility to free fatty acid-induced insulin resistance. *J. Gerontol. A. Biol. Sci. Med. Sci.* 65:800–808.

Eisenberg, T., H. Knauer, A. Schauer, S. Büttner, C. Ruckenstuhl, D. Carmona-Gutierrez, J. Ring, S. Schroeder, C. Magnes, L. Antonacci, H. Fussi, L. Deszcz, R. Hartl, E. Schraml, A. Criollo, E. Megalou, D. Weiskopf, P. Laun, G. Heeren, M. Breitenbach, B. Grubeck-Loebenstein, E. Herker, B. Fahrenkrog, K. U. Fröhlich, F. Sinner, N. Tavernarakis, N. Minois, G. Kroemer, and F. Madeo. 2009. Induction of autophagy by spermidine promotes longevity. *Nat. Cell Biol.* 11:1305–1314.

Eizirik, D. L., A. K. Cardozo, and M. Cnop. 2008. The role for endoplasmic reticulum stress in diabetes mellitus. *Endocr. Rev.* 29:42–61.

Ejaz, A., D. Wu, P. Kwan, and M. Meydani. 2009. Curcumin inhibits adipogenesis in 3T3-L1 adipocytes, and angiogenesis, and obesity in C57/BL mice. *J. Nutr.* 139:919–925.

Engel, N. and U. Mahlknecht. 2008. Aging, and anti-aging: unexpected side effects of everyday medication through sirtuin1 modulation. *Int. J. Mol. Med.* 21:223–232.

Engin, F. and G. S. Hotamisligil. 2010. Restoring endoplasmic reticulum function by chemical chaperones: an emerging therapeutic approach for metabolic diseases. *Diabetes Obes. Metab.* 12 Suppl 2:108–115.

Ernst, M. C., M. Issa, K. B. Goralski, and C. J. Sinal. 2010. Chemerin exacerbates glucose intolerance in mouse models of obesity and diabetes. *Endocrinology* 151:1998–2007.

Esposito, K., A. Pontillo, C. Di Palo, G. Giugliano, M. Masella, R. Marfella, and D. Giugliano. 2003. Effect of weight loss and lifestyle changes on vascular inflammatory markers in obese women – a randomized trial. *JAMA* 289:1799–1804.

Evangelopoulos, A. A., N. G. Vallianou, D. B. Panagiotakos, A. Georgiou, G. A. Zacharias, A. N. Alevra, G. J. Zalokosta, E. D. Vogiatzakis, and P. C. Avgerinos. 2008. An inverse relationship between cumulating components of the metabolic syndrome, and serum magnesium levels. *Nutr. Res.* 28:659–663.

Eyre, H., R. Kahn, R. M. Robertson, and ACS/ADA/AHA Collaborative Writing Committee. 2004. Preventing cancer, cardiovascular disease, and diabetes: a common agenda for the American Cancer Society, the American Diabetes Association, and the American Heart Association. *CA Cancer J. Clin.* 54:190–207.

Fang, D. L., Y. Wan, W. Shen, J. Cao, Z. X. Sun, H. H. Yu, Q. Zhang, W. H. Cheng, J. Chen, and B. Ning. 2013. Endoplasmic reticulum stress leads to lipid accumulation through upregulation of SREBP-1c in normal hepatic, and hepatoma cells. *Mol. Cell. Biochem.* 381:127–137.

Fantuzzi, G. and R. Faggioni. 2000. Leptin in the regulation of immunity, inflammation, and hematopoiesis. *J. Leukoc. Biol.* 68:437–446.

Farb, M. G., L. Ganley-Leal, M. Mott, Y. Liang, B. Ercan, M. E. Widlansky, S. J. Bigornia, A. J. Fiscale, C. M. Apovian, B. Carmine, D. T. Hess, J. A. Vita, and N. Gokce. 2012. Arteriolar function in visceral adipose tissue is impaired in human obesity. *Arterioscler. Thromb. Vasc. Biol.* 32:467–473.

Feige, J. N., M. Lagouge, C. Canto, A. Strehle, S. M. Houten, J. C. Milne, P. D. Lambert, C. Mataki, P. J. Elliott, and J. Auwerx. 2008. Specific SIRT1 activation mimics low energy levels and protects against diet-induced metabolic disorders by enhancing fat oxidation. *Cell Metab.* 8:347–358.

Ferguson, M., B. H. Sohal, M. J. Forster, and R. S. Sohal. 2007. Effect of long-term caloric restriction on oxygen consumption and body temperature in two different strains of mice. *Mech. Ageing Dev.* 128:539–545.

Ferrario, A., F. Villa, A. Malovini, F. Araniti, and A. A. Puca. 2012. The application of genetics approaches to the study of exceptional longevity in humans: potential, and limitations. *Immun. Ageing* 9:7.

Finkel, T., C. X. Deng, and R. Mostoslavsky. 2009. Recent progress in the biology, and physiology of sirtuins. *Nature* 460:587–591.

Fischer-Posovszky, P., V. Kukulus , D. Tews, T. Unterkircher, K. M. Debatin, S. Fulda, and M. Wabitsch. 2010. Resveratrol regulates human adipocyte number, and function in a Sirt1-dependent manner. *Am. J. Clin. Nutr.* 92:5–15.

Flachs, P., V. Mohamed-Ali, O. Horakova, M. Rossmeisl, M. J. Hosseinzadeh-Attar, M. Hensler, J. Ruzickova, and J. Kopecky. 2006. Polyunsaturated fatty acids of marine origin induce adiponectin in mice fed a high-fat diet. *Diabetologia* 49:394–397.

Fleenor, B. S., A. L. Sindler, N. K. Marvi, K. L. Howell, M. L. Zigler, M. Yoshizawa, and D. R. Seals. 2013. Curcumin ameliorates arterial dysfunction, and oxidative stress with aging. *Exp. Gerontol.* 48:269–276.

Fonseca, S. G., J. Gromada, and F. Urano. 2011. Endoplasmic reticulum stress, and pancreatic beta-cell death. *Trends Endocrinol. Metab.* 22:266–274.

Fontana, L. 2009. Neuroendocrine factors in the regulation of inflammation: Excessive adiposity and calorie restriction. *Exp. Gerontol.* 44:41–45.

Fontana, L. and S. Klein. 2007. Aging, adiposity and calorie restriction. *JAMA* 297:986–994.

Fontana, L., T. E. Meyer, S. Klein, and J. O. Holloszy. 2004. Long-term calorie restriction is highly effective in reducing the risk for atherosclerosis in humans. *Proc. Natl Acad. Sci. USA* 101:6659–6663.

Fontana, L., S. Klein, J. O. Holloszy, and B. N. Premachandra. 2006. Effect of long-term calorie restriction with adequate protein and micronutrients on thyroid hormones. *J. Clin. Endocrinol. Metab.* 91:3232–3235.

Fontana, L., D. T. Villareal, E. P. Weiss, S. B. Racette, K. Steger-May, S. Klein, and J. O. Holloszy. 2007. Calorie restriction or exercise: effects on coronary heart disease risk factors a randomized, controlled trial. *Am. J. Physiol. Endocrinol. Metabol.* 293:E197–E202.

Fontana, L., E. P. Weiss, D. T. Villareal, S. Klein, and J. O. Holloszy. 2008. Long-term effects of calorie or protein restriction on serum IGF-1, and IGFBP-3 concentration in humans. *Aging Cell* 7:681–687.

Fontana, L., S. Klein, and J. O. Holloszy. 2010a. Effects of long-term calorie restriction and endurance exercise on glucose tolerance, insulin action, and adipokine production. *Age (Dordr.)* 32:97–108.

Fontana, L., L. Partridge, and V. D. Longo. 2010b. Dietary restriction, growth factors and aging: from yeast to humans. *Science* 328:321–326.

Ford, E., R. Voit, G. Liszt, C. Magin, I. Grummt, and L. Guarente. 2006. Mammalian Sir2 homolog SIRT7 is an activator of RNA polymerase I transcription. *Genes Dev.* 20:1075–1080.

Fox, C. S., J. M. Massaro, U. Hoffmann, K. M. Pou, P. Maurovich-Horvat, C. Y. Liu, R. S. Vasan, J. M. Murabito, J. B. Meigs, L. A. Cupples, R. B. D'Agostino, and C. J. O'Donnell. 2007. Abdominal visceral and subcutaneous adipose tissue compartments: association with metabolic risk factors in the Framingham Heart Study. *Circulation* 116:39–48.

Fox, C. S., J. M. Massaro, C. L. Schlett, S. J. Lehman, J. B. Meigs, C. J. O'Donnell, U. Hoffmann, and J. M. Murabito. 2010. Periaortic fat deposition is associated with peripheral arterial disease: the Framingham Heart Study. *Circul. Cardiovasc. Imag.* 3:515–519.

Frescas, D., L. Valenti, and D. Accili. 2005. Nuclear trapping of the forkhead transcription factor FoxO1 via Sirt-dependent deacetylation promotes expression of glucogenetic genes. *J. Biol. Chem.* 280:20589–20595.

Friedrich, M., K. J. Petzke, D. Raederstorff, S. Wolfram, and S. Klaus. 2012. Acute effects of epigallocatechin gallate from green tea on oxidation, and tissue incorporation of dietary lipids in mice fed a high-fat diet. *Int. J. Obes.* 36:735–743.

Fruehwald-Schultes, B., K. M. Oltmanns, B. Toschek, S. Sopke, W. Kern, J. Born, H. L. Fehm, and A. Peters. 2002. Short-term treatment with metformin decreases serum leptin concentration without affecting body weight, and body fat content in normal-weight healthy men. *Metabolism* 51:531–536.

Fu, C., M. Hickey, M. Morrison, R. McCarter, and E. S. Han. 2006. Tissue specific, and non-specific changes in gene expression by aging, and by early stage CR. *Mech. Ageing Dev.* 127:905–916.

Fu, S., L. Yang, P. Li, O. Hofmann, L. Dicker, W. Hide, X. Lin, S. M. Watkins, A. R. Ivanov, and G. S. Hotamisligil. 2011. Aberrant lipid metabolism disrupts calcium homeostasis causing liver endoplasmic reticulum stress in obesity. *Nature* 473:528–531.

Fu, S., S. M. Watkins, and G. S. Hotamisligil. 2012. The role of endoplasmic reticulum in hepatic lipid homeostasis, and stress signaling. *Cell Metab.* 15:623–634.

Fuentes, E., F. Fuentes, G. Vilahur, L. Badimon, and I. Palomo. 2013. Mechanisms of chronic state of inflammation as mediators that link obese adipose tissue, and metabolic syndrome. *Mediators Inflamm.* 2013:136584.

Fukuda, S. and H. Ohno. 2014. Gut microbiome, and metabolic diseases. *Semin. Immunopathol.* 36:103–114.

Furuyashiki, T., H. Nagayasu, Y. Aoki, H. Bessho, T. Hashimoto, K. Kanazawa, and H. Ashida. 2004. Tea catechin suppresses adipocyte differentiation accompanied by down-regulation of PPARgamma2, and C/EBPalpha in 3T3-L1 cells. *Biosci. Biotechnol. Biochem.* 68:2353–2359.

Gamerdinder, M., P. Hajieva, A. M. Kaya, U. Wolfrum, F. U. Hartl, and C. Behl. 2009. Protein quality control during aging involves recruitment of the macroautophagy pathway by BAG3. *EMBO J.* 28:889 –901.

Garcia-Fuentes, E., J. M. Garcia-Almeida, J. Garcia-Arnes, S. Garcia-Serrano, J. Rivas-Marin, J. L. Gallego-Perales, G. Rojo-Martínez, L. Garrido-Sánchez, F. J. Bermudez-Silva, F. Rodríguez de Fonseca, and F. Soriguer. 2007. Plasma visfatin concentrations in severely obese subjects are increased after intestinal bypass. *Obesity (Silver Spring)* 15:2391–2395.

Gealekman, O., N. Guseva, C. Hartigan, S. Apotheker, M. Gorgoglione, K. Gurav, K. V. Tran, J. Straubhaar, S. Nicoloro, M. P. Czech, M. Thompson, R. A. Perugini, and S. Corvera. 2011. Depot-specific differences and insufficient subcutaneous adipose tissue angiogenesis in human obesity. *Circulation* 123:186–194.

Gelino, S. and M. Hansen. 2012. Autophagy – an emerging anti-aging mechanism. *J. Clin. Exp. Pathol. Suppl* 4:006.

Gertz, M. and C. Steegborn. 2010. Function, and regulation of the mitochondrial sirtuin isoform Sirt5 in Mammalia. *Biochim. Biophys. Acta* 1804:1658–1665.

Ghosh, H. S., M. McBurney, and P. D. Robbins. 2010. SIRT1 negatively regulates the mammalian target of rapamycin. *PLoS One* 5:e9199.

Gil, R., S. Barth, Y. Kanfi, and H. Y. Cohen. 2013. SIRT6 exhibits nucleosome-dependent deacetylase activity. *Nucleic Acids Res.* 41:8537–8545.

Golubović, M. V., D. Dimić, S. Antić, S. Radenković, B. Djindjić, and M. Jovanović. 2013. Relationship of adipokine to insulin sensitivity and glycemic regulation in obese women – the effect of body weight reduction by caloric restriction. *Vojnosanit Pregl.* 70:284–291.

Gomez-Cabello, A., G. V. Rodriguez, S. Vila-Maldonado, J. A. Casajus, and I. Ara. 2012. Aging and body composition: the sarcopenic obesity in Spain. *Nutr. Hosp.* 27:22–30.

Gomez-Zorita, S., K. Tréguer, J. Mercader, and C. Carpéné. 2013. Resveratrol directly affects in vitro lipolysis, and glucose transport in human fat cells. *J. Physiol. Biochem.* 69:585–593.

Gonzalez, A. A., R. Kumar, J. D. Mulligan, A. J. Davis, R. Weindruch, and K. W. Saupe. 2004. Metabolic adaptations to fasting, and chronic caloric restriction in heart, muscle, and liver do not include changes in AMPK activity. *Am. J. Physiol. Endocrinol. Metab.* 287:E1032–E1037.

Goodrick, C. L., D. K. Ingram, M. A. Reynolds, J. R. Freeman, and N. Cider. 1990. Effects of intermittent feeding upon body weight, and lifespan in inbred mice: interaction of genotype, and age. *Mech. Ageing Dev.* 55:69–87.

Goralski, K. B., T. C. McCarthy, E. A. Hanniman, B. A. Zabel, E. C. Butcher, S. D. Parlee, S. Muruganandan, and C. J. Sinal. 2007. Chemerin, a novel adipokine that regulates adipogenesis and adipocyte metabolism. *J. Biol. Chem.* 282:28175–28188.

Greer, E. L., P. R. Oskoui, M. R. Banko, J. M. Maniar, M. P. Gygi, S. P. Gygi, and A. Brunet. 2007. The energy sensor AMP-activated protein kinase directly regulates the mammalian FOXO3 transcription factor. *J. Biol. Chem.* 282:30107–30119.

Gregor, M. F. and G. S. Hotamisligil. 2007. Thematic review series: Adipocyte Biology. Adipocyte stress: the endoplasmic reticulum, and metabolic disease. J. *Lipid Res.* 48:1905–1914.

Gregor, M. F. and G. S. Hotamisligil. 2011. Inflammatory mechanisms in obesity. *Annu. Rev. Immunol.* 29:415–445.

Guarani, V. and M. Potente. 2010. SIRT1 – a metabolic sensor that controls blood vessel growth. *Curr. Opin. Pharmacol.* 10:139–145.

Guarente, L. 2011. Sirtuins, aging, and metabolism. *Cold Spring Harb. Symp. Quant. Biol.* 76:81–90.

Gullestad, L., M. Nes, R. Ronneberg, K. Midtvedt, D. Falch, and J. Kjekshus. 1994. Magnesium status in healthy free-living elderly Norwegians. *J. Am. Coll. Nutr.* 13:45–50.

Guo, Z., A. Heydari, and A. Richardson. 1998. Nucleotide excision repair of actively transcribed versus nontranscribed DNA in rat hepatocytes: effect of age, and dietary restriction. *Exp. Cell Res.* 245:228–238.

Guo, K. Y., P. Halo, R. L. Leibel, and Y. Zhang. 2004. Effects of obesity on the relationship of leptin mRNA expression and adipocyte size in anatomically distinct fat depots in mice. *Am. J. Physiol. Regul. Integr. Comp. Physiol.* 287:R112–R119.

Haider, D. G., K. Schindler, G. Schaller, G. Prager, M. Wolzt, and B. Ludvik. 2006. Increased plasma visfatin concentrations in morbidly obese subjects are reduced after gastric banding. *J. Clin. Endocrinol. Metab.* 91:1578–1581.

Haigis, M. C. and L. P. Guarente. 2006. Mammalian sirtuins – emerging roles in physiology, aging, and calorie restriction. *Genes & Dev.* 20:2913–2921.

Haigis, M. C., R. Mostoslavsky, K. M. Haigis, K. Fahie, D. C. Christodoulou, A. J. Murphy, D. M. Valenzuela, G. D. Yancopoulos, M. Karow, G. Blander, C. Wolberger, T. A. Prolla, R. Weindruch, F. W. Alt, and L. Guarente. 2006. SIRT4 inhibits glutamate dehydrogenase, and opposes the effects of calorie restriction in pancreatic beta cells. *Cell* 126:941–954.

Halberg, N., T. Khan, M. E. Trujillo, I. Wernstedt-Asterholm, A. D. Attie, S. Sherwani, Z. V. Wang, S. Landskroner-Eiger, S. Dineen, U. J. Magalang, R. A. Brekken, and P. E. Scherer. 2009. Hypoxia-inducible factor 1alpha induces fibrosis and insulin resistance in white adipose tissue. *Mol. Cell Biol.* 29:4467–4483.

Hallows, W. C., S. Lee, and J. M. Denu. 2006. Sirtuins deacetylate, and activate mammalian acetyl-CoA synthetases. *Proc. Natl Acad. Sci. USA* 103:10230–10235.

Hallows, W. C., W. Yu, B. C. Smith, M. K. Devries, J. J. Ellinger, S. Someya, M. R. Shortreed, T. Prolla, J. L. Markley, L. M. Smith, S. Zhao, K. L. Guan, and J. M. Denu. 2011. Sirt3 promotes the urea cycle, and fatty acid oxidation during dietary restriction. *Mol. Cell* 41:139–149.

Hambly, C. and J. R. Speakman. 2005. Contribution of different mechanisms to compensation for energy restriction in the mouse. *Obes. Res.* 13:1548–1557.

Hambly, C., J. S. Duncan, Z. A. Archer, K. M. Moar, J. G. Mercer, and J. R. Speakman. 2012. Repletion of TNFα or leptin in calorically restricted mice suppresses post-restriction hyperphagia. *Dis. Model. Mech.* 5:83–94.

Hammar, M. and C. J. Östgren. 2013. Healthy aging and age-adjusted nutrition and physical fitness. *Best Pract. Res. Clin. Obstet. Gynaecol.* 27:741–752.

Han, E. S. and M. Hickey. 2005. Microarray evaluation of dietary restriction. *J. Nutr.* 135:1343–1346.

Han, E. S., T. R. Evans, J. H. Shu, S. Lee, and J. F. Nelson. 2001. Food restriction enhances endogenous and corticotropin-induced plasma elevations of free but not total corticosterone throughout life in rats. *J. Gerontol. A Biol. Sci. Med. Sci.* 56:B391–B397.

Han, X., S. Turdi, N. Hu, R. Guo, Y. Zhang, and J. Ren. 2012. Influence of long-term caloric restriction on myocardial, and cardiomyocyte contractile function, and autophagy in mice. *J. Nutr. Biochem.* 23:1592–1599.

Hannigan, A. M. and S. M. Gorski. 2009. Macroautophagy. The key ingredient to a healthy diet? *Autophagy* 5:140–151.

Hansen, M., A. Chandra, L. L. Mitic, B. Onken, M. Driscoll, and C. Kenyon. 2008. A role for autophagy in the extension of lifespan by dietary restriction in C. elegans. *PLoS Genet.* 4:e24.

Hardie, D. G. 2011. Sensing of energy, and nutrients by AMP-activated protein kinase. *Am. J. Clin. Nutr.* 93:891S–896S.

Hardie, D. G., F. A. Ross, and S. A. Hawley. 2012. AMPK: a nutrient, and energy sensor that maintains energy homeostasis. *Nature Ver.* 13:251–262.

Hariharan, N., Y. Maejima, J. Nakae, J. Paik, R. A. Depinho, and J. Sadoshima. 2010. Deacetylation of FoxO by Sirt1 plays an essential role in mediating starvation-induced autophagy in cardiac myocytes. *Circul. Res.* 107:1470–1482.

Harmon, A. W., Y. M. Patel, and J. B. Harp. 2002. Genistein inhibits CCAAT/enhancer-binding protein beta (C/EBPbeta) activity, and 3T3-L1 adipogenesis by increasing C/EBP homologous protein expression. *Biochem. J.* 367:203–208.

Harrison, D. E., J. R. Archer, and C. M. Astle. 1984. Effects of food restriction on aging: separation of food intake and adiposity. *Proc. Natl Acad. Sci. USA* 81:1835–1838.

Harrison, D. E., R. Strong, Z. D. Sharp, J. F. Nelson, C. M. Astle, K. Flurkey, N. L. Nadon, J. E. Wilkinson, K. Frenkel, C. S. Carter, M. Pahor, M. A. Javors, E. Fernandez, and R. A. Miller. 2009. Rapamycin fed late in life extends lifespan in genetically heterogeneous mice. *Nature* 460:392–395.

Hauck, S. J., W. S. Hunter, N. Danilovich, J. J. Kopchick, and A. Bartke. 2001. Reduced levels of thyroid hormones, insulin, and glucose, and lower body core temperature in the growth hormone receptor/binding protein knockout mouse. *Exp. Biol. Med. (Maywood)* 226:552–558.

Hayes, J. D. and A. T. Dinkova-Kostova. 2014. The Nrf2 regulatory network provides an interface between redox and intermediary metabolism. *Trends Biochem. Sci.* 39:199–218.

Heilbronn, L. K., L. de Jonge, M. I. Frisard, J. P. DeLany, D. E. Larson-Meyer, J. Rood, T. Nguyen, C. K. Martin, J. Volaufova, M. M. Most, F. L. Greenway, S. R. Smith, W. A. Deutsch, D. A. Williamson, E. Ravussin and Pennington CALERIE Team. 2006. Effect of 6-month calorie restriction on biomarkers of longevity, metabolic adaptation, and oxidative stress in overweight individuals: a randomized controlled trial. *J. A. M. A.* 295:1539–1548.

Hetz, C. 2012. The unfolded protein response: controlling cell fate decisions under ER stress, and beyond. *Nat. Rev. Mol. Cell Biol.* 13:89–102.

Hetz, C., F. Martinon, D. Rodriguez, and L. H. Glimcher. 2011. The unfolded protein response: integrating stress signals through the stress sensor IRE1alpha. *Physiol. Rev.* 91:1219–1243.

Heydari, A. R., A. Unnikrishnan, L. V. Lucente, and A. Richardson. 2007. Caloric restriction, and genomic stability. *Nucleic Acids Res.* 35:7485–7496.

Hida, K., J. Wada, J. Eguchi, H. Zhang, M. Baba, A. Seida, I. Hashimoto, T. Okada, A. Yasuhara, A. Nakatsuka, K. Shikata, S. Hourai, J. Futami, E. Watanabe, Y. Matsuki, R. Hiramatsu, S. Akagi, H. Makino, and Y. S. Kanwar. 2005. Visceral adipose tissue-derived serine protease inhibitor: a unique insulin-sensitizing adipocytokine in obesity. *Proc. Natl Acad. Sci. USA* 102:10610–10615.

Hill, A. M., A. M. Coates, J. D. Buckley, R. Ross, and F. Thielecke. 2007. Can EGCG reduce abdominal fat in obese subjects? *J. Am. Coll. Nutr.* 26:396S–402S.

Hine, C. M. and J. R. Mitchell. 2012. NRF2 and the Phase II response in acute stress resistance induced by dietary restriction. *J. Clin. Exp. Pathol.* S4.

Hirosumi, J., G. Tuncman, L. Chang, C. Z. Gorgun, K. T. Uysal, K. Maeda, M. Karin, and G. S. Hotamisligil. 2002. A central role for JNK in obesity, and insulin resistance. *Nature* 420:333–336.

Hofer, T., L. Fontana, S. D. Anton, E. P. Weiss, D. Villareal, B. Malayappan, and C. Leeuwenburgh. 2008. Long-term effects of caloric restriction or exercise on DNA, and RNA oxidation levels in white blood cells, and urine in humans. *Rejuvenation Res.* 11:793–799.

Holloszy, J. O. and L. Fontana. 2007. Caloric restriction. *Exp. Gerontol.* 42:709–712.

Holloszy, J. O., E. K. Smith, M. Vining, and S. Adams. 1985. Effect of voluntary exercise on longevity of rats. *J. Appl. Physiol.* 59:826–831.

Holmström, K. M., L. Baird, Y. Zhang, I. Hargreaves, A. Chalasani, J. M. Land, L. Stanyer, M. Yamamoto, A. T. Dinkova-Kostova and A. Y. Abramov. 2013. Nrf2 impacts cellular bioenergetics by controlling substrate availability for mitochondrial respiration. *Biol. Open* 2:761–770.

Holzenberger, M., J. Dupont, B. Ducos, P. Leneuve, A. Géloën, P. C. Even, P. Cervera, and Y. Le Bouc. 2003. IGF-1 receptor regulates lifespan and resistance to oxidative stress in mice. *Nature* 421:182–187.

Hotamisligil, G. S. 2008. Inflammation, and endoplasmic reticulum stress in obesity, and diabetes. *Int. J. Obes. Lond.* 32 Suppl 7:S52–54.

Hotamisligil, G. S. 2010. Endoplasmic reticulum stress, and the inflammatory basis of metabolic disease. *Cell* 140:900–917.

Hsu, C. L. and G. C. Yen. 2006. Induction of cell apoptosis in 3T3-L1 pre-adipocytes by flavonoids is associated with their antioxidant activity. *Mol. Nutr. Food Res.* 50:1072–1079.

Hsu, T. F., A. Kusumoto, K. Abe, K. Hosoda, Y. Kiso, M. F. Wang, and S. Yamamoto. 2006. Polyphenol-enriched oolong tea increases fecal lipid excretion. *Eur. J. Clin. Nutr.* 60:1330–1336.

Hu, P., Z. Han, A. D. Couvillon, R. J. Kaufman, and J. H. Exton. 2006. Autocrine tumor necrosis factor alpha links endoplasmic reticulum stress to the membrane death receptor pathway through IRE1alpha-mediated NF-kappaB activation, and down-regulation of TRAF2 expression. *Mol. Cell. Biol.* 26:3071–3084.

Hu, Y., J. Liu, J. Wang, and Q. Liu. 2011. The controversial links among calorie restriction, SIRT1, and resveratrol. *Free Radic. Biol. Med.* 51:250–256.

Huang, J. H., Y. F. Lu, F. C. Cheng, J. N. Lee, and L. C. Tsai. 2012. Correlation of magnesium intake with metabolic parameters, depression, and physical activity in elderly type 2 diabetes patients: a cross-sectional study. *Nutr. J.* 11:41.

Hubbi, M. E., H. Hu, Kshitiz, D. M. Gilkes, and G. L. Semenza. 2013. Sirtuin-7 inhibits the activity of hypoxia-inducible factors. *J. Biol. Chem.* 288:20768–20775.

Huerta, M. G., J. N. Roemmich, M. L. Kington, V. E. Bovbjerg, A. L. Weltman, V. F. Holmes, J. T. Patrie, A. D. Rogol, and J. L. Nadler. 2005. Magnesium deficiency is associated with insulin resistance in obese children. *Diabetes Care* 28:1175–1181.

Hulbert, A. J., R. Pamplona, R. Buffenstein, and W. A. Buttemer. 2007. Life and death: metabolic rate, membrane composition, and life span of animals. *Physiol. Rev.* 87:1175–1213.

Hunter, W. S., W. B. Croson, A. Bartke, M. V. Gentry, and C. J. Meliska. 1999. Low body temperature in long-lived Ames dwarf mice at rest and during stress. *Physiol. Behav.* 67:433–437.

Hurt, R. T. and T. Wilson. 2012. Geriatric obesity: evaluating the evidence for the use of flavonoids to promote weight loss. *J. Nutr. Gerontol. Geriatr.* 31:269–289.

Hussain, S. G. and K. V. Ramaiah. 2007. Reduced eIF2alpha phosphorylation, and increased proapoptotic proteins in aging. *Biochem. Biophys. Res. Commun.* 355:365–370.

Ikeno, Y., G. B. Hubbard, S. Lee, L. A. Cortez, C. M. Lew, C. R. Webb, D. E. Berryman, E. O. List, J. J. Kopchick, and A. Bartke. 2009. Reduced incidence and delayed occurrence of fatal neoplastic diseases in growth hormone receptor/binding protein knockout mice. *J. Gerontol. A. Biol. Sci. Med. Sci.* 64:522–529.

Ikeno, Y., G. B. Hubbard, S. Lee, S. M. Dube, L. C. Flores, M. G. Roman, and A. Bartke. 2013. Do Ames dwarf, and calorie-restricted mice share common effects on age-related pathology? *Pathobiol. Aging Age Relat. Dis.* 3:20833.

Ikeyama, S., X. T. Wang, J. Li, A. Podlutsky, J. L. Martindale, G. Kokkonen, R. van Huizen, M. Gorospe, and N. J. Holbrook. 2003. Expression of the pro-apoptotic gene gadd153/chop is elevated in liver with aging, and sensitizes cells to oxidant injury. *J. Biol. Chem.* 278:16726–16731.

Inagi, R. 2009. Endoplasmic reticulum stress in the kidney as a novel mediator of kidney injury. *Nephron Exp. Nephrol.* 112:e1–9.

Ingram, D. K., M. Zhu, J. Mamczarz, S. Zou, M. A. Lane, G. S. Roth, and R. deCabo. 2006. Calorie restriction mimetics: an emerging research field. *Aging Cell* 5:97–108.

Ito, Y., T. Ichikawa, Y. Morohoshi, T. Nakamura, Y. Saegusa, and K. Ishihara. 2008. Effect of tea catechins on body fat accumulation in rats fed a normal diet. *Biomed. Res.* 29:27–32.

Jafari M., B. Khodayari, J. Felgner, I. I. Bussel, M. R. Rose, and L. D. Mueller. 2007. Pioglitazone: an anti-diabetic compound with anti-aging properties. *Biogerontology* 8:639–651.

Jiang, T., S. E. Liebman, M. S. Lucia, C. L. Phillips, and M. Levi. 2005. Calorie restriction modulates renal expression of sterol regulatory element binding proteins, lipid accumulation, and age-related renal disease. *J. Am. Soc. Nephrol.* 16:2385–2394.

Jiang, C., A. Qu, T. Matsubara, T. Chanturiya, W. Jou, O. Gavrilova, Y. M. Shah, and F. J. Gonzalez. 2011. Disruption of hypoxia-inducible factor 1 in adipocytes improves insulin sensitivity and decreases adiposity in high-fat diet-fed mice. *Diabetes* 60:2484–2495.

Jorgensen, F. B., H. M. O'Neill, L. Sylow, J. Honeyman, K. A. Hewitt, R. Palanivel, M. D. Fullerton, L. Öberg, A. Balendran, S. Galic, C. van der Poel, I. A. Trounce, G. S. Lynch, J. D. Schertzer, and G. R. Steinberg. 2013. Deletion of skeletal muscle SOCS-3 prevents insulin resistance in obesity. *Diabetes* 62:56–64.

Jung, S. H., H. S. Park, K. S. Kim, W. H. Choi, C. W. Ahn, B. T. Kim, S. M. Kim, S. Y. Lee, S. M. Ahn, Y. K. Kim, H. J. Kim, D. J. Kim, and K. W. Lee. 2008. Effect of weight loss on some serum cytokines in human obesity: increase in IL-10 after weight loss. *J. Nutr. Biochem.* 19:371–375.

Jung, C. H., I. Cho, J. Ahn, T. I. Jeon, and T. Y. Ha. 2013. Quercetin reduces high-fat diet-induced fat accumulation in the liver by regulating lipid metabolism genes. *Phytother. Res.* 27:139–143.

Kadowaki, T., T. Yamauchi, N. Kubota, K. Hara, K. Ueki, and K. Tobe. 2006. Adiponectin and adiponectin receptors in insulin resistance, diabetes, and the metabolic syndrome. *J. Clin. Invest.* 116:1784–1792.

Kaess, B. M., A. Pedley, J. M. Massaro, M. G. Larson, E. Corsini, U. Hoffmann, H. M. Smith, D. B. Sawyer, R. S. Vasan, and C. S. Fox. 2012. Relation of vascular growth factors with CT-derived measures of body fat distribution: the Framingham Heart Study. *J. Clin. Endocrinol. Metab.* 97:987–994.

Kagawa, Y. 1978. Impact of westernization on the nutrition of Japanese: changes in physique, longevity, and centenarians. *Prev. Med.* 7:205–217.

Kalender, A., A. Selvaraj, S. Y. Kim, P. Gulati, S. Brule, B. Viollet, B. E. Kemp, N. Bardeesy, P. Dennis, J. J. Schlager, A. Marette, S. C. Kozma, and G. Thomas. 2010. Metformin, independent of AMPK, inhibits mTORC1 in a rag GTPase-dependent manner. *Cell Metab.* 11:390–401.

Kammoun, H. L., H. Chabanon, I. Hainault, S. Luquet, C. Magnan, T. Koike, P. Ferre, and F. Foufelle. 2009. GRP78 expression inhibits insulin, and ER stress-induced SREBP-1c activation, and reduces hepatic steatosis in mice. *J. Clin. Invest.* 119:1201–1215.

Kanazawa, T., I. Taneike, R. Akaishi, F. Yoshizawa, N. Furuya, S. Fujimura, and M. Kadowaki. 2004. Amino acids, and insulin control autophagic proteolysis through different signaling pathways in relation to mTOR in isolated rat hepatocytes. *J. Biol. Chem.* 279:8452–8459.

Kanfi, Y., R. Shalman, V. Peshti, S. N. Pilosof, Y. M. Gozlan, K. J. Pearson, B. Lerrer, D. Moazed, J. C. Marine, R. de Cabo, and H. Y. Cohen. 2008. Regulation of SIRT6 protein levels by nutrient availability. *FEBS Lett.* 582:543–548.

Kanfi, Y., S. Naiman, G. Amir, V. Peshti, G. Zinman, L. Nahum, Z. Bar-Joseph, and H. Y. Cohen. 2012. The sirtuin SIRT6 regulates lifespan in male mice. *Nature* 483:218–221.

Kang, Q. and A. Chen. 2009. Curcumin suppresses expression of low-density lipoprotein (LDL) receptor, leading to the inhibition of LDL-induced activation of hepatic stellate cells. *Br. J. Pharmacol.* 157:1354–1367.

Kang, Y. S. 2013. Obesity Associated Hypertension: New Insights into Mechanism. *Electrolyte Blood Press.* 11:46–52.

Kao, Y. H., R. A. Hiipakka, and S. Liao. 2000. Modulation of endocrine systems, and food intake by green tea epigallocatechin gallate. *Endocrinology* 141:980–987.

Kaufman, R. J. 2002. Orchestrating the unfolded protein response in health, and disease. *J. Clin. Invest.* 110:1389–1398.

Kaufman, R. J., S. H. Back, B. Song, J. Han, and J. Hassler. 2010. The unfolded protein response is required to maintain the integrity of the endoplasmic reticulum, prevent oxidative stress, and preserve differentiation in beta-cells. *Diabetes Obes. Metab.* 12:99–107.

Kaur, J. 2014. A Comprehensive Review on Metabolic Syndrome. *Cardiol. Res. Pract.* 943162.

Kawahara, T. L., E. Michishita, A. S. Adler, M. Damian, E. Berber, M. Lin, R. A. McCord, K. C. Ongaigui, L. D. Boxer, H. Y. Chang, and K. F. Chua. 2009. SIRT6 links histone H3 lysine 9 deacetylation to NF-kappaB-dependent gene expression, and organismal life span. *Cell* 136:62–74.

Kawakami, T., R. Inagi, H. Takano, S. Sato, J. R. Ingelfinger, T. Fujita, and M. Nangaku. 2009. Endoplasmic reticulum stress induces autophagy in renal proximal tubular cells. *Nephrol. Dial. Transplant.* 24:2665–2672.

Kawakami, K., A. Nakamura, and S. Goto. 2012. Dietary restriction increases site-specific histone H3 acetylation in rat liver: possible modulation by sirtuins. *Biochem. Biophys. Res. Commun.* 418:836–840.

Kawamata, T., Y. Kamada, Y. Kabeya, T. Sekito, and Y. Ohsumi. 2008. Organization of the pre-autophagosomal structure responsible for autophagosome formation. *Mol. Biol. Cell* 19:2039–2050.

Kayo, T., D. B. Allison, R. Weindruch, and T. A. Prolla. 2001. Influences of aging, and caloric restriction on the transcriptional profile of skeletal muscle from rhesus monkeys. *Proc. Natl Acad. Sci. USA* 98:5093–5098.

Kealy, R. D., D. F. Lawler, J. M. Ballam, S. L. Mantz, D. N. Biery, E. H. Greeley, G. Lust, M. Segre, G. K. Smith, and H. D. Stowe. 2002. Effects of diet restriction on life span, and age-related changes in dogs. *J. Am. Vet. Med. Assoc.* 220:1315–1320.

Kelishadi, R. 2007. Childhood overweight, obesity, and the metabolic syndrome in developing countries. *Epidemiol. Rev.* 29:62–76.

Kennedy, B. K., K. K. Steffen, and M. Kaeberlein. 2007. Ruminations on dietary restriction and aging. *Cell. Mol. Life Sci.* 64:1323–1328.

Kenyon, C. J. 2010. The genetics of ageing. *Nature* 464:504–512.

Kenyon, C., J. Chang, E. Gensch, A. Rudner, and R. Tabtiang. 1993. A C. elegans mutant that lives twice as long as wild type. *Nature* 366:461–464.

Ketonen, J., T. Pilvi, and E. Mervaala. 2010. Caloric restriction reverses high-fat diet-induced endothelial dysfunction and vascular superoxide production in C57Bl/6 mice. *Heart Vessels* 25:254–262.

Kim, C. Y., T. T. Le, C. Chen, J. X. Cheng, and K. H. Kim. 2011a. Curcumin inhibits adipocyte differentiation through modulation of mitotic clonal expansion. *J. Nutr. Biochem.* 22:910–920.

Kim, D., M. D. Nguyen, M. M. Dobbin, A. Fischer, F. Sananbenesi, J. T. Rodgers, I. Delalle, J. A. Baur, G. Sui, S. M. Armour, P. Puigserver, D. A. Sinclair, and L. H. Tsai. 2007. SIRT1 deacetylase protects against neurodegeneration in models for Alzheimer's disease, and amyotrophic lateral sclerosis. *EMBO J.* 26:3169–3179.

Kim, H. and K. Sakamoto. 2012. (−)-Epigallocatechin gallate suppresses adipocyte differentiation through the MEK/ERK, and PI3K/Akt pathways. Cell Biol. *Int.* 36:147–153.

Kim, H. K., C. Nelson-Dooley, M. A. Della-Fera, J. Y. Yang, W. Zhang, J. Duan, D. L. Hartzell, M. W. Hamrick, and C. A. Baile. 2006. Genistein decreases food intake, body weight, and fat pad weight, and causes adipose tissue apoptosis in ovariectomized female mice. *J. Nutr.* 136:409–414.

Kim, J. and D. J. Klionsky. 2000. Autophagy, cytoplasm-to-vacuole targeting pathway, and pexophagy in yeast, and mammalian cells. *Annu. Rev. Biochem.* 69:303–342.

Kim, J., M. Kundu, B. Viollet, and K. L. Guan. 2011b. AMPK, and mTOR regulate autophagy through direct phosphorylation of Ulk1. *Nat. Cell Biol.* 13:132–141.

Kim, J. Y., D. H. Kim, J. Choi., J. K. Park, K. S. Jeong, C. Leeuwenburgh, B. P. Yu, and H. Y. Chung. 2009. Changes in lipid distribution during aging and its modulation by calorie restriction. *Age (Dordr.)* 31:127–142.

Kim, M. H., J. S. Park, M. S. Seo, J. W. Jung, Y. S. Lee, and K. S. Kang. 2010. Genistein, and daidzein repress adipogenic differentiation of human adipose tissue-derived mesenchymal stem cells via Wnt/β-catenin signalling or lipolysis. *Cell Prolif.* 43:594–605.

Kim, S., Y. Jin, Y. Choi, and T. Park. 2011c. Resveratrol exerts anti-obesity effects via mechanisms involving down-regulation of adipogenic and inflammatory processes in mice. *Biochem. Pharmacol.* 81:1343–1351.

Kirpichnikov, D., S. I. McFarlane, and J. R. Sowers. 2002. Metformin: an update. *Ann. Intern. Med.* 137:25–33.

Kitamura, M. 2008. Endoplasmic reticulum stress, and unfolded protein response in renal pathophysiology: Janus faces. *Am. J. Physiol. Renal Physiol.* 295:F323–334.

Kitamura, T. and Y. I. Kitamura. 2007. Role of FoxO proteins in pancreatic beta cells. *Endocr. J.* 54:507–515.

Kitteringham, N. R., A. Abdullah, J. Walsh, L. Randle, R. E. Jenkins, R. Sison, C. E. Goldring, H. Powell, C. Sanderson, S. Williams, L. Higgins, M. Yamamoto, J. Hayes and B. K. Park. 2010. Proteomic analysis of Nrf2 deficient transgenic mice reveals cellular defence and lipid metabolism as primary Nrf2-dependent pathways in the liver. *J. Proteomics* 73:1612–1631.

Klein, S., L. Fontana, V. L. Young, A. R. Coggan, C. Kilo, B. W. Patterson, and B. S. Mohammed. 2004. Absence of an effect of liposuction on insulin action and risk factors for coronary heart disease. *New Engl. J. Med.* 350:2549–2557.

Klionsky, D. J. and S. D. Emr. 2000. Autophagy as a regulated pathway of cellular degradation. *Science* 290:1717–1721.

Klöting, N., J. Berndt, S. Kralisch, P. Kovacs, M. Fasshauer, M. R. Schön, M. Stumvoll, and M. Blüher. 2006. Vaspin gene expression in human adipose tissue: association with obesity and type 2 diabetes. *Biochem. Biophys. Res. Commun.* 339:430–436.

Klöting N., P. Kovacs, M. Kern, J. T. Heiker, M. Fasshauer, M. R. Schön, M. Stumvoll, A. G. Beck-Sickinger, and M. Blüher. 2011. Central vaspin administration acutely reduces food intake and has sustained blood glucose-lowering effects. *Diabetologia* 54:1819–1823.

Kluth, D., A. Banning, I. Paur, R. Blomhoff and R. Brigelius-Flohe. 2007. Modulation of pregnane X receptor- and electrophile responsive element-mediated gene expression by dietary polyphenolic compounds. *Free Radic. Biol. Med.* 42:315–325.

Knab, A. M., R. A. Shanely, F. Jin, M. D. Austin, W. Sha, and D. C. Nieman. 2011. Quercetin with vitamin C, and niacin does not affect body mass or composition. *Appl. Physiol. Nutr. Metab.* 36:331–338.

Kobori, M., S. Masumoto, Y. Akimoto, and H. Oike. 2011. Chronic dietary intake of quercetin alleviates hepatic fat accumulation associated with consumption of a Western-style diet in C57/BL6J mice. *Mol. Nutr. Food Res.* 55:530–540.

Koizumi, A., Y. Wada, M. Tuskada, T. Kayo, M. Naruse, K. Horiuchi, T. Mogi, M. Yoshioka, M. Sasaki, Y. Miyamaura, T. Abe, K. Ohtomo, and R. L. Walford. 1996. A tumor preventive effect of dietary restriction is antagonized by a high housing temperature through deprivation of torpor. *Mech. Ageing Dev.* 92:67–82.

Kojima, T., H. Kamei, T. Aizu, Y. Arai, M. Takayama, S. Nakazawa, Y. Ebihara, H. Inagaki, Y. Masui, Y. Gondo, Y. Sakaki, and N. Hirose. 2004. Association analysis between longevity in the Japanese population, and polymorphic variants of genes involved in insulin, and insulin-like growth factor 1 signaling pathways. *Exp. Gerontol.* 39:1595–1598.

Koltai, E., Z. Szabo, M. Atalay, I. Boldogh, H. Naito, S. Goto, C. Nyakas, and Z. Radak. 2010. Exercise alters SIRT1, SIRT6, NAD, and NAMPT levels in skeletal muscle of aged rats. *Mech. Ageing Dev.* 131:21–28.

Kondo, M., R. Shibata, R. Miura, M. Shimano, K. Kondo, P. Li, T. Ohashi, S. Kihara, N. Maeda, K. Walsh, N. Ouchi, and T. Murohara. 2009. Caloric restriction stimulates revascularization in response to ischemia via adiponectin-mediated activation of endothelial nitric-oxide synthase. *J. Biol. Chem.* 284:1718–1724.

Kourtis, N. and N. Tavernarakis. 2011. Cellular stress response pathways, and ageing: intricate molecular relationships. *EMBO J.* 30:2520–2531.

Koutsari, C. and M. D. Jensen. 2006. Free fatty acid metabolism in human obesity. *J. Lipid Res.* 47:1643–1650.

Kovacikova, M., M. Vitkova, E. Klimcakova, J. Polak, J. Hejnova, M. Bajzova, Z. Kovacova, N. Viguerie, D. Langin, and V. Stich. 2008. Visfatin expression in subcutaneous adipose tissue of pre-menopausal women: relation to hormones and weight reduction. *Eur. J. Clin. Invest.* 38:516–522.

Kraft C., M. Peter, and K. Hofmann. 2010. Selective autophagy: ubiquitin-mediated recognition, and beyond. *Nat. Cell Biol.* 12:836–841.

Krishnan, J., C. Danzer, T. Simka, J. Ukropec, K. M. Walter, S. Kumpf, P. Mirtschink, B. Ukropcova, D. Gasperikova, T. Pedrazzini, and W. Krek. 2012. Dietary obesity-associated Hif1alpha activation in adipocytes restricts fatty acid oxidation and energy expenditure via suppression of the Sirt2-NAD+ system. *Genes Dev.* 26:259–270.

Krist, J., K. Wieder, N. Klöting, A. Oberbach, S. Kralisch, T. Wiesner, M. R. Schön, D. Gärtner, A. Dietrich, E. Shang, T. Lohmann, M. Dreßler, M. Fasshauer, M. Stumvoll, and M. Blüher. 2013. Effects of weight loss and exercise on apelin serum concentrations and adipose tissue expression in human obesity. *Obes. Facts.* 6:57–69.

Kristan, D. M. 2008. Caloric restriction and susceptibility to intact pathogens. *Age (Dordr.)* 30:147–156.

Krzyzanowska, K., F. Mittermayer, W. Krugluger, H. P. Kopp, and G. Schernthaner. 2006. Increase in visfatin after weight loss induced by gastroplastic surgery. *Obesity* 14:1886–1889.

Kuba, K., L. Zhang, Y. Imai, S. Arab, M. Chen, Y. Maekawa, M. Leschnik, A. Leibbrandt, M. Markovic, J. Schwaighofer, N. Beetz, R. Musialek, G. G. Neely, V. Komnenovic, U. Kolm, B. Metzler, R. Ricci, H. Hara, A. Meixner, M. Nghiem, X. Chen, F. Dawood, K. M. Wong, R. Sarao, E. Cukerman, A. Kimura, L. Hein, J. Thalhammer, P. P. Liu, and J. M. Penninger. 2007. Impaired heart contractility in apelin gene-deficient mice associated with aging and pressure overload. *Circul. Res.* 101:e32–e42.

Kuk, J. L. and C. I. Ardern. 2009. Are metabolically normal but obese individuals at lower risk for all-cause mortality? *Diabetes Care* 32:2297–2299.

Kurosu, H., M. Yamamoto, J. D. Clark, J. V. Pastor, A. Nandi, P. Gurnani, O. P. McGuinness, H. Chikuda, M. Yamaguchi, H. Kawaguchi, I. Shimomura, Y. Takayama, J. Herz, C. R. Kahn, K. P. Rosenblatt, and M. Kuro-o. 2005. Suppression of aging in mice by the hormone Klotho. *Science* 309:1829–1833.

Kursawe, R., S. Caprio, C. Giannini, D. Narayan, A. Lin, E. D'Adamo, M. Shaw, B. Pierpont, S. W. Cushman, and G. I. Shulman. 2013. Decreased transcription of ChREBP-alpha/beta isoforms in abdominal subcutaneous adipose tissue of obese adolescents with prediabetes or early type 2 diabetes: associations with insulin resistance and hyperglycemia. *Diabetes* 62:837–844.

Kusminski, C. M., P. G. McTernan, and S. Kumar. 2005. Role of resistin in obesity, insulin resistance and type II diabetes. *Clin. Sci.* 109:243–256.

Kwak, M. K., N. Wakabayashi, K. Itoh, H. Motohashi, M. Yamamoto and T. W. Kensler. 2003. Modulation of gene expression by cancer chemopreventive dithiolethiones through the Keap1-Nrf2 pathway. Identification of novel gene clusters for cell survival. *J. Biol. Chem.* 278:8135–8145.

Kwon, J. Y., S. G. Seo, S. Yue, J. X. Cheng, K. W. Lee, and K. H. Kim. 2012. An inhibitory effect of resveratrol in the mitotic clonal expansion, and insulin signaling pathway in the early phase of adipogenesis. *Nutr. Res.* 32:607–616.

Lafontan, M. 2014. Adipose tissue and adipocyte dysregulation. *Diabetes Metab.* 40:16–28.

Lagouge, M., C. Argmann, Z. Gerhart-Hines, H. Meziane, C. Lerin, F. Daussin, N. Messadeq, J. Milne, P. Lambert, P. Elliott, B. Geny, M. Laakso P., Puigserver, and J. Auwerx. 2006. Resveratrol improves mitochondrial function, and protects against metabolic disease by activating SIRT1, and PGC-1alpha. *Cell* 127:1109–1122.

Landry, J., A. Sutton, S. T. Tafrov, R. C. Heller, J. Stebbins, L. Pillus, and R. Sternglanz. 2000. The silencing protein SIR2, and its homologs are NAD-dependent protein deacetylases. *Proc. Natl Acad. Sci. USA* 97:5807–5811.

Lane, M. A., D. J. Baer, W. V. Rumpler, R. Weindruch, D. K. Ingram, E. M. Tilmont, R. G. Cutler, and G. S. Roth. 1996. Calorie restriction lowers body temperature in rhesus monkeys, consistent with a postulated anti-aging mechanism in rodents. *Proc. Natl Acad. Sci. USA* 93:4159–4164.

Lane, M. A., A. Black, A. M. Handy, S. A. Shapses, E. M. Tilmont, T. L. Kiefer, D. K. Ingram, and G. S. Roth. 2001. Energy restriction does not alter bone mineral metabolism or reproductive cycling and hormones in female rhesus monkeys. *J. Nutr.* 131:820–827.

Lanza, I. R., P. Zabielski, K. A. Klaus, D. M. Morse, C. J. Heppelmann, H. R. Bergen 3rd, S. Dasari, S. Walrand, K. R. Short, M. L. Johnson, M. M. Robinson, J. M. Schimke, D. R. Jakaitis, Y. W. Asmann, Z. Sun, and K. S. Nair. 2012. Chronic caloric restriction preserves mitochondrial function in senescence without increasing mitochondrial biogenesis. *Cell Metab.* 16:777–788.

Larson-Meyer, D. E., L. K. Heilbronn, L. M. Redman, B. R. Newcomer, M. I. Frisard, S. Anton, S. R. Smith, A. Alfonso, and E. Ravussin. 2006. Effect of calorie restriction with or without exercise on insulin sensitivity, beta-cell function, fat cell size, and ectopic lipid in overweight subjects. *Diabetes Care* 29:1337–1344.

Leal, V. O. and D. Mafra. 2013. Adipokines in obesity. *Clin. Chim. Acta* 419:87–94.

Lee, A. H., K. Heidtman, G. S. Hotamisligil, and L. H. Glimcher. 2011a. Dual, and opposing roles of the unfolded protein response regulated by IRE1alpha, and XBP1 in proinsulin processing, and insulin secretion. *Proc. Natl Acad. Sci. USA* 108:8885–8890.

Lee, C. K., R. G. Klopp, R. Weindruch, and T. A. Prolla. 1999. Gene expression profile of aging, and its retardation by caloric restriction. *Science* 285:1390–1393.

Lee, H., S. Bae, and Y. Yoon. 2013. The anti-adipogenic effects of (−)epigallocatechin gallate are dependent on the WNT/β-catenin pathway. *J. Nutr. Biochem.* 24:1232–1240.

Lee, I. H., L. Cao, R. Mostoslavsky, D. B. Lombard, J. Liu, N. E. Bruns, M. Tsokos, F. W. Alt, and T. Finkel. 2008. A role for the NAD-dependent deacetylase Sirt1 in the regulation of autophagy. *Proc. Natl Acad. Sci. USA* 105:3374–3379.

Lee, J. and U. Ozcan. 2014. Unfolded Protein Response Signaling, and Metabolic Diseases. *J. Biol. Chem.* 289:1203–1211.

Lee, J. E., J. I. Heo, S. H. Park, J. H. Kim, Y. J. Kho, H. J. Kang, H. Y. Chung, J. L. Yoon, and J. Y. Lee. 2011b. Calorie restriction (CR) reduces age-dependent decline of non-homologous end joining (NHEJ) activity in rat tissues. *Exp. Gerontol.* 46:891–896.

Lee, J. S., Z. Zheng, R. Mendez, S. W. Ha, Y. Xie, and K. Zhang. 2012. Pharmacologic ER stress induces non-alcoholic steatohepatitis in an animal model. *Toxicol. Lett.* 211:29–38.

Lee, M. S., C. T. Kim, and Y. Kim. 2009. Green tea (−)-epigallocatechin-3-gallate reduces body weight with regulation of multiple genes expression in adipose tissue of diet-induced obese mice. *Ann. Nutr. Metab.* 54:151–157.

Lee, Y., R. H. Naseem, L. Duplomb, B. H. Park, D. J. Garry, J. A. Richardson, J. E. Schaffer, and R. H. Unger. 2004. Hyperleptinemia prevents lipotoxic cardiomyopathy in acyl CoA synthase transgenic mice. *Proc. Natl Acad. Sci. USA* 101:13624–13629.

Lee, Y. M., J. S. Choi, M. H. Kim, M. H. Jung, Y. S. Lee, and J. Song. 2006. Effects of dietary genistein on hepatic lipid metabolism, and mitochondrial function in mice fed high-fat diets. *Nutrition* 22:956–964.

Lefevre, M., L. M. Redman, L. K. Heilbronn, J. V. Smith, C. K. Martin, J. C. Rood, F. L. Greenway, D. A. Williamson, S. R. Smith, E. Ravussin and Pennington CALERIE team. 2009. Caloric restriction alone, and with exercise improves CVD risk in healthy non-obese individuals. *Atherosclerosis* 203:206–213.

Lemasters, J. J. 2005. Selective mitochondria autophagy, or mitophagy, as a targetd defense against oxidative stress, mitochondrial dysfunction, and aging. *Rejuvenation Res.* 8:3–5.

Lesser, S., R. Cermak, and S. Wolffram. 2004. Bioavailability of quercetin in pigs is influenced by the dietary fat content. *J. Nutr.* 134:1508–1511.

Lhoták, S., S. Sood, E. Brimble, R. E. Carlisle, S. M. Colgan, A. Mazzetti, J. G. Dickhout, A. J. Ingram, and R. C. Austin. 2012. ER stress contributes to renal proximal tubule injury by increasing SREBP-2-mediated lipid accumulation, and apoptotic cell death. *Am. J. Physiol. Renal Physiol.* 303:F266–278.

Li, J. and N. J. Holbrook. 2004. Elevated gadd153/chop expression, and enhanced c-Jun N-terminal protein kinase activation sensitizes aged cells to ER stress. *Exp. Gerontol.* 39:735–744.

Li, X. J. and S. Li. 2011. Proteasomal dysfunction in aging, and Huntington disease. *Neurobiol. Dis.* 43:35–42.

Liao, C. Y., B. A. Rikke, T. E. Johnson, V. Diaz, and J. F. Nelson. 2010. Genetic variation in the murine lifespan response to dietary restriction: from life extension to life shortening. *Aging Cell* 9:92–95.

Lieb, W., R. Safa, E. J. Benjamin, V. Xanthakis, X. Yin, L. M. Sullivan, M. G. Larson, H. M. Smith, J. A. Vita, G. F. Mitchell, D. B. Sawyer, and R. S. Vasan. 2009. Vascular endothelial growth factor, its soluble receptor, and hepatocyte growth factor: clinical and genetic correlates and association with vascular function. *Eur. Heart J.* 30:1121–1127.

Lieb, W., J. P. Zachariah, V. Xanthakis, R. Safa, M. H. Chen, L. M. Sullivan, M. G. Larson, H. M. Smith, Q. Yang, G. F. Mitchell, J. A. Vita, D. B. Sawyer, and R. S. Vasan. 2010. Clinical and genetic correlates of circulating angiopoietin-2 and soluble Tie-2 in the community. *Circul. Cardiovasc. Genet.* 3:300–306.

Liesa, M., and O. S. Shirihai. 2013. Mitochondrial dynamics in the regulation of nutrient utilization and energy expenditure. *Cell Metab.* 17:491–506.

Lim, J. H., Y. M. Lee, Y. S. Chun, J. Chen, J. E. Kim, and J. W. Park. 2010. Sirtuin 1 modulates cellular responses to hypoxia by deacetylating hypoxia-inducible factor 1alpha. *Mol. Cell* 38:864–878.

Lim, J. H., Z. Gerhart-Hines, J. E. Dominy, Y. Lee, S. Kim, M. Tabata, Y. K. Xiang, and P. Puigserver. 2013. Oleic acid stimulates complete oxidation of fatty acids through protein kinase A-dependent activation of SIRT1-PGC1α complex. *J. Biol. Chem.* 288:7117–7126.

Lim, S. Y., S. M. Davidson, A. J. Paramanathan, C. C. Smith, D. M. Yellon, and D. J. Hausenloy. 2008. The novel adipocytokine visfatin exerts direct cardioprotective effects. *J. Cell. Mol. Med.* 12:1395–1403.

Lima, C. F., C. Pereira-Wilson, and S. I. Rattan. 2011. Curcumin induces heme oxygenase-1 in normal human skin fibroblasts through redox signaling: relevance for anti-aging intervention. *Mol. Nutr. Food Res.* 55:430–442.

Lin, J., M. A. Della-Fera, and C. A. Baile. 2005. Green tea polyphenol epigallocatechin gallate inhibits adipogenesis, and induces apoptosis in 3T3-L1 adipocytes. *Obes. Res.* 13:982–990.

Lind, L., L. Berglund, A. Larsson, and J. Sundstrom 2011. Endothelial function in resistance and conduit arteries and 5-year risk of cardiovascular disease. *Circulation* 123:1545–1551.

Liszt, G., E. Ford, M. Kurtev, and L. Guarente. 2005. Mouse Sir2 homolog SIRT6 is a nuclear ADP-ribosyltransferase. *J. Biol. Chem.* 280:21313–21320.

Liu, J., C. S. Fox, D. Hickson, D. Sarpong, L. Ekunwe, W. D. May, G. W. Hundley, J. J. Carr, and H. A. Taylor. 2010. Pericardial adipose tissue, atherosclerosis, and cardiovascular disease risk factors: the Jackson Heart Study. *Diabetes Care* 33:1635–1639.

Llaneza P., C. Gonzalez, J. Fernandez-Inarrrea, A. Alonso, F. Diaz, I. Arnott, and J. Ferrer-Barriendos. 2011. Soy isoflavones,diet, and physical exercise modify serum cytokines in healthy obese postmenopausal women. *Phytomedicine* 18:245–250.

Loebig, M., J. Klement, A. Schmoller, S. Betz, N. Heuck, U. Schweiger, A. Peters, B. Schultes, and K. M. Oltmanns. 2010. Evidence for a relationship between VEGF and BMI independent of insulin sensitivity by glucose clamp procedure in a homogenous group healthy young men. *PLoS One* 5:e12610.

Longo, V. D. and L. Fontana. 2010. Calorie restriction and cancer prevention: metabolic and molecular mechanisms. *Trends Pharmacol. Sci.* 31:89–98.

Lundgren, M., M. Svensson, S. Lindmark, F. Renström, T. Ruge, and J. W. Eriksson. 2007. Fat cell enlargement is an independent marker of insulin resistance and "hyperleptinaemia". *Diabetologia* 50:625–633.

Luo, J., A. Y. Nikolaev, S. Imai, D. Chen, F. Su, A. Shiloh, L. Guarente, and W. Gu. 2001. Negative control of p53 by Sir2alpha promotes cell survival under stress. *Cell* 107:137–148.

Macarulla, M. T., G. Alberdi, S. Gómez, I. Tueros, C. Bald, V. M. Rodríguez, J. A. Martínez, and M. P. Portillo. 2009. Effects of different doses of resveratrol on body fat, and serum parameters in rats fed a hypercaloric diet. *J. Physiol. Biochem.* 65:369–376.

Madeo, F., N. Tavernarakis, and G. Kroemer. 2010. Can autophagy promote longevity? *Nat. Cell Biol.* 12:842–846.

Malhi, H. and R. J. Kaufman. 2011. Endoplasmic reticulum stress in liver disease. *J. Hepatol.* 54:795–809.

Malhotra, J. D. and R. J. Kaufman. 2007. Endoplasmic reticulum stress, and oxidative stress: a vicious cycle or a double-edged sword? *Antioxid. Redox Signal.* 9:2277–2293.

Malhotra, J. D., H. Miao, K. Zhang, A. Wolfson, S. Pennathur, S. W. Pipe, and R. J. Kaufman. 2008. Antioxidants reduce endoplasmic reticulum stress, and improve protein secretion. *Proc. Natl Acad. Sci. USA* 105:18525–18530.

Malloy, V. L., R. A. Krajcik, S. J. Bailey, G. Hristopoulos, J. D. Plummer, and N. Orentreich. 2006. Methionine restriction decreases visceral fat mass, and preserves insulin action in aging male Fischer 344 rats independent of energy restriction. *Aging Cell* 5:305–314.

Malovini, A., M. Illario, G. Iaccarino, F. Villa, A. Ferrario, R. Roncarati, C. V. Anselmi, V. Novelli, E. Cipolletta, E. Leggiero, A. Orro, M. R. Rusciano, L. Milanesi, A. S. Maione, G. Condorelli, R. Bellazzi, and A. A. Puca. 2011. Association study on long-living individuals from Southern Italy identifies rs10491334 in the CAMKIV gene that regulates survival proteins. *Rejuvenation Res.* 14:283–291.

Manolopoulos, K. N., F. Karpe, and K. N. Frayn. 2010. Gluteofemoral body fat as a determinant of metabolic health. *Int. J. Obes. (Lond.)* 34:949–959.

Manzoni, M. S., E. A. Rossi, I. Z. Carlos, R. C. Vendramini, A. C. Duarte, and A. R. Dâmaso. 2005. Fermented soy product supplemented with isoflavones affected fat depots in juvenile rats. *Nutrition* 21:1018–1024.

Marino, M., C. Dolfi, C. Paradiso, G. Cavallini, M. Masini, Z. Gori, M. Pollera, A. Trentalance, and E. Bergamini. 1998. Age-dependent accumulation of dolichol in rat liver: is tissue dolichol a biomarker of aging? *J. Gerontol. A. Biol. Sci. Med. Sci.* 53:B87–B93.

Marchal, J., S. Blanc, J. Epelbaum, F. Aujard, and F. Pifferi. 2012. Effects of chronic calorie restriction or dietary resveratrol supplementation on insulin sensitivity markers in a primate, Microcebus murinus. *PLoS One* 7:e34289.

Marchal, J., A. Dal-Pan, J. Epelbaum, S. Blanc, S. Mueller, M. Wittig Kieffer, F. Metzger, F. Aujard, and RESTRIKAL Consortium. 2013. Calorie restriction, and resveratrol supplementation prevent age-related DNA, and RNA oxidative damage in a non-human primate. *Exp. Gerontol.* 48:992–1000.

Marciniak, S. J., C. Y. Yun, S. Oyadomari, I. Novoa, Y. Zhang, R. Jungreis, K. Nagata, H. P. Harding, and D. Ron. 2004. CHOP induces death by promoting protein synthesis, and oxidation in the stressed endoplasmic reticulum. *Genes Dev.* 18:3066–3077.

Martin-Montalvo, A., E. M. Mercken, S. J. Mitchell, H. H. Palacios, P. L. Mote, M. Scheibye-Knudsen, A. P. Gomes, T. M. Ward, R. K. Minor, M. J. Blouin, M. Schwab, M. Pollak, Y. Zhang, Y. Yu, K. G. Becker, V. A. Bohr, D. K. Ingram, D. A. Sinclair, N. S. Wolf, S. R. Spindler, M. Bernier, and R. de Cabo. 2013. Metformin improves healthspan, and lifespan in mice. *Nat. Commun.* 4:2192.

Masoro, E. J. 2002. *Caloric Restriction: A Key to Understand, and Modulating Aging*, Vijg, J. (ed.). Elsevier: Amsterdam.

Masoro, E. J. 2005. Overview of caloric restriction and ageing. *Mech. Ageing Dev.* 126:913–922.

Massey, A., R. Kiffin, and A. M. Cuervo. 2004. Pathophysiology of chaperone-mediated autophagy. *Int. J. Biochem. Cell Biol.* 36:2420–2434.

Massudi, H., R. Grant, N. Braidy, J. Guest, B. Farnsworth, and G. J. Guillemin. 2012. Age-associated changes in oxidative stress, and NAD+ metabolism in human tissue. *PLoS One* 7:e42357.

Mattagajasingh, I., C. S. Kim, A. Naqvi, T. Yamamori, T. A. Hoffman, S. B. Jung, J. DeRicco, K. Kasuno, and K. Irani. 2007. SIRT1 promotes endothelium-dependent vascular relaxation by activating endothelial nitric oxide synthase. *Proc. Natl Acad. Sci. USA* 104:14855–14860.

Mattison, J. A., M. A. Lane, G. S. Roth, and D. K. Ingram. 2003. Calorie restriction in rhesus monkeys. *Exp. Gerontol.* 38:35–46.

Mattison, J. A., G. S. Roth, T. M. Beasley, E. M. Tilmont, A. M. Handy, R. L. Herbert, D. L. Longo, D. B. Allison, J. E. Young, M. Bryant, D. Barnard, W. F. Ward, W. Qi, D. K. Ingram, and R. de Cabo. 2012. Impact of caloric restriction on health, and survival in rhesus monkeys from the NIA study. *Nature* 489:318–321.

Mattson, M. P. 2000. Neuroprotective signaling and the aging brain: take away my food and let me run. *Brain Res.* 886:47–53.

Mattson, M. P. and R. Wan. 2005. Beneficial effects of intermittent fasting, and caloric restriction on the cardiovascular, and cerebrovascular systems. *J. Nutr. Biochem.* 16:129–137.

Mattson, M. P., W. Duan, and Z. Guo. 2003. Meal size and frequency affect neuronal plasticity and vulnerability to disease: cellular and molecular mechanisms. *J. Neurochem.* 84:417–431.

Mattu, H. S. and H. S. Randeva. 2013. Role of adipokines in cardiovascular disease. *J. Endocrinol.* 216:T17–T36.

McCarter, R. J. and J. Palmer. 1992. Energy metabolism, and aging: a lifelong study of Fischer 344 rats. *Am. J. Physiol.* 263:E448–E452.

McCay, C. M., M. F. Crowell, and L. A. Maynard. 1935. The effect of retarded growthupon length of lifespan, and upon ultimate body size. *J. Nutr.* 10:63–79.

McKee A. J., M. A. DePetrillo, A. M. Gluesenkamp, A. C. Hartley, S. V. Verhoff, K. L. Zavodni, and T. P. Combs. 2010. Calorie restriction and dwarf mice in gerontological research. *Gerontology* 56:404–409.

McKiernan, S. H., R. J. Colman, M. Lopez, T. M. Beasley, J. M. Aiken, R. M. Anderson, and R. Weindruch. 2010. Caloric restriction delays aging-induced cellular phenotypes in rhesus monkey skeletal muscle. *Exp. Gerontol.* 46:23–29.

McLaughlin, T., C. Lamendola, A. Liu, and F. Abbasi. 2011. Preferential fat deposition in subcutaneous versus visceral depots is associated with insulin sensitivity. *J. Clin. Endocrinol. Metab.* 96:E1756–E1760.

Mercader, J., A. Palou, and M. L. Bonet. 2011. Resveratrol enhances fatty acid oxidation capacity, and reduces resistin, and Retinol-Binding Protein 4 expression in white adipocytes. *J. Nutr. Biochem.* 22:828–834.

Mercken, E. M., S. D. Crosby, D. W. Lamming, L. JeBailey, S. Krzysik-Walker, D. T. Villareal, M. Capri, C. Franceschi, Y. Zhang, K. Becker, D. M. Sabatini, R. de Cabo, and L. Fontana. 2013. Calorie restriction in humans inhibits the PI3K/AKT pathway, and induces a younger transcription profile. *Aging Cell* 12:645–651.

Merry, B. J. 2005. Dietary restriction in rodents – delayed or retarded ageing? *Mech. Ageing Dev.* 126:951–959.

Messaoudi, I., J. Warner, M. Fischer, B. Park, B. Hill, J. Mattison, M. A. Lane, G. S. Roth, D. K. Ingram, L. J. Picker, D. C. Douek, M. Mori, and J. Nikolich-Zugich. 2006. Delay of T cell senescence by caloric restriction in aged long-lived nonhuman primates. *Proc. Natl Acad. Sci. USA* 103:19448–19453.

Meydani, M. and S. T. Hasan. 2010. Dietary polyphenols, and obesity. *Nutrients* 2:737–751.

Meydani, M., S. Das, M. Band, S. Epstein, and S. Roberts. 2011. The effect of caloric restriction, and glycemic load on measures of oxidative stress, and antioxidants in humans: results from the CALERIE Trial of Human Caloric Restriction. *J. Nutr. Health Aging* 15:456–460.

Meyer, T. E., S. J. Kovács, A. A. Ehsani, S. Klein, J. O. Holloszy, and L. Fontana. 2006. Long-term caloric restriction ameliorates the decline in diastolic function in humans. *J. Am. Coll. Cardiol.* 47:398–402.

Miani, M., M. L. Colli, L. Ladriere, M. Cnop, and D. L. Eizirik. 2012. Mild endoplasmic reticulum stress augments the proinflammatory effect of IL-1beta in pancreatic rat beta-cells via the IRE1alpha/XBP1s pathway. *Endocrinology* 153:3017–3028.

Michishita, E., J. Y. Park, J. M. Burneskis, J. C. Barrett, and I. Horikawa. 2005. Evolutionarily conserved, and nonconserved cellular localizations, and functions of human SIRT proteins. *Mol. Biol. Cell* 16: 4623–4635.

Michishita, E., R. A. McCord, E. Berber, M. Kioi, H. Padilla-Nash, M. Damian, P. Cheung, R. Kusumoto, T. L. Kawahara, J. C. Barrett, H. Y. Chang, V. A. Bohr, T. Ried, O. Gozani, and K. F. Chua. 2008. SIRT6 is a histone H3 lysine 9 deacetylase that modulates telomeric chromatin. *Nature* 452:492–496.

Miller R. A., D. E. Harrison, C. M. Astle, J. A. Baur, A. R. Boyd, R. de Cabo, E. Fernandez, K. Flurkey, M. A. Javors, J. F. Nelson, C. J. Orihuela, S. Pletcher, Z. D. Sharp, D. Sinclair, J. W. Starnes, J. E. Wilkinson, N. L. Nadon, and R. Strong. 2011. Rapamycin, but not resveratrol or simvastatin, extends life span of genetically heterogeneous mice. *J. Gerontol. A. Biol. Sci. Med. Sci.* 66:191–201.

Milne, J. C., P. D. Lambert, S. Schenk, D. P. Carney, J. J. Smith, D. J. Gagne, L. Jin, O. Boss, R. B. Perni, C. B. Vu, J. E. Bemis, R. Xie, J. S. Disch, P. Y. Ng, J. J. Nunes, A. V. Lynch, H. Yang, H. Galonek, K. Israelian, W. Choy, A. Iffland, S. Lavu, O. Medvedik, D. A. Sinclair, J. M. Olefsky, M. R. Jirousek, P. J. Elliott, and C. H. Westphal. 2007. Small molecule activators of SIRT1 as therapeutics for the treatment of type 2 diabetes. *Nature* 450:712–716.

Minor, R. K., J. W. Chang, and R. de Cabo. 2009. Hungry for life: how the arcuate nucleus and neuropeptide Y may play a critical role in mediating the benefits of calorie restriction. *Mol. Cell. Endocrinol.* 299:79–88.

Mohammadi, A., A. Sahebkar, M. Iranshahi, M. Amini, R. Khojasteh, M. Ghayour-Mobarhan, and G. A. Ferns. 2013. Effects of supplementation with curcuminoids on dyslipidemia in obese patients: a randomized crossover trial. *Phytother. Res.* 27:374–379.

Monteiro R., M. Assunção, J. P. andrade, D. Neves, C. Calhau, and I. Azevedo. 2008. Chronic green tea consumption decreases body mass, induces aromatase expression, and changes proliferation, and apoptosis in adult male rat adipose tissue. *J. Nutr.* 138:2156–2163.

Moreno-Navarrete, J. M., F. Ortega, A. Castro, M. Sabater, W. Ricart, and J. M. Fernández-Real. 2011. Circulating omentin as a novel biomarker of endothelial dysfunction. *Obesity (Silver Spring)* 19:1552–1559.

Moschen, A. R., A. Kaser, B. Enrich, B. Mosheimer, M. Theurl, H. Niederegger, and H. Tilg. 2007. Visfatin, an adipocytokine with proinflammatory and immunomodulating properties. *J. Immunol.* 178:1748–1758.

Morselli, E., M. C. Maiuri, M. Markaki, E. Megalou, A. Pasparaki, K. Palikaras, A. Criollo, L. Galluzzi, S. A. Malik, I. Vitale, M. Michaud, F. Madeo, N. Tavernarakis, and G. Kroemer. 2010. The life span-prolonging effect of sirtuin-1 is mediated by autophagy. *Autophagy* 6:186–188.

Mostoslavsky, R., K. F. Chua, D. B. Lombard, W. W. Pang, M. R. Fischer, L. Gellon, P. Liu, G. Mostoslavsky, S. Franco, M. M. Murphy, K. D. Mills, P. Patel, J. T. Hsu, A. L. Hong, E. Ford, H. L. Cheng, C. Kennedy, N. Nunez, R. Bronson, D. Frendewey, W. Auerbach, D. Valenzuela, M. Karow, M. O. Hottiger, S. Hursting, J. C. Barrett, L. Guarente, R. Mulligan, B. Demple, G. D. Yancopoulos, and F. W. Alt. 2006. Genomic instability, and aging-like phenotype in the absence of mammalian SIRT6. *Cell* 124:315–329.

Mouton, P. R., M. E. Chachich, C. Quigley, E. Spangler, and D. K. Ingram. 2009. Caloric restriction attenuates amyloid deposition in middle-aged dtg APP/PS1 mice. *Neurosci. Lett.* 464:184–187.

Moynihan, K. A., A. A. Grimm, M. M. Plueger, E. Bernal-Mizrachi, E. Ford, C. Cras-Méneur, M. A. Permutt, and S. Imai. 2005. Increased dosage of mammalian Sir2 in pancreatic beta cells enhances glucose-stimulated insulin secretion in mice. *Cell Metab.* 2:105–117.

Murano, I., G. Barbatelli, V. Parisani, C. Latini, G. Muzzonigro, M. Castellucci, and S. Cinti. 2008. Dead adipocytes, detected as crown-like structures, are prevalent in visceral fat depots of genetically obese mice. *J. Lipid Res.* 49:1562–1568.

Muzumdar, R., D. B. Allison, D. M. Huffman, X. Ma, G. Atzmon, F. H. Einstein, S. Fishman, A. D. Poduval, T. Mcvei, S. W. Keith, and N. Barzilai. 2008. Visceral adipose tissue modulates mammalian longevity. *Aging Cell* 7:438–440.

Na, X. L., J. Ezaki, F. Sugiyama, H. B. Cui, and Y. Ishimi. 2008. Isoflavone regulates lipid metabolism via expression of related genes in OVX rats fed on a high-fat diet. *Biomed. Environ. Sci.* 21:357–364.

Nadler, J. and S. Scott. 1994. Evidence that pioglitazone increases intracellular free magnesium concentration in freshly isolated rat adipocytes. *Biochem. Biophys. Res. Commun.* 202:416–421.

Naidoo, N. 2009a. The endoplasmic reticulum stress response, and aging. *Rev. Neurosci.* 20:23–37.

Naidoo, N. 2009b. ER, and aging – protein folding, and the ER stress response. *Ageing Res. Rev.* 8:150–159.

Naidoo, N., M. Ferber, M. Master, Y. Zhu, and A. I. Pack. 2008. Aging impairs the unfolded protein response to sleep deprivation, and leads to proapoptotic signaling. *J. Neurosci.* 28:6539–6548.

Nair, U., A. Jotwani, J. Geng, N. Gammoh, D. Richerson, W. L. Yen, J. Griffith, S. Nag, K. Wang, T. Moss, M. Baba, J. A. McNew, X. Jiang, F. Reggiori, T. J. Melia, and D. J. Klionsky. 2011. SNARE proteins are required for macroautophagy. *Cell* 146:290–302.

Nakagawa, T., D. J. Lomb, M. C. Haigis, and L. Guarente. 2009. SIRT5 Deacetylates carbamoyl phosphate synthetase 1, and regulates the urea cycle. *Cell* 137:560–570.

Nakahata, Y., M. Kaluzova, B. Grimaldi, S. Sahar, J. Hirayama, D. Chen, L. P. Guarente, and P. Sassone-Corsi. 2008. The NAD+-dependent deacetylase SIRT1 modulates CLOCK-mediated chromatin remodeling, and circadian control. *Cell* 134:329–340.

Nakai, A., O. Yamaguchi, T. Takeda, Y. Higuchi, S. Hikoso, M. Taniike, S. Omiya, I. Mizote, Y. Matsumura, M. Asahi, K. Nishida, M. Hori, N. Mizushima, and K. Otsu. 2007. The role of autophagy in cardiomyocytes in the basal state, and in response to hemodynamic stress. *Nat. Med.* 13:619–624.

Neves, D., M. Assunção, F. Marques, J. P. andrade, and H. Almeida. 2008. Does regular consumption of green tea influence VEGF, and its receptors expression in aged rat erectile tissue? Possible implications in vasculogenic erectile dysfunction progression. *Age* 30:217–228.

Nielsen, F. H. 2010. Magnesium, inflammation, and obesity in chronic disease. *Nutr. Rev.* 68:333–340.

Niemann, B., R. E. Silber, and S. Rohrbach. 2008. Age-specific effects of short and long-term caloric restriction on the expression of adiponectin and adiponectin receptors: influence of intensity of food restriction. *Exp. Gerontol.* 43:706–713.

Nishimura, S., I. Manabe, M. Nagasaki, Y. Hosoya, H. Yamashita, H. Fujita, M. Ohsugi, K. Tobe, T. Kadowaki, R. Nagai, and S. Sugiura. 2007. Adipogenesis in obesity requires close interplay between differentiating adipocytes, stromal cells, and blood vessels. *Diabetes* 56:1517–1526.

Nisoli, E., C. Tonello, A. Cardile, V. Cozzi, R. Bracale, L. Tedesco, S. Falcone, A. Valerio, O. Cantoni, E. Clementi, S. Moncada, and M. O. Carruba. 2005. Calorie restriction promotes mitochondrial biogenesis by inducing the expression of eNOS. *Science* 310:314–317.

North, B. J. and E. Verdin. 2004. Sirtuins: Sir2-related NAD-dependent protein deacetylases. *Genome Biol.* 5:224.

North, B. J., B. L. Marshall, M. T. Borra, J. M. Denu, and E. Verdin. 2003. The human Sir2 ortholog, SIRT2, is an NAD+-dependent tubulin deacetylase. *Mol. Cell* 11:437–444.

Novoa, I., H. Zeng, H. P. Harding, and D. Ron. 2001. Feedback inhibition of the unfolded protein response by GADD34-mediated dephosphorylation of eIF2alpha. *J. Cell Biol.* 153:1011–1022.

Nuss, J. E., K. B. Choksi, J. H. DeFord, and J. Papaconstantinou. 2008. Decreased enzyme activities of chaperones PDI, and BiP in aged mouse livers. *Biochem. Biophys. Res. Commun.* 365:355–361.

Oberdoerffer, P., S. Michan, M. McVay, R. Mostoslavsky, J. Vann, S. K. Park, A. Hartlerode, J. Stegmuller, A. Hafner, P. Loerch, S. M. Wright, K. D. Mills, A. Bonni, B. A. Yankner, R. Scully, T. A. Prolla, F. W. Alt, and D. A. Sinclair. 2008. SIRT1 redistribution on chromatin promotes genomic stability but alters gene expression during aging. *Cell* 135:907–918.

O'Callaghan, N. J., P. M. Clifton, M. Noakes, and M. Fenech. 2009. Weight loss in obese men is associated with increased telomere length and decreased a basic sites in rectal mucosa. *Rejuvenation Res.* 12:169–176.

Ogata, M., S. Hino, A. Saito, K. Morikawa, S. Kondo, S. Kanemoto, T. Murakami, M. Taniguchi, I. Tanii, K. Yoshinaga, S. Shiosaka, J. A. Hammarback, F. Urano, and K. Imaizumi. 2006. Autophagy is activated for cell survival after endoplasmic reticulum stress. *Mol. Cell. Biol.* 26:9220–9231.

Ogihara, T., T. Asano, H. Katagiri, H. Sakoda, M. Anai, N. Shojima, H. Ono, M. Fujishiro, A. Kushiyama, Y. Fukushima, M. Kikuchi, N. Noguchi, H. Aburatani, Y. Gotoh, I. Komuro, and T. Fujita. 2004. Oxidative stress induces insulin resistance by activating the nuclear factor-kappa B pathway, and disrupting normal subcellular distribution of phosphatidylinositol 3-kinase. *Diabetologia* 47:794–805.

Ognjanovic, S., S. Bao, S. Y. Yamamoto, J. Garibay-Tupas, B. Samal, and G. D. Bryant-Greenwood. 2001. Genomic organization of the gene coding for human pre-B cell colony-enhancing factor and expression in human fetal membranes. *J. Mol. Endocrinol.* 26:107–117.

Ognjanovic, S. and G. D. Bryant-Greenwood. 2002. Pre-B cell colony-enhancing factor, a novel cytokine of human fetal membranes. *Am. J. Obstet. Gynecol.* 187:1051–1058.

Okazaki, N., J. Yan, S. Yuasa, T. Ueno, E. Kominami, Y. Masuho, H. Koga, and M. Muramatsu. 2000. Interaction of the Unc-51-like kinase, and microtubule-associated protein light chain 3 related proteins in the brain: possible role of vesicular transport in axonal elongation. *Brain Res. Mol. Brain Res.* 85:1–12.

Olholm, J., S. K. Paulsen, K. B. Cullberg, B. Richelsen, and S. B. Pedersen. 2010. Anti-inflammatory effect of resveratrol on adipokine expression, and secretion in human adipose tissue explants. *Int. J. Obes. (Lond.)* 34:1546–1553.

Oliveira, J. L., M. H. Aguiar-Oliveira, A. D'Oliveira, R. M. Pereira, C. R. Oliveira, C. T. Farias, J. A. Barreto-Filho, F. D. Anjos-Andrade, C. Marques-Santos, A. C. Nascimento-Junior, E. O. Alves, F. T. Oliveira, V. C. Campos, R. Ximenes, A. Blackford, G. Parmigiani, and R. Salvatori. 2007. Congenital growth hormone (GH) deficiency and atherosclerosis: effects of GH replacement in GH-naive adults. *J. Clin. Endocrinol. Metab.* 92:4664–4670.

Omodei, D. and L. Fontana. 2011. Calorie restriction and prevention of age-associated chronic disease. *FEBS Lett.* 585:1537–1542.

Ooka, H., P. E. Segall, and P. S. Timiras. 1988. Histology, and survival in age-delayed low-tryptophan-fed rats. *Mech. Ageing Dev.* 43:79–98.

Orentreich, N., J. R. Matias, A. DeFelice, and J. A. Zimmerman. 1993. Low methionine ingestion by rats extends life span. *J. Nutr.* 123:269–274.

Ørgaard, A. and L. Jensen. 2008. The effects of soy isoflavones on obesity. *Exp. Biol. Med.* 233:1066–1080.

Osborne, T. B., L. B. Mendel, and E. L. Ferry. 1917. The effect of retardation of growth upon the breeding period and duration of life of rats. *Science* 45:294–295.

Oslowski, C. M. and F. Urano. 2010. A switch from life to death in endoplasmic reticulum stressed beta cells. *Diabetes Obes. Metab.* 12 Suppl 2:58–65.

Ota, H., M. Eto, M. R. Kano, T. Kahyo, M. Setou, S. Ogawa, K. Iijima, M. Akishita, and Y. Ouchi. 2010. Induction of endothelial nitric oxide synthase, SIRT1, and catalase by statins inhibits endothelial senescence through the Akt pathway. *Arterioscler. Thromb. Vasc. Biol.* 30:2205–2211.

Otabe, S., X. Yuan, T. Fukutani, N. Wada, T. Hashinaga, H. Nakayama, N. Hirota, M. Kojima, and K. Yamada. 2007. Overexpression of human adiponectin in transgenic mice results in suppression of fat accumulation and prevention of premature death by high-calorie diet. *Am. J. Physiol. Endocrinol. Metab.* 293:E210–E218.

Otero, M., R. Lago, R. Gomez, F. Lago, C. Dieguez, J. J. Gómez-Reino, and O. Gualillo. 2006. Changes in fat-derived hormones plasma concentrations: adiponectin, leptin, resistin and visfatin in rheumatoid arthritis subjects. *Ann. Rheum. Dis.* 65:1198–1201.

Ouchi N., S. Kihara, Y. Arita, Y. Okamoto, K. Maeda, H. Kuriyama, K. Hotta, M. Nishida, M. Takahashi, M. Muraguchi, Y. Ohmoto, T. Nakamura, S. Yamashita, T. Funahashi, and Y. Matsuzawa. 2000. Adiponectin, an adipocyte-derived plasma protein, inhibits endothelial NF-kappaB signaling through a camp-dependent pathway. *Circulation* 102:1296–1301.

Ouchi, N., S. Kihara, Y. Arita, M. Nishida, A. Matsuyama, Y. Okamoto, M. Ishigami, H. Kuriyama, K. Kishida, H. Nishizawa, K. Hotta, M. Muraguchi, Y. Ohmoto, S. Yamashita, T. Funahashi, and Y. Matsuzawa. 2001. Adipocyte-derived plasma protein, adiponectin, suppresses lipid accumulation in class A scavenger receptors expression in human monocyte-derived macrophages. *Circulation* 103:1057–1063.

Ouchi, N., S. Kihara, T. Funahashi, Y. Matsuzawa, and K. Walsh. 2003. Obesity, adiponectin and vascular inflammatory disease. *Curr. Opin. Lipidol.* 14:561–566.

Ouchi, N., J. L. Parker, J. J. Lugus, and K. Walsh. 2011. Adipokines in inflammation and metabolic disease. *Nat. Rev. Immunol.* 11:85–97.

Owen, M. R., E. Doran, and A. P. Halestrap. 2000. Evidence that metformin exerts its anti-diabetic effects through inhibition of complex 1 of the mitochondrial respiratory chain. *Biochem. J.* 348:607–614.

Oyadomari, S. and M. Mori. 2004. Roles of CHOP/GADD153 in endoplasmic reticulum stress. *Cell Death Differ.* 11:381–389.

Ozcan, L. and I. Tabas. 2012. Role of endoplasmic reticulum stress in metabolic disease, and other disorders. *Annu. Rev. Med.* 63:317–328.

Ozcan, U., Q. Cao, E. Yilmaz, A. H. Lee, N. N. Iwakoshi, E. Ozdelen, G. Tuncman, C. Gorgun, L. H. Glimcher, and G. S. Hotamisligil. 2004. Endoplasmic reticulum stress links obesity, insulin action, and type 2 diabetes. *Science* 306:457–461.

Ozcan, U., E. Yilmaz, L. Ozcan, M. Furuhashi, E. Vaillancourt, R. O. Smith, C. Z. Gorgun, and G. S. Hotamisligil. 2006. Chemical chaperones reduce ER stress, and restore glucose homeostasis in a mouse model of type 2 diabetes. *Science* 313:1137–1140.

Pachikian, B. D., A. M. Neyrinck, L. Deldicque, F. C. De Backer, E. Catry, E. M. Dewulf, F. M. Sohet, L. B. Bindels, A. Everard, M. Francaux, Y. Guiot, P. D. Cani, and N. M. Delzenne. 2010. Changes in intestinal bifidobacteria levels are associated with the inflammatory response in magnesium-deficient mice. *J. Nutr.* 140:509–514.

Pagano, C., C. Pilon, M. Olivieri, P. Mason, R. Fabris, R. Serra, G. Milan, M. Rossato, G. Federspil, and R. Vettor. 2006. Reduced plasma visfatin/pre-B cell colony-enhancing factor in obesity is not related to insulin resistance in humans. *J. Clin. Endocrinol. Metab.* 91:3165–3170.

Palacios, O. M., J. J. Carmona, S. Michan, K. Y. Chen, Y. Manabe, J. L. Ward 3rd, L. J. Goodyear, and Q. Tong. 2009. Diet, and exercise signals regulate SIRT3, and activate AMPK, and PGC-1alpha in skeletal muscle. *Aging* 1:771–783.

Pamplona, R. and G. Barja. 2006. Mitochondrial oxidative stress, aging, and caloric restriction: the protein, and methionine connection. *Biochim. Biophys. Acta* 1757:496–508.

Pamplona, R., M. Portero-Otín, J. Requena, R. Gredilla, and G. Barja. 2002. Oxidative, glycoxidative, and lipoxidative damage to rat heart mitochondrial proteins is lower after 4 months of caloric restriction than in age-matched controls. *Mech. Ageing Dev.* 123:1437–1446.

Pan, J., S. R. Short, S. A. Goff, and J. F. Dice. 1993. Ubiquitin pools, ubiquitin mRNA levels, and ubiquitin-mediated proteolysis in human fibroblasts. *Exp. Gerontol.* 28:39–49.

Pan, M. H., C. S. Lai, M. L. Tsai, J. C. Wu, and C. T. Ho. 2012. Molecular mechanisms for anti-aging by natural dietary compounds. *Mol. Nutr. Food Res.* 56:88–115.

Panchal, S. K., H. Poudyal, and L. Brown. 2012. Quercetin ameliorates cardiovascular, hepatic, and metabolic changes in diet-induced metabolic syndrome in rats. *J. Nutr.* 142:1026–1032.

Parentini, I., G. Cavallini, A. Donati, Z. Gori, and E. Bergamini. 2005. Accumulation of dolichol in older tissues satisfies the proposed criteria to be qualified a biomarker of aging. *J. Gerontol. A. Biol. Sci. Med. Sci.* 60:39–43.

Park, S. K. and T. A. Prolla. 2005. Lessons learned from gene expression profile studies of aging, and caloric restriction. *Ageing Res. Rev.* 4:55–65.

Park, S. J., F. Ahmad, A. Philp, K. Baar, T. Williams, H. Luo, H. Ke, H. Rehmann, R. Taussig, A. L. Brown, M. K. Kim, M. A. Beaven, A. B. Burgin, V. Manganiello, and J. H. Chung. 2012. Resveratrol ameliorates aging-related metabolic phenotypes by inhibiting cAMP phosphodiesterases. *Cell* 148:421–433.

Pasarica, M., O. R. Sereda, L. M. Redman, D. C. Albarado, D. T. Hymel, L. E. Roan, J. C. Rood, D. H. Burk, and S. R. Smith. 2009. Reduced adipose tissue oxygenation in human obesity. *Diabetes* 58:718–725.

Patel, P. and N. Abate. 2013. Role of subcutaneous adipose tissue in the pathogenesis of insulin resistance. *J. Obes.* 2013:489187.

Paz Gavilan, M., J. Vela, A. Castano, B. Ramos, J. C. del Rio, J. Vitorica, and D. Ruano. 2006. Cellular environment facilitates protein accumulation in aged rat hippocampus. *Neurobiol. Aging* 27:973–982.

Pearson, K. J., K. N. Lewis, N. L. Price, J. W. Chang, E. Perez, M. V. Cascajo, K. L. Tamashiro, S. Poosala, A. Csiszar, Z. Ungvari, T. W. Kensler, M. Yamamoto, J. M. Egan, D. L. Longo, D. K. Ingram, P. Navas, and R. de Cabo. 2008a. Nrf2 mediates cancer protection but not prolongevity induced by caloric restriction. *Proc. Natl Acad. Sci. USA* 105:2325–2330.

Pearson, K. J., J. A. Baur, K. N. Lewis, L. Peshkin, N. L. Price, N. Labinskyy, W. R. Swindell, D. Kamara, R. K. Minor, E. Perez, H. A. Jamieson, Y. Zhang, S. R. Dunn, K. Sharma, N. Pleshko, L. A. Woollett, A. Csiszar, Y. Ikeno, D. Le Couteur, P. J. Elliott, K. G. Becker, P. Navas, D. K. Ingram, N. S. Wolf, Z. Ungvari, D. A. Sinclair, and R. de Cabo. 2008b. Resveratrol delays age-related deterioration, and mimics transcriptional aspects of dietary restriction without extending life span. *Cell Metab.* 8:157–168.

Peino, R., F. Cordido, A. Penalva, C. V. Alvarez, C. Dieguez, and F. F. Casanueva. 1996. Acipimox-mediated plasma free fatty acid depression per se stimulates growth hormone (GH) secretion in normal subjects, and potentiates the response to other GH-releasing stimuli. *J. Clin. Endocrinol. Metab.* 81:909–913.

Peng, C. H., Y. L. Chang, C. L. Kao, L. M. Tseng, C. C. Wu, Y. C. Chen, C. Y. Tsai, L. C. Woung, J. H. Liu, S. H. Chiou, and S. J. Chen. 2010. SirT1 – a sensor for monitoring self-renewal, and aging process in retinal stem cells. *Sensors* 10:6172–6194.

Penza, M., C. Montani, A. Romani, P. Vignolini, B. Pampaloni, A. Tanini, M. L. Brandi, P. Alonso-Magdalena, A. Nadal, L. Ottobrini, O. Parolini, E. Bignotti, S. Calza, A. Maggi, P. G. Grigolato, and D. Di Lorenzo. 2006. Genistein affects adipose tissue deposition in a dose-dependent, and gender-specific manner. *Endocrinology* 147:5740–5751.

Pfaffenbach, K. T. and A. S. Lee. 2011. The critical role of GRP78 in physiologic, and pathologic stress. *Curr. Opin. Cell Biol.* 23:150–156.

Pfeuffer, M., A. Auinger, U. Bley, I. Kraus-Stojanowic, C. Laue, P. Winkler, C. E. Rüfer, J. Frank, C. Bösch-Saadatmandi, G. Rimbach, and J. Schrezenmeir. 2013. Effect of quercetin on traits of the metabolic syndrome, endothelial function, and inflammation in men with different APOE isoforms. *Nutr. Metab. Cardiovasc. Dis.* 23:403–409.

Phalitakul, S., M. Okada, Y. Hara, and H. Yamawaki. 2011. Vaspin prevents TNF-α-induced intracellular adhesion molecule-1 via inhibiting reactive oxygen species-dependent NF-KB and PKCθ activation in cultured rat vascular smooth muscle cells. *Pharmacol. Res.* 64:493–500.

Picard, F., M. Kurtev, and N. Chung. 2004. Sirt1 promotes fat mobilization in white adipocytes by repressing PPAR-gamma. *Nature* 429:771–776.

Pierce, G. L., S. D. Beske, B. R. Lawson, K. L. Southall, F. J. Benay, A. J. Donato, and D. R. Seals. 2008. Weight loss alone improves conduit and resistance artery endothelial function in young and older overweight/obese adults. *Hypertension* 52:72–79.

Pinney, D. O., D. F. Stephens, and L. S. Pope. 1972. Lifetime effects of winter supplemental feed level, and age at first parturition on range beef cows. *J. Anim. Sci.* 34:1067–1074.

Piper, M. D. and A. Bartke. 2008. Diet and aging. *Cell Metab.* 8:99–104.

Polyzos, S. A., J. Kountouras, C. Zavos, and E. Tsiaousi. 2010. The role of adiponectin in the pathogenesis and treatment of non-alcoholic fatty liver disease. *Diabetes Obes. Metab.* 12:365–383.

Poulsen, M. M., P. F. Vestergaard, B. F. Clasen, Y. Radko, L. P. Christensen, H. Stødkilde-Jørgensen, N. Møller, N. Jessen, S. B. Pedersen, and J. O. Jørgensen. 2013. High-dose resveratrol supplementation in obese men: an investigator-initiated, randomized, placebo-controlled clinical trial of substrate metabolism, insulin sensitivity, and body composition. *Diabetes* 62:1186–1195.

Pugh, T. D., T. D. Oberley, and R. Weindruch. 1999 Dietary intervention at middle age: caloric restriction but not dehydroepiandrosterone sulfate increases lifespan and lifetime cancer incidence in mice. *Cancer Res.* 59:1642–1648.

Puri, P., F. Mirshahi, O. Cheung, R. Natarajan, J. W. Maher, J. M. Kellum, and A. J. Sanyal. 2008. Activation, and dysregulation of the unfolded protein response in nonalcoholic fatty liver disease. *Gastroenterology* 134:568–576.

Purushotham, A., T. T. Schug, Q. Xu, S. Surapureddi, X. Guo, and X. Li. 2009. Hepatocyte-specific deletion of SIRT1 alters fatty acid metabolism, and results in hepatic steatosis, and inflammation. *Cell Metab.* 9:327–338.

Qiao, L. P., B. Lee, B. Kinney, H. S. Yoo, and J. H. Shao. 2011. Energy intake and adiponectin gene expression. *Am. J. Physiol. Endocrinol. Metab.* 300:E809–E816.

Qiu, X., K. Brown, M. D. Hirschey, E. Verdin, and D. Chen. 2010. Calorie restriction reduces oxidative stress by SIRT3-mediated SOD2 activation. *Cell Metab* 12:662–667.

Rabek, J. P., W. H. Boylston, 3rd, and J. Papaconstantinou. 2003. Carbonylation of ER chaperone proteins in aged mouse liver. *Biochem Biophys Res Commun* 305:566–572.

Racette, S. B., E. P. Weiss, D. T. Villareal, H. Arif, K. Steger-May, K. B. Schechtman, L. Fontana, S. Klein, J. O. Holloszy, and Washington University School of Medicine CALERIE Group. 2006. One year of caloric restriction in humans: feasibility, and effects on body composition, and abdominal adipose tissue. *J. Gerontol. A. Biol. Sci. Med. Sci.* 61:943–950.

Rahbar, S., R. Natarajan, K. Yerneni, S. Scott, N. Gonzales, and J. L. Nadler. 2000. Evidence that pioglitazone, metformin, and pentoxifylline are inhibitors of glycation. *Clin. Chim. Acta* 301:65–77.

Raitakari, M., T. Ilvonen, M. Ahotupa, T. Lehtimäki, A. Harmoinen, P. Suominen, J. Elo, J. Hartiala, and O. T. Raitakari. 2004. Weight reduction with very-low-caloric diet and endothelial function in overweight adults: role of plasma glucose. *Arterioscler. Thromb. Vasc. Biol.* 24:124–128.

Rajala, M. W., Y. Qi, H. R. Patel, N. Takahashi, R. Banerjee, U. B. Pajvani, M. K. Sinha, R. L. Gingerich, P. E. Scherer, and R. S. Ahima. 2004. Regulation of resistin expression and circulating levels in obesity, diabetes, and fasting. *Diabetes* 53:1671–1679.

Rajawat, Y. S., Z. Hilioti, and I. Bossis. 2009. Aging: central role for autophagy and the lysosomal degradative system. *Ageing Res. Rev.* 8:199–213.

Ravikumar, B., C. Vacher, Z. Berger, J. E. Davies, S. Luo, L. G. Oroz, F. Scaravilli, D. F. Easton, R. Duden, C. J. O'Kane, and D. C. Rubinsztein. 2004. Inhibition of mTOR induces autophagy, and reduces toxicity of polyglutamine expansions in fly, and mouse models of Huntington disease. *Nat. Genet.* 36:585–595.

Ravikumar, B., S. Sarkar, J. E. Davies, M. Futter, M. Garcia-Arencibia, Z. W. Green-Thompson, M. Jimenez-Sanchez, V. I. Korolchuk, M. Lichtenberg, S. Luo, D. C. Massey, F. M. Menzies, K. Moreau, U. Narayanan, M. Renna, F. H. Siddiqi, B. R. Underwood, A. R. Winslow, and D. C. Rubinsztein. 2010. Regulation of mammalian autophagy in physiology, and pathophysiology. *Physiol. Rev.* 90:1383–1435.

Rayalam, S., J. Y. Yang, S. Ambati, M. A. Della-Fera, and C. A. Baile. 2008. Resveratrol induces apoptosis, and inhibits adipogenesis in 3T3-L1 adipocytes. *Phytother. Res.* 22:1367–1371.

Rayssiguier, Y., E. Gueux, W. Nowacki, E. Rock, and A. Mazur. 2006. High fructose consumption combined with low dietary magnesium intake may increase the incidence of the metabolic syndrome by inducing inflammation. *Magnes. Res.* 19:237–243.

Rector, R. S., E. M. Morris, S. Ridenhour, G. M. Meers, F. F. Hsu, J. Turk, and J. A. Ibdah. 2013. Selective hepatic insulin resistance in mice heterozygous for a mitochondrial trifunctional protein defect. *Hepatology* 57:2213–2223.

Redman, L. M., L. K. Heilbronn, C. K. Martin, A. Alfonso, S. R. Smith, E. Ravussin and Pennington CALERIE Team. 2007. Effect of calorie restriction with or without exercise on body composition, and fat distribution. *J. Clin. Endocrinol. Metab.* 92:865–872.

Redman, L. M., L. K. Heilbronn, C. K. Martin, L. de Jonge, D. A. Williamson, J. P. Delany, E. Ravussin and Pennington CALERIE Team. 2009. Metabolic and behavioral compensations in response to caloric restriction: implications for the maintenance of weight loss. *PLoS One* 4:e4377.

Reed, M. J., P. E. Penn, Y. Li, R. Birnbaum, R. B. Vernon, T. S. Johnson, W. R. Pendergrass, E. H. Sage, I. B. Abrass, and N. S. Wolf. 1996. Enhanced cell proliferation and biosynthesis mediate improved wound repair in refed, caloric-restricted mice. *Mech. Ageing Dev.* 89:21–43.

Rehman, J., R. V. Considine, J. E. Bovenkerk, J. Li, C. A. Slavens, R. M. Jones, and K. L. March. 2003. Obesity is associated with increased levels of circulating hepatocyte growth factor. *J. Am. Coll. Cardiol.* 41:1408–1413.

Reznick, R. M., H. Zong, J. Li, K. Morino, I. K. Moore, H. J. Yu, Z. X. Liu, J. Dong, K. J. Mustard, S. A. Hawley, D. Befroy, M. Pypaert, D. G. Hardie, L. H. Young, and G. I. Shulman. 2007. Aging-associated reductions in AMP-activated protein kinase activity, and mitochondrial biogenesis. *Cell Metab.* 5:151–156.

Rhen, T. and J. A. Cidlowski. 2005. Antiinflammatory action of glucocorticoids – new mechanisms for old drugs. *New Engl. J. Med.* 353:1711–1723.

Ribot, J., A. M. Rodríguez, E. Rodríguez, and A. Palou. 2008. Adiponectin and resistin response in the onset of obesity in male and female rats. *Obesity (Silver Spring)* 16:723–730.

Richard, C., M. M. Royer, P. Couture, K. Cianflone, R. Rezvani, S. Desroches, and B. Lamarche. 2013. Effect of the Mediterranean diet on plasma adipokine concentrations in men with metabolic syndrome. *Metabolism* 62:1803–1810.

Rikke, B. A., J. E. Yerg, M. E. Battaglia, T. R. Nagy, D. B. Allison, and T. E. Johnson. 2003. Strain variation in the response of body temperature to dietary restriction. *Mech. Ageing Dev.* 124:663–678.

Rippe, C., L. Lesniewski, M. Connell, T. LaRocca, A. J. Donato, and D. Seals. 2010. Short-term calorie restriction reverses vascular endothelial dysfunction in old mice by increasing nitric oxide and reducing oxidative stress. *Aging Cell* 9:304–312.

Rizza, W., N. Veronese, and L. Fontana. 2014. What are the roles of calorie restriction and diet quality in promoting healthy longevity? Ageing Res. *Rev.* 13:38–45.

Robert, L. 2010. Aging in the 21st century. *Pathol. Biol.* 58:185–186.

Rochon, J., C. W. Bales, E. Ravussin, L. M. Redman, J. O. Holloszy, S. B. Racette, S. B. Roberts, S. K. Das, S. Romashkan, K. M. Galan, E. C. Hadley, W. E. Kraus, and CALERIE Study Group. 2011. Design, and conduct of the CALERIE study: comprehensive assessment of the long-term effects of reducing intake of energy. *J. Gerontol. A. Biol. Sci. Med. Sci.* 66:97–108.

Rodgers, J. T., C. Lerin, W. Haas, S. P. Gygi, B. M. Spiegelman, and P. Puigserver. 2005. Nutrient control of glucose homeostasis through a complex of PGC-1alpha, and SIRT1. *Nature* 434:113–118.

Rodriguez-Mañas, L., M. El-Assar, S. Vallejo, P. Lopez-Doriga, J. Solis, R. Petidier, M. Montes, J. Nevado, M. Castro, C. Gomez-Guerrero, C. Peiro, and C. F. Sanchez-Ferrer. 2009. Endothelial dysfunction in aged humans is related with oxidative stress and vascular inflammation. *Aging Cell* 8:226–238.

Rodriguez-Moran, M. and F. Guerrero-Romero. 2004. Elevated concentrations of TNF-alpha are related to low serum magnesium levels in obese subjects. *Magnes. Res.* 17:189–196.

Rogina, B. and S. L. Helfand. 2004. Sir2 mediates longevity in the fly through a pathway related to calorie restriction. *Proc. Natl Acad. Sci. USA* 101:15998–16003.

Roman, A. A., S. D. Parlee, and C. J. Sinal. 2012. Chemerin: a potential endocrine link between obesity and type 2 diabetes. *Endocrine* 42:243–251.

Romero-Corral A., V. K. Somers, J. Sierra-Johnson, Y. Korenfeld, S. Boarin, J. Korinek, M. D. Jensen, G. Parati, and F. Lopez-Jimenez. 2010. Normal weight obesity: a risk factor for cardiometabolic dysregulation and cardiovascular mortality. *Eur. Heart J.* 31:737–746.

Ron, D. 2002. Translational control in the endoplasmic reticulum stress response. *J. Clin. Invest.* 110:1383–1388.

Ron, D. and P. Walter. 2007. Signal integration in the endoplasmic reticulum unfolded protein response. *Nat. Rev. Mol. Cell Biol.* 8:519–529.

Rosanoff, A., C. M. Weaver, and R. K. Rude. 2012. Suboptimal magnesium status in the United States: are the health consequences underestimated? *Nutr. Rev.* 70:153–164.

Rosenow, A., J. P. Noben, J. Jocken, S. Kallendrusch, P. Fischer-Posovszky, E. C. Mariman, and J. Renes. 2012. Resveratrol-induced changes of the human adipocyte secretion profile. *J. Proteome Res.* 11:4733–4743.

Rosenquist, K. J., A. Pedley, J. M. Massaro, K. E. Therkelsen, J. M. Murabito, U. Hoffmann, and C. S. Fox. 2013. Visceral and subcutaneous fat quality and cardiometabolic risk. *JACC Cardiovasc. Imag.* 6:762–771.

Rosito, G. A., J. M. Massaro, U. Hoffmann, F. L. Ruberg, A. A. Mahabadi, R. S. Vasan, C. J. O'Donnell, and C. S. Fox. 2008. Pericardial fat, visceral abdominal fat, cardiovascular disease risk factors, and vascular calcification in a community-based sample: the Framingham Heart Study. *Circulation* 117:605–613.

Roth, G. S., M. A. Lane, D. K. Ingram, J. A. Mattison, D. Elahi, J. D. Tobin, D. Muller, and E. J. Metter. 2002. Biomarkers of caloric restriction may predict longevity in humans. *Science* 297:811.

Roth, L. W. and A. J. Polotsky. 2012. Can we live longer by eating less? A review of caloric restriction and longevity. *Maturitas* 71:315–319.

Rowe, W. J. 2012. Correcting magnesium deficiencies may prolong life. *Clin. Interv. Aging* 7:51–54.

Rutkowski, D. T. and R. J. Kaufman. 2007. That which does not kill me makes me stronger: adapting to chronic ER stress. *Trends Biochem. Sci.* 32:469–476.

Rutkowski, J. M., K. E. Davis, and P. E. Scherer. 2009. Mechanisms of obesity and related pathologies: the macro- and microcirculation of adipose tissue. *FEBS J.* 276:5738–5746.

Sahebkar A. 2013. Why it is necessary to translate curcumin into clinical practice for the prevention, and treatment of metabolic syndrome? *Biofactors* 39:197–208.

Sahu, R., S. Kaushik, C. C. Clement, E. S. Cannizzo, B. Scharf, A. Follenzi, I. Potolicchio, E. Nieves, A. M. Cuervo, and L. Santambrogio. 2011. Microautophagy of cytosolic proteins by late endosomes. *Dev. Cell.* 20:131–139.

Sales, C. H., A. R. Santos, D. E. Cintra, and C. Colli. 2014. Magnesium-deficient high-fat diet: effects on adiposity, lipid profile, and insulin sensitivity in growing rats. *Clin. Nutr.* 33:879–888.

Salih, D. A. and A. Brunet. 2008. FoxO transcription factors in the maintenance of cellular homeostasis during aging. *Curr. Opin. Cell. Biol.* 20:126–136.

Salminen, A. and K. Kaarniranta. 2010. ER stress, and hormetic regulation of the aging process. *Ageing Res. Rev.* 9:211–217.

Samaras, K., A. Viardot, P. N. Lee, A. Jenkins, N. K. Botelho, A. Bakopanos, R. V. Lord, and C. S. Hayward. 2013. Reduced arterial stiffness after weight loss in obese type 2 diabetes and impaired glucose tolerance: the role of immune cell activation and insulin resistance. *Diab. Vasc. Dis. Res.* 10:40–48.

Sandoo, A., J. J. van Zanten, G. S. Metsios, D. Carroll, and G. D. Kitas. 2010. The endothelium and its role in regulating vascular tone. *Open Cardiovasc. Med. J.* 4:302–312.

Santarpia, L., F. Contaldo, and F. Pasanisi. 2013. Body composition changes after weight-loss interventions for overweight and obesity. *Clin. Nutr.* 32:157–161.

Sanz, A., P. Caro, and G. Barja. 2004. Protein restriction without strong caloric restriction decreases mitochondrial oxygen radical production, and oxidative DNA damage in rat liver. *J. Bioenerg. Biomembr.* 36:545–552.

Sanz, A., P. Caro, J. G. Sanchez, and G. Barja. 2006a. Effect of lipid restriction on mitochondrial free radical production, and oxidative DNA damage. *Ann. NY Acad. Sci.* 1067:200–209.

Sanz, A., J. Gómez, P. Caro, and G. Barja. 2006b. Carbohydrate restriction does not change mitochondrial free radical generation, and oxidative DNA damage. *J. Bioenerg. Biomembr.* 38:327–333.

Sanz, A., R. Pamplona, and G. Barja. 2006c. Is the mitochondrial free radical theory of aging intact? *Antioxid. Redox Signal.* 8:582–599.

Sato, N., K. Kobayashi, T. Inoguchi, N. Sonoda, M. Imamura, N. Sekiguchi, N. Nakashima, and H. Nawata. 2005. Adenovirus-mediated high expression of resistin causes dyslipidemia in mice. *Endocrinology* 146:273–279.

Sato, K., K. Tsuchihara, S. Fujii, M. Sugiyama, T. Goya, Y. Atomi, T. Ueno, A. Ochiai, and H. Esumi. 2007. Autophagy is activated in colorectal cancer cells, and contributes to the tolerance to nutrient deprivation. *Cancer Res.* 67:9677–9684.

Sasaki, S., Y. Higashi, K. Nakagawa, M. Kimura, K. Noma, S. Sasaki, K. Hara, H. Matsuura, C. Goto, T. Oshima, and K. Chayama. 2002. A low-calorie diet improves endothelium-dependent vasodilation in obese patients with essential hypertension. *Am. J. Hypertens.* 15:302–309.

Schächter, F., L. Faure-Delanef, F. Guénot, H. Rouger, P. Froguel, L. Lesueur-Ginot, and D. Cohen. 1994. Genetic associations with human longevity at the APOE, and ACE loci. *Nat. Genet.* 6:29–32.

Scher, M. B., A. Vaquero, and D. Reinberg. 2007. SirT3 is a nuclear NAD+-dependent histone deacetylase that translocates to the mitochondria upon cellular stress. *Genes Dev.* 21:920–928.

Scherz-Shouval, R. and Z. Elazar. 2011. Regulation of autophagy by ROS: physiology, and pathology. *Trends Biochem. Sci.* 36:30–38.

Schmeisser, S., S. Priebe, M. Groth, S. Monajembashi, P. Hemmerich, R. Guthke, M. Platzer, and M. Ristow. 2013. Neuronal ROS signaling rather than AMPK/sirtuin-mediated energy sensing links dietary restriction to lifespan extension. *Mol. Metab.* 2:92–102.

Schroder, M. and R. J. Kaufman. 2005. ER stress, and the unfolded protein response. *Mutat. Res.* 569:29–63.

Schwer, B., B. J. North, R. A. Frye, M. Ott, and E. Verdin. 2002. The human silent information regulator (Sir)2 homologue hSIRT3 is a mitochondrial nicotinamide adenine dinucleotide-dependent deacetylase. *J. Cell Biol.* 158:647–657.

Schwer, B., J. Bunkenborg, R. O. Verdin, J. S. andersen, and E. Verdin. 2006. Reversible lysine acetylation controls the activity of the mitochondrial enzyme acetyl-CoA synthetase 2. *Proc. Natl Acad. Sci. USA* 103:10224–10229.

Scrofano, M. M., F. Shang, T. R. Nowell Jr., S. Gong, D. E. Smith, M. Kelliher, J. Dunning, C. V. Mura, and A. A. Taylor. 1998. Aging, calorie restriction, and ubiquitin-dependent proteolysis in the livers of Emory mice. *Mech. Aging Dev.* 101:277–296.

Seals, D. R., K. L. Jablonski, and A. J. Donato. 2011. Aging and vascular endothelial function in humans. *Clin. Sci. (Lond.)* 120:357–375.

Selman, C., S. Lingard, A. I. Choudhury, R. L. Batterham, M. Claret, M. Clements, F. Ramadani, K. Okkenhaug, E. Schuster, E. Blanc, M. D. Piper, H. Al-Qassab, J. R. Speakman, D. Carmignac, I. C. Robinson, J. M. Thornton, D. Gems, L. Partridge, and D. J. Withers. 2008. Evidence for lifespan extension and delayed age-related biomarkers in insulin receptor substrate 1 null mice. *FASEB J.* 22:807–818.

Sell, H., J. Laurencikiene, A. Taube, K. Eckardt, A. Cramer, A. Horrighs, P. Arner, and J. Eckel. 2009. Chemerin is a novel adipocyte-derived factor inducing insulin resistance in primary human skeletal muscle cells. *Diabetes* 58:2731–2740.

Sell, H., A. Divoux, A. Poitou, A. Basdevant, J. L. Bouillot, P. Bedossa, J. Tordjman, J. Eckel, and K. Clément. 2010. Chemerin correlates with markers for fatty liver in morbidly obese patients and strongly decreases after weight loss induced by bariatric surgery. *J. Clin. Endocrinol. Metab.* 95:2892–2896.

Seo, H. A. and I. K. Lee. 2013. The role of Nrf2: adipocyte differentiation, obesity, and insulin resistance. *Oxid. Med. Cell. Longev.* 184598.

Shao, W., Z. Yu, Y. Chiang, Y. Yang Y, T. Chai, W. Foltz, H. Lu, I. G. Fantus, and T. Jin. 2012. Curcumin prevents high fat diet induced insulin resistance, and obesity via attenuating lipogenesis in liver, and inflammatory pathway in adipocytes. *PLoS One* 7:e28784.

Shen P., M. H. Liu, T. Y. Ng, Y. H. Chan, and E. L. Yong. 2006. Differential effects of isoflavones, from Astragalus membranaceus, and Pueraria thomsonii, on the activation of PPARalpha, PPARgamma, and, and adipocyte differentiation in vitro. *J. Nutr.* 136:899–905.

Shen, L. R., F. Xiao, P. Yuan, Y. Chen, Q. K. Gao, L. D. Parnell, M. Meydani, J. M. Ordovas, D. Li, and C. Q. Lai. 2013. Curcumin-supplemented diets increase superoxide dismutase activity, and mean lifespan in Drosophila. *Age* 35:1133–1142.

Sheng, C. H., J. Di, Y. Jin, Y. C. Zhang, M. Wu, Y. Sun, and G. Z. Zhang. 2008. Resistin is expressed in human hepatocytes and induces insulin resistance. *Endocrine* 33:135–143.

Shi, T., F. Wang, E. Stieren, and Q. Tong. 2005. SIRT3, a mitochondrial sirtuin deacetylase, regulates mitochondrial function, and thermogenesis in brown adipocytes. *J. Biol. Chem.* 280:13560–13567.

Shi, F. H., Y. Wu, D. Z. Dai, X. D. Cong, Y. M. Zhang, and Y. Dai. 2013. Hepatosteatosis, and hepatic insulin resistance are blunted by argirein, an anti-inflammatory agent, through normalizing endoplasmic reticulum stress, and apoptosis in diabetic liver. *J. Pharm. Pharmacol.* 65:916–927.

Shibata, R., N. Ouchi, R. Takahashi, Y. Terakura, K. Ohashi, N. Ikeda, A. Higuchi, H. Terasaki, S. Kihara, and T. Murohara. 2012. Omentin as a novel biomarker of metabolic risk factors. *Diabetol. Metabol. Syndr.* 26:37.

Shimokawa, I. and Y. Higami. 2001. Leptin and anti-aging action of caloric restriction. *J. Nutr. Health Aging* 5:43–48.

Shin, S., J. Wakabayashi, M. S. Yates, N. Wakabayashi, P. M. Dolan, S. Aja, K. T. Liby, M. B. Sporn, M. Yamamoto and T. W. Kensler. 2009. Role of Nrf2 in prevention of high-fat diet-induced obesity by synthetic triterpenoid CDDO-imidazolide. *Eur. J. Pharmacol.* 620:138–144.

Shinmura, K., K. Tamaki, K. Saito, Y. Nakano, T. Tobe, and R. Bolli. 2007. Cardioprotective effects of short-term caloric restriction are mediated by adiponectin via activation of AMP-activated protein kinase. *Circulation* 116:2809–2817.

Shinmura, K., K. Tamaki, and R. Bolli. 2008. Impact of 6-mo caloric restriction on myocardial ischemic tolerance: possible involvement of nitric oxide-dependent increase in nuclear Sirt1. *Am. J. Physiol. Heart Circul. Physiol.* 295:H2348–H2355.

Sierra-Johnson, J., A. Romero-Corral, F. Lopez-Jimenez, A. S. Gami, F. H. Sert Kuniyoshi, R. Wolk, and V. K. Somers. 2007. Relation of increased leptin concentrations to history of myocardial infarction and stroke in the United States population. *Am. J. Cardiol.* 100:234–239.

Silha, J. V., M. Krsek, J. V. Skrha, P. Sucharda, B. L. Nyomba, and L. J. Murphy. 2003. Plasma resistin, adiponectin and leptin levels in lean and obese subjects: correlations with insulin resistance. *Eur. J. Endocrinol.* 149:331–335.

Silha, J. V., M. Krsek, P. Sucharda, and L. J. Murphy. 2005. Angiogenic factors are elevated in overweight and obese individuals. *Int. J. Obes. (Lond.)* 29:1308–1314.

Smith, J., M. Al-Amri, A. Sniderman, and K. Cianflone. 2006. Visfatin concentration in Asian Indians is correlated with high density lipoprotein cholesterol and apolipoprotein A1. *Clin. Endocrinol.* 65:667–672.

Smith, J. J., R. D. Kenney, D. J. Gagne, B. P. Frushour, W. Ladd, H. L. Galonek, K. Israelian, J. Song, G. Razvadauskaite, A. V. Lynch, D. P. Carney, R. J. Johnson, S. Lavu, A. Iffland, P. J. Elliott, P. D. Lambert, K. O. Elliston, M. R. Jirousek, J. C. Milne, and O. Boss. 2009. Small molecule activators of SIRT1 replicate signaling pathways triggered by calorie restriction in vivo. *BMC Syst. Biol.* 3:31.

Soare, A., R. Cangemi, D. Omodei, J. O. Holloszy, and L. Fontana. 2011. Long-term calorie restriction, but not endurance exercise, lowers core body temperature in humans. *Aging* 3:374–379.

Soare, A., E. P. Weiss, and P. Pozzilli. 2014. Benefits of caloric restriction for cardiometabolic health, including type 2 diabetes mellitus risk. *Diabetes Metab. Res. Rev.* 30(Suppl 1):41–47.

Soerensen, M., K. Christensen, T. Stevnsner, and L. Christiansen. 2009. The Mn-superoxide dismutase single nucleotide polymorphism rs4880, and the glutathione peroxidase 1 single nucleotide polymorphism rs1050450 are associated with aging, and longevity in the oldest old. *Mech. Ageing Dev.* 130:308–314.

Soerensen, M., M. Thinggaard, M. Nygaard, S. Dato, Q. Tan, J. Hjelmborg, K. Andersen-Ranberg, T. Stevnsner, V. A. Bohr, M. Kimura, A. Aviv, K. Christensen, and L. Christiansen. 2012. Genetic variation in TERT, and TERC, and human leukocyte telomere length, and longevity: a cross-sectional, and longitudinal analysis. *Aging Cell* 11:223–227.

Sohal R. S. and B. H. Sohal. 1991. Hydrogen peroxide release by mitochondria increases during aging. *Mech. Ageing Dev.* 57:187–202.

Solinas, G. and M. Karin. 2010. JNK1, and IKKbeta: molecular links between obesity, and metabolic dysfunction. *Faseb J.* 24:2596–2611.

Someya, S., W. Yu, W. C. Hallows, J. Xu, J. M. Vann, C. Leeuwenburgh, M. Tanokura, J. M. Denu, and T. A. Prolla. 2010. Sirt3 mediates reduction of oxidative damage, and prevention of age-related hearing loss under caloric restriction. *Cell* 143:802–812.

Sone, H., H. Shimano, Y. Sakakura, N. Inoue, M. Amemiya-Kudo, N. Yahagi, M. Osawa, H. Suzuki, T. Yokoo, A. Takahashi, K. Iida, H. Toyoshima, A. Iwama, and N. Yamada. 2002. Acetyl-coenzyme A synthetase is a lipogenic enzyme controlled by SREBP-1, and energy status. *Am. J. Physiol. Endocrinol. Metab.* 282:E222–E230.

Speakman, J. R. and S. E. Mitchell. 2011. Caloric restriction. *Mol. Aspects Med.* 31:159–221.

Stadtman, E. R. 2001. Protein oxidation in aging, and age-related diseases. *Ann. NY Acad. Sci.* 928:22–38.

Stein, P. K., A. Soare, T. E. Meyer, R. Cangemi, J. O. Holloszy, and L. Fontana. 2012. Caloric restriction may reverse age-related autonomic decline in humans. *Aging Cell* 11:644–650.

Stevens, G. A., G. M. Singh, Y. Lu, G. Danaei, J. K. Lin, M. M. Finucane, A. N. Bahalim, R. K. McIntire, H. R. Gutierrez, M. Cowan, C. J. Paciorek, F. Farzadfar, L. Riley, M. Ezzati, and Global Burden of Metabolic Risk Factors of Chronic Diseases Collaborating Group (Body Mass Index). 2012. National, regional, and global trends in adult overweight and obesity prevalences. *Popul. Health Metr.* 20:22.

Stewart, L. K., J. L. Soileau, D. Ribnicky, Z. Q. Wang, I. Raskin, A. Poulev, M. Majewski, W. T. Cefalu, and T. W. Gettys. 2008. Quercetin transiently increases energy expenditure but persistently decreases circulating markers of inflammation in C57BL/6J mice fed a high-fat diet. *Metabolism* 57:S39–S46.

Strong R., R. A. Miller, C. M. Astle, J. A. Baur, R. de Cabo, E. Fernandez, W. Guo, M. Javors, J. L. Kirkland, J. F. Nelson, D. A. Sinclair, B. Teter, D. Williams, N. Zaveri, N. L. Nadon, and D. E. Harrison. 2013. Evaluation of resveratrol, green tea extract, curcumin, oxaloacetic acid, and medium-chain triglyceride oil on life span of genetically heterogeneous mice. *J. Gerontol. A. Biol. Sci. Med. Sci.* 68:6–16.

Suchankova, G., L. E. Nelson, Z. Gerhart-Hines, M. Kelly, M. S. Gauthier, A. K. Saha, Y. Ido, P. Puigserver, and N. B. Ruderman. 2009. Concurrent regulation of AMP-activated protein kinase, and SIRT1 in mammalian cells. *Biochem. Biophys. Res. Commun.* 378:836–841.

Sugimoto, H., K. Okada, J. Shoda, E. Warabi, K. Ishige, T. Ueda, K. Taguchi, T. Yanagawa, A. Nakahara, I. Hyodo, T. Ishii and M. Yamamoto. 2010. Deletion of nuclear factor-E2-related factor-2 leads to rapid onset and progression of nutritional steatohepatitis in mice. *Am. J. Physiol. Gastrointest. Liver Physiol.* 298: G283–G294.

Suh, Y., G. Atzmon, M. O. Cho, D. Hwang, B. Liu, D. J. Leahy, N. Barzilai, and P. Cohen. 2008. Functionally significant insulin-like growth factor I receptor mutations in centenarians. *Proc. Natl Acad. Sci. USA* 105:3438–3442.

Suliburska, J., P. Bogdanski, M. Szulinska, M. Stepien, D. Pupek-Musialik, and A. Jablecka. 2012. Effects of green tea supplementation on elements, total antioxidants, lipids, and glucose values in the serum of obese patients. *Biol. Trace Elem. Res.* 149:315–322.

Sun, L., A. A. Sadighi Akha, R. A. Miller, and J. M. Harper. 2009. Life-span extension in mice by preweaning food restriction, and by methionine restriction in middle age. *J. Gerontol. A. Biol. Sci. Med. Sci.* 64:711–722.

Sun, K., N. Halberg, M. Khan, U. J. Magalang, and P. E. Scherer. 2013. Selective inhibition of hypoxia-inducible factor 1alpha ameliorates adipose tissue dysfunction. *Mol. Cell Biol.* 33:904–917.

Sundaresan, N. R., S. A. Samant, V. B. Pillai, S. B. Rajamohan, and M. P. Gupta. 2008. SIRT3 is a stress-responsive deacetylase in cardiomyocytes that protects cells from stress-mediated cell death by deacetylation of Ku70. *Mol. Cell Biol.* 28:6384–6401.

Sundaresan, N. R., M. Gupta, G. Kim, S. B. Rajamohan, A. Isbatan, and M. P. Gupta. 2009. Sirt3 blocks the cardiac hypertrophic response by augmenting Foxo3a-dependent antioxidant defense mechanisms in mice. *J. Clin. Invest.* 119:2758–2771.

Sutter, N. B., C. D. Bustamante, K. Chase, M. M. Gray, K. Zhao, L. Zhu, B. Padhukasahasram, E. Karlins, S. Davis, P. G. Jones, P. Quignon, G. S. Johnson, H. G. Parker, N. Fretwell, D. S. Mosher, D. F. Lawler, E. Satyaraj, M. Nordborg, K. G. Lark, R. K. Wayne, and E. A. Ostrander. 2007. A single IGF1 allele is a major determinant of small size in dogs. *Science* 316:112–115.

Suzuki, K. and Y. Ohsumi. 2007. Molecular machinery of autophagosome formation in yeast, *Saccharomyces cerevisiae*. *FEBS Lett.* 581:2156–2161.

Swarbrick, M. M., K. L. Stanhope, I. T. Austrheim-Smith, M. D. Van Loan, M. R. Ali, B. M. Wolfe, and P. J. Havel. 2008. Longitudinal changes in pancreatic and adipocyte hormones following Roux-en-Y gastric bypass surgery. *Diabetologia* 51:1901–1911.

Sykiotis, G. P., I. G. Habeos, A. V. Samuelson, D. Bohmann. 2011. The role of the antioxidant and longevity-promoting Nrf2 pathway in metabolic regulation. *Curr. Opin. Clin. Nutr. Metab. Care* 14:41–48.

Szegezdi, E., D. C. Macdonald, T. Ni Chonghaile, S. Gupta, and A. Samali. 2009. Bcl-2 family on guard at the ER. *Am. J. Physiol. Cell. Physiol.* 296:C941–C953.

Taguchi, A. and M. F. White. 2008. Insulin-like signaling, nutrient homeostasis, and life span. *Annu. Rev. Physiol.* 70:191–212.

Taguchi, A., L. M. Wartschow, and M. F. White. 2007. Brain IRS2 signaling coordinates life span and nutrient homeostasis. *Science* 317:369–372.

Takaya, J., H. Higashino, and Y. Kobayashi. 2004. Intracellular magnesium, and insulin resistance. *Magnes. Res.* 17:126–136.

Takebayashi, K., M. Suetsugu, S. Wakabayashi, Y. Aso, and T. Inukai. 2007. Association between plasma visfatin and vascular endothelial function in patients with type 2 diabetes mellitus. *Metabolism* 56:451–458.

Tan, B. K., J. Chen, J. E. Digby, S. D. Keay, R. Kennedy, and H. S. Randeva. 2006. Increased visfatin messenger ribonucleic acid and protein levels in adipose tissue and adypocites in women with polycystic ovary syndrome: parallel increase in plasma visfatin. *J. Clin. Endocrinol. Metab.* 91:5022–5028.

Tanaka, Y., L. M. Aleksunes, R. L. Yeager, M. A. Gyamfi, N. Esterly, G. L. Guo and C. D. Klaassen. 2008. NF-E2-related factor 2 inhibits lipid accumulation and oxidative stress in mice fed a high-fat diet. *J. Pharmacol. Exp. Ther.* 325:655–664.

Tang, W., D. Zeve, J. M. Suh, D. Bosnakovski, M. Kyba, R. E. Hammer, M. D. Tallquist, and J. M. Graff. 2008. White fat progenitor cells reside in the adipose vasculature. *Science* 322:583–586.

Tchernof, A. and J. P. Després. 2013. Pathophysiology of human visceral obesity: an update. *Physiol. Rev.* 93:359–404.

Terman, A., B. Gustafsson, and U. T. Brunk. 2007. Autophagy, organelles, and ageing. *J. Pathol.* 211:134–143.

Testa, G., F. Biasi, G. Poli, and E. Chiarpotto. 2014. Calorie restriction and dietary restriction mimetics: a strategy for improving healthy aging and longevity. *Curr. Pharm. Des.* 20:2950–2977.

Thielecke, F., G. Rahn, J. Böhnke, F. Adams, A. L. Birkenfeld, J. Jordan, and M. Boschmann. 2010. Epigallocatechin-3-gallate, and postprandial fat oxidation in overweight/obese male volunteers: a pilot study. *Eur. J. Clin. Nutr.* 64:704–713.

Timmers, S., E. Konings, L. Bilet, R. H. Houtkooper, T. van de Weijer, G. H. Goossens, J. Hoeks, S. van der Krieken, D. Ryu, S. Kersten, E. Moonen-Kornips, M. K. Hesselink, I. Kunz, V. B. Schrauwen-Hinderling, E. E. Blaak, J. Auwerx, and P. Schrauwen. 2011. Calorie restriction-like effects of 30 days of resveratrol supplementation on energy metabolism, and metabolic profile in obese humans. *Cell Metab.* 14:612–622.

Tissenbaum, H. A. and L. Guarente. 2001. Increased dosage of a sir-2 gene extends lifespan in Caenorhabditis elegans. *Nature* 410:227–230.

To, K., H. Yamaza, T. Komatsu, T. Hayashida, H. Hayashi, H. Toyama, T. Chiba, Y. Higami, and I. Shimokawa. 2007. Down-regulation of AMP-activated protein kinase by calorie restriction in rat liver. *Exp. Gerontol.* 42:1063–1071.

Tomada, I., N. Tomada, H. Almeida, and D. Neves. 2013a. Androgen depletion in humans leads to cavernous tissue reorganization, and upregulation of Sirt1–eNOS axis. *Age* 35:35–47.

Tomada, I., D. Fernandes, J. T. Guimarães, H. Almeida, and D. Neves. 2013b. Energy restriction ameliorates metabolic syndrome-induced cavernous tissue structural modifications in aged rats. *Age* 35:1721–1739.

Tomada, I., R. Negrão, H. Almeida, and D. Neves. 2014. Long term high-fat consumption leads to downregulation of Akt phosphorylation of eNOS at Ser1177, and upregulation of Sirtuin-1 expression in rat cavernous tissue. *Age* 36:597–611.

Trepanowski, J. F., R. E. Canale, K. E. Marshall, M. M. Kabir, and R. J. Bloomer. 2011. Impact of caloric and dietary restriction regimens on markers of health and longevity in humans and animals: a summary of available findings. *Nutr. J.* 10:107.

Tsao, J. L., S. Dudley, B. Kwok, A. E. Nickel, P. W. Laird, K. D. Siegmund, R. M. Liskay, and D. Shibata. 2002. Diet, cancer, and aging in DNA mismatch repair deficient mice. *Carcinogenesis* 23:1807–1810.

Unger, R. H., G. O. Clark, P. E. Scherer, and L. Orci. 2010. Lipid homeostasis, lipotoxicity and the metabolic syndrome. *Biochim. Biophys. Acta* 1801:209–214.

Ungvari, Z., C. Parrado-Fernandez, A. Csiszar, and R. de Cabo. 2008. Mechanisms underlying caloric restriction and lifespan regulation: implications for vascular aging. *Circul. Res.* 102:519–528.

Ungvari, Z., G. Kaley, R. de Cabo, W. E. Sonntag, and A. Csiszar. 2010. Mechanisms of vascular aging: new perspectives. *J. Gerontol. A. Biol. Sci. Med. Sci.* 65:1028–1041.

Unno, T., C. Osada, Y. Motoo, Y. Suzuki, M. Kobayashi, and A. Nozawa. 2009. Dietary tea catechins increase fecal energy in rats. *J. Nutr. Sci. Vitaminol.* 55:447–451.

Urano, F., X. Wang, A. Bertolotti, Y. Zhang, P. Chung, H. P. Harding, and D. Ron. 2000. Coupling of stress in the ER to activation of JNK protein kinases by transmembrane protein kinase IRE1. *Science* 287:664–666.

Vakhrusheva, O., C. Smolka, P. Gajawada, S. Kostin, T. Boettger, T. Kubin, T. Braun, and E. Bober. 2008a. Sirt7 increases stress resistance of cardiomyocytes, and prevents apoptosis, and inflammatory cardiomyopathy in mice. *Circul. Res.* 102:703–710.

Vakhrusheva, O., D. Braeuer, Z. Liu, T. Braun, and E. Bober. 2008b. Sirt7-dependent inhibition of cell growth, and proliferation might be instrumental to mediate tissue integrity during aging. *J. Physiol. Pharmacol.* 59:201–212.

van Heemst, D., M. Beekman, S. P. Mooijaart, B. T. Heijmans, B. W. Brandt, B. J. Zwaan, P. E. Slagboom, and R. G. Westendorp. 2005. Reduced insulin/IGF-1 signalling and human longevity. *Aging Cell* 4:79–85.

van Herpen, N. A. and V. B. Schrauwen-Hinderling. 2008. Lipid accumulation in non-adipose tissue and lipotoxicity. *Physiol. Behav.* 94:231–241.

Vaquero, A. and D. Reinberg. 2009. Calorie restriction, and the exercise of chromatin. *Genes Dev.* 23:1849–1869.

Vaquero, A., M. Scher, D. Lee, H. Erdjument-Bromage, P. Tempst, and D. Reinberg. 2004. Human SirT1 interacts with histone H1, and promotes formation of facultative heterochromatin. *Mol. Cell* 16:93–105.

Vaquero A., M. B. Scher, D. H. Lee, A. Sutton, H. L. Cheng, F. W. Alt, L. Serrano, R. Sternglanz, and D. Reinberg. 2006. SirT2 is a histone deacetylase with preference for histone H4 Lys 16 during mitosis. *Genes Dev.* 20:1256–1261.

Venu, L., Y. D. Kishore, and M. Raghunath. 2005. Maternal, and perinatal magnesium restriction predisposes rat pups to insulin resistance, and glucose intolerance. *J. Nutr.* 135:1353–1358.

Venu, L., I. J. Padmavathi, Y. D. Kishore, N. V. Bhanu, K. R. Rao, P. B. Sainath, M. Ganeshan, and M. Raghunath. 2008. Long-term effects of maternal magnesium restriction on adiposity, and insulin resistance in rat pups. *Obesity (Silver Spring)* 16:1270–1276.

Vera, E., B. Bernardes de Jesus, M. Foronda, J. M. Flores, and M. A. Blasco. 2013. Telomerase reverse transcriptase synergizes with calorie restriction to increase health span, and extend mouse longevity. *PLoS One* 8:e53760.

Vergara, M., M. Smith-Wheelock, J. M. Harper, R. Sigler, and R. A. Miller. 2004. Hormone-treated snell dwarf mice regain fertility but remain long lived and disease resistant. *J. Gerontol. A. Biol. Sci. Med. Sci.* 59:1244–1250.

Verma, S., S. H. Li, C. H. Wang, P. W. Fedak, R. K. Li, R. D. Weisel, and D. A. Mickle. 2003. Resistin promotes endothelial cell activation: further evidence of adipokine–endothelial interaction. *Circulation* 108:736–740.

Vidal, H., D. Auboeuf, P. De Vos, B. Staels, J. P. Riou, J. Auwerx, and M. Laville. 1996. The expression of ob gene is not acutely regulated by insulin and fasting in human abdominal subcutaneous adipose tissue. *J. Clin. Invest.* 98:521–525.

Vieira, S. A. E., C. H. Schwanke, I. Gomes, and M. G. V. Valle. 2012. Effect of green tea (Camellia sinensis) consumption on the components of metabolic syndrome in elderly. *J. Nutr. Health Aging* 16:738–742.

Vielma, S. A., R. L. Klein, C. A. Levingston, and M. R. Young. 2013. Adipocytes as immune regulatory cells. *Int. Immunopharmacol.* 16:224–231.

Villalba, J. M. and F. J. Alcaín. 2012. Sirtuin activators, and inhibitors. *Biofactors* 38:349–359.

Vincent, A. M., K. Kato, L. L. McLean, M. E. Soules and E. L. Feldman. 2009. Sensory neurons and schwann cells respond to oxidative stress by increasing antioxidant defense mechanisms. *Antioxid. Redox Signal.* 11:425–438.

von Zglinicki, T. 2002. Oxidative stress shortens telomeres. *Trends Biochem. Sci.* 27:339–344.

Vytla, V. S. and R. S. Ochs. 2013. Metformin increases mitochondrial energy formation in l6 muscle cell cultures. *J. Biol. Chem.* 288:20369–20377.

Walford, R. L. and S. R. Spindler. 1997. The response to calorie restriction in mammals shows features also common to hibernation: a cross-adaptation hypothesis. *Gerontol. A. Biol. Sci. Med. Sci.* 52:B179–B183.

Wan Hasan, W. N., M. K. Kwak, S. Makpol, W. Z. Wan Ngah and Y. A. Mohd Yusof. 2014. Piper betle induces phase I & II genes through Nrf2/ARE signaling pathway in mouse embryonic fibroblasts derived from wild type and Nrf2 knockout cells. *BMC Complement. Altern. Med.* 14:72.

Wang, C., Y. Cui, C. Li, Y. Zhang, S. Xu, X. Li, H. Li and X. Zhang. 2013a. Nrf2 deletion causes "benign" simple steatosis to develop into nonalcoholic steatohepatitis in mice fed a high-fat diet. *Lipids Health Dis.* 12:165.

Wang, F., M. Nguyen, F. X. Qin, and Q. Tong. 2007. SIRT2 deacetylates FOXO3a in response to oxidative stress, and caloric restriction. *Aging Cell* 6:505–514.

Wang, F. and Q. Tong. 2009. SIRT2 suppresses adipocyte differentiation by deacetylating FOXO1, and enhancing FOXO1's repressive interaction with PPARgamma. *Mol. Biol. Cell* 20:801–808.

Wang, J., S. M. Vanegas X., Du, T. Noble, J. M. Zingg, M. Meydani, S. N. Meydani, and D. Wu. 2013b. Caloric restriction favorably impacts metabolic, and immune/inflammatory profiles in obese mice but curcumin/piperine consumption adds no further benefit. *Nutr. Metab. (Lond.)* 10:29.

Wang, M. Y., P. Grayburn, S. Chen, M. Ravazzola, L. Orci, and R. H. Unger. 2008a. Adipogenic capacity and the susceptibility to type 2 diabetes and metabolic syndrome. *Proc. Natl Acad. Sci. USA* 105:6139–6144.

Wang, R. H., Y. Zheng, H. S. Kim, X. Xu, L. Cao, T. Luhasen, M. H. Lee, C. Xiao, A. Vassilopoulos, W. Chen, K. Gardner, Y. G. Man, M. C. Hung, T. Finkel, and C. X. Deng. 2008b. Interplay among BRCA1, SIRT1, and Survivin during BRCA1-associated tumorigenesis. *Mol. Cell* 32:11–20.

Wang, R. H., K. Sengupta, C. Li, H. S. Kim, L. Cao, C. Xiao, S. Kim, X. Xu, Y. Zheng, B. Chilton, R. Jia, Z. M. Zheng, E. Appella, X. W. Wang, T. Ried, and C. X. Deng. 2008c. Impaired DNA damage response, genome instability, and tumorigenesis in SIRT1 mutant mice. *Cancer Cell* 14:312–323.

Wang, S. and R. J. Kaufman. 2012. The impact of the unfolded protein response on human disease. *J. Cell Biol.* 197:857–867.

Wang, S., S. Noh, and S. Koo. 2006. Green tea cathechins inhibit pancreatic phospholipase A(2), and intestinal absorption of lipids in ovariectomized rats. *J. Nutr. Biochem.* 17:492–498.

Wannamethee, S. G., J. Tchernova, P. Whincup, G. D. Lowe, A. Kelly, A. Rumley, A. M. Wallace, and N. Sattar. 2007. Plasma leptin: associations with metabolic, inflammatory and haemostatic risk factors for cardiovascular disease. *Atherosclerosis* 191:418–426.

Ward, W. F. 2002. Protein degradation in the aging organism. *Prog. Mol. Subcell. Biol.* 29:35–42.

Weindruch, R. 1992. Effect of caloric restriction on age-associated cancers. *Exp. Gerontol.* 27:575–581.

Weindruch, R., J. A. Kirstie, K. E. Cheney, and R. L. Walford. 1979. Influence of controlled dietary restriction on immunologic function and aging. *Fed. Proc.* 38:2007–2016.

Weindruch, R., R. L. Walford, S. Fligiel, and D. Guthrie. 1986. The retardation of aging in mice by dietary restriction: longevity, cancer, immunity, and lifetime energy intake. *J. Nutr.* 116:641–654.

Weir, R. A., K. S. Chong, J. R. Dalzell, C. J. Petrie, C. A. Murphy, T. Steedman, P. B. Mark, T. A. McDonagh, H. J. Dargie, and J. J. McMurray. 2009. Plasma apelin concentration is depressed following acute myocardial infarction in man. *Eur. J. Heart Fail.* 11:551–558.

Weisberg, S. P., R. Leibel, and D. V. Tortoriello. 2008. Dietary curcumin significantly improves obesity-associated inflammation, and diabetes in mouse models of diabesity. *Endocrinology* 149:3549–3558.

Weiss, E. P., S. B. Racette, D. T. Villareal, L. Fontana, K. Steger-May, K. B. Schechtman, S. Klein, J. O. Holloszy, and Washington University School of Medicine CALERIE Group. 2006. Improvements in glucose tolerance, and insulin action induced by increasing energy expenditure or decreasing energy intake: a randomized controlled trial. *Am. J. Clin. Nutr.* 84:1033–1042.

Weiss E. P., S. B. Racette, D. T. Villareal, L. Fontana, K. Steger-May, K. B. Schechtman, S. Klein, A. A. Ehsani, J. O. Holloszy, and Washington University School of Medicine CALERIE Group. 2007. Lower extremity muscle size and strength and aerobic capacity decrease with caloric restriction but not with exercise-induced weight loss. *J. Appl. Physiol.* 102:634–640.

Werner, C., C. Gensch, J. Pöss, J. Haendeler, M. Böhm, and U. Laufs. 2011. Pioglitazone activates aortic telomerase, and prevents stress-induced endothelial apoptosis. *Atherosclerosis* 216:23–34.

Westbrook, R., M. S. Bonkowski, O. Arum, A. D. Strader, and A. Bartke. 2014. Metabolic alterations due to caloric restriction, and every other day feeding in normal, and growth hormone receptor knockout mice. *J. Gerontol. A. Biol. Sci. Med. Sci.* 69:25–33.

Westerterp-Plantenga, M. S., M. P. Lejeune, and E. M. Kovacs. 2005. Body weight loss, and weight maintenance in relation to habitual caffeine intake, and green tea supplementation. *Obes. Res.* 13:1195–1204.

Weyer, C., J. E. Foley, C. Bogardus, P. A. Tataranni, and R. E. Pratley. 2000. Enlarged subcutaneous abdominal adipocyte size, but not obesity itself, predicts type II diabetes independent of insulin resistance. *Diabetologia* 43:1498–1506.

Wiernsperger, N. F. and C. J. Bailey. 1999. The antihyperglycaemic effect of metformin: therapeutic, and cellular mechanisms. *Drugs* 58:31–39.

Willcox, B. J., T. A Donlon., Q. He, R. Chen, J. S. Grove, K. Yano, K. H. Masaki, D. C. Willcox, B. Rodriguez, and J. D. Curb. 2008. FOXO3A genotype is strongly associated with human longevity. *Proc. Natl Acad. Sci. U. S. A.* 105:13987–13992.

Willcox, B. J., D. C. Willcox, H. Todoriki, A. Fujiyoshi, K. Yano, Q. He, J. D. Curb, and M. Suzuki. 2007. Caloric restriction, the traditional Okinawan diet, and healthy aging: the diet of the world's longest-lived people, and its potential impact on morbidity, and life span. *Ann. NY Acad. Sci.* 1114:434–455.

Willcox, D. C., B. J. Willcox, H. Todoriki, J. D. Curb, and M. Suzuki. 2006. Caloric restriction, and human longevity: what can we learn from the Okinawans? *Biogerontology* 7:173–177.

Wolfram, S., D. Raederstorff, Y. Wang, S. R. Teixeira, V. Elste, and P. Weber. 2005. TEAVIGO (epigallocatechin gallate) supplementation prevents obesity in rodents by reducing adipose tissue mass. *Ann. Nutr. Metab.* 49:54–63.

Wong, R. H., P. R. Howe, J. D. Buckley, A. M. Coates, I. Kunz, and N. M. Berry. 2011. Acute resveratrol supplementation improves flow-mediated dilatation in overweight/obese individuals with mildly elevated blood pressure. *Nutr. Metab. Cardiovasc. Dis.* 21:851–856.

Wong, R. H., N. M. Berry, A. M. Coates, J. D. Buckley, J. Bryan, I. Kunz, and P. R. Howe. 2013. Chronic resveratrol consumption improves brachial flow-mediated dilatation in healthy obese adults. *J. Hypertens.* 31:1819–1827.

Wood, J. G., B. Rogina, S. Lavu, K. Howitz, and S. L. Helfand. 2004. Sirtuin activators mimic caloric restriction, and delay ageing in metazoans. *Nature* 430:686–689.

Wu, J., R. Zhang, M. Torreggiani, A. Ting, H. Xiong, G. E. Striker, H. Vlassara, and F. Zheng. 2010. Induction of diabetes in aged C57B6 mice results in severe nephropathy: an association with oxidative stress, endoplasmic reticulum stress, and inflammation. *Am. J. Pathol.* 176:2163–2176.

Xia, E., G. Rao, H. Van Remmen, A. R. Heydari, and A. Richardson. 1995. Activities of antioxidant enzymes in various tissues of male Fischer 344 rats are altered by food restriction. *J. Nutr.* 125:195–201.

Xiang, L. and G. He. 2011. Calorie restriction and antiaging effects. *Ann. Nutr. Metab.* 58:42–48.

Xiao, X. and B. L. Song. 2013. SREBP: a novel therapeutic target. *Acta Biochim. Biophys. Sin. Shanghai* 45:2–10.

Xie, Z., K. Lau, B. Eby, P. Lozano, C. He, B. Pennington, H. Li, S. Rathi, Y. Dong, R. Tian, D. Kem, and M. H. Zou. 2011. Improvement of cardiac functions by chronic metformin treatment is associated with enhanced cardiac autophagy in diabetic OVE26 mice. *Diabetes* 60:1770–1778.

Xiong, S., G. Salazar, N. Patrushev, M. Ma, F. Forouzandeh, L. Hilenski, and R. W. Alexander. 2013. Peroxisome proliferator-activated receptor γ coactivator-1α is a central negative regulator of vascular senescence. *Arterioscler. Thromb. Vasc. Biol.* 33:988–998.

Xue, B., Z. Yang, X. Wang, and H. Shi. 2012. Omega-3 polyunsaturated fatty acids antagonize macrophage inflammation via activation of AMPK/SIRT1 pathway. *PLoS One* 7:e45990.

Xydakis, A. M., C. C. Case, P. H. Jones, R. C. Hoogeveen, M. Y. Liu, E. O. Smith, K. W. Nelson, and C. M. Ballantyne. 2004. Adiponectin, inflammation, and the expression of the metabolic syndrome in obese individuals: the impact of rapid weight loss through caloric restriction. *J. Clin. Endocrinol. Metabol.* 89:2697–2703.

Yamagishi, S. I., D. Edelstein, X. L. Du, Y. Kaneda, M. Guzmán, and M. Brownlee. 2001. Leptin induces mitochondrial superoxide production and monocyte chemoattractant protein-1 expression in aortic endothelial cells by increasing fatty acid oxidation via protein kinase A. *J. Biol. Chem.* 276:25096–25100.

Yamawaki, H., N. Tsubaki, M. Mukohda, M. Okada, and Y. Hara. 2010. Omentin, a novel adipokine, induces vasodilation in rat isolated blood vessels. *Biochem. Biophys. Res. Commun.* 393:668–672.

Yang, H., T. Yang, J. A. Baur, E. Perez, T. Matsui, J. J. Carmona, D. W. Lamming, N. C. Souza-Pinto, V. A. Bohr, A. Rosenzweig, R. de Cabo, A. A. Sauve, and D. A. Sinclair. 2007. Nutrient-sensitive mitochondrial NAD^+ levels dictate cell survival. *Cell* 130:1095–1107.

Yang, J. Y., S. J. Lee, H. W. Park, and Y. S. Cha. 2006a. Effect of genistein with carnitine administration on lipid parameters, and obesity in C57Bl/6J mice fed a high-fat diet. *J. Med. Food* 9:459–467.

Yang, L., P. Li, S. Fu, E. S. Calay, and G. S. Hotamisligil. 2010. Defective hepatic autophagy in obesity promotes ER stress, and causes insulin resistance. *Cell Metab.* 11:467–478.

Yang, R. Z., M. J. Lee, H. Hu, J. Pray, H. B. Wu, B. C. Hansen, A. R. Shuldiner, S. K. Fried, J. C. McLenithan, and D. W. Gong. 2006b. Identification of omentin as a novel depot-specific adipokine in human adipose tissue: possible role in modulating insulin action. *Am. J. Physiol. Endocrinol. Metab.* 290:E1253–E1261.

Yang, Z., M. Hulver, R. P. McMillan, L. Cai, E. E. Kershaw, L. Yu, B. Xue, and H. Shi. 2012. Regulation of insulin and leptin signaling by muscle suppressor of cytokine signaling 3 (SOCS3). *PLoS One* 7:e47493.

Yen, W. L. and D. J. Klionsky. 2008. How to live long, and prosper: autophagy, mitochondria, and aging. *Physiology (Bethesda)* 23:248–262.

Yeung, F., J. E. Hoberg, C. S. Ramsey, M. D. Keller, D. R. Jones, R. A. Frye, and M. W. Mayo. 2004. Modulation of NF-kappaB-dependent transcription, and cell survival by the SIRT1 deacetylase. *EMBO J.* 23:2369–2380.

Yoshimori T. 2004. Macroautophagy: a regulated bulk degradation process inside cells. *Biochem. Biophys. Res. Commun.* 313:453–458.

Yoshino, J., C. Conte, L. Fontana, B. Mittendorfer, S. Imai, K. B. Schechtman, C. Gu, I. Kunz, F. Rossi Fanelli, B. W. Patterson, and S. Klein. 2012. Resveratrol supplementation does not improve metabolic function in nonobese women with normal glucose tolerance. *Cell Metab.* 16:658–664.

Young, A. R., E. Y. Chan, X. W. Hu, R. Köchl, S. G. Crawshaw, S. High, D. W. Hailey, J. Lippincott-Schwartz, and S. A. Tooze. 2006. Starvation, and ULK1-dependent cycling of mammalian Atg9 between the TGN, and endosomes. *J. Cell Sci.* 119:3888–3900.

Yu, A., Y. Zheng, R. Zhang, J. Huang, Z. Zhu, R. Zhou, D. Jin, and Z. Yang. 2013. Resistin impairs SIRT1 function and induces senescence-associated phenotype in hepatocytes. *Mol. Cell Endocrinol.* 377:23–32.

Yuan, R., S. W. Tsaih, S. B. Petkova, C. Marin de Evsikova, S. Xing, M. A. Marion, M. A. Bogue, K. D. Mills, L. L. Peters, C. J. Bult, C. J. Rosen, J. P. Sundberg, D. E. Harrison, G. A. Churchill, and B. Paigen. 2009. Aging in inbred strains of mice: study design, and interim report on median lifespans, and circulating IGF1 levels. *Aging Cell* 8:277–287.

Yue, P., H. Jin, M. Aillaud, A. C. Deng, J. Azuma, T. Asagami, R. K. Kundu, G. M. Reaven, T. Quertermous, and P. S. Tsao. 2010. Apelin is necessary for the maintenance of insulin sensitivity. *Am. J. Physiol. Endocrinol. Metab.* 298:E59–E67.

Zámbó, V., L. Simon-Szabó, P. Szelényi, E. Kereszturi, G. Bánhegyi, and M. Csala. 2013. Lipotoxicity in the liver. *World J. Hepatol.* 5:550–557.

Zanetti, M., G. Gortan Cappellari, I. Burekovic, R. Barazzoni, M. Stebel, and G. Guarnieri. 2010. Caloric restriction improves endothelial dysfunction during vascular aging: effects on nitric oxide synthase isoforms and oxidative stress in rat aorta. *Exp. Gerontol.* 45:848–855.

Zeier, Z., I. Madorsky, Y. Xu, W. O. Ogle, L. Notterpek, and T. C. Foster. 2011. Gene expression in the hippocampus: regionally specific effects of aging, and caloric restriction. *Mech. Ageing Dev.* 132:8–19.

Zha, J. M., W. J. Di, T. Zhu, Y. Xie, J. Yu, J. Liu, P. Chen, and G. Ding. 2009. Comparison of gene transcription between subcutaneous and visceral adipose tissue in Chinese adults. *Endocr. J.* 56:935–944.

Zhang, K. 2010. Integration of ER stress, oxidative stress, and the inflammatory response in health, and disease. *Int. J. Clin. Exp. Med.* 3:33–40.

Zhang, K. and R. J. Kaufman. 2008. From endoplasmic-reticulum stress to the inflammatory response. *Nature* 454:455–462.

Zhang, K., X. Shen, J. Wu, K. Sakaki, T. Saunders, D. T. Rutkowski, S. H. Back, and R. J. Kaufman. 2006. Endoplasmic reticulum stress activates cleavage of CREBH to induce a systemic inflammatory response. *Cell* 124:587–599.

Zhang, X. H., B. Huang, S. K. Choi, and J. S. Seo. 2012. Anti-obesity effect of resveratrol-amplified grape skin extracts on 3T3-L1 adipocytes differentiation. *Nutr. Res. Pract.* 6:286–293.

Zhang, X. Q., C. F. Xu, C. H. Yu, W. X. Chen, and Y. M. Li. 2014. Role of endoplasmic reticulum stress in the pathogenesis of nonalcoholic fatty liver disease. *World J. Gastroenterol.* 20:1768–1776.

Zhang, Y., T. Lei, J. F. Huang, S. B. Wang, L. L. Zhou, Z. Q. Yang, and X. D. Chen. 2011. The link between fibroblast growth factor 21, and sterol regulatory element binding protein 1c during lipogenesis in hepatocytes. *Mol. Cell. Endocrinol.* 342:41–47.

Zhang, Y. K., K. C. Wu and C. D. Klaassen. 2013. Genetic activation of Nrf2 protects against fasting-induced oxidative stress in livers of mice. *PLoS One* 8: e59122.

Zhao, J., X. B. Sun, F. Ye, and W. X. Tian. 2011. Suppression of fatty acid synthase, differentiation, and lipid accumulation in adipocytes by curcumin. *Mol. Cell. Biochem.* 351:19–28.

Zhong, L., J. K. Furne, and M. D. Levitt. 2006. An extract of black, green, and mulberry teas causes malabsorption of carbohydrate but not of triacylglycerol in healthy volunteers. *Am. J. Clin. Nutr.* 84:551–555.

Zhong, X., X. Li, F. Liu, H. Tan, and D. Shang. 2012. Omentin inhibits TNF-α-induced expression of adhesion molecules in endothelial cells via ERK/NF-κB pathway. *Biochem. Biophys. Res. Commun.* 425:406–410.

Zhou, G., R. Myers, Y. Li, Y. Chen, X. Shen, J. Fenyk-Melody, M. Wu, J. Ventre, T. Doebber, N. Fujii, N. Musi, M. F. Hirshman, L. J. Goodyear, and D. E. Moller. 2001. Role of AMP-activated protein kinase in mechanism of metformin action. *J. Clin. Invest.* 108:1167–1174.

Zhou, J., W. Liao, J. Yang, K. Ma, X. Li, Y. Wang, D. Wang, L. Wang, Y. Zhang, Y. Yin, Y. Zhao, and W. G. Zhu. 2012. FOXO3 induces FOXO1-dependent autophagy by activating the AKT1 signaling pathway. *Autophagy* 8:1712–1723.

Zhu, M., J. Miura, L. X. Lu, M. Bernier, R. DeCabo, M. A. Lane, G. S. Roth, and D. K. Ingram. 2004. Circulating adiponectin levels increase in rats on caloric restriction: the potential for insulin sensitization. *Exp. Gerontol.* 34:1049–1059.

Zong, H., J. M. Ren, L. H. Young, M. Pypaert, J. Mu, M. J. Birnbaum, and G. I. Shulman. 2002. AMP kinase is required for mitochondrial biogenesis in skeletal muscle in response to chronic energy deprivation. *Proc. Natl Acad. Sci. USA* 99:15983–15987.

CHAPTER 3

Nutrition, epigenetics and ageing

Jill Ann McKay[1] and Luisa Anne Wakeling[2]
[1] Sir James Spence Institute, Royal Victoria Infirmary, Queen Victoria Road, Newcastle upon Tyne, UK
[2] School of Dental Sciences, Newcastle University, Newcastle upon Tyne, UK

3.1 Introduction

As Westernized populations are becoming increasingly old, it has become more important to understand how we age in order to promote lifestyle choices that will lead to healthy ageing. There has therefore been a growing interest in understanding the biological basis for ageing, and the influence of environmental factors. One set of biological mechanisms modifiable by environmental factors while also having the potential to influence variation in life expectancy and health are epigenetic marks, including DNA methylation, histone modifications and noncoding RNAs (ncRNA). Although a variety of environmental factors have been shown to alter epigenetic patterns, the influence of diet and nutrition on these marks is widely documented. Furthermore, the consequences of early life nutrition on epigenetic mechanisms are hypothesized to be life-long with potential impacts on health, disease and longevity.

Here we explore the potential for nutrition and dietary factors to modulate the epigenetic marks associated with ageing and comment on how this may lead to further understanding of chronic diseases and/or longevity in humans.

3.2 Epigenetics

Epigenetics refers to a series of marks on and around the genome that are copied from one cell generation to the next, without alteration of the primary DNA sequence. Three distinct types of epigenetic marks exist that closely interact to form the "epigenome". These marks include DNA methylation, histone modifications and noncoding microRNAs (miRNA) (Goldberg *et al.*, 2007; Link *et al.*, 2010). Collectively the epigenome is involved in gene regulation during embryonic and *in utero* development, playing a key role in cellular and organ-specific differentiation (Reik, 2007). The stability of epigenetic marks is also important throughout the life course in maintaining cellular and overall health, with aberrations or "epimutations" thought to influence the risk of noncommunicable diseases and to be involved in the ageing processes.

Anti-Ageing Nutrients: Evidence-Based Prevention of Age-Associated Diseases, First Edition. Edited by Delminda Neves.

3.2.1 DNA methylation

DNA methylation refers to the addition of a methyl group to dinucleotide residues of DNA. Although other types of DNA methylation exist, the vast majority of methylation marks on DNA are found on the 5′ position of cytosine residues where the cytosine is followed by a guanine residue in the 5′ to 3′ direction. Methylation at these CpG dinucleotide sites is the most widely investigated methylation mark. In the human genome, CpG sites occur less frequently than expected (Jones & Liang, 2009), and tend to either cluster in dense "CpG-rich" regions or be dispersed throughout the genome in "CpG-poor" regions. While cytosines within CpG-poor regions tend to be methylated, CpG-rich regions, termed CpG islands (CGI), tend to be positioned within the promoter regions of actively transcribed house-keeping and tumour suppressor genes, and are usually unmethylated. In contrast, some silent genes do contain CGI within the promoters that are predominantly methylated (Bird, 2002). Both hypermethylation of usually unmethylated CGI and hypomethylation of non-CGI regions are a frequent observation in cancers, emphasizing the importance of maintaining the integrity of these marks (Jones and Baylin, 2002, 2007). Growing evidence suggests the tissue specificity of DNA methylation patterns (Ollikainen *et al.*, 2010; Schneider *et al.*, 2010), supporting the role of this epigenetic mark in gene regulation for cellular and organ-specific differentiation during development. Furthermore, DNA methylation is involved in several key physiological processes, including inactivation of the X chromosome, genomic imprinting and the silencing of germline-specific genes and repetitive elements.

DNA methyltransferases (DNMTs) are the family of enzymes responsible for establishing and maintaining DNA methylation (Table 3.1). These enzymes utilize the universal methyl donor *S*-adenosylmethionine (SAM) as a substrate to add a methyl group to DNA. Mouse models have demonstrated that Dnmt1, Dnmt3a and Dnmt3b are essential for normal embryo development (Li *et al.*, 1992; Okano *et al.*, 1999), underscoring the significance of DNA methylation in development. During embryogenesis, methylation patterns are established ("*de novo*") by Dnmt3a and Dnmt3b. While DNMT3L has no catalytic

Table 3.1 Function of the different DNA methyltransferases (DNMT)

Human DNA Methyltransferase	Mouse DNA Methyltransferase	Function	Reference
DNMT1	Dnmt1	Maintenance of DNA methylation patterns during mitosis	Maunakea *et al.* (2010)
DNMT3A DNMT3B	Dnmt3a Dnmt3b	Essential for normal embryo development in establishing methylation patterns and involved in maintenance of methylation	Li *et al.* (1992); Okano *et al.* (1999); Jones and Liang (2009)
DNMT3L	Dnmt3L	Lacks methyltransferase activity, regulates DNMT3 for allele-specific methylation in imprinted regions	Bourc'his *et al.* (2001)

activity, it is responsible for the activation of DNMT3A to establish allele-specific methylation in imprinted regions of the genome (Bourc'his *et al.*, 2001). Maintenance of DNA methylation patterns during mitosis is primarily achieved by the DNMT1 enzyme, whereby methylation marks are copied from the parental to the daughter strand soon after replication (Maunakea *et al.*, 2010) owing to the high affinity of DNMT1 for hemimethylated DNA (Pradhan *et al.*, 1999). More recently it has been suggested that DNMT3A and DNMT3B complete the maintenance methylation process, in particular, by correcting errors left by DNMT1 (Jones and Liang, 2009).

A further DNA methylation mark, 5-hydroxymethyl-2′deoxycytidine, has been recently discovered. Although currently little is known about it, including its origin, it may be particularly important in the brain. It has been reported to constitute 0.6% of total nucleotides in Purkinje cells (Kriaucionis & Heintz, 2009) and may play a role in epigenetic control of neuronal function.

3.2.2 Histone modifications

DNA is packaged into chromatin by wrapping around an octamer core of histone proteins. This nucleosome core contains two copies of each of the four core histones – H3, H4, H2A and H2B (Kouzarides, 2007) – which provides structure and stability for the DNA and a mechanism for regulation of gene expression. Histone tails protrude from the core proteins, which can have a number of post-translational modifications of specific amino acid residues. These epigenetic modifications include acetylation and ubiquitination of lysine residues, phosphorylation of serines and methylation of lysine and arginines (Berger, 2007). Further modifications include ADP-ribosylation, proline isomerization, citrullination, butyrylation, propionylation and glycosylation (Gardner *et al.*, 2011). Over 100 distinct post-translational modifications of histones exist (Kouzarides, 2007), which comprise the histone code (Jenuwein & Allis, 2001). Together with the other epigenetic marks, this complex series of histone modifications regulates the expression of associated genes (Bernstein *et al.*, 2007) by orchestrating the chromatin structure to be active or repressive. As with the other epigenetic mechanism, DNA methylation, this sophisticated control of gene expression via histone modification is cell and tissue specific with major consequences for cell fate decisions, but is also responsive to the environment, which therefore has consequences for both normal and pathological development (Jenuwein & Allis, 2001) as well as ageing (Mathers, 2006).

3.2.3 Noncoding RNAs

Only around 3% of all eukaryotic transcripts encode proteins, with the majority of transcripts being for ncRNA [The ENCODE (ENCyclopedia Of DNA Elements) Project, 2004]. Noncoding RNAs have a regulatory function in gene expression via roles in transcription, mRNA degradation, splicing and translation (Kaikkonen *et al.*, 2011). Small interfering RNAs induce heterochromatin to recruit histone deacetylase complexes, leading to post-transcriptional silencing (Grewal, 2010), while long ncRNAS help establish cell-specific epigenetic patterns by guiding chromatin-modifying complexes to specific loci in the genome (Guttman *et al.*, 2009; Khalil *et al.*, 2009).

MicroRNA comprises a large family of small (18–24 nucleotide long) single-stranded RNAs. These miRNA bind to RNA in a sequence-specific manner to regulate transcription of approximately 30% of all protein-encoding genes, therefore influencing almost all genetic pathways by targeting transcription factors, secreted factors, receptors and transporters (Esquela-Kerscher & Slack, 2006). Target mRNA expression is suppressed by influencing mRNA stability and/or targeting the mRNA for degradation (Esquela-Kerscher & Slack, 2006). Furthermore miRNA are able to bind to DNA regulatory regions and recruit chromatin modifying complexes, leading to altered chromatin conformation and resulting in altered gene expression (Chuang & Jones, 2007). Genomic sequences encoding miRNA have been reported to be polymorphic (Ryan *et al.*, 2010), adding complexity to the interactions between the genome and the epigenetic machinery responsible for regulating gene expression.

3.2.4 The function of epigenetic mechanisms

The major function of epigenetic mechanisms lies in the ability to control and orchestrate the regulation of gene expression. In general, gene silencing is associated with the methylation of DNA and miRNA signals, while specific histone modifications are characteristic of either gene silencing or gene expression. While the implications of many histone marks remain uncertain, evidence suggests that the combination of histone deacetylation with the methylation of lysine residue 9 on histone H3 (H3K9) and lysine 27 (H3K27) is associated with gene silencing, whereas overall histone acetylation, H3K9 and H3K27 demethylation combined with H3K4 methylation, is observed in active gene transcription (Delage & Dashwood, 2008). Together these individual epigenetic mechanisms unite to provide a robust and responsive system for gene regulation. Additionally, epigenetic mechanisms are responsible for the suppression of viral genomes (Jaenisch & Bird, 2003) and other potentially hazardous sequences that have become integrated into the human genome over evolutionary time.

The maintenance of these epigenetic mechanisms is vital for optimal cell function to ensure that gene regulation is (a) characteristic of that cell lineage, (b) appropriate for the developmental state of the organism and (c) responsive to intrinsic and environmental signals (Jaenisch & Bird, 2003). While the function of these mechanisms demands that they are modifiable, the inherent plasticity of epigenetic marks means that they are susceptible to changes over time and through environmental cues. Indeed, increasing evidence demonstrates epigenetic drift over time/with age (Bjornsson *et al.*, 2008; Bocklandt *et al.*, 2011) and alterations in epigenetic marks in response to a range of environmental factors, including diet and nutrition (reviewed in Bollati & Baccarelli, 2010; Mathers *et al.*, 2010; McKay & Mathers, 2011; Cortessis *et al.*, 2012). Although there is now convincing proof of the function of epigenetic marks (Jaenisch & Bird, 2003), there are still considerable areas of ignorance about the roles of specific marks and proteins and their interactions between one another and with external environmental factors.

Despite the degree of plasticity, it is imperative that epigenetic control is largely maintained, with aberrations of epigenetic marks implicated in the aetiology of noncommunicable diseases, including cancers and metabolic and neurodegenerative disorders (reviewed in Cortessis *et al.*, 2012). Many of these diseases are age-related, suggesting that a gradual loss of epigenetic control with age may be causal. If such epigenetic control could be maintained through environmental factors such as diet and nutrition, disease prevention and healthy ageing may therefore be plausible.

3.3 Epigenetics and ageing

3.3.1 DNA methylation profiles and ageing

Normal cellular function is governed by the interplay between genetics, epigenetics and the environment. Epigenetic patterns are not permanent and are susceptible to changes across tissues; these changes are not necessarily the same in all cells, therefore tissue is susceptible to epigenetic drift over time. Maintenance of epigenetic homeostasis is therefore important to reduce cell diversity that may affect function across the tissue, thus contributing to the ageing process.

Alteration in DNA methylation with age involves a global loss of 5-methyl cytosine content across the genome. First identified in salmon (Berdyshev *et al.*, 1967), further study revealed that methylation is mainly reduced with age in highly methylated, repetitive short and long interspersed elements of the genome, such as Alu and LINE1 respectively (Fraga *et al.*, 2007; Rodriguez *et al.*, 2008). Methylation of Alu in DNA from lymphocytes was shown, over a period of 8 years, to significantly decline in individuals (Bollati *et al.*, 2009). The implications of methylation loss are important and contribute to instability of the chromosome and tumour formation (Eden *et al.*, 2003; discussed in Chapter 4).

In addition, typically unmethylated domains can undergo an age-related increase in methylation. Detection of age-related, gene-specific hypermethylation of the oestrogen receptor *ESR1* in normal human colonic and prostate tissue (Issa *et al.*, 1994; Kwabi-Addo *et al.*, 2007) coincides with a similar change observed owing to cancer. The occurrence of hypermethylation in CGI of promoter regions is believed to decrease the expression of genes, although this inverse correlation is not always the case (van Eijk *et al.*, 2012). Loss of function of hypermethylated genes in aged or age-related diseased tissue supports the idea that aberrant methylation can contribute to an ageing cellular phenotype.

DNMT enzymes are directly responsible for the addition of methyl groups and so a loss of genome methylation during ageing has been attributed to a decrease in expression and activity of the maintenance methyltransferase, DNMT1 (Lopatina *et al.*, 2002; Casillas *et al.*, 2003). Conversely an increase in gene-specific methylation is proposed by increased activity of the *de novo* methyltransferase, DNMT3b (Casillas *et al.*, 2003). Conservation of DNMT level is important in controlling the integrity of telomeres (Gonzalo *et al.*, 2006), a well-known marker of biological ageing.

We have evidence that alterations in DNA methylation are associated with normal and accelerated ageing processes (Heyn *et al.*, 2013), but changes have been mainly identified with age-associated diseases, primarily cancer (Kulis and Esteller, 2010). However, the challenge remains to distinguish if a change in DNA methylation is causal in disease or a consequence of the disease itself. As technology moves forward, techniques such as epigenome-wide association studies may move towards discovering the key epigenetic determinants of disease. These techniques are still in their infancy (Rakyan *et al.*, 2011), but may eventually be used to uncover the epigenetic changes required to initiate the complex process of ageing.

3.3.2 Histone modifications and ageing

Amino acid residues of histone tails that protrude from the nucleosome complex can be altered by post-translational modifications such as acetylation, methylation and phosphorylation and form a complex process (Berger, 2007). Changes with ageing are apparent: histone acetylation status between older monozygous twins is remarkably different when, in the early years of life, monozygous twins are generally epigenetically indistinguishable (Fraga *et al.*, 2005). An increase in the trimethylation of lysine 20 residue of histone 4 (H4-K20) was observed in the kidney and liver of older rats (Sarg *et al.*, 2002) and in humans a gradual dephosphorylation of histone H1 was observed in peripheral blood lymphocytes over the compared age groups (23–30, 38–50 and 60–65 years; Happel *et al.*, 2008). Outcomes from a change in these modifications with the ageing process are currently unclear.

3.3.3 MicroRNAs and ageing

The study of the relationship between miRNAs and ageing is a rapidly expanding area of research. MicroRNAs post-transcriptionally regulate genes connected with many cellular processes, including cell development, proliferation and death. The first, discovered in *Caenorhabditis elegans*, was lin-4 (Lau *et al.*, 2001) and a mutation in this miRNA showed that it determined lifespan, involving insulin/insulin-like signalling, a pathway concerned with ageing. Various miRNAs are differentially expressed across various tissues during ageing (reviewed in Smith-Vikos & Slack, 2012). MicroRNAs are also involved in regulating senescence, effecting the expression of p53 and p21, important factors involved in DNA damage response-induced senescence (reviewed in Chen *et al.*, 2010). Many age-related targets and pathways are shown to be regulated by miRNAs and are proposed to act positively or negatively towards lifespan (Chen *et al.*, 2010), but with the multiple targets that one miRNA can affect, and also the fact that many miRNAs can target one gene, those miRNAs that are critical in the ageing process will be difficult to disentangle in *in vitro* systems and yet more complex *in vivo*.

3.4 Influence of nutrition on epigenetic modifications

Growing evidence supports the role of dietary factors, including specific nutrients, in shaping the epigenome (Davis & Uthus, 2004; Mathers & Ford, 2009). Currently there is evidence that dietary habits in humans or diet strategies in animal models (i.e. high fat, low protein or energy restriction) can alter a range of epigenetic marks (Hass *et al.*, 1993; Miyamura *et al.*, 1993; Rees *et al.*, 2000; Lillycrop *et al.*, 2005, 2008; Brait *et al.*, 2009; van Straten *et al.*, 2010; Widiker *et al.*, 2010). Furthermore, variation of specific micronutrient or non-nutrient dietary components (i.e. folate, selenium or polyphenols) alone can alter the epigenome (Jacob *et al.*, 1998; Davis *et al.*, 2000; Rampersaud *et al.*, 2000; Demary *et al.*, 2001; Day *et al.*, 2002; Davis & Uthus, 2003; Fang *et al.*, 2003, 2005; Waterland & Jirtle, 2003; Druesne *et al.*, 2004; Dolinoy *et al.*, 2006; Niculescu *et al.*, 2006; Kovacheva *et al.*, 2007; Xiang *et al.*, 2008; Steegers-Theunissen *et al.*, 2009; Pandey *et al.*, 2010; McKay *et al.*, 2011a–d, 2012).

While Gabory *et al.* (2009) postulate that activation of nuclear receptor by ligands and membrane receptor signalling cascades may be indirect mechanisms by which environmental factors may influence epigenetic marks, they also suggest that direct activation/inhibition of chromatin machinery by environmental factors is a third mechanism. The latter may be broadly achieved in two major ways: (a) altering the abundance and/or efficacy of the enzymes responsible for epigenetic modification; and (b) altering the availability of the enzyme substrate. Although there is emerging evidence demonstrating that a range of nutrients can influence ncRNA expression (reviewed by Mathers *et al.*, 2010), the mechanisms by which this occurs is currently not well understood. However, the direct mechanisms by which DNA methylation and certain histone modifications are altered through nutritional factors are more clearly defined and will be discussed later.

3.4.1 Nutritional modulation of epigenetic enzyme activity

There are many enzymes responsible for the establishment and maintenance of epigenetic patterns. Factors that have the ability to influence the efficacy of any one of these enzymes therefore have the capacity to alter epigenetic patterning.

Given their fundamental role in forming methylcytosine, altering the activity of the DNMT enzymes is the one mechanism by which dietary factors have been postulated to alter DNA methylation (Fig. 3.1A). Selenium has been reported to reduce DNMT expression, which would be expected to reduce the capacity for DNA methylation (Xiang *et al.*, 2008). Furthermore, selenite inhibits the binding of the activator protein 1 (AP-1) transcription factor to DNA. Since DNMT1 normally binds to DNA at DNA-AP-1 transcription factor complexes, the ability of DNMT1 to bind to DNA is reduced, which in turn could lead to reduced DNA methylation (Handel *et al.*, 1995; Spyrou *et al.*, 1995). Epigallocatechin-3-*O*-gallate (EGCG) from green tea has been reported to inhibit DNMT1 directly by fitting to the binding pocket of the DNMT1, thus reducing its ability to methylate DNA (Fang *et al.*, 2003; Lee *et al.*, 2005). Genistein, however, has been implicated in increasing DNMT activity (and thus DNA methylation) via its effect on oestrogen receptor-dependent processes (Fang *et al.*, 2005). Membrane-mediated oestrogenic actions inducing c-fos are hypothesized to be triggered by genistein, leading to direct up-regulation of DNMT1 transcription (Hyder *et al.*, 1992; Bakin & Curran, 1999).

Several enzymes are known to be involved in the modification of histones. Histone acetyltransferases (HATs) and histone methyltransferases (HMTs) add acetyl and methyl groups to histones respectively, while histone deacetylases (HDACs) and histone demethylases (HDMs) remove these groups. These enzymes can be inhibited by several nutritional and dietary components (Fig. 3.1B). HDAC inhibitors include butyrate (a short-chain carboxylic acid produced in the colon by bacterial fermentation of carbohydrates) and dietary polyphenols (from e.g. garlic, soya and cinnamon; Demary *et al.*, 2001; Druesne *et al.*, 2004; Kida *et al.*, 2006; Rada-Iglesias *et al.*, 2007; Wang *et al.*, 2007; Link *et al.*, 2010), while green tea polyphenols and copper inhibit the HAT enzymes (Kang *et al.*, 2005; Lin *et al.*, 2005; Choi *et al.*, 2009). EGCG and a reduced availability of dietary methyl donors have been reported to inhibit HMT (Balasubramanian *et al.*, 2010; Pogribny *et al.*, 2007).

In addition to influencing the key enzymes involved in the formation of epigenetic marks, various nutrients act as co-factors to enzymes involved in the associated pathways. The most well-defined pathway known to influence epigenetic patterns is the one-carbon metabolism, which, owing to the culmination in production of SAM, can influence the methylation of both DNA and histones. Some of the micronutrients that are co-factors for enzymes in this pathway include folate, vitamin B_6, vitamin B_{12}, choline and methionine (see Fig. 3.2). In addition, dietary zinc intake may modulate DNA and histone methylation via its structural and functional role for metalloproteins. For example, betaine-homocysteine *S*-methyltransferase and cystathionine synthase are zinc metalloenzymes; therefore changes in zinc availability may affect the activity of these enzymes and thus may alter homocysteine concentrations (Fig. 3.2; Mathers & Ford, 2009).

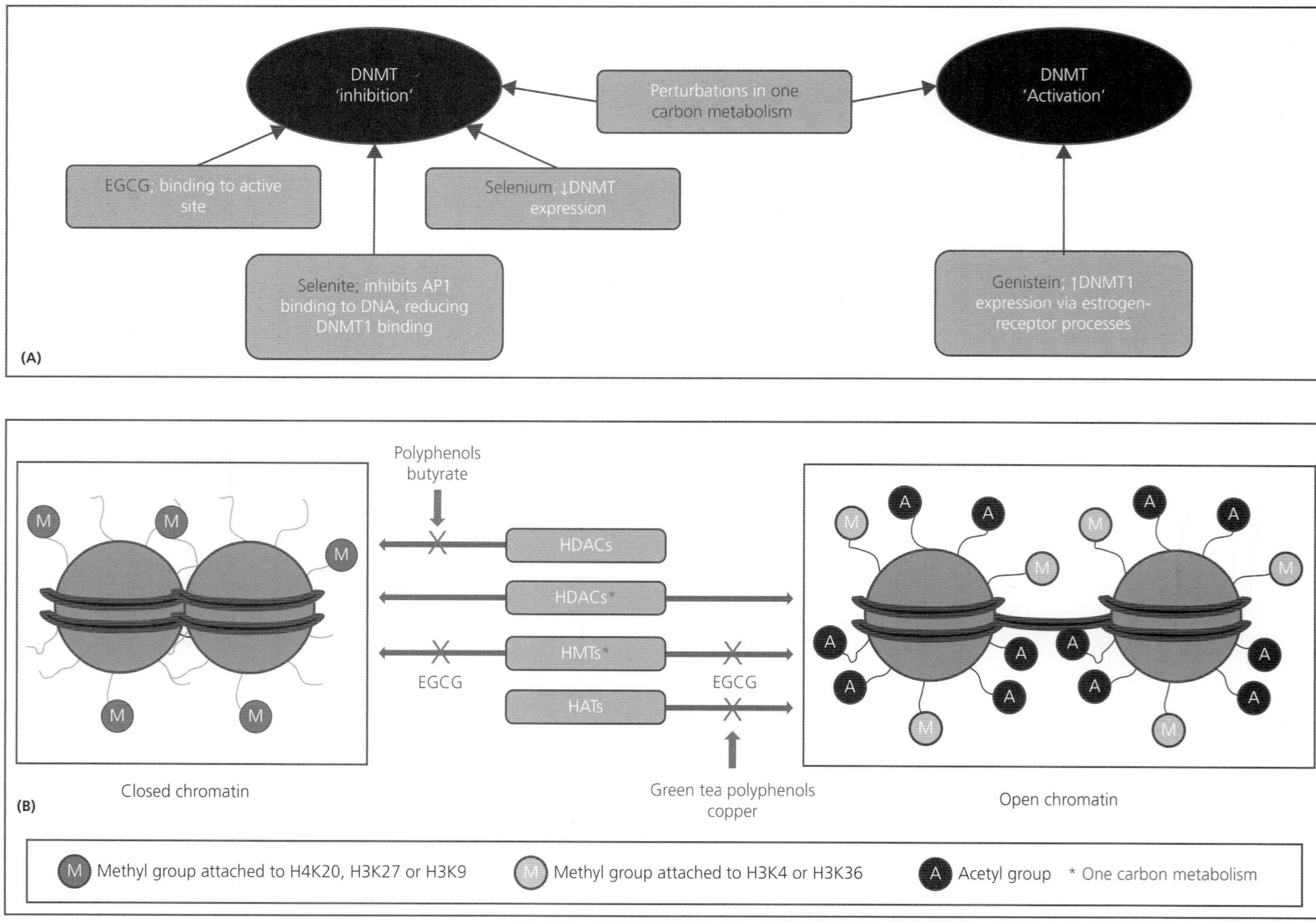

Figure 3.1 Overview of nutritional influence on key enzymes involved in the establishment and maintenance of epigenetic marks. (A) Overview of nutrients or pathways (illustrated in red) that may influence the efficacy of the DNA methyltransferase enzymes (DNMT), potentially affecting DNA methylation patterns. (B) Overview of nutrients or pathways (illustrated in red) that may influence the efficacy of some enzymes involved in the modification of histones [histone deacetylases (HDACs), histone demethylases (HDMs), histone methylatransfereases (HMTs)] and histone acetyltransferases (HATs), and therefore influence chromatin configuration, i.e. open or closed. (Color version of the figure is available in the online version.)

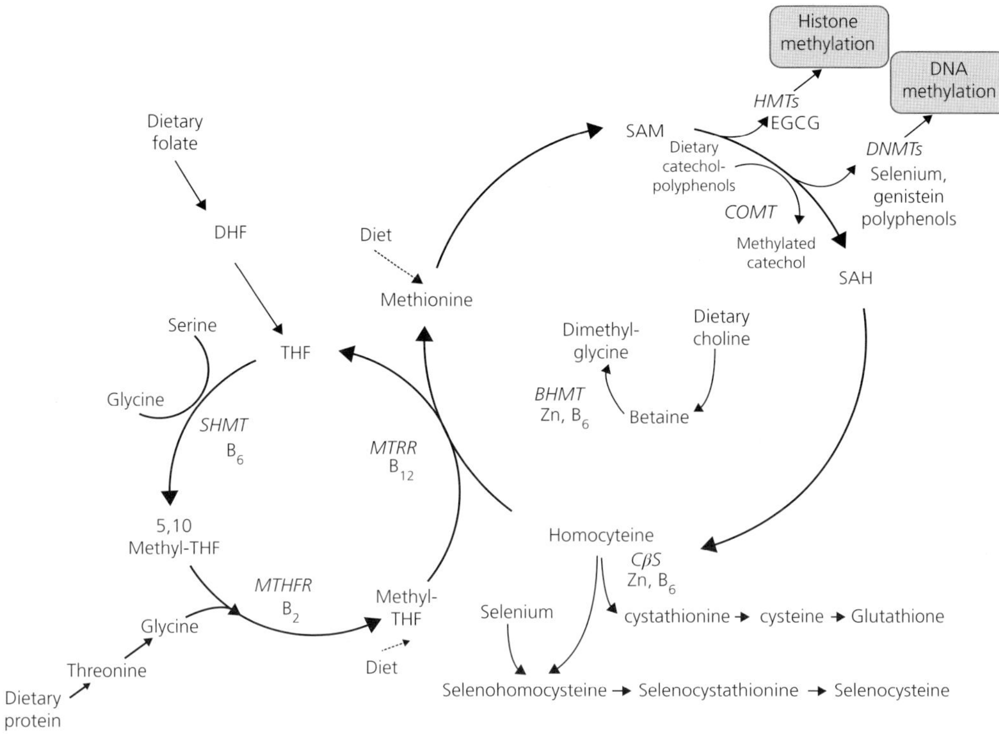

Figure 3.2 Summary of the main pathways involved in cellular one-carbon metabolism, which includes the production of *S*-adenosylmethionine (SAM) for the methylation of DNA and histones. The nutrients, and other dietary components, that have potential to modulate epigenetic marks through affecting the availability of SAM are illustrated in red, while the enzymes involved in the processes are shown in blue. Briefly, ingested dietary folates are reduced to tetrahydrofolate (THF) in the gut via di- and tetrahydrofolate reductases. THF is then absorbed from the small intestine and actively transported into enterocytes by the reduced folate carrier. Following absorption into the enterocyte, THF is converted to methyl-THF, via 5,10-methylTHF. This is through serine to glycine conversion by serine hydroxymethyltransferase (SHMT) followed by the reduction of 5,10-methylTHF to methylTHF by methylenetetrahydrofolate reductase (MTHFR). Methionine synthase reductase (MTRR) then utilizes methylTHF as a carbon donor in order to convert homocysteine to methionine, thus reducing methylTHF to THF and donating a carbon molecule to the one-carbon cycle. Methionine is subsequently converted to SAM, which is used in the process of methylating biological molecules such as DNA or histones. Modified from McKay & Mathers (2011). DHF, Dihydrofolate; EGCG, epigallocatechin-3-*O*-gallate; SAH, *S*-adenosylhomocysteine; HMTs, histone methyltransferases; DNMTs, DNA methyltransferases; COMT, catechol-*O*-methyl transferase; BHMT, betaine-homocysteine *S*-methyltransferase; CbS, cystathionine synthase. (Color version of the figure is available in the online version.)

3.4.2 Influence of nutrition on substrate availability for epigenetic modifications

The availability of substrates for enzymes that generate epigenetic marks is important in determining epigenetic patterns, that is, lack or abundance of substrate (such as methyl, acetyl, phosphate groups etc) availability for these enzymes is likely to influence the epigenetic profile. In this context the most widely investigated substrate is methyl group supply for one-carbon metabolism (Fig. 3.2), central to the methylation of DNA and histones (Fig. 3.2). Any dietary factors that can influence this pathway may affect the methylation of DNA and histone proteins through SAM availability. Strong evidence suggests that several nutrients can affect DNA methylation in this way (reviewed in Johnson & Belshaw, 2008; Mathers & Ford, 2009). The main group of nutrients thought to influence methylation via this mechanism are the methyl donors, that is, folate, vitamin B_6, vitamin B_{12}, choline and methionine. A deficiency or excess of any of these micronutrients could alter the availability of SAM in the methionine cycle, and therefore directly influence both histone and DNA methylation.

However, other nutrients and other dietary components can affect one-carbon metabolism indirectly. Dietary selenium has been reported to cause an imbalance in the methylation cycle by decreasing homocysteine concentrations in rats (Davis & Uthus, 2003). It was proposed that, in the presence of selenium, homocysteine is converted to selenohomocysteine, cystathionine, selenocystathionine, glutathione and selenocysteine, thus reducing homocysteine availability for methionine cycle and therefore reducing global DNA methylation (Davis *et al.*, 2000; Fig. 3.2). Dietary protein intake can influence the methylation of biological molecules by altering threonine concentrations, which leads to changes in the SAM:SAH (*S*-adenosylhomocysteine) ratio, via altered threonine>glycine>methylTHF conversion (van Straten *et al.*, 2010). Green tea polyphenols are also thought to alter the SAM:SAH ratio through induction of catechol-*O*-methyl transferase (COMT)-mediated *O*-methylation, for which catechol-containing polyphenols such as EGCG are excellent substrates (Zhu *et al.*, 1994, 2000, 2001; Zhu & Liehr, 1996). Since COMT-mediated *O*-methylation also utilizes SAM as a substrate, when *O*-methylation is increased owing to an abundance of these polyphenols, there is a subsequent decrease in available SAM (Lee *et al.*, 2005).

A wide range of dietary and nutritional factors have now been reported to alter epigenetic marks, which has previously been reviewed elsewhere (Mathers & Ford, 2009; McKay & Mathers, 2011; Park *et al.*, 2012). The impact that nutritional influences have on epigenomic markers is however highly dependent on a number of factors, including the specific nutrient itself, nutrient dose, target tissue of interest, the target epigenetic mark under investigation and the timing and duration of exposure. In particular, there are periods during early development that are critical in establishing epigenetic patterns, which if disturbed may influence long-term health.

3.4.3 Critical windows and the developmental origins hypothesis

Although, nutrition and diet are likely to play an important role throughout the lifecourse in influencing epigenetic patterns, there are critical periods of development during which all environmental factors, including nutrition, are likely to play a major role in shaping the epigenetic landscape. The developmental origins of health and disease hypothesis proposes that exposures during early life modulate the risk of developing noncommunicable diseases in adulthood. Indeed, there is substantial evidence for an association between lower birth weight and increased risk of type 2 diabetes, coronary heart disease and hypertension, which has been attributed to poor nutrition *in utero* (Barker, 2004). These observations indicate the potential for a degree of plasticity during development, in which the foetal phenotype may be altered in response to environment cues (Bateson *et al.*, 2004) in ways that may prepare it for the anticipated postnatal environment (Gluckman *et al.*, 2005). In order to persist into adulthood and affect disease risk, the foetus must be "marked" at the molecular, cellular or tissue level by these environmentally orchestrated programming events. These marks must then be sustained for much of the life course and impact on the processes leading to disease development. Although the mechanistic basis of such programming events is poorly understood, there is evidence to suggest that epigenetic mechanisms are attractive potential candidates as mediators of the long-term effects of early life exposures such as nutrition.

The best documented examples of this are the studies investigating epigenetic regulation of metastable epialleles in rodent models. In their initial pivotal experiment using the agouti mouse model, Waterland and Jirtle reported that the maternal diet had a profound influence on offspring phenotype via epigenetic regulation. In this mouse model, an intracisternal A-particle is inserted into the promoter region of the agouti viable gene (A^{vy}) which is responsible for coat colour, resulting in a metastable epiallele (Waterland & Jirtle, 2003). The expression of the A^{vy} gene is then under the control of the newly formed promoter region, and is determined by the degree of DNA methylation within the promoter region (Rakyan *et al.*, 2002), that is, when hypomethylated the gene is expressed, resulting in yellow fur, along with increased susceptibility to obesity, diabetes and tumours, whereas when hypermethylated the gene is repressed, resulting a brown coat colour and a more long-lived phenotype. When pregnant dams were fed diets supplemented with methyl donors (i.e. folic acid, choline, methionine, vitamin B_{12}), their offspring tended to have brown coats and the A^{vy} gene promoter tended to be methylated in comparison with unsupplemented dams, which were likely to have offspring with yellow coats and to be unmethylated at the A^{vy} promoter locus (Waterland & Jirtle, 2003). Similar effects were observed when dams' diets were supplemented with genistein, suggesting that a variety of nutritional exposures may impact on phenotype via epigenetic mechanisms (Dolinoy *et al.*, 2006). Furthermore, the murine axin fused [*Axin(Fu)*] metastabile epiallele, which results in kinking of the tail, exhibits epigenetic plasticity to maternal diet (Waterland *et al.*, 2006). Methyl donor supplementation of female mice before and during pregnancy increased DNA methylation at *Axin(Fu)*, reducing the incidence of tail kinking in *Axin(Fu)*/+offspring by half (Waterland *et al.*, 2006). Thus this phenomenon is not exclusive to the agouti locus. Indeed there are numerous examples from the literature that suggest that nutritional exposures during development can influence the long-term epigenetic profile of the offspring (McKay *et al.*, 2011a, b; Hoile *et al.*, 2012; Langie *et al.*, 2013); however, the examples given examining the influence of maternal diet on metastable epialleles have the advantage of elegantly demonstrating the direct impact of changes in methylation at one locus on the phenotype of the offspring.

Another example of the impact of nutrition on phenotype via epigenetic mechanisms is the honey bee. Adult female bees can form two different castes, the queen and the worker. The queen is twice as large as the worker, has specialized anatomy, can actively reproduce (laying up to 2000 eggs per day) and lives up to 10 times longer, even though she is derived from fertilized eggs that are no different from those which form the workers (Wheeler, 1986; Page & Peng, 2001). The diet determines the developmental fate of the larvae – a nutritious concoction, royal jelly, produced by the digestion of pollen and nectar in the hypopharyngeal glands of nurse bees, is responsible for maintaining a queen phenotype (Winston, 1987). Larvae destined to become workers are switched from their initial diet of royal jelly to a of low-protein, high-carbohydrate diet on day 3 of their life course, a critical window of development (Nelson *et al.*, 1924). Royal jelly has yet to be completely assessed for its entire components but one component, royal actin, has been shown to be necessary for the development of the queen (Kamakura, 2011).

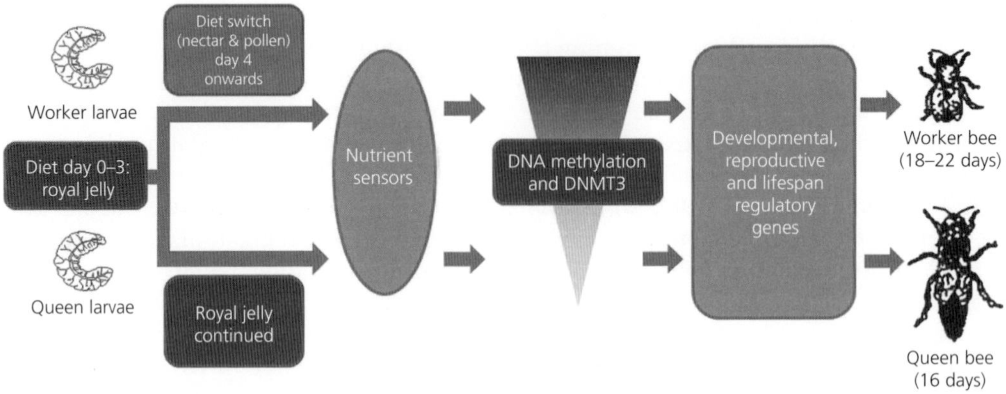

Figure 3.3 A schematic of the development of a female adult honeybee into the two potential castes. Larvae are fed royal jelly for the first 3 days by nurse bees of the hive. After the third day, in a period known as the fourth to fifth instar, larvae that are destined to become queens continue to be fed royal jelly in abundance and those larvae that are destined to become workers are switched to a more restricted diet of pollen and nectar. It is proposed that this change in diet will alter nutrient sensors, possibly through pathways such as insulin/insulin-like signalling and target of rapamycin signalling. Downstream of this will be an observed change in DNA methylation; it has been determined that there is less DNA methylation and less DNA methyltransferase (DNMT) activity in the brain of the queen. Characteristic of the queen phenotype is early emergence (16 vs 18–22 days), larger body size, specialized anatomy, active reproduction and a lifespan up to 10 times that of the worker bee. It is therefore likely that those methylation differences may occur in genes that are responsible for or feed into pathways of development, reproduction and longevity. Modified from Ford (2013).

The honeybee expresses all three DNMT enzymes and exhibits methylation at CpG dinucleotides; it is unusual to find such a fully functional system in insects (Wang *et al.*, 2006). Queens and workers differ in their DNA methylation profile with over 550 genes in the brain differentially methylated (Lyko *et al.*, 2010). Ground-breaking research revealed recently that royal jelly induces the queen phenotype through effects on DNA methylation. Larvae that were fed royal jelly the longest had significantly lower DNMT3 activities and mRNA expression, and significantly less methylation of a drosophila nutrient-sensing gene, dynactin p62 (Shi *et al.*, 2011). Silencing DNMT3 with RNA interference in honeybee larvae reduced methylation and also produced a higher proportion of queens (Kucharski *et al.*, 2008). Figure 3.3 shows the two pathways of female honeybee development driven by diet and featuring changes in methylation. This model system shows in a robust manner the link between diet, DNA methylation and lifespan and is the focus of current research to investigate further dietary components that can affect DNA methylation in longevity-related pathways (Ford, 2013).

3.5 Nutrition, epigenetics and ageing

3.5.1 Overview

Diet can influence lifespan in a number of ways: the dramatic effect of dietary restriction, a reduction in food intake, robustly extends the lifespan of many evolutionarily distinct species (discussed in Chapter 2); a dietary component of red wine, resveratrol, can also increase the lifespan of these species; and perhaps more subtle effects of dietary components may provide health benefits to reduce age-associated diseases and as a result may lengthen lifespan. We also know now that DNA methylation profiles change as we age, contributing to the ageing process, and that diet can influence DNA methylation, thus posing the question "Does diet influence the ageing process through effects on DNA methylation?"

3.5.2 Specific dietary regimens and nutrients that influence epigenetics and ageing

3.5.2.1 Dietary restriction

Mechanisms underpinning the lifespan extension effect of dietary restriction remain undetermined. With respect to epigenetic changes caused by dietary restriction, there remains limited published evidence; however, some effects on DNA methylation have been reported. Mice that were subjected to dietary restriction exhibited a transient global hypomethylation in the liver and fewer age-dependent changes in methylation of the *c-myc* oncogene (Miyamura *et al.*, 1993), and in dietary-restricted rats, hypermethylation of the *c-Ha-ras* oncogene in the pancreas was observed (Hass *et al.*, 1993). Lists of genes from published sources were shown to overlap significantly between genes that were differentially expressed in response to dietary restriction and genes altered in their methylation with increased age (Ions *et al.*, 2013). Genes identified as altered in their methylation and expression in dietary-restricted model organisms could provide links to crucial pathways involved in regulating lifespan and provide targets for other dietary interventions.

3.5.2.2 Dietary polyphenols

DNA methylation changes have been observed in the treatment of cell line models with dietary polyphenols. The major green tea polyphenol, epigallocatechin-3-gallate, has been shown to cause demethylation of numerous loci, in particular the retinoic acid receptor β gene (*RARβ*), O6-methylguanine methyltransferase gene (*MGMT*), *p16INK4a* and the human mutL homologue 1 gene (*hMLH1*) in many different cancer cell lines (Fang *et al.*, 2003; Lee *et al.*, 2005). Polyphenols from soya, the isoflavones, genistein, daidzein and biochanin A, have also been shown to reverse hypermethylation at the *RARβ* locus as well as effects on *MGMT* and *p16INK4a* (Fang *et al.*, 2005). The isoflavone genistein is also effective in influencing DNA methylation in mice, but in contrast to its effect in cell lines, by hypermethylating genes such as the A^{vy} promoter locus discussed previously (Dolinoy *et al.*, 2006). The influence of these polyphenols on DNA methylation in humans remains to be determined, as well as the subsequent effect on lifespan.

Resveratrol, a polyphenol found in the skin of red grapes, does however have an effect on lifespan, and when given to organisms such as yeast, worms, flies and honeybees has extended their lifespan (Bauer *et al.*, 2004; Jarolim *et al.*, 2004; Agarwal & Baur, 2011; Rascon *et al.*, 2012). With respect to epigenetic effects, resveratrol has been shown to demethylate the tumour suppressor gene, deleted in liver cancer 1 (*DLC-1)* and in oestrogen receptor (ER)+ breast cancer cells, and inhibit DNMTs in a dose-dependent manner (Qin *et al.*, 2005). Furthermore, a dose-dependent decrease in Ras-Association Domain Family 1a (*RASSF-1a*) methylation was associated with increasing levels of circulating *trans*-resveratrol and the glucuronide metabolite in a double-blind, randomized, placebo-controlled clinical trial of women at increased breast cancer risk (Zhu *et al.*, 2012). Since methylation of the *RASSF-1a* gene is an early indicator of tumorigenesis (Richter *et al.*, 2009), this could suggest that nutritional factors may influence epigenetic events leading to disease onset/progression. Targeting lifespan regulatory genes and measuring the effects of resveratrol on the methylation of these genes would provide more concrete evidence for epigenetics as a mechanism underling the lifespan extension effect of this polyphenol (Wakeling *et al.*, 2009).

3.5.2.3 One-Carbon metabolism

Given the involvement of one-carbon metabolism on the establishment and maintenance of epigenetic marks such as DNA methylation, and the body of evidence that implies that nutritional factors influencing this pathway can also alter epigenetic patterns (Waterland & Jirtle, 2003; Lillycrop *et al.*, 2005; Waterland *et al.*, 2006; Steegers-Theunissen *et al.*, 2009; McKay *et al.*, 2011a–d, 2012; Hoile *et al.*, 2012; Ono *et al.*, 2012; Langie *et al.*, 2013), it is not surprising that such nutritional factors may also influence these patterns during the ageing process.

In this context, folate has been most widely studied. In mice, decreased global and increased *p16* methylation have been reported in the colon of older mice compared with younger animals (Keyes *et al.*, 2007; Sauer *et al.*, 2010). However, in old, but not young mice, both genomic and *p16* methylation increased in a manner that was directly related to dietary folate, suggesting that the response to dietary folate in terms of DNA methylation is age dependant (Keyes *et al.*, 2007).

Similar relationships between folate status and ageing with regard to DNA methylation patterns have also been observed in human studies. Wallace *et al.* (2010) reported increased methylation in the normal colonic mucosa at the oestrogen receptor α and secreted frizzled related protein-1 (*SFRP1*) loci in relation to 10 year increases in age. Furthermore, erythrocyte folate levels were also found to be positively associated with methylation levels of these genes (Wallace *et al.*, 2010). More recently, Tapp *et al.* (2013) reported age-associated methylation in the normal mucosa within CGIs of nine genes. Furthermore, methylation of four of these CGI was found to be significantly positively associated with folate status (Tapp *et al.*, 2013). These observations therefore question the safety of folate supplementation in healthy adults, given that gene-specific hypermethylation of the normal colon may predispose to the development of colorectal neoplasia.

However, this may be in conflict to the reported potential beneficial effects of B vitamins, such as folate, on dementia in older adults. In particular, decreased plasma folate and increased plasma homocysteine levels, are common in Alzheimer disease (AD) and impaired SAM levels have been reported in AD brains (reviewed by Coppede, 2010). Furthermore, data from prospective cohort studies suggest that higher folate intake has been related to lower AD risk in the elderly (Ravaglia *et al.*, 2005; Luchsinger *et al.*, 2007) and more recently B-vitamin treatment of elderly subjects with increased dementia risk has been found to slow accelerated brain atrophy, shrinkage of the whole brain volume and cognitive and clinical decline (Smith *et al.*, 2010; de Jager *et al.*, 2012; Douaud *et al.*, 2013). Epigenetic mechanisms are thought to play a role in this protective effect, given that reduced levels of overall DNA methylation (Mastroeni *et al.*, 2009, 2010) and abnormal methylation of Presenilin-1 (*PSEN1*), Apolipoprotein E (*APOE*), Methylenetetrahydrofolate reductase (*MTHFR*) and *DNMT1* genes have been reported in the brains of AD patients (Wang *et al.*, 2008). Furthermore, in TgCRND8 and wild-type 129Sv mice, vitamin B deficiency was reported to lead to hypomethylation of the *PSEN1* gene, (a mutation in this gene causes familial AD, therefore suggesting an aetiological role in disease) with SAM supplementation reversing this effect (Fuso *et al.*, 2011), emphasizing a potential role for B-vitamin intake in the aetiology of the disease, which could be via epigenetic mechanisms.

It is therefore evident that further research is warranted, enabling us to understand in detail the interaction between ageing and nutritional factors on epigenetic marks, and the consequences of these effects upon the development of different disease types. In understanding more about these complex interactions, we may be able to move towards more personalized advice based on an individual's specific disease risk, enabling recommendations to be tailored appropriately, that is, an individual with higher risk of developing colorectal neoplasia may be discouraged from using supplemental folate, whereas those at risk or in the early stages of dementia may benefit from folate, and other B vitamin supplementation.

3.6 Conclusions and future perspective

In order to fully appreciate how epigenetic mechanisms can influence health, it will be essential to understand the complex interplay between the individual epigenetic mechanisms, and the interaction and influence that individual dietary factors have on these intricate, interwoven systems of regulation. Data from cell line experiments, using state-of-the-art next-generation sequencing techniques, may allow us to uncover the complex interplay between the epigenome in a highly controlled manner. However, in order to fully understand the impact of how dietary factors can manipulate the epigenome, and how these manifest themselves in terms of health, and healthy ageing, the use of model systems will be essential. While the study of ageing in rodent models is invaluable as a mammalian system, given the rodent lifespan, these studies can be both lengthy and costly. New emerging model systems such as the honeybee model may be more appropriate alternatives to investigate given the importance of epigenetic control in these organisms. Use of such model systems will be invaluable in pinpointing specific epigenetic markers to target as biomarkers in human cohorts to link epigenetics with nutrition and age-associated diseases. By using a combination of *in vivo, in vitro* and molecular epidemiological approaches, we will slowly be able to uncover the secrets of the epigenome, and its complex interaction with nutritional factors. Better understanding of the impact of diet and nutrition on the epigenome and the consequences for health and disease may enable us in the future to make public health recommendations to promote healthy ageing throughout the lifecourse.

References

Agarwal, B. and J. A. Baur. 2011. Resveratrol and life extension. *Ann. NY Acad. Sci.* 1215:138–143.

Bakin, A. V. and T. Curran. 1999. Role of DNA 5-methylcytosine transferase in cell transformation by fos. *Science* 283:387–390.

Balasubramanian, S., G. Adhikary, and R. L. Eckert. 2010. The Bmi-1 polycomb protein antagonizes the (−)-epigallocatechin-3-gallate-dependent suppression of skin cancer cell survival. *Carcinogenesis* 31:496–503.

Barker, D. J. 2004. The developmental origins of well-being. *Phil. Trans. R. Soc. Lond B Biol. Sci.* 359:1359–1366.

Bateson, P., D. Barker, T. Clutton-Brock, D. Deb, B. D'Udine, R. A. Foley, P. Gluckman, K. Godfrey, T. Kirkwood, M. M. Lahr, J. McNamara, N. B. Metcalfe, P. Monaghan, H. G. Spencer, and S. E. Sultan. 2004. Developmental plasticity and human health. *Nature* 430:419–421.

Bauer, J. H., S. Goupil, G. B. Garber, and S. L. Helfand. 2004. An accelerated assay for the identification of lifespan-extending interventions in *Drosophila melanogaster*. *Proc. Natl Acad. Sci. USA* 101: 12980–12985.

Berdyshev, G. D., G. K. Korotaev, G. V. Boiarskikh, and B. F. Vaniushin. 1967. Nucleotide composition of DNA and RNA from somatic tissues of humpback and its changes during spawning. *Biokhimiia* 32:988–993.

Berger, S. L. 2007. The complex language of chromatin regulation during transcription. *Nature* 447:407–412.

Bernstein, B. E., A. Meissner, and E. S. Lander. 2007. The mammalian epigenome. *Cell* 128:669–681.

Bird, A. 2002. DNA methylation patterns and epigenetic memory. *Genes Dev*,16:6–21.

Bjornsson, H. T., M. I. Sigurdsson, M. D. Fallin, R. A. Irizarry, T. Aspelund, H. Cui, W. Yu, M. A. Rongione, T. J. Ekstrom, T. B. Harris, L. J. Launer, G. Eiriksdottir, M. F. Leppert, C. Sapienza, V. Gudnason, and A. P. Feinberg. 2008. Intra-individual change over time in DNA methylation with familial clustering. *JAMA* 299:2877–2883.

Bocklandt, S., W. Lin, M. E. Sehl, F. J. Sanchez, J. S. Sinsheimer, S. Horvath, and E. Vilain. 2011. Epigenetic predictor of age. *PLoS One* 6: p. e14821.

Bollati, V. and A. Baccarelli. 2010. Environmental epigenetics. *Heredity (Edinb.)* 105:105–112.

Bollati, V., J. Schwartz, R. Wright, A. Litonjua, L. Tarantini, H. Suh, D. Sparrow, P. Vokonas, and A. Baccarelli. 2009. Decline in genomic DNA methylation through aging in a cohort of elderly subjects. *Mech. Ageing Dev.* 130:234–239.

Bourc'his, D., G. L. Xu, C. S. Lin, B. Bollman, and T. H. Bestor. 2001. Dnmt3L and the establishment of maternal genomic imprints. *Science* 294:2536–2539.

Brait, M., J. G. Ford, S. Papaiahgari, M. A. Garza, J. I. Lee, M. Loyo, L. Maldonado, S. Begum, L. McCaffrey, M. Howerton, D. Sidransky, M. R. Emerson, S. Ahmed, C. D. Williams, and M. O. Hoque. 2009. Association between lifestyle factors and CpG island methylation in a cancer-free population. *Cancer Epidemiol. Biomarkers Prev.* 18:2984–2991.

Casillas, M. A. Jr, N. Lopatina, L. G. Andrews, and T. O. Tollefsbol. 2003. Transcriptional control of the DNA methyltransferases is altered in aging and neoplastically-transformed human fibroblasts. *Mol. Cell. Biochem.* 252:33–43.

Chen, L. H., G. Y. Chiou, Y. W. Chen, H. Y. Li, and S. H. Chiou. 2010. MicroRNA and aging: a novel modulator in regulating the aging network. *Ageing Res. Rev.* 9 Suppl 1:S59–S66.

Choi, K. C., M. G. Jung, Y. H. Lee, J. C. Yoon, S. H. Kwon, H. B. Kang, M. J. Kim, J. H. Cha, Y. J. Kim, W. J. Jun, J. M. Lee, and H. G. Yoon. 2009. Epigallocatechin-3-gallate, a histone acetyltransferase inhibitor, inhibits EBV-induced B lymphocyte transformation via suppression of RelA acetylation. *Cancer Res.* 69:583–592.

Chuang, J. C. and P. A. Jones. 2007. Epigenetics and microRNAs. *Pediatr. Res.* 61:24R–29R.

Coppede, F. 2010. One-carbon metabolism and Alzheimer's disease: focus on epigenetics. *Curr. Genom.* 11, 246–260.

Cortessis, V. K., D. C. Thomas, A. J. Levine, C. V. Breton, T. M. Mack, K. D. Siegmund, R. W. Haile, and P. W. Laird. 2012. Environmental epigenetics: prospects for studying epigenetic mediation of exposure–response relationships. *Hum. Genet.* 131:1565–1589.

Davis, C. D. and E. O. Uthus. 2003. Dietary folate and selenium affect dimethylhydrazine-induced aberrant crypt formation, global DNA methylation and one-carbon metabolism in rats. *J. Nutr.* 133:2907–2914.

Davis, C. D. and E. O. Uthus. 2004. DNA methylation, cancer susceptibility, and nutrient interactions. *Exp. Biol. Med. (Maywood)* 229:988–995.

Davis, C. D., E. O. Uthus, and J. W. Finley. 2000. Dietary selenium and arsenic affect DNA methylation in vitro in Caco-2 cells and in vivo in rat liver and colon. *J. Nutr.* 130:2903–2909.

Day, J. K., A. M. Bauer, C. DesBordes, Y. Zhuang, B. E. Kim, L. G. Newton, V. Nehra, K. M. Forsee, R. S. MacDonald, C. Besch-Williford, T. H. Huang, and D. B. Lubahn. 2002. Genistein alters methylation patterns in mice. *J. Nutr.* 132 Suppl 8:2419S–2423S.

de Jager, C. A., A. Oulhaj, R. Jacoby, H. Refsum, and A. D. Smith. 2012. Cognitive and clinical outcomes of homocysteine-lowering B-vitamin treatment in mild cognitive impairment: a randomized controlled trial. *Int. J. Geriatr. Psychiat.* 27:592–600.

Delage, B. and R. H. Dashwood. 2008. Dietary manipulation of histone structure and function. *Annu. Rev. Nutr.* 28:347–366.

Demary, K., L. Wong, and R. A. Spanjaard. 2001. Effects of retinoic acid and sodium butyrate on gene expression, histone acetylation and inhibition of proliferation of melanoma cells. *Cancer Lett.* 163:103–107.

Dolinoy, D. C., J. R. Weidman, R. A. Waterland, and R. L. Jirtle. 2006. Maternal genistein alters coat color and protects Avy mouse offspring from obesity by modifying the fetal epigenome. *Environ. Health Perspect.*114:567–572.

Douaud, G., H. Refsum, C. A. de Jager, R. Jacoby, T. E. Nichols, S. M. Smith, and A. D. Smith. 2013. Preventing Alzheimer's disease-related gray matter atrophy by B-vitamin treatment. *Proc. Natl Acad. Sci. USA* 110:9523–9528.

Druesne, N., A. Pagniez, C. Mayeur, M. Thomas, C. Cherbuy, P. H. Duee, P. Martel, and C. Chaumontet. 2004. Diallyl disulfide (DADS) increases histone acetylation and p21(waf1/cip1) expression in human colon tumor cell lines. *Carcinogenesis* 25:1227–1236.

Eden, A., F. Gaudet, A. Waghmare, and R. Jaenisch. 2003. Chromosomal instability and tumors promoted by DNA hypomethylation. *Science* 300:455.

The ENCODE (ENCyclopedia Of DNA Elements) Project. 2004. *Science* 306:636–640.

Esquela-Kerscher, A. and F. J. Slack. 2006. Oncomirs – microRNAs with a role in cancer. *Nat. Rev. Cancer* 6:259–269.

Fang, M. Z., Y. Wang, N. Ai, Z. Hou, Y. Sun, H. Lu, W. Welsh, and C. S. Yang. 2003. Tea polyphenol (−)-epigallocatechin-3-gallate inhibits DNA methyltransferase and reactivates methylation-silenced genes in cancer cell lines. *Cancer Res.* 63:7563–7570.

Fang, M. Z., D. Chen, Y. Sun, Z. Jin, J. K. Christman, and C. S. Yang. 2005. Reversal of hypermethylation and reactivation of p16INK4a, RARbeta, and MGMT genes by genistein and other isoflavones from soy. *Clin. Cancer Res.* 11:7033–7041.

Ford, D. 2013. Honeybees and cell lines as models of DNA methylation and aging in response to diet. *Exp. Gerontol.* 48:614–619.

Fraga, M. F., R. Agrelo, and M. Esteller. 2007. Cross-talk between aging and cancer: the epigenetic language. *Ann. NY Acad. Sci.* 1100:60–74.

Fraga, M. F., E. Ballestar, M. F. Paz, S. Ropero, F. Setien, M. L. Ballestar, D. Heine-Suner, J. C. Cigudosa, M. Urioste, J. Benitez, M. Boix-Chornet, A. Sanchez-Aguilera, C. Ling, E. Carlsson, P. Poulsen, A. Vaag, Z. Stephan, T. D. Spector, Y. Z. Wu, C. Plass, and M. Esteller. 2005. Epigenetic differences arise during the lifetime of monozygotic twins. *Proc. Natl Acad. Sci. USA* 102:10604–10609.

Fuso, A., V. Nicolia, A. Pasqualato, M. T. Fiorenza, R. A. Cavallaro and S. Scarpa. 2011. Changes in Presenilin 1 gene methylation pattern in diet-induced B vitamin deficiency. *Neurobiol. Aging* 32:187–199.

Gabory, A., L. Attig, and C. Junien. 2009. Sexual dimorphism in environmental epigenetic programming. *Mol. Cell. Endocrinol.* 304:8–18.

Gardner, K. E., C. D. Allis, and B. D. Strahl. 2011. Operating on chromatin, a colorful language where context matters. *J. Mol. Biol.* 409:36–46.

Gluckman, P. D., M. A. Hanson, S. M. Morton, and C. S. Pinal. 2005. Life-long echoes – a critical analysis of the developmental origins of adult disease model. *Biol. Neonate* 87:127–139.

Goldberg, A. D., C. D. Allis, and E. Bernstein. 2007. Epigenetics: a landscape takes shape. *Cell* 128:635–638.

Gonzalo, S., I. Jaco, M. F. Fraga, T. Chen, E. Li, M. Esteller, and M. A. Blasco. 2006. DNA methyltransferases control telomere length and telomere recombination in mammalian cells. *Nat. Cell Biol.* 8:416–424.

Grewal, S. I. 2010. RNAi-dependent formation of heterochromatin and its diverse functions. *Curr. Opin. Genet. Dev.* 20:134–141.

Guttman, M., I. Amit, M. Garber, C. French, M. F. Lin, D. Feldser, M. Huarte, O. Zuk, B. W. Carey, J. P. Cassady, M. N. Cabili, R. Jaenisch, T. S. Mikkelsen, T. Jacks, N. Hacohen, B. E. Bernstein, M. Kellis, A. Regev, J. L. Rinn, and E. S. Lander. 2009. Chromatin signature reveals over a thousand highly conserved large non-coding RNAs in mammals. *Nature* 458:223–227.

Handel, M. L., C. K. Watts, A. deFazio, R. O. Day, and R. L. Sutherland. 1995. Inhibition of AP-1 binding and transcription by gold and selenium involving conserved cysteine residues in Jun and Fos. *Proc. Natl Acad. Sci. USA* 92:4497–4501.

Happel, N., D. Doenecke, K. E. Sekeri-Pataryas, and T. G. Sourlingas. 2008. H1 histone subtype constitution and phosphorylation state of the ageing cell system of human peripheral blood lymphocytes. *Exp. Gerontol.* 43:184–199.

Hass, B. S., R. W. Hart, M. H. Lu, and B. D. Lyn-Cook. 1993. Effects of caloric restriction in animals on cellular function, oncogene expression, and DNA methylation in vitro. *Mutat. Res.* 295:281–289.

Heyn, H., S. Moran, and M. Esteller. 2013. Aberrant DNA methylation profiles in the premature aging disorders Hutchinson–Gilford Progeria and Werner syndrome. *Epigenetics* 8:28–33.

Hoile, S. P., K. A. Lillycrop, L. R. Grenfell, M. A. Hanson, and G. C. Burdge. 2012. Increasing the folic acid content of maternal or post-weaning diets induces differential changes in phosphoenolpyruvate carboxykinase mRNA expression and promoter methylation in rats. *Br. J. Nutr.* 108:852–857.

Hyder, S. M., G. M. Stancel, Z. Nawaz, D. P. McDonnell, and D. S. Loose-Mitchell. 1992. Identification of an estrogen response element in the 3′-flanking region of the murine c-fos protooncogene. *J. Biol. Chem.* 267:18047–18054.

Ions, L. J., L. A. Wakeling, H. J. Bosomworth, J. E. Hardyman, S. M. Escolme, D. C. Swan, R. A. Valentine, J. C. Mathers, and D. Ford. 2013. Effects of Sirt1 on DNA methylation and expression of genes affected by dietary restriction. *Age (Dordr.)* 35:1835–1849.

Issa, J. P., Y. L. Ottaviano, P. Celano, S. R. Hamilton, N. E. Davidson, and S. B. Baylin. 1994. Methylation of the oestrogen receptor CpG island links ageing and neoplasia in human colon. *Nat. Genet.* 7:536–540.

Jacob, R. A., D. M. Gretz, P. C. Taylor, S. J. James, I. P. Pogribny, B. J. Miller, S. M. Henning, and M. E. Swendseid. 1998. Moderate folate depletion increases plasma homocysteine and decreases lymphocyte DNA methylation in postmenopausal women. *J. Nutr.* 128:1204–1212.

Jaenisch, R. and A. Bird. 2003. Epigenetic regulation of gene expression: how the genome integrates intrinsic and environmental signals. *Nat. Genet.* 33:245–254.

Jarolim, S., J. Millen, G. Heeren, P. Laun, D. S. Goldfarb, and M. Breitenbach. 2004. A novel assay for replicative lifespan in Saccharomyces cerevisiae. *FEMS Yeast Res.* 5:169–177.

Jenuwein, T. and C. D. Allis. 2001. Translating the histone code. *Science* 293:1074–1080.

Johnson, I. T. and N. J. Belshaw. 2008. Environment, diet and CpG island methylation: epigenetic signals in gastrointestinal neoplasia. *Food Chem. Toxicol.* 46:1346–1359.

Jones, P. A. and S. B. Baylin. 2002. The fundamental role of epigenetic events in cancer. *Nat. Rev. Genet.* 3:415–428.

Jones, P. A. and S. B. Baylin. 2007. The epigenomics of cancer. *Cell* 128:683–692.

Jones, P. A. and G. Liang. 2009. Rethinking how DNA methylation patterns are maintained. *Nat. Rev. Genet.* 10:805–811.

Kaikkonen, M. U., M. T. Lam, and C. K. Glass. 2011. Non-coding RNAs as regulators of gene expression and epigenetics. *Cardiovasc Res.* 90:430–440.

Kamakura, M. 2011. Royalactin induces queen differentiation in honeybees. *Nature*, 473:478–483.

Kang, J., J. Chen, Y. Shi, J. Jia, and Y. Zhang. 2005. Curcumin-induced histone hypoacetylation: the role of reactive oxygen species. *Biochem. Pharmacol.* 69:1205–1213.

Keyes, M. K., H. Jang, J. B. Mason, Z. Liu, J. W. Crott, D. E. Smith, S. Friso, and S. W. Choi. 2007. Older age and dietary folate are determinants of genomic and p16-specific DNA methylation in mouse colon. *J. Nutr.* 137:1713–1717.

Khalil, A. M., M. Guttman, M. Huarte, M. Garber, A. Raj, D. Rivea Morales, K. Thomas, A. Presser, B. E. Bernstein, A. van Oudenaarden, A. Regev, E. S. Lander, and J. L. Rinn. 2009. Many human large intergenic noncoding RNAs associate with chromatin-modifying complexes and affect gene expression. *Proc. Natl Acad. Sci. USA* 106:11667–11672.

Kida, Y., T. Shimizu, and K. Kuwano. 2006. Sodium butyrate up-regulates cathelicidin gene expression via activator protein-1 and histone acetylation at the promoter region in a human lung epithelial cell line, EBC-1. *Mol. Immunol.* 43:1972–1981.

Kouzarides, T. 2007.Chromatin modifications and their function. *Cell* 128:693–705.

Kovacheva, V. P., T. J. Mellott, J. M. Davison, N. Wagner, I. Lopez-Coviella, A. C. Schnitzler, and J. K. Blusztajn. 2007. Gestational choline deficiency causes global and Igf2 gene DNA hypermethylation by up-regulation of Dnmt1 expression. *J. Biol. Chem.* 282:31777–31788.

Kriaucionis, S. and N. Heintz. 2009. The nuclear DNA base 5-hydroxymethylcytosine is present in Purkinje neurons and the brain. *Science* 324:929–930.

Kucharski, R., J. Maleszka, S. Foret, and R. Maleszka. 2008. Nutritional control of reproductive status in honeybees via DNA methylation. *Science* 319:1827–1830.

Kulis, M. and M. Esteller. 2010. DNA methylation and cancer. *Adv. Genet.* 70:27–56.

Kwabi-Addo, B., W. Chung, L. Shen, M. Ittmann, T. Wheeler, J. Jelinek, and J. P. Issa. 2007. Age-related DNA methylation changes in normal human prostate tissues. *Clin. Cancer Res.* 13:3796–3802.

Langie, S. A., S. Achterfeldt, J. P. Gorniak, K. J. Halley-Hogg, D. Oxley, F. J. van Schooten, R. W. Godschalk, J. A. McKay, and J. C. Mathers. 2013. Maternal folate depletion and high-fat feeding from weaning affects DNA methylation and DNA repair in brain of adult offspring. *FASEB J* 27:3323–3334.

Lau, N. C., L. P. Lim, E. G. Weinstein, and D. P. Bartel. 2001. An abundant class of tiny RNAs with probable regulatory roles in *Caenorhabditis elegans*. *Science* 294:858–862.

Lee, W. J., J. Y. Shim, and B. T. Zhu. 2005. Mechanisms for the inhibition of DNA methyltransferases by tea catechins and bioflavonoids. *Mol. Pharmacol.* 68:1018–1030.

Li, E., T. H. Bestor, and R. Jaenisch. 1992. Targeted mutation of the DNA methyltransferase gene results in embryonic lethality. *Cell* 69:915–926.

Lillycrop, K. A., E. S. Phillips, A. A. Jackson, M. A. Hanson, and G. C. Burdge. 2005. Dietary protein restriction of pregnant rats induces and folic acid supplementation prevents epigenetic modification of hepatic gene expression in the offspring. *J. Nutr.* 135:1382–1386.

Lillycrop, K. A., E. S. Phillips, C. Torrens, M. A. Hanson, A. A. Jackson, and G. C. Burdge. 2008. Feeding pregnant rats a protein-restricted diet persistently alters the methylation of specific cytosines in the hepatic PPAR alpha promoter of the offspring. *Br. J. Nutr.* 100:278–282.

Lin, C., J. Kang, and R. Zheng. 2005. Oxidative stress is involved in inhibition of copper on histone acetylation in cells. *Chem. Biol. Interact.* 151:167–176.

Link, A., F. Balaguer, and A. Goel. 2010. Cancer chemoprevention by dietary polyphenols: promising role for epigenetics. *Biochem. Pharmacol.* 80:1771–1792.

Lopatina, N., J. F. Haskell, L. G. Andrews, J. C. Poole, S. Saldanha, and T. Tollefsbol. 2002. Differential maintenance and de novo methylating activity by three DNA methyltransferases in aging and immortalized fibroblasts. *J. Cell. Biochem.* 84:324–334.

Luchsinger, J. A., M. X. Tang, J. Miller, R. Green, and R. Mayeux. 2007. Relation of higher folate intake to lower risk of Alzheimer disease in the elderly. *Arch. Neurol.* 64:86–92.

Lyko, F., S. Foret, R. Kucharski, S. Wolf, C. Falckenhayn, and R. Maleszka. 2010. The honey bee epigenomes: differential methylation of brain DNA in queens and workers. *PLoS Biol.* 8: e1000506.

Mastroeni, D., A. Grover, E. Delvaux, C. Whiteside, P. D. Coleman, and J. Rogers. 2010. Epigenetic changes in Alzheimer's disease: decrements in DNA methylation. *Neurobiol. Aging* 31:2025–2037.

Mastroeni, D., A. McKee, A. Grover, J. Rogers, and P. D. Coleman. 2009. Epigenetic differences in cortical neurons from a pair of monozygotic twins discordant for Alzheimer's disease. *PLoS One* 4: e6617.

Mathers, J. C. 2006. Nutritional modulation of ageing: genomic and epigenetic approaches. *Mech. Ageing Dev.* 127:584–589.

Mathers, J. C. and D. Ford. 2009. Nutrition, epigenetics and aging. *In*: S. W. Choi and S.S. Friso (eds) *Nutrients and Epigenetics*. Boca Raton, FL: CRC Press.

Mathers, J. C., G. Strathdee, and C. L. Relton. 2010. Induction of epigenetic alterations by dietary and other environmental factors. *Adv. Genet.* 71:3–39.

Maunakea, A. K., I. Chepelev, and K. Zhao. 2010. Epigenome mapping in normal and disease states. *Circul. Res.* 107:327–339.

McKay, J. A. and J. C. Mathers. 2011. Diet induced epigenetic changes and their implications for health. *Acta Physiol. (Oxf.)* 202:103–118.

McKay, J. A., K. J. Waltham, E. A. Williams, and J. C. Mathers. 2011a. Folate depletion during pregnancy and lactation reduces genomic DNA methylation in murine adult offspring. *Genes Nutr.* 6:189–196.

McKay, J. A., E. A. Williams, and J. C. Mathers. 2011b. Effect of maternal and post-weaning folate supply on gene-specific DNA methylation in the small intestine of weaning and adult apc and wild type mice. *Front. Genet.* 2:23.

McKay, J. A., Y. K. Wong, C. L. Relton, D. Ford, and J. C. Mathers. 2011c. Maternal folate supply and sex influence gene-specific DNA methylation in the fetal gut. *Mol. Nutr. Food Res.* 55:1717–1723.

McKay, J. A., L. Xie, S. Harris, Y. K. Wong, D. Ford, and J. C. Mathers. 2011d. Blood as a surrogate marker for tissue-specific DNA methylation and changes due to folate depletion in post-partum female mice. *Mol. Nutr. Food Res.* 55:1026–1035.

McKay, J. A., A. Groom, C. Potter, L. J. Coneyworth, D. Ford, J. C. Mathers, and C. L. Relton. 2012. Genetic and non-genetic influences during pregnancy on infant global and site specific DNA methylation: role for folate gene variants and vitamin B12. *PLoS One* 7: p. e33290.

Miyamura, Y., R. Tawa, A. Koizumi, Y. Uehara, A. Kurishita, H. Sakurai, S. Kamiyama, and T. Ono. 1993 Effects of energy restriction on age-associated changes of DNA methylation in mouse liver. *Mutat. Res.* 295:63–69.

Nelson, J. A., A. P. Sturtevant, and B. Lineburg. 1924. Growth and feeding of honeybee larvae. *US Dept Agric. Bull.* 1222:37.

Niculescu, M. D., C. N. Craciunescu, and S. H. Zeisel. 2006. Dietary choline deficiency alters global and gene-specific DNA methylation in the developing hippocampus of mouse fetal brains. *FASEB J.* 20:43–49.

Okano, M., D. W. Bell, D. A. Haber, and E. Li. 1999.DNA methyltransferases Dnmt3a and Dnmt3b are essential for de novo methylation and mammalian development. *Cell* 99:247–257.

Ollikainen, M., K. R. Smith, E. J. Joo, H. K. Ng, R. Andronikos, B. Novakovic, N. K. Abdul Aziz, J. B. Carlin, R. Morley, R. Saffery, and J. M. Craig. 2010. DNA methylation analysis of multiple tissues from newborn twins reveals both genetic and intrauterine components to variation in the human neonatal epigenome. *Hum. Mol. Genet.* 19:4176–4188.

Ono, H., M. Iwasaki, A. Kuchiba, Y. Kasuga, S. Yokoyama, H. Onuma, H. Nishimura, R. Kusama, S. Ohnami, H. Sakamoto, T. Yoshida, and S. Tsugane. 2012. Association of dietary and genetic factors related to one-carbon metabolism with global methylation level of leukocyte DNA. *Cancer Sci.* 103:2159–2164.

Page R. E. Jr, and C. Y. Peng. 2001. Aging and development in social insects with emphasis on the honey bee, *Apis mellifera* L. *Exp. Gerontol.* 36:695–711.

Pandey, M., S. Shukla, and S. Gupta. 2010. Promoter demethylation and chromatin remodeling by green tea polyphenols leads to re-expression of GSTP1 in human prostate cancer cells. *Int. J. Cancer* 126:2520–2533.

Park, L. K., S. Friso, and S. W. Choi. 2012. Nutritional influences on epigenetics and age-related disease. *Proc. Nutr. Soc.* 71:75–83.

Pogribny, I. P., V. P. Tryndyak, L. Muskhelishvili, I. Rusyn, and S. A. Ross. 2007. Methyl deficiency, alterations in global histone modifications, and carcinogenesis. *J. Nutr.* 137 Suppl 1:216S–222S.

Pradhan, S., A. Bacolla, R. D. Wells, and R. J. Roberts. 1999. Recombinant human DNA (cytosine-5) methyltransferase. I. Expression, purification, and comparison of de novo and maintenance methylation. *J. Biol. Chem.* 274:33002–33010.

Qin, W., W. Zhu, and E. Sauter. 2005. Resveratrol induced DNA methylation in ER+ breast cancer. *In*: *Proceedings of the American Association of Cancer Research*, Cellular and Molecular Biology 36: Epigenetic Mechanisms 1, Abstract 2750.

Rada-Iglesias, A., S. Enroth, A. Ameur, C. M. Koch, G. K. Clelland, P. Respuela-Alonso, S. Wilcox, O. M. Dovey, P. D. Ellis, C. F. Langford, I. Dunham, J. Komorowski, and C. Wadelius. 2007. Butyrate mediates decrease of histone acetylation centered on transcription start sites and down-regulation of associated genes. *Genome Res.* 17:708–719.

Rakyan, V. K., M. E. Blewitt, R. Druker, J. I. Preis, and E. Whitelaw. 2002. Metastable epialleles in mammals. *Trends Genet.* 18:348–351.

Rakyan, V. K., T. A. Down, D. J. Balding, and S. Beck. 2011. Epigenome-wide association studies for common human diseases. *Nat. Rev. Genet.* 12:529–541.

Rampersaud, G. C., G. P. Kauwell, A. D. Hutson, J. J. Cerda, and L. B. Bailey. 2000. Genomic DNA methylation decreases in response to moderate folate depletion in elderly women. *Am. J. Clin. Nutr.* 72:998–1003.

Rascon, B., B. P. Hubbard, D. A. Sinclair, and G. V. Amdam. 2012. The lifespan extension effects of resveratrol are conserved in the honey bee and may be driven by a mechanism related to caloric restriction. *Aging (Albany NY)* 4:499–508.

Ravaglia, G., P. Forti, F. Maioli, M. Martelli, L. Servadei, N. Brunetti, E. Porcellini, and F. Licastro. 2005. Homocysteine and folate as risk factors for dementia and Alzheimer disease. *Am. J. Clin. Nutr.* 82:636–643.

Rees, W. D., S. M. Hay, D. S. Brown, C. Antipatis, and R. M. Palmer. 2000.Maternal protein deficiency causes hypermethylation of DNA in the livers of rat fetuses. *J. Nutr.* 130:1821–1826.

Reik, W. 2007. Stability and flexibility of epigenetic gene regulation in mammalian development. *Nature* 447:425–432.

Richter, A. M., G. P. Pfeifer, and R. H. Dammann. 2009. The RASSF proteins in cancer; from epigenetic silencing to functional characterization. *Biochim. Biophys. Acta* 1796:114–128.

Rodriguez, J., L. Vives, M. Jorda, C. Morales, M. Munoz, E. Vendrell, and M. A. Peinado. 2008. Genome-wide tracking of unmethylated DNA Alu repeats in normal and cancer cells. *Nucleic Acids Res.* 36:770–784.

Ryan, B. M., A. I. Robles, and C. C. Harris. 2010. Genetic variation in microRNA networks: the implications for cancer research. *Nat. Rev. Cancer* 10:389–402.

Sarg, B., E. Koutzamani, W. Helliger, I. Rundquist, and H. H. Lindner. 2002. Postsynthetic trimethylation of histone H4 at lysine 20 in mammalian tissues is associated with aging. *J. Biol. Chem.* 277:39195–39201.

Sauer, J., H. Jang, E. M. Zimmerly, K. C. Kim, Z. Liu, A. Chanson, D. E. Smith, J. B. Mason, S. Friso, and S. W. Choi. 2010. Ageing, chronic alcohol consumption and folate are determinants of genomic DNA methylation, p16 promoter methylation and the expression of p16 in the mouse colon. *Br. J. Nutr.* 104:24–30.

Schneider, E., G. Pliushch, N. El Hajj, D. Galetzka, A. Puhl, M. Schorsch, K. Frauenknecht, T. Riepert, A. Tresch, A. M. Muller, W. Coerdt, U. Zechner, and T. Haaf. 2010. Spatial, temporal and interindividual epigenetic variation of functionally important DNA methylation patterns. *Nucleic Acids Res.* 38:3880–3890.

Shi, Y. Y., Z. Y. Huang, Z. J. Zeng, Z. L. Wang, X. B. Wu, and W. Y. Yan. 2011. Diet and cell size both affect queen-worker differentiation through DNA methylation in honey bees (*Apis mellifera*, Apidae). *PLoS One* 6:e18808.

Smith, A. D., S. M. Smith, C. A. de Jager, P. Whitbread, C. Johnston, G. Agacinski, A. Oulhaj, K. M. Bradley, R. Jacoby, and H. Refsum. 2010. Homocysteine-lowering by B vitamins slows the rate of accelerated brain atrophy in mild cognitive impairment: a randomized controlled trial. *PLoS One* 5:e12244.

Smith-Vikos, T. and F. J. Slack. 2012. MicroRNAs and their roles in aging. *J. Cell Sci.* 125:7–17.

Spyrou, G., M. Bjornstedt, S. Kumar, and A. Holmgren. 1995. AP-1 DNA-binding activity is inhibited by selenite and selenodiglutathione. *FEBS Lett.* 368:59–63.

Steegers-Theunissen, R. P., S. A. Obermann-Borst, D. Kremer, J. Lindemans, C. Siebel, E. A. Steegers, P. E. Slagboom, and B. T. Heijmans. 2009. Periconceptional maternal folic acid use of 400 microg per day is related to increased methylation of the IGF2 gene in the very young child. *PLoS One* 4: e7845.

Tapp, H. S., D. M. Commane, D. M. Bradburn, R. Arasaradnam, J. C. Mathers, I. T. Johnson, and N. J. Belshaw. 2013. Nutritional factors and gender influence age-related DNA methylation in the human rectal mucosa. *Aging Cell* 12:148–155.

van Eijk, K. R., S. de Jong, M. P. Boks, T. Langeveld, F. Colas, J. H. Veldink, C. G. de Kovel, E. Janson, E. Strengman, P. Langfelder, R. S. Kahn, L. H. van den Berg, S. Horvath, and R. A. Ophoff. 2012. Genetic analysis of DNA methylation and gene expression levels in whole blood of healthy human subjects. *BMC Genom.* 13:636.

van Straten, E. M., V. W. Bloks, N. C. Huijkman, J. F. Baller, H. Meer, D. Lutjohann, F. Kuipers, and T. Plosch. 2010. The liver X-receptor gene promoter is hypermethylated in a mouse model of prenatal protein restriction. *Am. J. Physiol. Regul. Integr. Comp. Physiol.* 298:R275–282.

Wakeling, L. A., L. J. Ions, and D. Ford. 2009. Could Sirt1-mediated epigenetic effects contribute to the longevity response to dietary restriction and be mimicked by other dietary interventions? *Age (Dordr.)* 31:327–341.

Wallace, K., M. V. Grau, A. J. Levine, L. Shen, R. Hamdan, X. Chen, J. Gui, R. W. Haile, E. L. Barry, D. Ahnen, G. McKeown-Eyssen, J. A. Baron, and J. P. Issa. 2010. Association between folate levels and CpG Island hypermethylation in normal colorectal mucosa. *Cancer Prev. Res. (Phila)* 3:1552–1564.

Wang, L. G., A. Beklemisheva, X. M. Liu, A. C. Ferrari, J. Feng, and J. W. Chiao. 2007. Dual action on promoter demethylation and chromatin by an isothiocyanate restored GSTP1 silenced in prostate cancer. *Mol. Carcinog.* 46:24–31.

Wang, S. C., B. Oelze, and A. Schumacher. 2008. Age-specific epigenetic drift in late-onset Alzheimer's disease. *PLoS One* 3:e2698.

Wang, Y., M. Jorda, P. L. Jones, R. Maleszka, X. Ling, H. M. Robertson, C. A. Mizzen, M. A. Peinado, and G. E. Robinson. 2006.Functional CpG methylation system in a social insect. *Science* 314:645–647.

Waterland, R. A. and R. L. Jirtle. 2003. Transposable elements: targets for early nutritional effects on epigenetic gene regulation. *Mol. Cell. Biol.* 23:5293–5300.

Waterland, R. A., D. C. Dolinoy, J. R. Lin, C. A. Smith, X. Shi, and K. G. Tahiliani. 2006. Maternal methyl supplements increase offspring DNA methylation at Axin Fused. *Genesis* 44:401–406.

Wheeler, D. E. 1986. *Developmental and Physiological Determinants of Caste in Social Hymenoptera: Evolutionary Implications*. The University of Chicago Press for The American Society of Naturalists

Widiker, S., S. Karst, A. Wagener, and G. A. Brockmann. 2010. High-fat diet leads to a decreased methylation of the Mc4r gene in the obese BFMI and the lean B6 mouse lines. *J. Appl. Genet.* 51:193–197.

Winston, M. 1987. *The Biology of the Honey Bee*. Cambridge, MA: Harvard University Press:

Xiang, N., R. Zhao, G. Song, and W. Zhong. 2008. Selenite reactivates silenced genes by modifying DNA methylation and histones in prostate cancer cells. *Carcinogenesis* 29:2175–2181.

Zhu, B. T., E. L. Ezell, and J. G. Liehr. 1994. Catechol-*O*-methyltransferase-catalyzed rapid *O*-methylation of mutagenic flavonoids. Metabolic inactivation as a possible reason for their lack of carcinogenicity in vivo. *J. Biol. Chem.*269:292–299.

Zhu, B. T. and J. G. Liehr. 1996. Inhibition of catechol *O*-methyltransferase-catalyzed *O*-methylation of 2- and 4-hydroxyestradiol by quercetin. Possible role in estradiol-induced tumorigenesis. *J. Biol. Chem.* 271:1357–1363.

Zhu, B. T., U. K. Patel, M. X. Cai, and A. H. Conney. 2000. *O*-Methylation of tea polyphenols catalyzed by human placental cytosolic catechol-*O*-methyltransferase. *Drug. Metab. Dispos.* 28:1024–1030.

Zhu, B. T., U. K. Patel, M. X. Cai, A. J. Lee, and A. H. Conney. 2001. Rapid conversion of tea catechins to monomethylated products by rat liver cytosolic catechol-*O*-methyltransferase. *Xenobiotica* 31:879–890.

Zhu, W., W. Qin, K. Zhang, G. E. Rottinghaus, Y. C. Chen, B. Kliethermes, and E. R. Sauter. 2012. *Trans*-resveratrol alters mammary promoter hypermethylation in women at increased risk for breast cancer. *Nutr. Cancer* 64:393–400.

PART II

Nutritional modulation of age-related organ functional decline

CHAPTER 4

Nutritional interventions in age-related genetic and epigenetic instability and cancer

Thomas Prates Ong[1] and Ana Paula de Melo Loureiro[2]

[1] *Laboratory of Nutrigenomics and Programming, Food and Experimental Nutrition Department, Faculty of Pharmaceutical Sciences, and Food and Nutrition Research Center, University of São Paulo, São Paulo, Brazil*

[2] *Department of Clinical and Toxicological Analyses, Faculty of Pharmaceutical Sciences, University of São Paulo, São Paulo, Brazil*

4.1 Cancer as an age-associated disease

Ageing is a natural consequence of changes occurring in molecular, cellular, tissue and organ levels over the course of time. Although it is inevitable with increasing life expectancy, current knowledge states that its rate and the incidence of commonly associated chronic diseases can be influenced by lifestyle, diet, and behavior through life. A great challenge today is to understand the role of health factors and apply them in order to control the incidence of major chronic noncommunicable diseases – cancer, diabetes, obesity, ischemic heart disease and stroke. Efforts are currently being directed towards understanding biological pathways involved in the ageing rate, risk of age-associated disease and lifespan, which will offer tools for more precise intervention actions (Prasad *et al.*, 2012; Deelen *et al.*, 2013; Valdes *et al.*, 2013).

According to the "Global Burden of Diseases, Injuries, and Risk Factors Study", 8 million people died from cancer worldwide in 2010, representing 15.1% of all deaths, a number that had increased by 38% since 1990, accompanying both population growth and ageing. The 2010 age-standardized cancer mortality rates show an evident age-related rise in cancer deaths beyond the 35–40 year age, going from 30.28 deaths/100,000 for the 35–39 year age group to 1420.05 deaths/100,000 for the 80+ year age group (Lozano *et al.*, 2012). A parallel exponential increase has been shown for the incidence of invasive epithelial carcinomas with age (DePinho, 2000). Major age-increased death rates have been shown for lung, colorectal, stomach, prostate, liver, breast, pancreatic, bladder and esophageal cancer (Lozano *et al.*, 2012).

Cancer is the term used for a large number of tissue diseases in which cells change their energy metabolism, lose growth control, resist apoptosis, induce angiogenesis and gain the capacity to migrate and invade other adjacent and distant tissues. These hallmarks of cancer cells result from complex and heterogeneous genetic and epigenetic alterations that culminate in the activation of oncogene and/or inactivation of tumor suppressor gene networks (Hanahan & Weinberg, 2011; Hofree *et al.*, 2013). The time

Anti-Ageing Nutrients: Evidence-Based Prevention of Age-Associated Diseases, First Edition. Edited by Delminda Neves.

period elapsing in the presence of factors that promote these alterations, in combination with genetic features, helps in understanding the increased cancer incidence in the elderly. The predominance of epithelial carcinomas over cancers of mesenchymal or hematopoietic origin in the aged may be due in part to differences in the replicative index and susceptibility to DNA damage of different tissues (DePinho, 2000; Kennedy *et al.*, 2012). There is evidence that different tissue types accumulate different levels of mutations throughout life (Hill *et al.*, 2004). For example, by comparing mutation frequencies at the hypoxanthine phosphoribosyl transferase locus between human renal epithelial cells and T-lymphocytes during ageing, it was verified that the renal epithelial cells suffered an approximately 10-fold higher increase in mutation load (Cole & Skopek, 1994; Martin *et al.*, 1996; Kennedy *et al.*, 2012). In general, somatic mutations in human epithelia appear to increase exponentially with age (Martin *et al.*, 1996).

Molecular pathways altered with age in response to endogenous (e.g. hormonal changes, fat accumulation, inflammation) and exogenous (e.g. pollution, poor diet) stimuli seem to prompt cells to accumulate damage, driving gene mutations and genetic instability. On the other hand, accumulated mutations during a lifespan may guide cells to develop a "mutator phenotype", since mutations in genes that have some role in supporting genome stability will make the cells prone to augmented DNA damage and mutation rates, attaining levels that facilitate cancer development (DePinho, 2000; Kennedy *et al.*, 2012). This process occurs slowly over many years (an estimated 20 years from the initial event) and the final outcome is the result of continuous selection of cells able to bypass the barriers that limit unrestricted cell proliferation. Both nuclear and mitochondrial mutation burden have been shown to be amplified with age (Kennedy *et al.*, 2012). Moreover, somatic mutations in different gene networks that control cell survival, growth, DNA damage response and epigenetic features give rise to different tumor subtypes with different clinical outcomes reflected in patient survival, response to therapy and tumor histology (Hofree *et al.*, 2013). In addition to stressing the importance of mutations for tumor development and outcomes, current knowledge shows that characterizing tumor-mutated networks is a promising strategy to obtain molecular signatures that help in deciding the most effective therapy (Hofree *et al.*, 2013; Garraway & Lander, 2013). Given the importance of gene network mutations for tumor development, controlling the factors that increase the risk of these mutations over a lifetime seems to be one of the best strategies to manage cancer.

It is recognized, however, that not only DNA mutations, but also epigenetic marks, such as DNA methylation, histone modifications and microRNAs profiling (discussed in Chapter 3), drive changes in gene expression that contribute to tumor development and phenotype (DePinho, 2000). The existence of different levels of heritable control of gene expression that may be altered in carcinogenesis shows that the scenario is more complex than initially thought. Beyond mutagenic pathways, attention must also be given to cellular events and risk factors able to disrupt epigenetic marks. The roles of telomere dysfunction and stromal milieu in tumor development are also evidenced as other important pieces of the complex puzzle of carcinogenesis (DePinho, 2000).

It is now recognized that genetic predisposition alone accounts for only a very small percentage of cancer cases and that cancer development results from complex interactions involving the genome and its environment (70–90%; Colditz *et al.*, 2006). Therefore, gene–environment interactions must be considered in the analysis of different susceptibilities to cancer development. It is well known that single nucleotide polymorphisms occurring, for example, in protein-coding sequences may affect protein function, giving diverse capabilities for different individuals to deal with their environment (Kennedy *et al.*, 2012; Yuan *et al.*, 2012). Urgent action must be taken to avoid the known causes of cancer in order to contain its incidence (Clapp *et al.*, 2007).

One point of convergence for the risk factors linked to age-associated chronic diseases is the induction of chronic inflammation and oxidative stress. Tobacco use, excessive alcohol intake, poor diet, obesity, pollution, stress, infectious agents, occupational exposure to several xenobiotics and lack of physical activity are among the risk factors that together account for nearly 90% of all cancer cases and are able to activate inflammation-associated molecules and induce oxidative stress (Luch, 2005; Clapp *et al.*, 2007; Prasad *et al.*, 2012; Sethi *et al.*, 2012). Clear links exist between chronic inflammation, oxidative stress and cancer. Pro-inflammatory mediators, pro-inflammatory transcription factors and reactive oxygen species are shown to be involved in all phases of the neoplastic development (Sethi *et al.*, 2012).

Ageing is accompanied by increased levels of inflammatory markers and oxidative damage, as well as by a decline of mitochondrial function and energy metabolism (Kennedy *et al.*, 2012; discussed in Chapter 1). Overexpression of genes associated with inflammation, immune response and lysossome function have been evidenced as the main age-associated gene expression changes in a meta-analysis study performed with 27 microarray datasets from mice, rats and humans. Downregulation of collagen-, oxidative phosphorylation-, mitochondria-, and energy metabolism-related genes, as well as alterations in the expression of apoptosis, cell cycle and senescence genes have also been demonstrated to occur as a function of age (Magalhães *et al.*, 2009).

4.2 Genetic and epigenetic alterations as molecular mechanisms underlying carcinogenesis

Carcinogenesis is a chronic process in which successive and heritable alterations in diverse gene expression pathways take place, originating somatic cell clones with a growth advantage compared with normal adjacent cells. Despite its clonal nature, cancer progression occurs through changes in diverse pathways in different tumor cells, giving rise to a complex tissue with different cell types interacting with each other (Hanahan & Weinberg, 2011).

Classically, three phases are highlighted in neoplastic development: initiation, promotion, and progression. The *initiation phase* encompasses the emergence and survival of mutated cells within a tissue. As heritable suppression or induction of gene expression may also be controlled by the epigenome, the existence of nonmutated initiated cells within a tissue is increasingly being recognized (Luch, 2005; Shen & Laird, 2013). However, changes in the epigenome may be reverted by changes in the tissue microenvironment or therapeutic intervention, while mutations are invariably maintained in the subsequent cell generations.

Initiated cells will support tumor development if the rate of their division accelerates in response to replication signals. This step constitutes the *promotion phase*, which may be reversed if the signals for tumor growth are withdrawn. This means that, at the beginning of tumor development, its growth may be restricted and even reversed by changes in its microenvironment. However, if genetic and epigenetic changes intensify while cells proliferate, a threshold of gene expression alterations is attained and cells will gain the capacity to replicate even without external stimuli. This is the *progression phase*, characterized by genetic instability, loss of growth control and metastasis (Klaunig *et al.*, 2011). Nowadays, the tumor microenvironment is also being recognized as an important contributor for the survival of initiated cells, as well as for tumor promotion and progression (Barcellos-Hoff *et al.*, 2013; Parks *et al.*, 2013).

The importance of genetic lesions for cancer development may be shown by the study of some rare genetic syndromes in which DNA repair systems are deficient. Examples are the *Werner* and *Xeroderma Pigmentosum* (XP) syndromes, which are autosomal-recessive diseases. *Werner* syndrome (WRN) is characterized by the loss of WRN protein function owing to the mutated gene. WRN protein bears helicase and exonuclease activities, which are essential for the maintenance of genome stability and correct processing of transcription, replication and DNA repair. WRN patients are prone to increased incidence of genomic rearrangements and exhibit signs of ageing early in life, such as cataracts, scleroderma, thinning gray hair, atherosclerosis, diabetes, myocardial infarction, stroke, osteoporosis and increased incidence of certain types of cancer (Kennedy *et al.*, 2012). On the other hand, XP syndrome occurs as a result of mutations in one of eight genes (*XP-A, B, C, D, E, F, G* or *V*) that participate in the nucleotide excision repair (NER) pathway (*A–G*) or DNA damage tolerance/lesion bypass (*V*). XP patients present at least a 1000-fold increase in their susceptibility to developing skin cancer owing to the defective NER necessary to remove UV-induced DNA bulky lesions, such as the pyrimidine dimers. Increased frequencies of internal cancers are also observed in XP patients, which are attributed to the defective repair of oxidatively generated DNA lesions. Neuronal degeneration, sensorineural hearing loss, ataxia, areflexia and microcephaly have been also observed in XP patients (Berquist & Wilson, 2012).

Defective DNA repair combined with exposure to DNA damaging agents, such as reactive xenobiotics and endogenous substances, leads to the increased mutation rates necessary to induce cell malignant transformation (Poirier, 2004; Hecht, 2012). This assumption is also well demonstrated in mouse strains deficient in DNA repair, which present increased cancer rates in parallel to elevated mutation frequencies (Hasty *et al.*, 2003). Polymorphisms in DNA repair genes have been shown to be associated with increased cancer risk, although some controversies exist (Ricceri *et al.*, 2012). For example, an association between polymorphisms of the base-excision repair (BER) genes human 8-oxoguanine DNA N-glycosylase 1 (hOGG1) and X-ray repair cross-complementing protein 1 (XRCC1) and increased risk of hepatocellular carcinoma has been verified (Yuan *et al.*, 2012). Furthermore, there are data showing a decline in DNA repair capacity with age (Moriwaki *et al.*, 1996; Goukassian *et al.*, 2000), although it has not been fully demonstrated to be linked to carcinogenesis (DePinho, 2000).

Types of genetic alterations that are increased in aged cells include base substitutions, frameshifts, insertions, deletions, rearrangements, chromosome loss, chromosomal aberrations, micronuclei, sister chromatid exchanges and DNA strand breaks (Hill *et al.*, 2004; Kennedy *et al.*, 2012). It is estimated that thousands to hundreds of thousands of mutations are present in each tumor cell (Salk *et al.*, 2010; Kennedy *et al.*, 2012). Mutated genes affect cell signaling [e.g. mitogen-activated protein kinases (MAPK), phosphatidylinositol 3-kinase (PI3K), Notch, target of rapamycin (TOR), wingless-related integration site (Wnt)/β-catenin, transforming growth factor β, nuclear factor-kappaB (NF-κB) signaling pathways], cell cycle, genome integrity, telomere stability, the epigenome (DNA methylation, DNA hydroxymethylation, chromatin histone methyltransferases, demethylases and acetyltransferases), chromatin structure (SWItch/Sucrose NonFermentable complexes), RNA splicing, protein homeostasis, metabolism, apoptosis and cell differentiation (Garraway & Lander, 2013). Cancer genome projects, in conjunction with The Cancer Genome Atlas, the International Cancer Genome Consortium and the Slim Initiative for Genomic Medicine, are underway to systematically characterize the cancer genome in different tumor types of diverse anatomic sites (brain/central nervous system, head and neck, thoracic, breast, gastrointestinal, gynecologic, urologic, skin, soft tissue and hematologic; Garraway & Lander, 2013). These studies reveal prevalent mutations in genes of different samples of each tumor type, and the mutated pathways emerge as potential targets for therapy (Tsou *et al.*, 2002; Belinsky, 2004; Damiani *et al.*, 2008; Reck *et al.*, 2011; Scrima *et al.*, 2012). For example, serine/threonine-protein kinase B-raf mutations (oncogene, MAPK signaling) have been found in 50% of melanomas, phosphatidylinositol 4,5-bisphosphate 3-kinase catalytic subunit alpha isoform (PIK3CA) mutations (oncogene, PI3K signaling) in 25–30% of breast and colorectal cancers, and epidermal growth factor receptor mutations (receptor tyrosine kinase signaling) in 10–15% of nonsmall cell lung cancers (NSCLC) (Garraway & Lander, 2013).

Chronic inflammation and mitochondrial dysfunction are the major sources of a set of reactive oxygen and nitrogen species (ROS and RNS, respectively) that are multifunctional drivers in ageing and carcinogenesis (Kennedy *et al.*, 2012; Berquist & Wilson, 2012). Proteins, lipids, carbohydrates, nuclear DNA, mitochondrial DNA and RNAs are targets for the most reactive species generated. Among the possible targets, DNA and polyunsaturated fatty acids have been the most studied.

A variety of oxidized DNA bases, oxidized DNA sugar moiety, DNA–protein crosslinks, and DNA adducts from reaction of DNA bases with electrophylic lipid peroxidation products (etheno adducts, propane adducts, malonaldehyde adducts) have been described (Evans *et al.*, 2004; Medeiros, 2009; Berquist & Wilson, 2012). The highly reactive hydroxyl radical ($^{\bullet}OH$), for example, adds to double bonds of the four DNA bases and oxidizes the methyl group of thymine or the C–H bonds of 2′-deoxyribose and polyunsaturated fatty acids at diffusion-controlled rates. The diverse biomolecular radicals generated in this manner rearrange in several ways, giving rise to numerous oxidized products, in addition to DNA fragmentation. At least 24 major oxidized products of DNA bases have been identified (Evans *et al.*, 2004). The most studied one is 8-oxo-7,8-dihydro-2′-deoxyguanosine (8-oxodGuo), which is highlighted as a biomarker of DNA damage induced by oxidative stress. It is able to induce mainly GC → TA transversions in mammalian cells (Moriya, 1993). This type of mutation, although not specific for 8-oxodGuo, is frequently found in mutated tumor suppressor genes and oncogenes (Hussain and Harris, 1998). Other oxidized DNA bases, such as 8-oxo-7,8-dihydro-adenine, 2-hydroxyadenine, thymine glycol, 5-formyluracil, 5-formylcytosine, 5-hydroxyuracil, uracil glycol, 5-hydroxycytosine and the formamidopyrimidines FapyGua and FapyAde are also mutagenic lesions (Evans *et al.*, 2004). Elevated levels of oxidatively modified DNA bases have been observed in cancer tissues or urine of cancer patients in several studies (Evans *et al.*, 2004). These and other DNA lesions are removed from DNA by different repair pathways that act simultaneously. It is believed that their persistence in DNA is implicated in tumor initiation if damaged cells are not repaired or removed by apoptosis (Evans *et al.*, 2004; Berquist & Wilson, 2012). Thus, therapeutic and nutritional interventions to control oxidative stress, regulate cell metabolism, improve the fidelity of

DNA polymerases, induce apoptosis of damaged cells and enhance the performance of DNA repair pathways (BER, NER, strand break repair, homologous recombination and interstrand crosslink repair) are hopeful strategies to slow down mutation rates during ageing and, consequently, the development of age-associated diseases, including cancer (Berquist & Wilson, 2012; Kennedy *et al.*, 2012; Prasad *et al.*, 2012).

Beyond the induction of genetic lesions and mutations, it has been shown that ROS can modulate gene expression through nongenotoxic mechanisms, cooperating, for example, for the proliferation of initiated cells (*promotion phase*). The intracellular redox state influences the activity of diverse signaling networks [kinases, such as phosphatidylinositol 3-kinase/RAC-alpha serine/threonine-protein kinase (PI3K/Akt), protein kinase C and MAPKs] and transcription factors [e.g. NF-κB, activator protein 1, hypoxia inducible factor 1 (HIF1), p53 and nuclear factor erythroid 2-related factor 2 (Nrf2)], resulting in widely altered gene expression that will drive cells to their fate (senescence, death, growth or division), depending on ROS levels and nature (Leonarduzzi *et al.*, 2010; Indran *et al.*, 2010). ROS may also alter cell metabolism, epigenetic marks (such as DNA methylation and histone modifications) and telomerase [human telomerase reverse transcriptase (hTERT)] expression, activity and subcellular localization, leading to complex changes in gene expression pathways that did not originate from changes in DNA sequence (Fedotcheva *et al.*, 2006; Brookes *et al.*, 2006; Hitchler & Domann, 2009; Indran *et al.*, 2010).

The metabolism of cancer cells is emerging as a promising target for cancer therapy (Heiden *et al.*, 2009; Cairns *et al.*, 2011; Amoedo *et al.*, 2011; Parks *et al.*, 2013). The metabolic shift of cancer cells toward aerobic glycolysis (increased glucose oxidation to lactate even in the presence of high oxygen partial pressures), to the detriment of oxidative phosphorylation, was originally described in the 1920s by the Nobel Prize winner Otto Warburg, and is called the "Warburg effect" (Kroemer & Pouyssegur, 2008). These metabolic changes are coordinated by oncogenic signaling pathways, represented mainly by PI3K/AKT/mTOR (mechanistic target of rapamycin), HIF1, v-myc avian myelocytomatosis viral oncogene homolog and octamer-binding protein 1, which have the ability to activate the glycolytic pathway and/or inhibit the tricarboxylic acid cycle (Cairns *et al.*, 2011). Activation of these pathways by mutations, epigenetic mechanisms, intracellular metabolites or redox state will change the cell metabolism.

The PI3K/AKT/mTOR pathway is commonly altered in diverse types of human cancer, inducing biosynthesis and cell replication. Its aberrant activation is, for example, one of the most common molecular alterations in lung cancer, having an important role in both the initiation and progression of NSCLC, and emerging as an important target in therapy. However, *PIK3CA* mutations and the gain of gene copies explain only in part the pathway activation, suggesting the existence of other mechanisms regulating gene expression and protein activity (Gustafson *et al.*, 2010; Scrima *et al.*, 2012).

Activated PI3K/AKT/mTOR leads to the activation of different oncogenic transcription factors, among which is the HIF. HIF favors cell adaptation to low oxygen tensions, inducing neovascularization and glycolysis, along with other effects allied to the induction of more than 50 genes that are responsive to hypoxia. The complexes HIF1 and HIF2 are heterodimers composed of one constitutively expressed subunit, HIF1β, and the HIF1α or HIF2α subunits, which are rapidly stabilized under hypoxia. HIF1α is the most expressed subunit, with best characterized metabolic effects. Mutations or metabolic and epigenetic alterations that lead to HIF1α stabilization in the presence of oxygen make HIF protein active, altering cell metabolism under normoxia (Selak *et al.*, 2005; Serra-Pérez *et al.*, 2010; Cairns *et al.*, 2011).

How metabolic alterations contribute to the activation of signaling pathways and to epigenetic changes that favor tumor development is currently under careful investigation (Chia *et al.*, 2011; Cairns *et al.*, 2011). In this context, studies indicate that intermediates of the Krebs cycle regulate the activity of key enzymes involved in the control of cellular metabolism and maintenance of the epigenetic pattern.

The Krebs cycle intermediate α-ketoglutarate is a co-substrate of a family of dioxygenases that use molecular oxygen to hydroxylate their substrates, being, in turn, oxidized and decarboxylated directly to succinate. Among the enzymes dependent on α-ketoglutarate are the prolyl hydroxylases (PHD1-3) of HIFα, which also rely on oxygen, Fe(II) and ascorbate to be active, and are considered important sensors of oxygen in the cells. These enzymes catalyze the hydroxylation of the oxygen-dependent degradation domain of HIFα, leading to its degradation via proteasome (Selak *et al.*, 2005; Serra-Pérez *et al.*, 2010). Succinate, fumarate and oxaloacetate are intermediates of the tricarboxylic acid cycle capable of inhibiting oxygenases dependent on α-ketoglutarate, among which are PHD1-3. Thus, HIF activity may be increased in response to dysfunctions of the Krebs cycle (Selak *et al.*, 2005; Koivunen *et al.*, 2007). It has been reported that mutations that lead to inhibition of succinate dehydrogenase and fumarate hydratase, with subsequent increase in intracellular levels of succinate and fumarate, are related to an increased risk of developing tumors, such as pheochromocytoma, paraganglioma, renal carcinoma, gastric carcinoma, colon carcinoma and thyroid cancer. Increased levels of HIF1α and induction of hypoxia-responsive genes have been found in tumors containing these mutations (Selak *et al.*, 2005; Serra-Pérez *et al.*, 2010).

In addition to PHD1-3, other dioxygenases dependent on α-ketoglutarate and Fe(II) are the Jumonji C-terminal domain (JmjC) histone lysine demethylases and Ten-Eleven-Translocation (TET) protein methylcytosine hydroxylases, which are part of the epigenetic machinery for gene transcription regulation (Cyr & Domann, 2011). A link between Krebs cycle disruption and change in epigenetic marks may then exist, which could potentiate gene expression changes during carcinogenesis.

A fine control of gene expression is exerted by epigenetic marks in the genome, including DNA methylation and post-translational modifications of histones, without changing the primary sequence of DNA nucleotides (discussed in Chapter 3). The currently best characterized epigenetic mark is DNA methylation, which in association with modifications of histones and other proteins plays a regulatory role in chromatin structure maintenance. A fraction of 2–5% of cytosine levels in human DNA is in the methylated form 5-methyl-2′-deoxycytidine (5-mdC), which is the fifth most abundant deoxynucleoside in DNA (Robertson & Wolffe, 2000; Bender, 2004; Maganã *et al.*, 2007).

The pattern of 5-mdC in DNA is precisely preserved by mitotic inheritance via DNA methyltransferase (DNMT) activity. Three catalytically active members of this family of enzymes are found in mammalian cells – DNMT1, DNMT3a and DNMT3b. Methylation in mammalian somatic tissues occurs in cytosine preceding guanine bases (CpG dinucleotides) and its distribution in the genome is not random. A large fraction of 5-mdC is located on transposons, which represent more than 40% of the human genome and are a challenge for its function and stability. It is estimated that approximately 70% of the CpG dinucleotides in DNA are methylated, whereas nonmethylated CpGs are found primarily in "CpG islands". Such islands are regions of DNA more than 500 bp long with high relative densities of CpG dinucleotides. The majority of promoter regions of human genes (more than 60%) contain nonmethylated "CpG islands". Specific transcription factors and histone modifications determine the transcriptional activity or inactivity of these genes. Normally, methylated "CpG islands" are found in the promoter regions of imprinted genes, genes from the inactive X chromosome in females and tissue-specific genes (Sharma *et al.*, 2010; Brenet *et al.*, 2011; Dahl *et al.*, 2011; Williams *et al.*, 2011). Dense methylation of the promoter region is generally associated with gene silencing. Tumor cells typically exhibit a loss of global DNA methylation (hypomethylation) accompanied by focal hypermethylation, which can lead to genomic instability and transcriptional silencing of tumor suppressor genes, respectively (Irizarry *et al.*, 2009; Doi *et al.*, 2009; Dahl *et al.*, 2011).

Mechanisms responsible for the maintenance of nonmethylated "CpG islands" are poorly understood, and may be attended by TET protein methylcytosine hydroxylases. The hydroxylated form of 5-mdC, 5-hydroxymethyl-2′-deoxycytidine (5-hmdC), was first described in mammalian DNA in the early 1970s (Penn *et al.*, 1972), but only four decades later were its levels accurately determined in mouse tissues, ranging from 0.03 to 0.7% of the total deoxycytidine in DNA, depending on the tissue (Globisch *et al.*, 2010). Oxidation of 5-mdC to 5-hmdC is catalyzed by a family of dioxygenases dependent on α-ketoglutarate and Fe(II), named TET proteins, with three representatives in mammals – TET1, TET2 and TET3 (Tahiliani *et al.*, 2009; Ito *et al.*, 2010; Dahl *et al.*, 2011; Williams *et al.*, 2011). It is hypothesized that oxidation of 5-mdC to 5-hmdC via TET proteins is the first step toward the complete reaction of DNA demethylation (Tahiliani *et al.*, 2009; Globisch *et al.*, 2010; Nabel & Kohli, 2011). It is reported that proteins that bind to methyl-CpG have low affinity for 5-hmdC, resulting in alterations of transcriptional activity of genes with high levels of 5-hmdC in the promoter region (Valinluck & Sowers, 2007; Jin *et al.*, 2010; Dahl *et al.*, 2011). Such actions may have a biological significance that remains to be unraveled.

There is limited knowledge about mechanisms that lead to hypermethylation of CpG islands in promoter regions of genes in the carcinogenesis process. It is suggested that the loss of function of TET proteins can lead to hypermethylation of gene promoter regions, with consequent disruption of transcription and cell differentiation (Williams *et al.*, 2011). It is noteworthy that TET2 is frequently mutated in myeloid neoplasms and that TET1 and TET2 are frequently mutated in gliomas (Chia *et al.*, 2011; Pronier & Delhommeau, 2012). Since TET proteins are dependent on α-ketoglutarate for their catalytic activity, the relationship between changes in the tricarboxylic acid cycle and levels of 5-mdC and 5-hmdC in DNA must be investigated (Chia *et al.*, 2011). Indeed, it has been found that fumarate and succinate accumulation in cells mutated for fumarate hydratase and succinate dehydrogenase leads to inhibition of 5-mdC hydroxylation in DNA (Xiao *et al.*, 2012).

As evidence of the role of epigenetic changes in carcinogenesis, it is known that more than 60 genes are epigenetically silenced in lung tumors (Belinsky, 2004; Damiani *et al.*, 2008). Such silencing may occur in the early stages of carcinogenesis. For instance, methylation of tumor suppressor gene *p16* has been observed in alveolar hyperplasia, basal cell hyperplasia and bronchial epithelium of cancer-free smokers (Belinsky, 2004). Given the importance of promoter region methylation for gene silencing, the determination of methylation patterns of multiple genes is implicated as a highly sensitive and specific tool for the diagnosis of lung cancer and for screening individuals at increased risk of developing this type of cancer (Tsou *et al.*, 2002; Anglim *et al.*, 2008; Suzuki & Yoshino, 2010; Zhang *et al.*, 2011b; Kontic *et al.*, 2012).

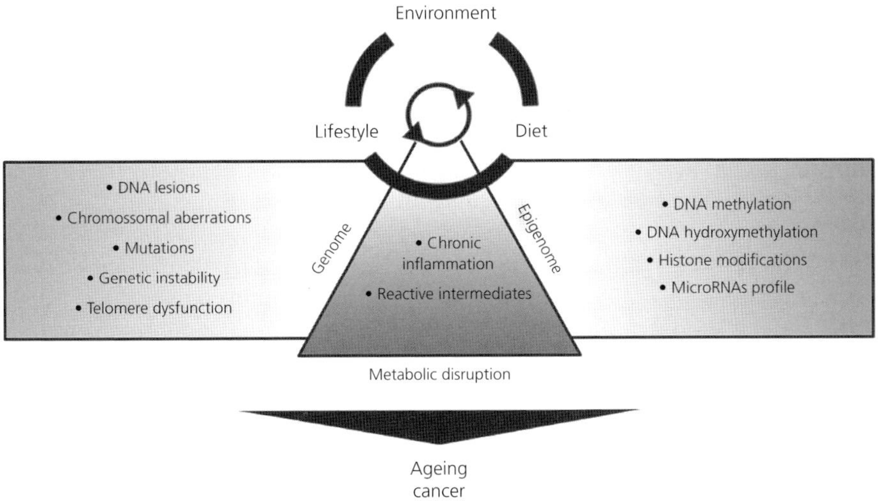

Figure 4.1 Ageing and cancer as the outcomes of detrimental changes occurring in genome, epigenome and metabolism in response to environment, lifestyle and diet over the course of time. Figure artwork by Tiago Franco de Oliveira, PhD.

In summary, key alterations that contribute to cell malignant transformation are gathered in Fig. 4.1.

4.3 Diet, nutrition and cancer

Interest in the complex relationship between nutritional factors and cancer has significantly increased in recent decades and it has attracted the attention of several stakeholders, including the public, the media and food regulators (Weed, 2013). Nutrition is one of the main environmental factors affecting cancer risk and it has been estimated that one-third of cancer deaths in the world could be prevented through a healthy lifestyle, including adequate dietary habits (Danaei *et al.*, 2005; World Cancer Research Fund/American Institute for Cancer Research, 2007; Duthie, 2011). Epidemiological studies conducted among populations that have migrated from less developed countries to highly industrialized ones have been vital in showing the importance of the environment, particularly diet, for cancer development (Shapira *et al.*, 2013). They show that, over several generations, migrants come to present the same cancer incidence as the native population in the Western host countries (Martin, 2013).

Because prevention remains the most promising strategy for reducing both cancer incidence and mortality (Umar *et al.*, 2012), identification of dietary factors that affect disease development is of utmost importance. Obesity is an inadequate nutritional condition that has been associated with increased risk of the disease, particularly breast, endometrial, colorectal, renal and prostate cancers (De Pergola & Silvestris, 2013). It is estimated that 20% of cancer cases are induced by obesity (Wolin *et al.*, 2010). Furthermore, excessive alcohol, red meat, sugar and salt represent dietary factors that promote carcinogenesis and consumption of these should be reduced (World Cancer Research Fund/American Institute for Cancer Research, 2007).

On the other hand, regular consumption of fruit and vegetables is strongly associated with reduced risk of developing cancer (Potter & Steinmetz, 1996; Martin *et al.*, 2013a). Based on these accumulated data, the general population should be educated to regularly eat at least nine servings of fruit and vegetables in all forms (fresh, cooked and processed) per day (Liu, 2003). In addition, the promotion of high intake of these foods through national campaigns and health policies is considered a preferable strategy to promote health and decrease the burden of noncommunicable diseases, including cancer (Boeing *et al.*, 2012).

The anticancer effects of fruit and vegetables is attributed to the presence of nutrients (vitamins and minerals), dietary fiber and bioactive food components (BFCs) also known as phytochemicals or nutraceuticals (polyphenolic compounds, sulfur-containing compounds and terpenoids, among others; Ong *et al.*, 2012; Liu, 2013). Particular interest has been directed towards the cancer preventive potential of BFCs that comprise secondary metabolites widely distributed in foods of plant origin. They represent promising natural agents for cancer prevention because they are commonly consumed in regular foods, display little or no toxicity and have the potential to be associated with standard chemotherapy (Li *et al.*, 2011b). It is estimated that a regular portion of vegetables contains more than 100 different BFCs and their metabolites (Surh, 2003). For example, more than 5000 individual flavonoids have been identified, which are distributed in at least 10 subgroups according to their structure (Kocic *et al.*, 2013). Thus the anticancer actions of fruit and vegetables have been suggested to be a reflection of their complex mixture of bioactive compounds that act through additive and synergistic interactions (Liu, 2003). However, important aspects of BFC anticancer actions still need to be better characterized, including the minimum quantity that should be consumed, the ideal time for intervention and the impact of genetics in determining the response (Kim *et al.*, 2009).

Vitamins, minerals and BFCs have been shown to influence every stage of cancer development by modulating different cellular and molecular processes during initiation, promotion and progression phases (Davis *et al.*, 2010; González-Vallinas *et al.*, 2013). Because several features of the cancer cell, including limitless replicative potential, evasion of apoptosis and sustained angiogenesis, are ultimately underpinned by genomic instability induced by environmental stress and ageing, maintenance of DNA integrity emerges as a central mechanism for cancer prevention by nutritional factors (Tan *et al.*, 2011). DNA repair, carcinogen detoxification and anti-oxidant and anti-inflammatory effects illustrate some of the beneficial effects through which nutritional factors protect the genome (Milner, 2008; Ong *et al.*, 2012; González-Vallinas *et al.*, 2013). The identification of dietary compounds and regimens that inhibit cellular and molecular changes that lead to age-associated diseases, including cancer, may ultimately contribute to slowing of the ageing process and the extension of life expectancy (Dabhade & Kotwal, 2013; Fig. 4.1).

Although cancer and ageing are suggested to be inexorably linked, there are still no established approaches for ameliorating them in concert (Sharp *et al.*, 2013). Because ageing and cancer can be understood as distinct manifestations of the same underlying process represented by accumulation of cellular damage (López-Otín *et al.*, 2013), which display common molecular pathways and regulatory mechanisms, it has been proposed that cancer-preventive strategies are likely to have an impact on slowing the ageing process and vice-versa. That is, anti-ageing therapies are likely to contribute to cancer risk reduction (Chobotova, 2009; De Magalhães, 2013). Thus the importance of vitamins, minerals, bioactive compounds from fruit and vegetables and energy restriction has been highlighted for both anti-ageing and cancer-prevention interventions (Chobotova, 2009; Dabhade & Kotwal, 2013).

Both genomic instability and epigenetic drift represent interconnected primary hallmarks of ageing that play a central role in cellular damage induction (López-Otín *et al.*, 2013). The epigenetic changes that accumulate over time can indeed be considered "chromatin damage" (Sedivy *et al.*, 2008). Several compounds found in the human diet and/or environment have been suggested to modify the epigenome and chromatin architecture and affect processes related to the carcinogenesis processes, including increased susceptibility to carcinogen attack. These compounds, which include ethanol and heavy metals, have been termed "epigens" (Martin, 2013).

Although the importance of epigenetic alterations in cancer was first recognized more than three decades ago, it was only more recently that interest emerged concerning the impact of nutritional modulation of epigenetic marks on health outcomes, including cancer prevention and longevity (Ong & Pérusse, 2011). Diet can modulate both the ageing process and carcinogenesis by regulating epigenetic processes, including DNA methylation, to affect the functionality of the genetic blueprint (Liu *et al.*, 2003). Thus it has been proposed that epigenetic mechanisms could mediate the interactions between genes, ageing and disease susceptibility (Park *et al.*, 2012)

Diet may affect epigenetic processes, including DNA methylation and histone modifications, through several complex mechanisms (McKay & Mathers, 2011). Nutrients and BFCs modulate DNA methylation through at least four mechanisms: some dietary factors are important sources of methyl groups necessary for trans-methylation reactions; dietary factors can affect methyl group utilization by processes including shifts in DNMT activity; a third plausible mechanism could be related to DNA demethylation, although direct evidence is still lacking; and finally, DNA methylation leading to activation or repression of genes related to carcinogenesis could modulate the response to dietary interventions (Ross, 2003). Histone post-translational modifications, including acetylation and methylation, can be altered by dietary components through modulation of several members of the epigenetic machinery (i.e. histone deacetylases, histone acetyltransferases, histone methytransfersases, members of co-activator and co-repressor complexes; Huang *et al.*, 2011). Because epigenetic deregulation occurs early in carcinogenesis and is potentially reversible, intervention strategies targeting the epigenome with nutrients and BFCs have been proposed for cancer prevention (Ong *et al.*, 2011). Dietary components with cancer-preventive potential that have been shown to modulate epigenetic processes include folate, butyric acid, vitamin A, selenium, polyphenols, isothiocyanates and allyl compounds (Ong *et al.*, 2011; Chagas *et al.*, 2012).

4.4 Targeting age-related genomic and epigenomic alterations with nutritional interventions for cancer prevention

Among the diverse types of dietary compounds and interventions with cancer preventive potential, emphasis should be directed toward folate, energy restriction and polyphenol compounds, especially resveratrol, because they have also been shown to play an important role in the ageing process. In particular, their ability to target age-related genomic and epigenomic alterations is of great interest in this context.

4.4.1 Folate

Folate comprises a vitamin of the B Complex group present in high concentrations in green leafy vegetables that exerts a central role in one-carbon metabolism (Baggott *et al.*, 2012). Through this network of biochemical reactions, folate coenzymes in association with other nutrients, including riboflavin (vitamin B_2), pyridoxine (vitamin B_6), cobalamin (vitamin B_{12}), methionine and choline, participate in the biosynthesis of purine and thymine nucleotides, as well as of *S*-adenosyl-L-methionine (SAM), the universal methyl donor for DNA and histone methylation (Stefanska *et al.*, 2012). Folate maintains genomic stability by donating one-carbon units for cellular metabolism and by regulating DNA biosynthesis, repair and methylation (Duthie, 2011). Thus DNA synthesis and DNA methylation represent plausible mechanisms through which folate could affect cancer risk (Williams, 2012), and determination of the proper status of this vitamin is needed to prevent age-associated cancer development (Kim *et al.*, 2009)

The association between folate and cancer, particularly colorectal cancer, is however complex. Although epidemiological studies show a role for dietary folate in the prevention of colorectal cancer, experimental studies have brought conflicting results (Rosati *et al.*, 2012). The impact of folate deficiency and supplementation on cancer development varies according to cell and target organ, level of consumption and stage of the carcinogenic process (Van Engeland & Herman, 2010). A dual modulatory effect on colon carcinogenesis has been reported. Protective effects were observed when folic acid was administered to animals at physiological doses before the appearance of colonic preneoplastic lesions. On the other hand, higher levels promoted the expansion and progression of established preneoplastic lesions (Kim, 2007; Mason, 2011). The association between folate and cancer risk is further complicated because folate dietary intake and polymorphisms in its associated genes influence the metabolism of this vitamin (Nazki *et al.*, 2014).

Cellular alterations induced by ageing have been proposed to lead to low folate tissue levels, impairing one-carbon metabolism and promoting cancer development (Jang *et al.*, 2005). Folate deficiency has been suggested to promote carcinogenesis through two main mechanisms: (a) by promoting uracil misincorporation during DNA synthesis, an alteration that is associated with DNA strand breakage and other chromosomal aberrations; and/or (b) by inducing global genomic hypomethylation and proto-oncogene activation (Lee, 2009). More specifically, folate deficiency results in decreased intracellular 5,10-methylenetetrahydrofolate levels, which retard conversion of deoxyuridine monophosphate to deoxythymidine monophosphate, leading to cellular thymidine depletion and uracil misincorporation into DNA. It also impacts purine biosynthesis by inhibiting 10-formyltetrahydrofolate-mediated production of adenosine and guanosine. Reduced levels of 5-methyltetrahydrofolate limit remethylation of S-adenosylhomocysteine (SAH) to SAM in the methionine cycle, leading to cytosine demethylation and global DNA hypomethylation (Duthie *et al.*, 2010).

Folate homeostasis is altered during ageing and this has been associated with increased DNA damage. More specifically, it was observed in mice that age-associated spontaneous loss of folate in the colon was accompanied by accumulation of uracil into colon DNA. Interestingly, these results show that increased expression of folate-absorption and retention genes (reduced folate carrier, multidrug resistance protein 3 and γ-glutamyl hydrolase) within the colonocyte is not enough to fully restore folate status during ageing (Simon *et al.*, 2012). In addition to high levels of 8-oxodGuo in lymphocyte DNA, folate-deficient rats presented increased activity of the DNA repair enzymes 8-oxoguanine DNA

N-glycosylase 1 and *O*-6-methylguanine-DNA methyltransferase in the liver, but not in the colon (Duthie *et al.*, 2010). The inability of colon tissue to respond to folate deficiency (i.e. elevated DNA damage or an imbalance in the nucleotide precursor pool) could increase the potential for malignant transformation (Duthie *et al.*, 2010).

The importance of folate and other components of the one-carbon metabolism for epigenetic processes is illustrated by classical studies that showed that a diet deficient in methyl-donors can be carcinogenic *per se* (Poirier, 1994). Folate, choline and methionine deficiency promote decreased hepatic SAM levels, global DNA hypomethylation, hepatic steatosis, cirrhosis and ultimately hepatocarcinogenesis in rodents (Esfandiari *et al.*, 2003). These hepatocarcinogenic effects are mediated by alteration of the expression of several components of the epigenetic machinery, including DNMTs and methyl CpG binding proteins (methyl CpG binding protein 2 and methyl-CpG binding domain protein 1, 2 and 4; Ghoshal *et al.*, 2006). It has been proposed that ageing and folate deficiency would synergistically provide an epigenetic milieu toward cancer development, as each is associated with altered DNA methylation (Kim *et al.*, 2009). More specifically, ageing-associated decreased DNMT activity accompanied by reduced methyl group availability would lead to lower genomic DNA methylation, tumor suppressor gene hypermethylation and histone modifications (Kim *et al.*, 2009). In old but not young mice, global DNA methylation and p16 promoter methylation in colon tissue were susceptible to modulation by dietary folate (Keyes *et al.*, 2007). Results from a cross-sectional study, in which rectal biopsies from 185 patients free from gastrointestinal inflammatory or neoplastic diseases were analyzed, show that ageing is the main factor affecting methylation status of a panel of genes involved in the Wnt signaling pathway, which has been implicated in colorectal pathogenesis (Tapp *et al.*, 2013). In addition, folate has also been identified as a relevant nutritional modulator of methylation of these genes in normal mucosa of healthy individuals (Tapp *et al.*, 2013). Red blood cell folate levels and advanced age were positively associated with methylation levels of the promoter regions of estrogen receptor α and secreted frizzled related protein-1 in normal colorectal mucosa, suggesting the need for caution when considering supplementing healthy individuals with folic acid as increased methylation of specific promoters could increase the risk of colorectal neoplasia (Wallace *et al.*, 2010).

Polymorphisms in one-carbon metabolism genes could also influence epigenetic processes. For example, the C677T variation in the methylenetetrahydrofolate reductase gene, which codes for an enzyme that plays a central role in this metabolism, is associated with increased global DNA hypomethylation in human leukocytes and lymphocytes, especially under folate deficient status (Kim, 2007).

Results from *in vivo* studies have highlighted that maintenance of genomic stability is a central mechanism associated with folate cancer chemoprevention effects. Inhibition of hepatic preneoplastic lesions development was observed in rats treated with folic acid during early hepatocarcinogenesis (Chagas *et al.*, 2011). These effects were accompanied by decreased DNA damage but no alterations in global methylation pattern, although hepatic SAM/SAH ratio was increased (Chagas *et al.*, 2011). Progressive DNA strand breaks within exons 5–8 of the p53 gene were observed in colon tissue of rats consuming a folate-deficient diet (Kim *et al.*, 2000). Conversely, dietary folate supplementation increased p53 integrity and expression (Kim *et al.*, 2000). Folic acid supplementation increased rectal mucosa genomic DNA methylation in patients with colon cancer and adenoma (Cravo *et al.*, 1994; Kim *et al.*, 2001).

Timing is also a fundamental aspect to consider when designing nutritional intervention strategies for cancer prevention. As also described for other chronic diseases, including diabetes and obesity, some cancers may have a developmental origin (Hilakivi-Clarke & de Assis, 2006). During embryogenesis and fetal development, folate is needed for DNA methylation processes that regulate transcriptional programs involved in cell proliferation, death and differentiation (Guéant *et al.*, 2013). Some studies have shown that increased folate consumption by mothers during gestation can modify epigenetic marks and the phenotype of the adult offspring (Wollf *et al.*, 1998; Sie *et al.*, 2013). In the context of cancer prevention, care should be taken, however, regarding maternal interventions with increased folic acid levels. In rats, maternal folic acid supplementation at levels equivalent to those recommended for women of reproductive age protected against the development of colorectal cancer in the offspring (Sie *et al.*, 2011). This protective effect was accompanied by increased global DNA methylation and decreased epithelial proliferation and DNA damage in the colorectum (Sie *et al.*, 2011). On the other hand, maternal and postweaning folic acid supplementation increased the risk of mammary tumor development in the offspring, and this deleterious effect was associated with decreased global DNA methylation and DNMT activity in the mammary gland (Ly *et al.*, 2011).

4.4.2 Energy restriction

Energy restriction without malnutrition (discussed in Chapter 2), the most-studied nutritional intervention able to increase longevity, presents significant effects on spontaneous and carcinogen-induced tumors in rodents (Omodei & Fontana, 2011; de Magalhães, 2013). Energy restriction has been suggested to increase longevity and to prevent age-associated cancer by promoting increased DNA stability. This hypothesis is supported by results from several experimental studies conducted during recent years showing that this nutritional intervention reduces DNA damage, including 8-oxodGuo, 5-hydroxymethyl uracil, formamidopyrimidine-DNA glycosylase and endonuclease III sensitive oxidized bases, single-strand breaks and mtDNA deletions, in different tissues and rodent strains (Heydari *et al.*, 2007). In addition to inducing DNA repair systems, energy restriction also inhibits DNA damage by modulating carcinogen activation enzymes and inducing endogenous anti-oxidant systems, including glutathione levels (Heydari *et al.*, 2007; Walsh *et al.*, 2014). These protective effects are likely to be mediated by the modulation of gene expression associated with several pathways, including NRF2 (Longo & Fontana, 2010; Martín-Montalvo *et al.*, 2011).

In fact, energy restriction prevention of chemically induced skin carcinogenesis in mice requires NRF2 transcription factor and is also associated with an increase in the hepatic expression of the anti-oxidant enzyme NAD(P)H:quinone oxireductase 1 (Pearson *et al.*, 2008). Treatment of MCF-7 human breast cancer cells with low levels of glucose reversed the tumor-promoting effects induced by the C-terminal binding protein (CtBP), an NADH-dependent transcriptional factor (Di *et al.*, 2013). This energy restriction inhibited CtBP activity, reversed CtBP-associated gene expression and increased DNA repair. Promoter analysis showed that increased expression of breast cancer 1 early onset gene (BRACA1), also verified in this experiment, was associated with decreased levels of CtBP loading and compensatory increase in H4 acetylation (Di *et al.*, 2013). Obese men who lost an average of 10.6 kg through an energy-restricted diet showed increased telomere length and decreased levels of abasic sites in DNA in the rectal mucosa (O´Callaghan *et al.*, 2009).

The impact of energy restriction on the chromatin is complex and occurs at different levels. It involves activation of the DNA repair system and the ROS detoxification system and increased fidelity of DNA replication. In addition, protection of genome integrity and chromatin structure by energy restriction has also been suggested to involve several mediators, including poly(ADP-ribose) polymerases (PARPs), CtBP, glyceraldehyde-3-phosphate dehydrogenase, TOR and sirtuins (SIRT). It has been proposed that the energetic imbalance induced by energy restriction would downregulate PARPs and activate SIRTs through changes in the $NAD^+/NADH$ ratio (Vaquero & Reinberg, 2009).

Because SIRTs deacetylate not only histones but also other components of the machinery involved in the regulation of the epigenome, including transcription factors, histone methyltransferases and histone acetyltransferases, much interest has been directed toward the role of this family of proteins in the context of energy restriction, ageing and cancer (Mostoslavsky *et al.*, 2010). While SIRT1 induction has been associated with the longevity-promoting effects of energy restriction, the meaning of its induction for cancer prevention is still controversial as studies show both cancer-promoting and cancer-suppressing activities (Hall *et al.*, 2013) and, on the other hand, histone deacetylase inhibitors represent promising agents for cancer prevention and treatment (Zhu *et al.*, 2013). Delay of the progression of lesions to pancreatic cancer by energy restriction was accompanied by the inhibition of cell proliferation and increased SIRT1 expression in mice (Lanza-Jacoby *et al.*, 2013). Similarly, the inhibition of carcinogen-induced colon preneoplastic lesions by energy restriction also involved the inhibition of cell proliferation and increased SIRT1 expression in colonic tissue (Tomita, 2012). However, it was observed in rats that treatment with the histone deacetylase inhibitor suberoylanilide hydroxamic acid did not alter the anti-breast cancer effects elicited by energy restriction (Zhu *et al.*, 2013). Furthermore, p53-heterozygous mice presented the same level of protection against tumor formation after energy restriction regardless of the genetic overexpression of SIRT1, suggesting that this histone deacetylase plays no role, or a limited role, in energy restriction-induced cancer protection (Herranz *et al.*, 2011).

Although activation of gate-keeping tumor suppressor genes, such as p53, after DNA damage is an important response mediating cancer prevention, it may increase ageing through apoptosis or senescence induction (Zhang *et al.*, 2011a). This indicates the existence of a delicate balance between ageing and cancer and it was proposed that targeting care-taking tumor supressors would maintain the stability of the genome and simultaneously slow ageing and prevent cancer (van Heemst *et al.*, 2007; Zhang *et al.*, 2011a). SIRT3 has been pointed out as one such potential care-taking tumor suppressor (Zhang *et al.*, 2011a). It has been proposed that this deacetylase is needed for activation of mitochondrial manganese superoxide dismutase (SOD2), one of the main anti-oxidant enzymes that controls the levels of ROS and inhibits DNA damage associated with cancer development (Shih & Donmez, 2013). Protection elicited by energy restriction against oxidative stress in mice required SIRT3-mediated SOD2 deacetylation that significantly increased this mitochondrial anti-oxidant enzyme activity (Qiu *et al.*, 2010). However, as also pointed out for SIRT1, care should be taken when considering SIRT3 as a target for cancer prevention, as this deacetylase has also shown tumor-promoting effects depending on the context (Shih & Donmez, 2013).

Epigenetic deregulation during ageing involves progressive loss of global DNA methylation that is accompanied by specific gene promoter hypermethylation (McKay & Mathers, 2011). It has been proposed that energy restriction anti-ageing effects would involve the reversal of age-related DNA methylation abnormalities, leading to the maintenance of genomic stability (Li *et al.*, 2011a). Examples of genes regulated by DNA methylation during energy restriction include runt-related transcription factor 3 (RUNX3), a transcription factor involved in development (Kim *et al.*, 2004), and the proto-oncogene *ras*, which decreased expression through increased DNA methylation, has been associated with energy-restriction anticarcinogenic effects (Hass *et al.*, 1993). It was also shown that glucose restriction extended the lifespan of normal cells and decreased precancerous cell growth. These effects were mediated by DNA methylation and chromatin remodeling of the promoter regions of hTERT and p16 genes, suggesting that epigenetic marks may represent common molecular targets for cancer chemoprevention and anti-ageing strategies focused on energy restriction interventions (Li *et al.*, 2010). Importantly, the detailed methylation-regulated pathways and target genes that may be responsible for energy restriction-induced longevity and disease prevention need to be further elucidated (Li *et al.*, 2011a).

Because energy restriction and BFCs share common cancer preventive and anti-ageing mechanisms, the combination of both nutritional interventions has been suggested to represent an attractive strategy for health and longevity promotion (Martin *et al.*, 2013b).

4.4.3 Bioactive food components

BFCs comprise compounds consumed in the regular diet that are not essential for cellular and metabolic function, but display health-promoting effects (Choi & Friso, 2010). The consumption of the Mediterranean diet has been associated with increased longevity and reduced risk of cancer. This diet is rich in fruit and vegetables that provide several BFCs, including anti-oxidant vitamins, glucosinolates and polyphenols. In particular, these latter compounds share common anti-ageing mechanisms, including SIRT activation with energy restriction, and have thus been classified as energy restriction mimetics (Pallauf *et al.*, 2013) (discussed in Chapter 2). Resveratrol is one such polyphenolic energy restriction mimetic that has been the subject of intense research in both the ageing and cancer prevention fields.

Resveratrol is a stilbene produced in plants by the enzyme stilbene synthase under stress conditions such as vicissitudes in climate, exposure to ozone, sunlight and heavy metals, and infection by pathogenic microorganisms. This polyphenolic compound is primarily found in the skin of grapes as well as in other fruits and plants, such as raspberries, blueberries, mulberries and Scots pine (Athar *et al.*, 2009). There are strong *in vitro* and *in vivo* data supporting a protective role by resveratrol against several malignancies, including melanoma and breast, lung, esophageal, gastric, colorectal and prostate cancers (Athar *et al.*, 2007). It has been reported that this polyphenolic compound can interfere with mechanisms involved in all stages of carcinogenesis (initiation, promotion and progression). These include the modulation of carcinogen bioactivation, inhibition of inflammatory responses and cell proliferation, apoptosis induction and the prevention of oxidative damage of DNA (Brisdelli *et al.*, 2009). Resveratrol anticancer effects involve the modulation of several molecular targets, including aryl hydrocarbon receptor, p53, NFkappaB and Nrf2 (Whitlock & Baek, 2012).

The initiation effects of estrogen and 2,3,7,8-tetrachlorodibenzo-*p*-dioxin (TCDD) in MCF-10F normal breast cells were prevented by resveratrol. These effects involved the modulation of estrogen metabolism, the inhibition of TCDD-induced cytochrome P450, family 1, subfamily B and polypeptide 1 (CYP1B1) expression and decreased adduct formation (Lu *et al.*, 2008). *In vivo* resveratrol inhibited peripheral blood cell DNA damage and increased the anti-oxidant status when provided to rats before and after initiation with the carcinogen 1,2-dimethylhydrazine (Sengottuvelan *et al.*, 2009). These results provide a mechanistic basis to explain resveratrol's preventive effects against colon carcinogenesis (Sengottuvelan *et al.*, 2006). Furthermore, previous treatment with resveratrol inhibited kidney oxidative DNA damage (8-oxodGuo) induced by the carcinogen $KBrO_3$ (Cadenas & Barja, 1999). Although anti-oxidant actions by resveratrol have been reported in several investigations, in some contexts this polyphenolic compound can behave as a pro-oxidant. This is particularly important in tumor cells, where the low-pH environment owing to the "Warburg effect" is associated with pro-oxidant-induced DNA damage that triggers apoptosis. More specifically, low pH-induced altered DNA conformation favors resveratrol attack of exposed DNA-bound copper, reducing it and thus generating ROS, leading to oxidative DNA cleavage (Muqbil *et al.*, 2012).

Epigenetic modulation has been suggested to represent a relevant feature of cancer preventive actions by dietary polyphenolic compounds. These BFCs have been shown to inhibit the activity of DNMT *in vitro* and *in vivo* and this could be due to allosteric regulation or inhibition of the enzyme expression (Vanden Berghe, 2012). In breast cancer cells, resveratrol-mediated deacetylation of the oncogenic transcription factor signal transducer and activator of transcription 3 (STAT-3) led to demethylation and activation of the *estrogen receptor-α* gene, sensitizing the tumor cells to antiestrogens that compete with estrogen for binding this receptor (Lee *et al.*, 2012). Furthermore, also in breast cancer cells, resveratrol prevented TCDD-mediated BRCA1 gene promoter-increased CpG methylation and decreased expression (Papoutsis *et al.*, 2012). Similar effects were observed when resveratrol was offered to rats exposed to TCDD *in utero* (Papoutsis *et al.*, 2013). One recent human study showed that women at increased breast cancer risk who consumed high levels of resveratrol presented reduced methylation levels of the tumor suppressor gene Ras association (RalGDS/AF-6) domain family member 1(RASSF-1A) in mammary tissue (Zhu *et al.*, 2012).

The energy restriction mimetic and anti-ageing mechanisms of resveratrol have been suggested to contribute to its effects against cancer (Bishayee, 2009). Resveratrol has been shown to be an indirect activator of SIRT1 *in vitro* and *in vivo* (Herranz & Serrano, 2010). This could represent a relevant mechanism associated with this BFC's life-extending activity and its protective activity against several chronic diseases, including cancer (Chung *et al.*, 2010; Subramanian *et al.*, 2010). For example, the chemopreventive effect of resveratrol against chemically induced skin papillomas is lost in SIRT1-null mice. This indicates that the protective effects of this polyphenol are mediated at least in part by SIRT1 (Boily *et al.*, 2009). The strong *in vitro* and *in vivo* inhibition of BRCA1 mutant tumors by resveratrol involved upregulation of SIRT1 activity that was followed by reduction of Survivin expression, leading to growth arrest and apoptosis (Wang *et al.*, 2008). It has been proposed that increasing SIRT1 activity with resveratrol would represent an interesting opportunity to "kill two birds with one stone", that is, extend lifespan and inhibit cancer development (Fernández & Fraga, 2011).

4.5 Conclusions and perspectives

Cancer and ageing represent related processes that share common mechanisms and pathways. One central mechanism to both processes is DNA damage. Another relevant one is epigenetic deregulation. Thus they comprise interesting targets to intervene with dietary compounds or regimens in order to reduce the risk of disease and promote longevity.

Although this represents an attractive concept, there are still no established nutritional interventions capable of simultaneously impact cancer and ageing. Accumulating data show that folate, energy restriction and BFCs, including the polyphenolic compound resveratrol, play a relevant role in the ageing process and can target age-related genomic and epigenomic alterations with positive consequences for cancer prevention. However, before these promising dietary compounds and regimens can be routinely used, their efficacy should be validated in clinical trials and their underlying cancer-preventive mechanisms deeply investigated.

Acknowledgment

We thank Tiago Franco de Oliveira for the artwork of Fig. 4.1. The authors' laboratories are supported by grants and fellowships from Fundação de Amparo à Pesquisa do Estado de São Paulo (FAPESP), Conselho Nacional de Desenvolvimento Científico e Tecnológico (CNPq), and Coordenação de Aperfeiçoamento de Pessoal de Nível Superior (CAPES).

References

Amoedo, N. D., T. El-Bacha, M. F. Rodrigues, and F. D. Rumjanek. 2011. Cell cycle and energy metabolism in tumor cells: strategies for drug therapy. *Recent Patents Anti-Cancer Drug Discov.* 6:15–25.

Anglim, P. P., T. A. Alonzo, and I. A. Laird-Offringa. 2008. DNA methylation-based biomarkers for early detection of non-small cell lung cancer: an update. *Mol Cancer* 7:81.

Athar, M., J. H. Back, X. Tang, K. H. Kim, L. Kopelovich, D. R. Bickers, and A. L. Kim. 2007. Resveratrol: a review of preclinical studies for human cancer prevention. *Toxicol. Appl. Pharmacol.* 224:274–283.

Athar, M., J. H. Back, L. Kopelovich, D. R. Bickers, and A. L. Kim. 2009. Multiple molecular targets of resveratrol: anti-carcinogenic mechanisms. *Arch. Biochem. Biophys.* 486:95–102.

Baggott, J. E., R. A. Oster, and T. Tamura. 2012. Meta-analysis of cancer risk in folic acid supplementation trials. *Cancer Epidemiol.* 36:78–81.

Barcellos-Hoff, M. H., D. Lyden, and T. C. Wang. 2013. The evolution of the cancer niche during multistage carcinogenesis. *Nat. Rev. Cancer* 13:511–518.

Belinsky, S. A. 2004. Gene-promoter hypermethylation as a biomarker in lung cancer. *Nat. Rev. Cancer* 4:707–717.

Bender, J. 2004. DNA methylation and epigenetics. *Annu. Rev. Plant Biol.* 55:41–68.

Berquist, B. R. and D. M. Wilson III. 2012. Pathways for repairing and tolerating the spectrum of oxidative DNA lesions. *Cancer Lett.* 327:61–72.

Bishayee, A. 2009. Cancer prevention and treatment with resveratrol: from rodent studies to clinical trials. *Cancer Prev. Res.* 2:409–418.

Boeing, H., A. Bechthold, A. Bub, S. Ellinger, D. Haller, A. Kroke, E. Leschik-Bonnet, M. J. Müller, H. Oberritter, M. Schulze, P. Stehle, and B. Watzl. 2012. Critical review: vegetables and fruit in the prevention of chronic diseases. *Eur. J. Nutr.* 51:637–663.

Boily, G., X. H. He, B. Pearce, K. Jardine, and M. W. McBurney. 2009. SirT1-null mice develop tumors at normal rates but are poorly protected by resveratrol. *Oncogene* 28:2882–2893.

Brenet, F., M. Moh, P. Funk, E. Feierstein, A. J. Viale, N. D. Socci, and J. M. Scandura. 2011. DNA methylation of the first exon is tightly linked to transcriptional silencing. *PLoS One* 6:e14524.

Brisdelli, F., G. D'Andrea, and A. Bozzi. 2009. Resveratrol: a natural polyphenol with multiple chemopreventive properties. *Curr. Drug Metabol.* 10:530–546.

Brookes, P. S., R. S. Freeman, and M. C. Barone. 2006. A shortcut to mitochondrial signaling and pathology: a commentary on "Nonenzymatic formation of succinate in mitochondria under oxidative stress". *Free Radic. Biol. Med.* 41:41–45.

Cadenas, S. and G. Barja. 1999. Resveratrol, melatonin, vitamin E, and PBN protect against renal oxidative DNA damage induced by the kidney carcinogen $KBrO_3$. *Free Radic. Biol. Med.* 26:1531–1537.

Cairns, R. A., I. S. Harris, and T. W. Mak. 2011. Regulation of cancer cell metabolism. *Nat. Rev. Cancer* 11:85–95.

Chagas, C. E., B. K. Bassoli, C. A. de Souza, R. Deminice, A. A. Jordão Júnior, S. A. Paiva, M. L. Dagli, T. P. Ong, and F. S. Moreno. 2011. Folic acid supplementation during early hepatocarcinogenesis: cellular and molecular effects. *Int. J. Cancer.* 129:2073–2082.

Chia, N., L. Wang, X. Lu, M. C. Senut, C. Brenner, and D. M. Ruden. 2011. Hypothesis: environmental regulation of 5-hydroxymethylcytosine by oxidative stress. *Epigenetics* 6:853–856.

Chobotova, K. 2009. Ageing and cancer: converging routes to disease prevention. *Integr. Cancer Ther.* 8:115.

Choi, S. W. and S. Friso. 2010. Epigenetics: a new bridge between nutrition and health. *Adv Nutr.* 1(1): 8–16.

Chung, S., H. Yao, S. Caito, J-W. Hwang, G. Arunachalam, and I. Rahman. 2010. Regulation of SIRT1 in cellular functions: Role of polyphenols. *Arch. Biochem. Biophys* 501:79–90.

Clapp, R. W., G. K. Howe, and M. M. Jacobs. 2007. Environmental and occupational causes of cancer: A call to act on what we know. *Biomed. Pharmacother.* 61:631–639.

Colditz, G. A., T. A. Sellers, and E. Trapido. 2006. Epidemiology – identifying the causes and preventability of cancer? *Nat. Rev. Cancer* 6:75–83.

Cole, J. and T. R. Skopek. 1994. Somatic mutant frequency, mutation rates and mutational spectra in the human population in vivo. *Mutat. Res.* 304:33–105.

Cravo, M., P. Fidalgo, A. D. Pereira, A. Gouveia-Oliveira, P. Chaves, J. Selhub, J. B. Mason, F. C. Mira, and C. N. Leitao. 1994. DNA methylation as an intermediate biomarker in colorectal cancer: modulation by folic acid supplementation. *Eur. J. Cancer Prev.* 3:473–479.

Cyr, A. R. and F. E. Domann. 2011. The redox basis of epigenetic modifications: from mechanisms to functional consequences. *Antioxid. Redox Signal.* 15:551–589.

Dabhade, P. and S. Kotwal. 2013. Tackling the ageing process with bio-molecules: a possible role for caloric restriction, food-derived nutrients, vitamins, amino acids, peptides, and minerals. *J. Nutr. Gerontol. Geriatr.*, 32:24–40.

Dahl, C., K. Grønbæk, and P. Guldberg. 2011. Advances in DNA methylation: 5-hydroxymethyl-cytosine revisited. *Clin. Chim. Acta* 412:831–836.

Damiani, L. A., C. M. Yingling, S. Leng, P. E. Romo, J. Nakamura, S. A. Belinsky. 2008. Carcinogen-induced gene promoter hypermethylation is mediated by DNMT1 and causal for transformation of immortalized bronchial epithelial cells. *Cancer Res.* 68:9005–9014.

Danaei, G., S. Vander Hoorn, A. D. Lopez,C. J. Murray, M. Ezzati, and Comparative Risk Assessment collaborating group. 2005. Causes of cancer in the world: comparative risk assessment of nine behavioral and environmental risk factors. *Lancet* 366:1784–1793.

Davis, C. D., N. J. Emenaker, and J. A. Milner. 2010. Cellular proliferation, apoptosis and angiogenesis: molecular targets for nutritional preemption of cancer. *Semin. Oncol.* 37:243–257.

Deelen, J., M. Beekman, M. Capri, C. Franceschi, and P. E. Slagboom. 2013. Identifying the genomic determinants of ageing and longevity in human population studies: progress and challenges. *Bioessays* 35:386–396.

de Magalhães, J. P. 2013. How ageing processes influence cancer. *Nat. Rev. Cancer* 13:357–365.

De Pergola, G. and F. Silvestris. 2013. Obesity as a major risk factor for cancer. *J Obes.* 2013:291546.

DePinho, R. A. 2000. The age of cancer. *Nature* 408:248–254.

Di, L. J., J. S. Byun, M. M. Wong, C. Wakano, T. Taylor, S. Bilke, S. Baek, K. Hunter, H. Yang, M. Lee, C. Zvosec, G. Khramtsova, F. Cheng, C. M. Perou, C. R. Miller, R. Raab, O. I. Olopade, and K. Gardner. 2013. Genome-wide profiles of CtBP link metabolism with genome stability and epithelial reprogramming in breast cancer. *Nat. Commun.* 4:1449.

Doi, A., I. H. Park, B. Wen, P. Murakami, M. J. Aryee, R. Irizarry, B. Herb, C. Ladd-Acosta, J. Rho, S. Loewer, J. Miller, T. Schlaeger, G. Q. Daley, and A. P. Feinberg. 2009. Differential methylation of tissue- and cancer-specific CpG island shores distinguishes human induced pluripotent stem cells, embryonic stem cells and fibroblasts. *Nat. Genet.* 41:1350–1353.

Duthie, S. J. 2011. Folate and cancer: how DNA damage, repair and methylation impact on colon carcinogenesis. *J. Inherit. Metab. Dis.* 34:101–109.

Duthie, S. J., G. Grant, L. P. Pirie, A. J. Watson, and G. P. Margison. 2010. Folate deficiency alters hepatic and colon MGMT and OGG-1 DNA repair protein expression in rats but has no effect on genome-wide DNA methylation. *Cancer Prev. Res.* 3:92–100.

Esfandiari, F., R. Green, R. F. Cotterman, I. P. Pogribny, S. J. James, and J. W. Miller. 2003. Methyl deficiency causes reduction of the methyl-CpG-binding protein, MeCP2, in rat liver. *Carcinogenesis* 24:1935–1940.

Evans, M. D., M. Dizdaroglu, and M. S. Cooke. 2004. Oxidative DNA damage and disease: induction, repair and significance. *Mutat. Res.* 567:1–61.

Fedotcheva, N. I., A. P. Sokolov, and M. N. Kondrashova. 2006. Nonezymatic formation of succinate in mitochondria under oxidative stress. *Free Radic. Biol. Med.* 41:56–64.

Fernández A. F. and M. F. Fraga. 2011. The effects of the dietary polyphenol resveratrol on human healthy ageing and lifespan. *Epigenetics* 6:870–874.

Garraway, L. A. and E. S. Lander. 2013. Lessons from the cancer genome. *Cell* 153:17–37.

Ghoshal, K., X. Li, J. Datta, S. Bai, I. Pogribny, M. Pogribny, Y. Huang, D. Young, S. T. Jacob. 2006. A folate- and methyl-deficient diet alters the expression of DNA methyltransferases and methyl CpG bindingproteins involved in epigenetic gene silencing in livers of F344 rats. *J Nutr.* 136:1522–1527.

Globisch, D., M. Münzel, M. Müller, S. Michalakis, M. Wagner, S. Koch, T. Brückl, M. Biel, and T. Carell. 2010. Tissue distribution of 5-hydroxymethylcytosine and search for active demethylation intermediates. *PLoS One* 5:e15367.

González-Vallinas, M., M. González-Castejón, A. Rodríguez-Casado, and A. R. de Molina. 2013. Dietary phytochemicals in cancer prevention and therapy: a complementary approach with promising perspectives. *Nutr. Rev.* 71:585–599.

Goukassian, D., F. Gad, M. Yaar, M. S. Eller, U. S. Nehal, and B. A. Gilchrest. 2000. Mechanisms and implications of the age-associated decrease in DNA repair capacity. *FASEB J.* 14:1325–1334.

Guéant, J. L., F. Namour, R. M. Guéant-Rodriguez, and J. L. Daval. 2013. Folate and fetal programming: a play in epigenomics? *Trends Endocrinol. Metab.* 24:279–289.

Gustafson, A. M., R. Soldi, C. Anderlind, M. B. Scholand, J. Qian, X. Zhang, K. Cooper, D. Walker, A. McWilliams, G. Liu, E. Szabo, J. Brody, P. P. Massion, M. E. Lenburg, S. Lam, A. H. Bild, and A. Spira. 2010. Airway PI3K pathway activation is an early and reversible event in lung cancer development. *Sci. Transl. Med.* 2:26ra25.

Hall, J. A., J. E. Dominy, Y. Lee, and P. Puigserver. 2013. The sirtuin family's role in ageing and age-associated pathologies. *J. Clin. Invest.*123:973–979.

Hanahan, D. and R. A. Weinberg. 2011. Hallmarks of cancer: the next generation. *Cell* 144:646–674.

Hass, B. S., R. W. Hart, M. H. Lu, and B. D. Lyn-Cook. 1993. Effects of caloric restriction in animals on cellular function, oncogene expression, and DNA methylation in vitro. *Mutat. Res.* 295:281–289.

Hasty, P., J. Campisi, J. Hoeijmakers, H. van Steeg, and J. Vijg. 2003. Ageing and genome maintenance: lessons from the mouse? *Science* 299:1355–1359.

Hecht, S. S. 2012. Lung carcinogenesis by tobacco smoke. *Int. J. Cancer* 131:2724–2732.

Heiden, M. G. V., L. C. Cantley, and C. B. Thompson. 2009. Understanding the Warburg effect: the metabolic requirements of cell proliferation. *Science* 324:1029–1033.

Herranz, D. and M. Serrano. 2010. SIRT1: recent lessons from mouse models. *Nat. Rev. Cancer.*10:819–823.

Herranz, D., G. Iglesias, M. Muñoz-Martín, and M. Serrano. 2011. Limited role of Sirt1 in cancer protection by dietary restriction. *Cell Cycle* 10:2215–2217.

Heydari, A. R., A. Unnikrishnan, L. V. Lucente, and A. Richardson. 2007. Caloric restriction and genomic stability. *Nucleic Acids Res.* 35:7485–7496.

Hilakivi-Clarke, L. and S. de Assis. 2006. Fetal origins of breast cancer. *Trends Endocrinol. Metab.* 17:340–348.

Hill, K. A., V. L. Buettner, A. Halangoda, M. Kunishige, S. R. Moore, J. Longmate, W. A. Scaringe, and S. S. Sommer. 2004. Spontaneous mutation in Big Blue® mice from fetus to old age: tissue-specific time courses of mutation frequency but similar mutation types. *Environ. Mol. Mutagen.* 43:110–120.

Hitchler, M. J. and F. E. Domann. 2009. Metabolic defects provide a spark for the epigenetic switch in cancer. *Free Radic. Biol. Med.* 47:115–127.

Hofree, M., J. P. Shen, H. Carter, A. Gross, and T. Ideker. 2013. Network-based stratification of tumor mutations. *Nat. Meth.* 10:1108–1115.

Huang, J., C. Plass, and C. Gerhauser. 2011. Cancer chemoprevention by targeting the epigenome. *Curr. Drug Targets* 12:1925–1956.

Hussain, S. P. and C. C. Harris. 1998. Molecular epidemiology of human cancer: contribution of mutation spectra studies of tumor suppressor genes. *Cancer Res.* 58:4023–4037.

Indran, I. R., M. P. Hande, and S. Pervaiz. 2010. Tumor cell redox state and mitochondria at the center of the non-canonical activity of telomerase reverse transcriptase. *Mol. Aspects of Med.* 31:21–28.

Irizarry, R. A., C. Ladd-Acosta, B. Wen, Z. Wu, C. Montano, P. Onyango, H. Cui, K. Gabo, M. Rongione, M. Webster, H. Ji, J. B. Potash, S. Sabunciyan, and A. P. Feinberg. 2009. The human colon cancer methylome shows similar hypo- and hypermethylation at conserved tissue-specific CpG island shores. *Nat. Genet.* 41:178–186.

Ito, S., A. C. D'Alessio, O. V. Taranova, K. Hong, L. C. Sowers, and Y. Zhang. 2010. Role of Tet proteins in 5mC to 5hmC conversion, ES-cell self-renewal and inner cell mass specification. *Nature* 466:1129–1133.

Jang, H., J. B. Mason, and S. W. Choi. 2005. Genetic and epigenetic interactions between folate and ageing in carcinogenesis. *J. Nutr.* 135:2967S–2971S.

Jin, S. G., S. Kadam, and G. P. Pfeifer. 2010. Examination of the specificity of DNA methylation profiling techniques towards 5-methylcytosine and 5-hydroxymethylcytosine. *Nucleic Acids Res.* 38:e125.

Kennedy, S. R., L. A. Loeb, and A. J. Herr. 2012. Somatic mutations in ageing, cancer and neurodegeneration. *Mech. Ageing Dev.* 133:118–126.

Keyes, M. K., H. Jang, J. B. Mason, Z. Liu, J. W. Crott, D. E. Smith, S. Friso, and S. W. Choi. 2007. Older age and dietary folate are determinants of genomic and p16-specific DNA methylation in mouse colon. *J Nutr.*137:1713–1717.

Kim, K. C., S. Friso, and S. W. Choi. 2009a. DNA methylation, an epigenetic mechanism connecting folate to healthy embryonic development and ageing. *J. Nutr. Biochem.* 20:917–926.

Kim, T. Y., H. J. Lee, K. S. Hwang, M. Lee, J. W. Kim, Y. J. Bang, and G. H. Kang. 2004. Methylation of RUNX3 in various types of human cancers and premalignant stages of gastric carcinoma. *Lab. Invest.* 84:476–484.

Kim Y-I. 2007. Folate and colorectal cancer: an evidence-based critical review. *Mol. Nutr. Food Res.* 51:267–292.

Kim, Y. I., S. Shirwadkar, S. W. Choi, M. Puchyr, Y. Wang, and J. B. Mason. 2000. Effects of dietary folate on DNA strand breaks within mutation-prone exons of the p53 gene in rat colon. *Gastroenterology* 119:151–161.

Kim, Y. I., H. W. Baik, K. Fawaz, T. Knox, Y. M. Lee, R. Norton, E. Libby, and J. B. Mason. 2001. Effects of folate supplementation on two provisional molecular markers of colon cancer: a prospective, randomized trial. *Am. J Gastroenterol.*96:184–195.

Kim, Y. S., M. R. Young, G. Bobe, N. H. Colburn, and J. A. Milner. 2009. Bioactive food components, inflammatory targets, and cancer prevention. *Cancer Prev. Res.* 2:200–208.

Klaunig, J. E., Z. Wang, X. Pu, and S. Zhou. 2011. Oxidative stress and oxidative damage in chemical carcinogenesis. *Toxicol. Appl. Pharmacol.* 254:86–99.

Kocic, B., D. Kitic, and S. Brankovic. 2013. Dietary flavonoid intake and colorectal cancer risk: evidence from human population studies. *J. BUON* 18:34–43.

Koivunen, P., M. Hirsilä, A. M. Remes, I. E. Hassinen, K. I. Kivirikko, and J. Myllyharju. 2007. Inhibition of hypoxia-inducible factor (HIF) hydroxylases by citric acid cycle intermediates: possible links between cell metabolism and stabilization of HIF. *J. Biol. Chem.* 282:4524–4532.

Kontic, M., J. Stojsic, D. Jovanovic, V. Bunjevacki, S. Ognjanovic, J. Kuriger, S. Puumala, and H. H. Nelson. 2012. Aberrant promoter methylation of CDH13 and MGMT genes is associated with clinicopathologic characteristics of primary non-small-cell lung carcinoma. *Clin. Lung Cancer* 13:297–303.

Kroemer, G. and J. Pouyssegur. 2008. Tumor cell metabolism: cancer's Achilles' heel. *Cancer Cell* 13: 472–482.

Lanza-Jacoby, S., G. Yan, G. Radice, C. LePhong, J. Baliff, and R. Hess. 2013. Calorie restriction delays the progression of lesions to pancreatic cancer in the LSL-KrasG12D; Pdx-1/Cre mouse model of pancreatic cancer. *Exp. Biol. Med.* 238:787–797.

Lee H., P. Zhang, A. Herrmann, C. Yang, H. Xin, Z. Wang, D. S. B. Hoon, S. J. Forman, R. Jove, A. D. Riggs, and H. Yu. 2012. Acetylated STAT3 is crucial for methylation of tumor-suppressor gene promoters and inhibition by resveratrol results in demethylation. *Proc. Natl Acad. Sci. USA* 109:7765–7769.

Lee, S. A. 2009. Gene–diet interaction on cancer risk in epidemiological studies. *J. Prev. Med. Public Health* 42:360–370.

Leonarduzzi, G., B. Sottero, and G. Poli. 2010. Targeting tissue oxidative damage by means of cell signaling modulators: the antioxidant concept revisited. *Pharmacol. Therapeut.* 128:336–374.

Li Y, L. Liu, and T. O. Tollefsbol TO. 2010. Glucose restriction can extend normal cell lifespan and impair precancerous cell growth through epigenetic control of hTERT and p16 expression. *FASEB J.* 24: 1442–1453.

Li, Y., M. Daniel, and T. O. Tollefsbol. 2011a. Epigenetic regulation of caloric restriction in ageing. *BMC Med.* 9:98.

Li, Y., M. S. Wicha, S. J. Schwartz, and D. Sun. 2011b. Implications of cancer stem cell theory for cancer chemoprevention by natural dietary compounds. *J. Nutr. Biochem.* 22:799–806.

Liu, L., R. C. Wylie, L. G. Andrews, and T. O. Tollesfsbol. 2003. Ageing, cancer and nutrition: the DNA methylation connection. *Mech. Ageing Dev.* 124:989–998.

Liu, R. H. 2003. Health benefits of fruit and vegetables are from additive and synergistic combinations of phytochemicals. *Am. J. Clin. Nutr.* 78:517S–520S.

Liu, R. H. 2013. Dietary bioactive compounds and their health implications. *J. Food Sci.* 78:A18–25.

Longo, V. D. and L. Fontana. 2010. Calorie restriction and cancer prevention: metabolic and molecular mechanisms. *Trends Pharmacol. Sci.* 31:89–98.

López-Otín, C., M. A. Blasco, L. Partridge, M. Serrano, and G. Kroemer. 2013. The hallmarks of ageing. *Cell* 153:1194–1217.

Lozano, R., M. Naghavi, K. Foreman, S. Lim, K. Shibuya, V. Aboyans, J. Abraham, T. Adair, R. Aggarwal, S. Y. Ahn, *et al.* 2012. Global and regional mortality from 235 causes of death for 20 age groups in 1990 and 2010: a systematic analysis for the Global Burden of Disease Study 2010. *Lancet* 380:2095–2128.

Lu, F., M. Zahid, C. Wang, M. Saeed, E. L.Cavalieri, and E. G. Rogan. 2008. Resveratrol prevents estrogen–DNA adduct formation and neoplastic transformation in MCF-10F cells. *Cancer Prev. Res.* 1:135–145.

Luch, A. 2005. Nature and nurture – lessons from chemical carcinogenesis. *Nat. Rev. Cancer* 5:113–125.

Ly, A., H. Lee, J. Chen, K. K. Sie, R. Renlund, A. Medline, K. J. Sohn, R. Croxford, L. U. Thompson, and Y. I. Kim. 2011. Effect of maternal and postweaning folic acid supplementation on mammary tumor risk in the offspring. *Cancer Res.* 71:988–997.

Magalhães, J. P., J. Curado, and G. M. Church. 2009. Meta-analysis of age-related gene expression profiles identifies common signatures of ageing. *Bioinformatics* 25:875–881.

Magaña, A. A., K. Wrobel, Y. A. Caudillo, S. Zaina, G. Lund, and K. Wrobel. 2007. High-performance liquid chromatography determination of 5-methyl-2′-deoxycytidine, 2′-deoxycytidine, and other deoxynucleosides and nucleosides in DNA digests. *Anal. Biochem.* 374:378–385.

Martin, C., Y. Zhang, C. Tonelli, and K. Petroni. 2013a. Plants, diet, and health. *Annu. Rev. Plant Biol.* 64:19–46.

Martin, F. L. 2013. Epigenetic influences in the aetiology of cancers arising from breast and prostate: a hypothesised transgenerational evolution in chromatin accessibility. *ISRN Oncol.* 2013:624794.

Martin, G. M., C. E. Ogburn, L. M. Colgin, A. M. Gown, S. D. Edland, and R. J. Monnat, Jr. 1996. Somatic mutations are frequent and increase with age in human kidney epithelial cells. *Hum. Mol. Genet.* 5:215–221.

Martin, S. L., T. M. Hardy, and T. O. Tollefsbol. 2013b. Medicinal chemistry of the epigenetic diet and caloric restriction. *Curr. Med. Chem.* 20:4050–4059.

Martín-Montalvo, A., J. M. Villalba, P. Navas, and R. de Cabo R. 2011. NRF2, cancer and calorie restriction. *Oncogene* 30:505–520.

Mason, J. B. 2011. Unraveling the complex relationship between folate and cancer risk. *Biofactors* 37:253–260.

McKay, J. A. and J. C. Mathers. 2011. Diet induced epigenetic changes and their implications for health. *Acta Physiol.* 202:103–118.

Medeiros, M. H. G. 2009. Exocyclic DNA adducts as biomarkers of lipid oxidation and predictors of disease. Challenges in developing sensitive and specific methods for clinical studies. *Chem. Res. Toxicol.* 22:419–425.

Milner, J. A. 2008. Nutrition and cancer: essential elements for a roadmap. *Cancer Lett.* 269:189–198.

Moriwaki, S.-I., S. Ray, R. E. Tarone, K. H. Kraemer, and L. Grossman. 1996. The effect of donor age on the processing of UV-damaged DNA by cultured human cells: reduced DNA repair capacity and increased DNA mutability. *Mutat. Res.* 364:117–123.

Moriya, M. 1993. Single-stranded shuttle phagemid for mutagenesis studies in mammalian cells: 8-oxoguanine in DNA induces targeted G·C → T·A transversions in simian kidney cells. *Proc. Natl Acad. Sci. USA* 90:1122–1126.

Mostoslavsky, R., M. Esteller, and A. Vaquero. 2010. At the crossroad of lifespan, calorie restriction, chromatin and disease: meeting sirtuins. *Cell Cycle* 9:1907–1912.

Muqbil, I., F. W. J. Beck, B. Bao, F. H. Sarkar, R. M. Mohammad, S. M. Hadi, and A. S. Azmi. 2012. Old wine in a new bottle: the Warburg effect and anticancer mechanisms of resveratrol. *Curr. Pharm. Des.* 18:1645–1654.

Nabel, C. S. and R. M. Kohli. 2011. Molecular biology. Demystifying DNA demethylation. *Science* 333:1229–1230.

Nazki, F. H., A. S. Sameer, and B. A. Ganaie. 2014. Folate: metabolism, genes, polymorphisms and the associated diseases. *Gene* 533:11–20.

O'Callaghan, N. J., P. M. Clifton, M. Noakes, and M. Fenech. 2009. Weight loss in obese men is associated with increased telomere length and decreased abasic sites in rectal mucosa. *Rejuvenation Res.* 12:169–176.

Omodei, D. and L. Fontana. 2011. Calorie restriction and prevention of age-associated chronic disease. *FEBS Lett.* 585:1537–1542.

Ong, T. P. and L. Pérusse. 2011. Impact of nutritional epigenomics on disease risk and prevention: introduction. *J. Nutrigenet. Nutrigenom.* 4:245–247

Ong, T. P., F. S. Moreno, and Ross S. A. 2011. Targeting the epigenome with bioactive food components for cancer prevention. *J. Nutrigenet. Nutrigenom.* 4:275–292.

Ong, T. P., M. T. Cardozo, A. de Conti, and F. S. Moreno. 2012. Chemoprevention of hepatocarcinogenesis with dietary isoprenic derivatives: cellular and molecular aspects. *Curr. Cancer Drug Targets.* 12:1173–1190.

Pallauf K, K. Giller, P. Huebbe, and G.Rimbach. 2013. Nutrition and healthy ageing: calorie restriction or polyphenol-rich "mediterrasian" diet? *Oxid. Med. Cell. Longev.* 2013:707421.

Papoutsis, A. J., J. L. Borg, O. I. Selmin, and D. F. Romagnolo. 2012. BRCA-1 promoter hypermethylation and silencing induced by the aromatic hydrocarbon receptor–ligand TCDD are prevented by resveratrol in MCF-7 cells. *J. Nutr. Biochem.* 23:1324–1332.

Papoutsis, A. J., O. I. Selmin, J. L. Borg, and D. F. Romagnolo. 2013. Gestational exposure to the AhR agonist 2,3,7,8-tetrachlorodibenzo-p-dioxin induces BRCA-1 promoter hypermethylation and reduces BRCA-1 expression in mammary tissue of rat offspring: Preventive effects of resveratrol. *Mol Carcinog.;* epub ahead of print.

Park, L. K., Si. Friso, and S-W Choi. 2012. Symposium 4: vitamins, infectious and chronic disease during adulthood and ageing nutritional influences on epigenetics and age-related disease. *Proc. Nutr. Soc.* 71:75–83.

Parks, S. K., J. Chiche, and J. Pouysségur. 2013. Disrupting proton dynamics and energy metabolism for cancer therapy. *Nat. Rev. Cancer* 13:611–623.

Pearson, K. J., K. N. Lewis, N. L. Price, J. W. Chang, E. Perez, M. V. Cascajo, K. L. Tamashiro, S. Poosala, A. Csiszar, Z. Ungvari, T. W. Kensler, M. Yamamoto, J. M. Egan, D. L. Longo, D. K. Ingram, P. Navas, and R. de Cabo. 2008. Nrf2 mediates cancer protection but not prolongevity induced by caloric restriction. *Proc. Natl Acad. Sci. USA* 105:2325–2330.

Penn, N. W., R. Suwalski, C. O'Riley, K. Bojanowski, and R. Yura. 1972. The presence of 5-hydroxymethylcytosine in animal deoxyribonucleic acid. *Biochem. J.* 126:781–790.

Poirier, L. A. 1994. Methyl group deficiency in hepatocarcinogenesis. *Drug Metab. Rev.* 26:185–199.

Potter, J. D. and K. Steinmetz. 1996. Vegetables, fruit and phytoestrogens as preventive agents. *IARC Sci. Publ.* 139:61–90.

Prasad, S., B. Sung, and B. B. Aggarwal. 2012. Age-associated chronic diseases require age-old medicine: role of chronic inflammation. *Prev. Med.* 54:S29–S37.

Pronier, E. and F. Delhommeau. 2012. Role of TET2 mutations in myeloproliferative neoplasms. *Curr. Hematol. Malig. Rep.* 7:57–64.

Qiu, X., K. Brown, M. D. Hirschey, E. Verdin, and D. Chen. 2010. Calorie restriction reduces oxidative stress by SIRT3-mediated SOD2 activation. *Cell Metab.* 12:662–667.

Reck, M., A. Hermes, E. H. Tan, E. Felip, B. Klughammer, and J. Baselga. 2011. Tissue sampling in lung cancer: a review in light of the MERIT experience. *Lung Cancer* 74:1–6.

Ricceri, F., G. Matullo, and P. Vineis. 2012. Is there evidence of involvement of DNA repair polymorphisms in human cancer? *Mutat. Res.* 736:117–121.

Robertson, K. D. and A. P. Wolffe. 2000. DNA methylation in health and disease. *Nat. Rev. Genet.* 1:11–19.

Rosati, R., H. Ma, and D. C. Cabelof. 2012. Folate and colorectal cancer in rodents: a model of DNA repair deficiency. *J. Oncol.* 2012:105949.

Ross, S. A. 2003. Diet and DNA methylation interactions in cancer prevention. *Ann. NY Acad. Sci.* 983: 197–207.

Salk, J. J., E. J. Fox, and L. A. Loeb. 2010. Mutational heterogeneity in human cancers: origin and consequences. *Annu. Rev. Pathol. Mech. Dis.* 5:51–75.

Scrima, M., C. De Marco, F. Fabiani, R. Franco, G. Pirozzi, G. Rocco, M. Ravo, A. Weisz, P. Zoppoli, M. Ceccarelli, G. Botti, D. Malanga, and G. Viglietto. 2012. Signaling networks associated with AKT activation in non-small cell lung cancer (NSCLC): new insights on the role of phosphatydil-inositol-3 kinase. *PLoS One.* 7:e30427.

Sedivy, J. M., G. Banumathy, and P. D. Adams. 2008. Ageing by epigenetics – a consequence of chromatin damage? *Exp. Cell Res.* 314:1909–1917.

Selak, M. A., S. M. Armour, E. D. MacKenzie, H. Boulahbel, D. G. Watson, K. D. Mansfield, Y. Pan, M. C. Simon, C. B. Thompson, and E. Gottlieb. 2005. Succinate links TCA cycle dysfunction to oncogenesis by inhibiting HIF-alpha prolyl hydroxylase. *Cancer Cell* 7:77–85.

Sengottuvelan, M., P.Viswanathan, and N. Nalini. 2006. Chemopreventive effect of trans-resveratrol-a phytoalexin against colonic aberrant crypt foci and cell proliferation in 1,2-dimethylhydrazine induced colon carcinogenesis. *Carcinogenesis* 27:1038–1046.

Sengottuvelan, M., K. Deeptha, and N. Nalini. 2009. Resveratrol ameliorates DNA damage, prooxidant and antioxidant imbalance in 1,2-dimethylhydrazine induced rat colon carcinogenesis. *Chem. Biol. Interact.* 181:193–201.

Serra-Pérez, A., A. M. Planas, A. Núñez-O'Mara, E. Berra, J. García-Villoria, A. Ribes, and T. Santalucía. 2010. Extended ischemia prevents HIF1degradation at reoxygenation by impairing prolyl-hydroxylation. Role of Krebs cycle metabolites. *J. Biol. Chem.* 285:18217–18224.

Sethi, G., M. K. Shanmugam, L. Ramachandran, A. P. Kumar, and V. Tergaonkar. 2012. Multifaceted link between cancer and inflammation. *Biosci. Rep.* 32:1–15.

Shapira, I., K. Sultan, A. Lee, and E. Taioli. 2013. Evolving concepts: how diet and the intestinal microbiome act as modulators of breast malignancy. *SRN Oncol.* 2013:693920.

Sharma, S., T. K. Kelly, and P. A. Jones. 2010. Epigenetics in cancer. *Carcinogenesis* 31:27–36.

Sharp, Z. D., T. J. Curiel, and C. B. Livi. 2013. Chronic mechanistic target of rapamycin inhibition: preventing cancer to delay ageing, or vice versa? *Interdiscip. Top Gerontol.* 38:1–16.

Shen, H. and P. W. Laird. 2013. Interplay between the cancer genome and epigenome. *Cell* 153:38–55.

Shih, J. and G. Donmez. 2013. Mitochondrial sirtuins as therapeutic targets for age-related disorders. *Genes Cancer* 4:91–96.

Sie, K. K., J. Li, A. Ly, K. J. Sohn, R. Croxford, and Y. I. Kim. 2013. Effect of maternal and postweaning folic acid supplementation on global and gene-specific DNA methylation in the liver of the rat offspring. *Mol. Nutr. Food Res.* 57:677–685.

Simon, K. W., H. Ma, A. A. Dombkowski, and D. C. Cabelof. 2012. Ageing alters folate homeostasis and DNA damage response in colon. *Mech. Ageing Dev.* 133:75–82.

Stefanska, B., H. Karlic, F. Varga, K. Fabianowska-Majewska, and A. Haslberger. 2012. Epigenetic mechanisms in anti-cancer actions of bioactive food components – the implications in cancer prevention. *Br. J. Pharmacol.* 167:279–297.

Subramanian, L., S. Youssef, S. Bhattacharya, J. Kenealey, A. S. Polans, and P. R. van Ginkel. 2010. Resveratrol: challenges in translation to the clinic – a critical discussion. *Clin. Cancer Res.* 16:5942–5948.

Surh, Y. J. 2003. Cancer chemoprevention with dietary phytochemicals. *Nat. Rev. Cancer* 3:768–780.

Suzuki, M. and I. Yoshino. 2010. Aberrant methylation in non-small cell lung cancer. *Surg. Today* 40:602–607.

Tahiliani, M., K. P. Koh, Y. Shen, W. A. Pastor, H. Bandukwala, Y. Brudno, S. Agarwal, L. M. Iyer, D. R. Liu, L. Aravind, and A. Rao. 2009. Conversion of 5-methylcytosine to 5-hydroxymethylcytosine in mammalian DNA by MLL partner TET1. *Science* 324:930–935.

Tan, A. C., I. Konczak, D. M. Sze, and I. Ramzan. Molecular pathways for cancer chemoprevention by dietary phytochemicals. *Nutr Cancer* 2011;63(4):495–505.

Tapp, H. S., D. M. Commane, D. M. Bradburn, R. Arasaradnam, J. C. Mathers, I. T. Johnson, and N. J. Belshaw. 2013. Nutritional factors and gender influence age-related DNA methylation in the human rectal mucosa. *Ageing Cell* 12:148–155.

Tomita, M. 2012. Caloric restriction reduced 1, 2-dimethylhydrazine-induced aberrant crypt foci and induces the expression of Sirtuins in colonic mucosa of F344 rats. *J. Carcinog.* 11:10.

Tsou, J. A., J. A. Hagen, C. L. Carpenter, and I. A. Laird-Offringa. 2002. DNA methylation analysis: a powerful new tool for lung cancer diagnosis. *Oncogene* 21:5450–5461.

Umar, A., B. K. Dunn, and P. Greenwald. 2012. Future directions in cancer prevention. *Nat. Rev. Cancer.* 12:835–848.

Valdes, A. M., D. Glass, and T. D. Spector. 2013. Omics technologies and the study of human ageing. *Nat. Rev. Genet.* 14:601–607.

Valinluck, V. and L. C. Sowers. 2007. Endogenous cytosine damage products alter the site selectivity of human DNA maintenance methyltransferase DNMT1. *Cancer Res.* 67:946–950.

Vanden Berghe, W. 2012. Epigenetic impact of dietary polyphenols in cancer chemoprevention: Lifelong remodeling of our epigenomes. *Pharmacol. Res.* 65:565–576.

van Engeland, M. and J. G. Herman. 2010. Viewing the epigenetics of colorectal cancer through the window of folic acid effects. *Cancer Prev. Res.* 3:1509–1512.

van Heemst, D., P. M. den Reijer, and R. G. J. Westendorp. 2007. Ageing or cancer: a review on the role of caretakers and gatekeepers. *Eur. J. Cancer* 43:2144–2152.

Vaquero, A. and D. Reinberg. 2009. Calorie restriction and the exercise of chromatin. 2009. *Genes Dev.* 23:1849–1869.

Wallace, K., M. V. Grau, A. J. Levine, L. Shen, R. Hamdan, X. Chen, J. Gui, R. W. Haile, E. L. Barry, D. Ahnen, G. McKeown-Eyssen, J. A. Baron, and J. P. Issa. 2010. Association between folate levels and CpG Island hypermethylation in normal colorectal mucosa. *Cancer Prev. Res.* 3:1552–1564.

Walsh, M. E., Y. Shi, and H. Van Remmen. 2014. The effects of dietary restriction on oxidative stress in rodents. *Free. Radic. Biol. Med.* 66:88–99.

Wang, R. H., Y. Zheng, H. S. Kim, X. Xu, L. Cao, T. Luhasen, M. H. Lee, C. Xiao, A. Vassilopoulos, W. Chen, K. Gardner, Y. G Man, M. C. Hung, T. Finkel, and C. X. Deng. 2008. Interplay among BRCA1, SIRT1, and Survivin during BRCA1-associated tumorigenesis. *Mol. Cell* 32:11–20.

Weed, D. L. 2013. The quality of nutrition and cancer reviews: a systematic assessment. *Crit. Rev. Food Sci. Nutr.* 53:276–286.

Whitlock, N. C. and S. J. Baek. 2012. The anticancer effects of resveratrol: modulation of transcription factors. *Nutr. Cancer* 64:493–502.

Williams, E. A. 2012. Folate, colorectal cancer and the involvement of DNA methylation. *Proc. Nutr. Soc.* 71:592–597.

Williams, K., J. Christensen, and K. Helin. 2011. DNA methylation: TET proteins – guardians of CpG islands? *EMBO Rep.* 13:28–35.

Wolff, G. L., R. L. Kodell, S. R. Moore, and C. A. Cooney. 1998. Maternal epigenetics and methyl supplements affect agouti gene expression in Avy/a mice. *FASEB J.* 12:949–957.

Wolin, K. Y., K. Carson, and G. A. Colditz. 2010. Obesity and cancer. *Oncologist* 15:556–565.

World Cancer Research Fund/American Institute for Cancer Research. 2007. *Food, Nutrition, Physical Activity, and the Prevention of Cancer: a Global Perspective*. Washington, DC: American Institute for Cancer Research.

Xiao, M., H. Yang, W. Xu, S. Ma, H. Lin, H. Zhu, L. Liu, Y. Liu, C. Yang, Y. Xu, S. Zhao, D. Ye, Y. Xiong, and K. L. Guan. 2012. Inhibition of α-KG-dependent histone and DNA demethylases by fumarate and succinate that are accumulated in mutations of FH and SDH tumor suppressors. *Genes Dev.* 26:1326–1338.

Yuan, T., J. Wei, J. Luo, M. Liu, S. Deng and P. Chen. 2012. Polymorphisms of base-excision repair genes hOGG1 326cys and XRCC1 280His increase hepatocellular carcinoma risk. *Dig. Dis. Sci.* 57:2451–2457.

Zhang, D., Y. Liu, and D. Chen. 2011a. SIRT-ain relief from age-inducing stress. *Ageing* 3:158–161.

Zhang, J. J., L. Zhang, K. Zhou, X. Ye, C. Liu, L. Zhang, J. Kang, and C. Cai. 2011b. Analysis of global DNA methylation by hydrophilic interaction ultra-high-pressure liquid chromatography tandem mass spectrometry. *Anal. Biochem.* 413:164–170.

Zhu, W., W. Qin, K. Zhang, G. E. Rottinghaus, Y. C. Chen, B. Kliethermes, and E. R. Sauter. 2012. *Trans*-resveratrol alters mammary promoter hypermethylation in women at increased risk for breast cancer. *Nutr. Cancer* 64:393–400.

Zhu, Z., W. Jiang, J. N. McGinley, and H. J. Thompson. 2013. Defining the role of histone deacetylases in the inhibition of mammary carcinogenesis by dietary energy restriction (DER): effects of suberoylanilide hydroxamic acid (SAHA) and DER in a rat model. *Cancer Prev. Res.* 6:290–298.

CHAPTER 5
Nutraceuticals in immunosenescence

Thea Magrone and Emilio Jirillo
Department of Basic Medical Sciences Neuroscience and Sensory Organs, University of Bari, Bari, Italy

5.1 Introduction

Over the past few decades, longevity has significantly increased in Western and Westernized countries and, as a consequence, the health system is currently facing the growing emergence of age-associated diseases (Candore *et al.*, 2010; Magrone & Jirillo, 2013a). For example, genetic mutations accelerate the ageing process, such as in the case of patients carrying mutations in telomerase reverse transcriptase, telomerase RNA component or other telomerase-maintaining genes (Bernardes de Jesus & Blasco, 2013). All of these mutations are responsible for certain pathologies, such as congenital dyskeratosis, and the severity of pathology correlates with the number of short telomeres present in a given individual (Calado & Young, 2009). Food itself is a cause of age-associated disease since the production of reactive oxygen species (ROS), advanced glycation endproducts, advanced lipoxidation endproducts and inflammatory mediators leads to multiple tissue damage (Magrone *et al.*, 2013). On this basis, in free-living elderly subjects, ageing is characterized by low-grade inflammation, the so-called "inflammaging", which may evolve toward a chronic inflammatory status when the accumulation of metabolic products becomes excessive, thus aggravating tissue damage (Franceschi *et al.*, 2007). This is the case for amyloid plaques in Alzheimer disease (AD) where microglia maintains the inflammatory status (Meda *et al.*, 1995).

Immunosenescence indicates the decline with age of the immune response in humans and abnormal immunity contributes to the complications of age-associated disease. Immune abnormalities in the elderly have been detected in both the innate and the adaptive immune system. In particular, dysfunction of granulocytes, monocytes/macrophages ($M\theta$) and natural killer (NK) cells has been reported. On the other hand, alterations of both T and B lymphocytes have been described in senescence. Further details on immune cells will be provided in this chapter.

Easier access of pathogens into the aged host plays a pathogenic role in the aggravation of inflammatory and dysmetabolic conditions (obesity and diabetes), atherosclerosis and neurodegeneration (Li, 2013). In addition, in the elderly, imbalanced immune networks can account for the increased frequency of autoimmune disease and cancer, thus justifying therapeutic attempts to correct impaired immunity in the elderly (Candore *et al.*, 2010).

In this chapter, first an overview of the major alterations of the immune system in the elderly will be provided. Next, treatment of age-associated disease by nutraceuticals will be

Anti-Ageing Nutrients: Evidence-Based Prevention of Age-Associated Diseases, First Edition. Edited by Delminda Neves.

discussed. By definition, nutraceuticals currently employed in clinical trials are presented not as foods but in a medicine-like format, such as capsules or tablets. In contrast, functional foods are those such as fermented milk and orange juice that, in addition to providing the body with essential nutrients, including proteins, carbohydrates, fats and vitamins, also improve the general well-being or health status (Kalra, 2003).

Thus, novel therapeutic attempts to correct the aged immune responsiveness with nutraceuticals will be described. In particular, the mechanism(s) of action of specific bioactives in preventing or attenuating age-associated disease will be elucidated.

5.2 The immune response in ageing

5.2.1 Phagocytes

A very broad set of receptors is involved in the phagocytic process, such as Toll-like receptors, complement receptors, fragment crystallizable receptors and scavenger receptors in response to pathogens and autologous apoptotic cells (Napoli & Neumann, 2010). In aged people, both polymorphonuclear cells (PMN) and Mθ display impaired phagocytosis and oxidative burst (Tortorella *et al.*, 1999). Furthermore, in the case of Mθ, defective chemotaxis, antigen presentation and molecular histocompatibility class II molecule expression, respectively, have been reported (Solana *et al.*, 2012). With regard to phagocytosis of apoptotic cells, aged mice exhibited diminished phagocytic clearance of apoptotic cells and, in addition, serum from aged mice, when *in vitro* added to Mθ, abrogated their ability to phagocyte apoptotic cells (Aprahamian *et al.*, 2008). In elderly humans, dendritic cells also exhibited a reduced capacity to phagocyte apoptotic cells *in vitro* (Agrawal *et al.*, 2007). The above-mentioned abnormalities may explain the increased frequency of infectious events (e.g. winter infections) in ageing. On the other hand, reduced phagocytic clearance of apoptotic cells may lead to accumulation of debris which, in turn, triggers inflammation or autoimmune reactions into the aged host (Aprahamian *et al.*, 2008). Also an impaired signaling of immunosuppressive receptors such as phosphatidylserine and proto-oncogene tyrosine-protein kinase (MerTK) may render Mθ more pro-inflammatory in response to released intracellular contents (Freeman *et al.*, 2010).

5.2.2 Natural killer cells

With special reference to NK cells, evidence has been provided that these cells undergo age-related changes, which may explain the increased incidence of viral infections in the elderly (Hazeldine & Lord, 2013). In particular, aged NK cells display reduced perforin-mediated cytotoxicity and release of cytokines and chemokines. In addition, NK cells play an immunoregulatory role and, consequently, the impaired crosstalk between NK cells and dendritic cells may lead to a defective antigen presentation and T cell polarization in the elderly (Vitale *et al.*, 2005). This event may explain a diminished response to vaccines in older people. In this framework, the NK-mediated enhancement of Mθ functions has been shown to be depressed in the elderly, thus explaining the increased incidence and/or severity of bacterial and fungal infections (Vitale *et al.*, 2005). Furthermore, reactivation of latent tuberculosis in aged persons may be due to the defective Mθ functions regulated by NK cells (Hoursburg *et al.*, 2010).

5.2.3 T cells

Aged individuals are characterized by both qualitative and quantitative changes in T cells, including the loss of surface markers with an increase in stimulatory receptors, cytotoxicity and resistance to apoptosis (Lynch *et al.*, 2009). In particular, the T helper (Th)1/Th2 balance is rather pro-inflammatory in ageing, thus explaining the increased frequency of age-associated diseases. Interestingly, aged T cells lose the CD28 surface marker, and $CD28^-$ T cell activation does not depend on antigen-presenting cells but rather on pathogen product and stress-derived molecules stimulation (Vallejo, 2005). These terminally differentiated T cells are also abundant in younger patients affected by autoimmune disease. Also, in the case of T regulatory (Treg) cells, some alterations have been reported in ageing (Fessler *et al.*, 2013). For instance, in aged mice, $CD25^{low}$ Treg cells have been identified in the spleen (Lages *et al.*, 2008) as well as in patients with systemic lupus erythematosus, whose immune system prematurely ages (Bonelli *et al.*, 2009). In aged healthy individuals, $CD8^+CD25^+$ Treg cells have been characterized with a function overlapping that of $CD4^+$ Treg cells (Simone *et al.*, 2008). All of these modifications may account for an increased incidence of autoimmune diseases, cancer and infections in the elderly, even if their mechanism(s) of action needs more detailed investigations. In fact, the tuning of Treg cell-mediated immune suppression in ageing is very delicate and its imbalance may shift from a protective effect (anti-inflammatory activity) to a detrimental condition of disease outcome (immune inhibition).

Th17 cells polarize the immune response toward an inflammatory profile and play a major role in the development of autoimmune and chronic inflammatory disease, thus overcoming the anti-inflammatory effects exerted by Treg cells. Th17 cells are increased in ageing with a reduction of Treg cells (Schimtt *et al.*, 2013). However, after activation the Th17/Treg cell ratio tends to decrease with an increase in forkhead box (Fox)P3 and interleukin (IL)-10. Therefore, this ratio may represent an important target for controlling autoimmune and inflammatory disease in the elderly.

5.2.4 B cells

The decline in murine B cell lymphopoiesis with advancing age seems to depend on the inability of hemopoietic stem cells to generate B cells, thus causing a lack of early B cell-lineage precursors (Kogut *et al.*, 2012). In addition, IL-7 production by stromal cells of the bone marrow is reduced with increasing age, thus retarding B cell development in the early phase with a significant reduction of pre-B cell numbers. In aged mice, the reduced influx of B cells to the periphery is compensated by the increase in mature B cell lifespan and the emergence of B1 cell lineage (Dorshkind & Montecino-Rodriguez, 2007; Alter-Wolf *et al.*, 2009). In humans aged $CD19^+$ B cell number decreases (Ademokun *et al.*, 2010), while the ageing-associated B cell (ABC) subset can be detected in peripheral blood (Rubtsov *et al.*, 2011). In *in vitro* studies, ABCs have been shown to respond to innate stimuli with polarization toward Th17 cells and secretion of autoantibodies. Finally, age-associated modifications in somatic hypermutation and class switch recombination in both mice and humans may account for poor antibody response toward new antigens, the reduction of antibody repertoire and the extent of clonal expansion (Frasca & Blomberg, 2009). The main alterations of immune responses for each cell type in senescence are summarized in Table 5.1.

Table 5.1 Alterations of immune responses in senescence.

Cell type	Upregulation	Downregulation
	Innate immune response	
Neutrophils/macrophages	Increased release in pro-inflammatory cytokines	Oxidative burst, phagocytic capacity, bactericidal activity
Natural killer cells	Cell number	Response to IL-12
Dendritic cells		Antigen presentation to T cells, homing to secondary lymphoid organs
	Adaptive immune response	
T lymphocytes	Number of effector and memory cells, release of pro-inflammatory cytokines	Number of virgin T cells, diversity of T cell repertoire, expression of co-stimulatory molecules, proliferative capacity
B lymphocytes	Serum autoantibodies	Number of precursors and virgin B cells, diversity of B cell repertoire, isotype switch antibody affinity, expression of co-stimulatory molecules

5.3 Micronutrients that modulate immunosenescence

The daily intake of micronutrients is often insufficient in the elderly, owing many causes, such as poor socio-economic conditions, loss of appetite, lack of teeth, altered intestinal absorption of food and low requirement of energy (Kant, 2000). The major micronutrients with immunomodulating properties will be discussed later.

5.3.1 Zinc

Zinc (Zn) is a trace element that is fundamental for the growth and development of all organs, including the immune system. In humans, Zn deficiency leads to the impairment of various immune activities, causing thymus involution with reduction of Th1 functions (diminished release of IL-2) and, consequently, reduction of NK cell and Mθ activity as well as neutrophil performance (Mocchegiani *et al.*, 2012). Also antibody production is affected by Zn deficiency. Acrodermatitis enterophathica is a rare disease caused by Zn-specific malabsorption and characterized by thymic atrophy and lymphopenia as well as increased frequency of infections (Haase & Rink, 2009). Zn-mediated immune abnormalities and clinic manifestations in the course of acrodermatitis enterophathica are not dissimilar to those observed in elderly subjects. In particular, Th1 function downregulation in aged individuals with a predominant polarization of the immune response toward the Th2 subset leads to so-called “inflammaging”, as previously mentioned (Franceschi *et al.*, 2007; Franceschi, 2007). In this framework, alteration of Zn transporters Zip1, Zip2 and Zip3 as a result of chronic inflammation or DNA methylation-dependent repression of gene expression leads to reduced cellular Zn uptake in ageing (Giacconi *et al.*, 2012), which seriously compromises mechanisms that depend on Zn to function, as well as the synthesis of molecules that integrate Zn atoms in its structure, including transcription factors with Zn finger motifs. Among Zn finger motifs, the Kruppel Zn-finger (Klf) family is involved in the regulation of interferon (IFN)-γ and tumor necrosis factor (TNF)-α production (Das *et al.*, 2006). In particular, Klf2 controls the migration of mature T lymphocytes from thymus to periphery, also preserving them by apoptosis (Pearson *et al.*,

2008). In addition, the Zn-dependent thymic hormone thymulin also contributes to the migration of T lymphocytes from the thymus to the periphery (Mocchegiani *et al.*, 1998). On the other hand, the Klf5 influences the activity of the enzyme poly(ADP-ribose) polymerase-1, which, in turn, acts on DNA repair during oxidative stress and inflammation in the elderly (Mocchegiani *et al.*, 2000).

Supplementation of Zn to elderly people has been intensively investigated but results have been conflicting. Some groups have reported increased delayed-type hypersensitivity (DHT) responses, immunoglobulin (Ig)G production and number of circulating T cells as well as higher mRNA expression of interleukin 2 receptor (IL-2R) following Zn intake (Prasad *et al.*, 2006). Others, comparing immune responses between Zn-treated healthy elderly and their placebo-treated elderly counterparts, over a follow-up period of 12 months, showed fluctuations of cellular functions at different time points, while DHT was even greater in the placebo group (Bogden *et al.*, 1990). The same was also true in the case of lymphocyte subsets in terms of variation of $CD4^{+}$ and cytotoxic T lymphocytes following Zn supplementation (Kahmann *et al.*, 2006). Elderly subjects receiving Zn exhibited increased levels of thymulin in serum (Mocchegiani *et al.*, 2003). However, NK cell activity (Mocchegiani *et al.*, 2003), as a biomarker of thymulin activation, was increased in some studies, while in other studies NK cell function was elevated after 3 months and decreased between 6 and 12 months (Bogden *et al.*, 1988).

The differences observed may depend on the genetic background of the people examined. Elderly subjects carrying the GG genotype in the IL-6-174 G/C locus displayed some differences between concentration of Zn and immune responsiveness when compared with older individuals carrying GC and CC genotypes (Mocchegiani *et al.*, 2008). In the former group, low plasma Zn correlated with impaired NK cell activity. In this direction, in a subgroup analysis, those elderly subjects with Zn deficiency and carrying MT1a+647GC and IL-6-174GC/CC alleles received a greater advantage from Zn supplementation than individuals bearing other genotypes (Mariani *et al.*, 2008). In the individuals carrying MT1a+647GC and IL-6-174GC/CC alleles, higher levels of plasma Zn and NK activity with reduced levels of IL-6 and monocyte chemotactic protein (MCP)-1 were good indicators of the beneficial effects of Zn supplementation.

Protective effects of Zn administration against respiratory infections have been observed in institutionalized elderly people. For instance, increased antibody titers after vaccination, increased serum levels of Zn, fewer common colds and infections (e.g. pneumonia) and lower use of antibiotics were recorded in clinical trials (Girodon *et al.*, 1999).

In conclusion, Zn deficiency gives rise to immune alterations similar to those observed in the elderly. In this age group, immune response to Zn supplementation may vary in relation to genetic background and this fact should be taken into serious account in the evaluation of Zn efficacy in diminishing the frequency of infections in the elderly.

5.3.2 Copper

Copper (Cu) actively participates in a series of reactions promoting growth and development and its major source in food is meat (Hartmann *et al.*, 1993). The principal storage of Cu is in the liver, where it is contained in a membrane-bound form as metallothioneins. Ceruloplasmin, a blood protein synthesized by the liver, contains many molecules of Cu, thus representing a biomarker of Cu status in the body (Harvey *et al.*, 2009). Decreased Cu in the elderly seems to be related to a reduced intake of food and beverages, particularly milk, which promotes copper absorption at the intestinal level along with glucose (Wapnir, 1998). Cu supplied by dietary sources is not only distributed in the body but also facilitates iron (Fe) metabolism (conversion of Fe^{2+} to Fe^{3+} and facilitation of Fe efflux) (Osaki & Johnson, 1969).

Dietary Cu deficiency leads to a variety of immune abnormalities in animals and humans. For instance, neutropenia, impairment of $M\theta$ and NK cell functions and reduction of IL-2 production have been observed in Cu deficiency (Koller *et al.*, 1987). Interestingly, a full recovery of immune functions was attained following Cu supplementation in Cu-deficient individuals (Bala & Failla, 1992; Bonham *et al.*, 2002).

The role played by Cu in ageing has been little investigated. Since pro-inflammatory cytokines control synthesis and secretion of Cu-containing molecules by the liver, increased plasma Cu levels have been found in some age-associated diseases such as atherosclerosis and AD (Brewer, 2009). In atherosclerosis, Cu seems to be implicated in the generation of oxidized low-density lipoproteins (Stadler *et al.*, 2004), while evidence on the role of Cu in AD is still contradictory. On the other hand, in the case of severe Cu deficiency, impaired immune response as well as anti-oxidant activity and altered metabolism have been detected in elderly subjects, and supplementation of Cu seems to be essential for recovery of cellular functions, as reviewed by Mocchegiani *et al.* (2012).

5.3.3 Iron

Iron (Fe) is another essential element for the proliferation and differentiation of cells. In addition to oxygen transport, Fe is mostly involved in the catalyzation of hydroxyl radical formation, these radicals being implicated in the activity of transcription factors such as hypoxia inducible factor-1 or nuclear factor kappa-light-chain-enhancer of activated B cells (NF-κB) (Wang & Pantopoulos, 2011; Rosen *et al.*, 1995).

Fe deficiency causes a number of immune dysfunctions in the elderly and this condition is frequently associated with anemia (Guyatt *et al.*, 1990). Thymic atrophy, depletion of T cells and NK cells with a predominant polarization toward Th2 cells have been observed in Fe-deficient subjects (Ekiz *et al.*, 2005; Santos & Falcão, 1990). Therefore, Fe supplementation in anemic elderly patients seems to be essential for the maintenance of immune homeostasis and prevention of degenerative disease outcome. This was the case of centenarians characterized by normal levels of ferritin, reduced Fe stores and a low-grade inflammation. Clinical trials (Italian Multicentric Study on Centenarians, 1998) in healthy elderly subjects have demonstrated that Fe supplementation is beneficial in Fe-deficiency anemia to avoid Fe stores. Fe stores, in turn, have been shown to lead to chronic inflammation in age-associated disease, thus sustaining oxidative damage (Welch *et al.*, 2002).

5.3.4 Selenium

Selenium (Se) exhibits anti-oxidant activities in virtue of its incorporation into selenoproteins, which, in turn, control ROS and redox status and, ultimately, inflammation and immune responses (Huang *et al.*, 2012). In view of the increase in oxidative damage in senescence, Se has been used as supplement in the elderly. In aged persons, supplementation of Se alone or in association with β-carotene, led to an increase of $CD4^+$ T cells that persisted for 2 months following discontinuation of the administration regimen (Wood *et al.*, 2000). In other studies in aged humans, Se concentration positively correlated with an increase in the number of NK cells. Furthermore, a correlation was made between low levels of Se and severity of IL-6-mediated inflammation (Ershler & Keller, 2000).

Table 5.2 Impact of micronutrients on the immune ageing.

- Zinc, copper, iron and selenium deficits lead to impaired immune functions, thus aggravating the process of immunosenescence
- Micronutrient supplementation to aged people tends to reinforce the otherwise impaired immune response as well as the anti-oxidant status, even if results of clinical trials are sometimes conflicting
- Micronutrients may act upon genes that encode proteins involved in the maintenance of the inflammatory/anti-inflammatory ratio (nutrigenomic approach)
- The genetic inter-individual variability may affect the absorption and uptake of micronutrients. Low absorption of micronutrients results in imbalance of inflammatory/anti-inflammatory ratio (nutrigenetic approach)

Interestingly, in aged persons, several nutritional markers were evaluated for their correlation with proliferation of peripheral blood lymphocytes. Se was one of four nutrients that positively correlated with lymphocyte proliferation (Wardwell *et al.*, 2008). The interactions between micronutrients and immune ageing are summarized in Table 5.2.

5.4 Probiotics and prebiotics

Microbial communities, the so-called microbiota, are harbored in the human colon, thus providing the host with nutrients and energy via fermentation of nondigestible dietary components. A delicate balance among the components of the microbiota has been shown to regulate either metabolism or immune function (Magrone & Jirillo, 2013b). An imbalanced microbiota results in elevated inflammation and infection, which represent important cofactors in the ageing process and correlate to frailty (Magrone & Jirillo, 2013a). As previously discussed, so-called "inflammaging" (Franceschi *et al.*, 2007; Jirillo *et al.*, 2008) is characterized by a decline in viable counts of *Bacteroides* (Bartosch *et al.*, 2005) and in species diversity within the genus *Bacteroides* (Enck *et al.*, 2009). A reduction in *Bifidobacteria* species diversity in elderly people has also been also observed, which may depend on their weak adhesion to the intestinal mucosa as a consequence of chemical or structural modifications of bacteria or of changes in intestinal mucus (He *et al.*, 2001). On the other hand, an increase in *Fusobacteria* in elderly is common, which results in the generation of noxious products, such as ammonia and indoles (Potrykus *et al.*, 2008). The same holds true for an increase in *Clostridia* in elderly populations (Smith & Ratard, 2011).

Probiotics and prebiotics are currently used in elderly people for correcting their altered microbiota. Therefore, the characteristics and mechanisms of action of these dietary products will be outlined.

5.4.1 Probiotics

Probiotics are defined as "live bacteria which, when administered in adequate amounts confer a health benefit to the host" (Hume, 2011). As a general statement, probiotics mostly act through the regulation of pro- and anti-inflammatory cytokines (Meijerink & Wells, 2010), also increasing humoral immune responses (Yan & Polk, 2011; Hatakka & Saxelin, 2008). In this direction (Hoang *et al.*, 2010), phagocytic capacities and T lymphocyte and NK cell functions were increased in elderly subjects by the administration of *Bifidobacterium lactis* HN019 (Gill *et al.*, 2001). The same results were obtained after administration of *Lactobacillus rhamnosus* HN001 in the same subjects. Moreover, in a double-blind feeding trial in older individuals, supplementation of a symbiotic (a mix of of pre- and probiotics) containing *B. lactis* BL-01, *Bifidobacterium bifidum* BB-02 and inulin (a prebiotic) (Smith & Ratard, 2011) gave rise to a significant increase in *B. bifidum*, total *Bifidobacteria* and total *Lactobacilli* in comparison to the placebo group. Clinically, a reduction in winter infections was recorded in these subjects. We have recently reported that administration of a symbiotic (fermented cow milk containing *L. rhamnosus* GG and oligofructose as a prebiotic) to free-living elderly people for 1 month led to increased serum levels of IL-1, IL-6 and IL-8, while levels of IL-12, IL-10 and TNF-α remained unmodified. In particular, IL-12 and IL-10 serum concentrations were undetectable in these elderly subjects as an index of an imbalanced inflammatory/anti-inflammatory ratio. Our data also suggest that the observed increase in IL-8 release may facilitate the influx of neutrophils to lungs, thus offering protection against winter infections (Amati *et al.*, 2010).

In another trial (Mañè *et al.*, 2011), 50 elderly subjects were treated for 12 weeks with 5×10^8 cfu/day of *Lactobacillus plantarum* CECT7315/7316 ("low probiotic dose") or 5×10^9 cfu/day of the probiotic mixture ("high probiotic dose"). The high probiotic dose increased the percentages of $CD8^+CD25^+$ and NK cells, while the low probiotic dose increased $CD4^+CD25^+$ cells, B lymphocytes ($CD19^+$) and antigen-presenting cells by human leukocyte antigens ($HLA\text{-}DR^+$). Transforming growth factor-β1 plasma concentration significantly decreased with both doses. A lower incidence of infections and a lower trend for mortality was recorded in the high-probiotic-dose group.

Influenza vaccination in the elderly is currently performed in many countries, but since immune responses may be impaired with ageing, vaccination is often not effective. In a pilot and confirmatory study (Boge *et al.*, 2009), 86 and 222 elderly volunteers, respectively, were administered with a fermented dairy drink, containing the probiotic strain *Lactobacillus casei* DN-114 001 and yoghurt ferments (Actimel®), in comparison to a placebo group for a period of 7 weeks (pilot) or 13 weeks (confirmatory) and then vaccinated 4 weeks later. In both pilot study and confirmatory study, antibody titers against HIN1, H3N2 and B viral strains were determined after different intervals of time. Antibody titers against the B strain significantly increased in comparison to the placebo group, providing a health benefit in this population. The observed adjuvant effect of probiotics might be explained (Maassen & Claassen, 2008) by the stimulation of gut-associated lymphoid tissues cells with the release of IL-6, which boosts antigen-specific B cell responses, systemically, following influenza vaccination (Coombes & Powrie, 2008; Artis, 2008).

5.4.2 Prebiotics

The term "prebiotic" means "a non-digestible food ingredient that selectively stimulates growth and/or activity of one or a limited number of bacteria in the colon, thereby improving host health" (Roberfroid *et al.*, 2010). Prebiotics are naturally present in breast milk and in vegetables but can also be synthesized, as in the case of fructooligosaccharides (FOS) and galactooligosaccharides (GOS) (Rastall & Maitin, 2002). Few studies have been conducted with isolated prebiotics in the elderly population. In aged people supplementation of 8 g FOS daily for 3 weeks increased bifidobacterial levels and total lymphocyte count ($CD4^+$ and $CD8^+$ cells) (Guigoz *et al.*, 2002). Furthermore, an augmented phagocytosis exerted by PMN and Mθ was also reported. In one trial, the effects of GOS on the elderly were investigated. GOS administration increased levels of bifidobacteria in the gut, phagocytosis, NK cell activity and IL-10, while reducing the pro-inflammatory contingent of cytokines (e.g. IL-6, IL-1β and TNF-α); (Vulevic *et al.*, 2008).

Table 5.3 Probiotics and prebiotics effects on immune responsiveness in older people.

Administration of probiotics
• Increase in phagocyte, natural killer cell and T lymphocyte activities
• Increase in antibody titers against influenza viruses in vaccinated subjects
Administration of prebiotics
• Increase in Bifidobacterial levels
• Increase in phagocyte, natural killer cell and T lymphocyte count
• Decrease in pro-inflammatory cytokines
Administration of symbiotics (prebiotics + probiotics)
• Increase in *B. bifidum*, total *Bifidobacteria* and total *Lactobacilli*
• Increase in IL-8 serum levels
• Reduction of winter infections

The various effects exerted by prebiotics and probiotics on the aged immune system are summarized in Table 5.3.

5.5 Dietary lipids

Dietary lipids are nutrients that not only provide energy to the body but also regulate various cellular functions. Dietary fatty acids are classified as essential (omega-3 and omega-6 families), saturated, monounsaturated and polyunsaturated (PUFA). High caloric intake and dietary fat in Western diet correlate with aged-related disease development (Kau *et al.*, 2011). In a recent report Myles *et al.* (2013) found that parental fat intake leads to alteration of offspring microbiome and immunity, with increased levels of circulating lipopolysaccharides (LPS) in comparison to pups receiving a low-fat diet. Intake of long-chain omega-3 PUFA [eicosapentanoic acid (EPA) and docosahexaenoic acid (DHA)] or fish oil seems to exert beneficial anti-inflammatory effects on the outcome of cardiovascular, degenerative, neurological, inflammatory and autoimmune diseases as well as age-related macular degeneration. However, omega-3 PUFA suppresses both innate and adaptive immune responses and, therefore, its supplementation in the elderly population should carefully be assessed. In fact, omega-3 PUFA-mediated impairment of the immune response in the elderly may further increase the risk of infections and neoplastic diseases. There is evidence that omega-3 PUFA exert their anti-inflammatory activity by inhibiting the production of eicosanoids (prostaglandin E2, 4-series leukotrienes), cytokines (IL-1β, TNF-α, IL-6), chemokines (IL-8, MCP-1), adhesion molecules (intercellular adhesion molecule-1, vascular cell adhesion molecule-1, selectins), platelet activating factor and ROS as well as reactive nitrogen species (Galli & Calder, 2009; Fernandes, 2008; Fritsche, 2007; Sijben & Calder, 2007; Shaikh & Edidin, 2006; Kim *et al.*, 2010; Calder, 2010). They also display a pro-resolution effect on inflammation, acting as precursors of resolvins, protectins and marensins (Serhan *et al.*, 2008; Kohli & Levy, 2009). In general, T cell-mediated immunity is the major target of omega-3 PUFA. In this framework, consumption of fish oil or omega-3 PUFA was able to inhibit *ex vivo* CD4$^+$ T cell proliferation, IL-2 production and IL-2R expression, or specific antigen-driven CD4$^+$ T cell expansion both *ex vivo* and *in vivo* (Pompos & Fritsche, 2002; Zhang *et al.*, 2006); the

Table 5.4 Dietary omega-3 PUFA effects on the immune responsiveness in ageing.

- Reduction of both innate and adaptive immune responses
- Anti-inflammatory activity
- Decrease in neutrophil respiratory burst
- Decrease in T cell proliferation
- Decrease in IL-2 production
- Decrease in pro-inflammatory cytokine generation
- Data on reduction of infectious events are conflicting

same effects were seen for DHT (Meydani *et al.*, 1993). In particular, omega-3 PUFA can inhibit the mechanism of T cell receptor activation, including phosphorylation of signaling molecules and their translocation into the immunological synapse (Shaikh & Edidin, 2006; Kim *et al.*, 2010; Chapkin *et al.*, 2009). Meydani *et al.* (1991) reported that omega-3 PUFA supplementation (1.68 g EPA and 0.72 g DHA/day) in the elderly for 3 months significantly inhibited T cell mitogen-induced peripheral blood mononuclear cell (PBMC) proliferation, IL-2 production and inflammatory cytokine (IL-1β, IL-6, TNF-α) release. Bechoua *et al.* (2003) showed that, in elderly subjects (70–83 years old) consuming omega-3 PUFA (30 mg EPA and 150 mg DHA/day) for 6 weeks, a decreased lymphocyte proliferation was detected. Rees *et al.* (2006) found that EPA treatment in elderly subjects also decreased neutrophil respiratory burst.

In relation to the effects of omega-3 PUFA on the incidence of infections in humans, data are controversial. A prospective study of 83,165 participants (27–44 years old) demonstrated that women in the highest quintile of EPA and DHA intake exhibited a 24% higher risk of pneumonia in comparison to those in the lowest quintile (Alperovich *et al.*, 2007). However, in another study no association was found between EPA and DHA intakes and pneumonia risk (Merchant *et al.*, 2005). Also in animal studies, intake of omega-3 PUFA gave rise to controversial effects in terms of protection against infections (Anderson & Fritsche, 2002; Byleveld *et al.*, 1999, 2000; Schwerbrock *et al.*, 2009; Paul *et al.*, 1997; McFarland *et al.*, 2008; Jordao *et al.*, 2008; Bonilla *et al.*, 2010; Fritsche *et al.*, 1997; Chang *et al.*, 1992). Results on the effects of n-3 PUFA supplementation to elderly people are summarized in Table 5.4.

In conclusion, high omega-3 PUFA intake might be advantageous to treat inflammatory conditions such as inflammatory bowel disease, rheumatoid arthritis, cardiovascular disease, type 2 diabetes and AD rather than affording protection against pathogens. An association of omega-3 PUFA with vitamin E may result in a greater net effect in the improvement of aged host defenses against pathogens (Pae *et al.*, 2012).

5.6 Polyphenols

Polyphenols are broadly distributed in the plant kingdom and, in particular, vegetables, fruit and cereals abundantly contain these bioactive natural products. Structurally, we distinguish two major categories of polyphenols, flavonoids and nonflavonoids compounds (e.g. resveratrol) (Xiuzhen *et al.*, 2007; Holme & Pervaiz, 2007) (see Table 5.5). The antioxidant and anti-inflammatory properties of polyphenols have previously been described in several reports and, at present, mostly of their mechanisms of action are object of intensive investigation (Magrone & Jirillo, 2010; Nunes *et al.*, 2013; Stefenon *et al.*, 2014).

Table 5.5 Classification of polyphenols (flavonoids and stilbenes).

	Sources	Major flavonoid
Flavonoids *subclasess*		
Flavanol	Cocoa, barley, green tea	Cathechin; gallocatechin
Flavanol	Green tea, grape	Epicatechin-3-gallate
Flavanones	Lemon	Eriodyctyol
Flavones	Celery, parsley, artichokes, carrots	Apigenin; luteolin
Isoflavones	Soy, peanuts	Dadzein; genistein
Flavonols	Apples, cranberries, wine, tomatoes	Quercetin; kaemperol
Anthocyanins	Blueberry, red apples	Cyanidin; delphinidin
Nonflavonoid		
3,4 ,5-Trihidroxy-*trans*-stilbene	Wine, grape seed and skin, nuts	Resveratrol

Polyphenols contained in red wine were studied some decades ago and the so-called "French Paradox" (de Lorgeril & Salen, 1999; Criqui & Ringel, 1994) was based on the cardiovascular protection exerted by moderate consumption of Bordeaux wine. Such epidemiological evidence has initiated a series of experimental and clinical investigations into the mechanism(s) of action of polyphenols to assess their potential therapeutic use.

Our group has intensively explored the immunomodulating/anti-inflammatory activities of red wine or red grape polyphenols either *in vitro* or *in vivo*. Polyphenols directly extracted from the red wine *Vitis vinifera* Negroamaro were able to modulate immune response *in vitro* in terms of increased release of nitric oxide (NO) from circulating monocytes (Magrone *et al.*, 2007). In fact, NO as a vasodilator can, in part, explain the cardiovascular protection afforded by a moderate intake of red wine (discussed in Chapter 6).

In terms of adaptive immune response, both Th1 and Th2 type cytokines were released by *in vitro* polyphenol-stimulated PBMCs and the effects exerted by secreted cytokines were counterbalanced by the release of IL-10 (Magrone *et al.*, 2008a). Polyphenols also induced secretion of IgG and IgA, thus also affecting the humoral arm of the immune response (Magrone *et al.*, 2008b). In terms of their mechanisms of action, polyphenols, when co-incubated with LPS, attenuated the NF-κB pathway induced by LPS (Magrone *et al.*, 2008c). Therefore, reduced production of pro-inflammatory cytokines may explain the anti-inflammatory activity of polyphenols in septic conditions. Furthermore, we have also reported that p38 phosphorylated form is elevated in PBMC treated with LPS alone, while its expression decreases when PBMCs are co-incubated with LPS plus Negroamaro polyphenols. Considering that polyphenols downregulate the LPS-induced p38 phosphorylation pathway, this class of molecules may play a putative beneficial role in Gram-negative infections. In fact, inhibition of p38α activity by the inhibitor SB203580 reduced mortality in the course of LPS shock and collagen-induced arthritis (Pietersma *et al.*, 1997; Badger *et al.*, 1996). Also deletion of p38α (Mθ) has been shown to limit the noxious effects of LPS (Kang *et al.*, 2008).

On the other hand, treating PBMCs with fermented grape marc (FGM) obtained from *V. vinifera* Negroamaro and Koshu resulted in the synthesis of a plethora of cytokines, including IL-10, detected in supernatants (Marzulli *et al.*, 2014). In particular, the intracellular content of IL-10 in FGM-treated lymphocytes was higher than that of the pro-inflammatory cytokines. This result prompted studies on the ability of FGM to induce the development of Treg cells, through assessment of the expression of the FoxP3 marker in $CD4^{+}CD25^{+}$ cells. We found that FGM *in vitro* induced Treg cell activation and release of IL-10, thus explaining the anti-inflammatory activity of these compounds. In addition, FGM was also able to reduce the release of free radicals from both PMN and monocytes *in vitro*, thus contributing to the host protection against oxidative damage (Marzulli *et al.*, 2014). In *in vivo* studies, Kawaguchi *et al.* (2011) found attenuation of murine colitis exerted by FGM, which may rely on the presence of Treg cells in the immune milieu, as also suggested by decreased levels of TNF-α and IL-1β in inflamed colon homogenates (Kawaguchi *et al.*, 2011).

Taken together, all of these results prompted us to investigate the *in vivo* activity of polyphenols when administered to elderly people. In this direction, a recent report based on the supplementation of polyphenol-rich biscuits to mature and old mice evidenced a modulation of immune functions, in terms of the enhancement of phagocytic and proliferative performance of immune cells (De la Fuente *et al.*, 2011).

Our pilot study (Magrone *et al.*, 2014) was conducted on 20 aged, frail people. Ten subjects were treated for 1 month with Leucoselect®Phytosome® at a dosage of 300 mg/day. Leucoselect®Phytosome® is an extract of seed skin highly enriched in catechins [15% (+)-catechin and (−)-epicatechin; 80% (−)-epicatechin gallate, dimers, trimers, tetramers and their gallates; 5% pentamers, hexamers, heptamers and their gallate, with improved bioavailability by complexing with soy phospholipids (1:3 w/w)]. The other 10 subjects were treated with placebo only. Serum cytokines were detected before and after administration of Leucoselect®Phytosome®. Surprisingly, both treated and untreated older people did not exhibit major alterations of the immune response when compared with their younger counterparts. Mostly a condition of equilibrium between IL-10 and IL-17 was found in all subjects. We hypothesized that the Mediterranean-type diet adopted by these elderly subjects throughout life might account for the retarded decline of their immune response. In any case, Leucoselect®Phytosome® was able to upregulate Th1 function in a few subjects in comparison to the placebo group, as seen by increased levels of IL-2 and IFN-γ. It is well known that both cytokines are involved in the protection against viral infections and tumor development (Magrone *et al.*, 2014). In addition, IL-8 was increased in some subjects of the treated group, thus suggesting an increased recruitment of neutrophils, for example, to lungs during winter infections.

Neurodegenerative diseases, such as AD and Parkinson disease are age associated. Many *in vitro* and *in vivo* studies have emphasized the neuroprotective role of polyphenols in these pathologies (Candore *et al.*, 2010; Magrone & Jirillo, 2011; Magrone *et al.*, 2012). In particular, the evidence that FGM reduces the release of granzyme B from CD8$^+$ cells (Marzulli *et al.*, 2012), which exhibit neurotoxic activity in the process of neurodegeneration, suggests the potential therapeutic application of these compounds in neurodegenerative disease. The major effects of polyphenols on the aged immune cells are illustrated in Table 5.6.

Table 5.6 Major effects of polyphenols on immune response in senescence.

- Increased release in IL-2 and IFN-γ, thus conferring immune protection against viral infections and tumor development
- Increased release in IL-8 levels, thus augmenting recruitment of neutrophils
- Reduced release in granzyme B from CD8$^+$, thus inhibiting neurotoxicity
- Inhibition of LPS-induced release of pro-inflammatory cytokines by downregulation of NF-κB pathway
- Normalization of intestinal microbiota, thus promoting immune homeostasis at intestinal level
- Increased in IL-10 release by T regulatory cells

5.7 Conclusion and future directions

As discussed in the previous sections of this chapter plant-derived substances and natural extracts seem to represent a novel therapeutic approach to preventing or limiting the effect of the ageing process. Therefore, measurement of the anti-oxidant and anti-inflammatory activity (CAA) of natural compounds is critical in the selection of a bioactive product (Becker *et al.*, 2014). The oxygen radical absorbance capacity (ORAC) (Ou *et al.*, 2001) and the cell-based anti-oxidant activity (Wolfe & Liu, 2007) are currently used. However, a model of mitogen-stimulated PBMCs has recently been introduced (Jenny *et al.*, 2011) for assessing the anti-oxidant capacities of natural products. In particular, the PBMC assay based on neopterin production and tryptophan degradation represents a good indicator of Th1 type response. In conclusion, the contemporary application of ORAC, CAA and PBMC methods should allow better identification of natural as well as synthetic compounds in terms of their anti-oxidant and anti-inflammatory effects.

In this context, it is important to mention the age-related consequences of the decline in mitochondrial function for cell senescence (Lòpez-Lluch *et al.*, 2008). Peroxisome proliferator-activated receptor γ-coactivator-1 (PGC-1α) regulates transcription and translation in mitochondria (Scarpulla, 2008). Novel evidence has demonstrated that PGC-1α and sirtuin 1 (SIRT1), an NAD^+-dependent protein deacetylase, reside in mithocondria further to nucleus and cytoplasm, and control their biogenesis (Aquilano *et al.*, 2010). Therefore, the complex SIRT1/PGC-1α emerges as an important drug target for correcting mitochondrial dysfunction in ageing. In this respect, evidence has been provided that resveratrol (a polyphenol) ameliorates mitochondrial function in the course of metabolic disease via activation of PGC-1α and SIRT1 (Lagouge *et al.*, 2006). Moreover, Davinelli *et al.* (2013) reported that the combined effects of resveratrol and equol (another polyphenol) on SIRT1 induction in human umbilical vein endothelial cells led to an increase in mitochondrial mass and mitochondrial content.

In conclusion, polyphenols exert either anti-inflammatory effects or control of mitochondrial biogenesis in human ageing. We have discussed the anti-ageing effects of an array of dietary substances and live organisms able to recover impaired immune functions in the elderly. The future goal comprises more complex clinical trials based on a balanced mix of all of the nutraceuticals mentioned above in order to attain the maximum response and benefit of dietary association in elderly people.

Acknowledgments

Thea Magrone is a recipient of a contract in the context of the project "Bioscience and Health" (PONa3_00395).

References

Ademokun, A., Y. C. Wu, and D. Dunn-Walters. 2010. The ageing B cell population: composition and function. *Biogerontology.* 11:125–137.

Agrawal, A., S. Agrawal, J. N. Cao, H. Su, K. Osann, and S. Gupta. 2007. Altered innate immune functioning of dendritic cells in elderly humans: a role of phosphoinositide 3-kinase-signaling pathway. *J. Immunol.* 178:6912–6922.

Alperovich, M., M. I. Neuman, W. C. Willett, and G. C. Curhan. 2007. Fatty acid intake and the risk of community-acquired pneumonia in U.S. women. *Nutrition* 23:196–202.

Alter-Wolf, S., B. B. Blomberg, and R. L. Riley. 2009. Deviation of the B cell pathway in senescent mice is associated with reduced surrogate light chain expression and altered immature B cell generation, phenotype, and light chain expression. *J. Immunol.* 182:138–147.

Amati, L., G. Marzulli, M. Martulli, A. Tafaro, F. Jirillo, V. Pugliese, G. Martemucci, A. G. D'Alessandro, and E. Jirillo. 2010. Donkey and goat milk intake and modulation of the human aged immune response. *Curr. Pharm. Des.* 16:864–869.

Anderson, M. and K. L. Fritsche. 2002. (n-3) Fatty acids and infectious disease resistance. *J Nutr.* 132:3566–3576.

Aprahamian, T., Y. Takemura, D. Goukassian, and K. Walsh. 2008. Ageing is associated with diminished apoptotic cell clearance in vivo. *Clin. Exp. Immunol.* 152:448–455.

Aquilano, K., P. Vigilanza, S. B. G. Rotilio, and M. R. Ciriolo. 2010. Peroxisome proliferator-activated receptor gamma co-activator 1alpha (PGC-1alpha) and sirtuin 1 (SIRT1) reside in mitochondria: possible direct function in mitochondrial biogenesis. *J. Biol. Chem.* 285:21590–21599.

Artis, D. 2008 Epithelial-cell recognition of commensal bacteria and maintenance of immune homeostasis in the gut. *Nat. Rev. Immunol.* 8:411–420.

Badger, A. M., J. N. Bradbeer, B. Votta, J. C. Lee, J. K. Adams, and D. E. Griswold. 1996. Pharmacological profile of SB 203580, a selective inhibitor of cytokine suppressive binding protein/p38 kinase, in animal models of arthritis, bone resorption, endotoxin shock and immune function. *J. Pharmacol. Exp. Ther.* 279:1453–1461.

Bala, S. and M. L. Failla. 1992. Copper deficiency reversibly impairs DNA synthesis in activated T lymphocytes by limiting interleukin 2 activity. *Proc. Natl Acad. Sci. USA* 89:6794–6797.

Bartosch, S., E. J. Woodmansey, J. C. Paterson, M. E. McMurdo, and G. T. Macfarlane. 2005. Microbiological effects of consuming a symbiotic containing *Bifidobacterium bifidum, Bifidobacterium lactis,* and oligofructose in elderly persons, determined by real-time polymerase chain reaction and counting of viable bacteria. *Clin. Infect. Dis.* 40:28–37.

Bechoua, S., M. Dubois, E. Vericel, P. Chapuy, M. Lagarde, and A. F. Prigent. 2003. Influence of very low dietary intake of marine oil on some functional aspects of immune cells in healthy elderly people. *Br. J. Nutr.* 89:523–531.

Becker, K., S. Schroecksnadel, J. C. H. Schennach, F. Uberall, D. and Fuchs. 2014. Comparison of in vitro tests for antioxidant and immunomodulatory capacities of compounds. *Phytomedicine.* 21:164–171.

Bernardes de Jesus, B. and M. A. Blasco. 2013. Telomerase at the intersection of cancer and aging. *Trends in genetics.* 29:513–520.

Bogden, J. D., J. M. Oleske, M. A. Lavenhar, E. M. Munves, F. W. Kemp, K. S. Bruening, K. J. Holding, T. N. Denny, M. A. Guarino, L. M. Krieger, and B. K. Holland. 1988. Zinc and immunocompetence in elderly people: effects of zinc supplementation for 3 months. *Am. J. Clin. Nutr.* 48:655–663.

Bogden, J. D., J. M. Oleske, M. A. Lavenhar, E. M. Munves, F. W. Kemp, K. S. Bruening, K. J. Holding, T. N. Denny, M. A. Guarino, and B. K. Holland. 1990. Effects of one year of supplementation with zinc and other micronutrients on cellular immunity in the elderly. *J. Am. Coll. Nutr.* 9:214–225.

Boge, T., M. Rémigy, S. Vaudaine, J. Tanguy, R. Bourdet-Sicard, S. and van der Werf. 2009. A probiotic fermented dairy drink improves antibody response to influenza vaccination in the elderly in two randomised controlled trials. *Vaccine.* 27:5677–5684.

Bonelli, M., A. Savitskaya, C.W. Steiner, E. Rath, J.S. Smolen, and C. Scheinecker. 2009. Phenotypic and functional analysis of $CD4^{+}$ $CD25^{-}$ $Foxp3^{+}$ T cells in patients with systemic lupus erythematosus. *J. Immunol.* 182:1689–1695.

Bonham, M., J. M. O'Connor, B. M. Hannigan, and J. J. Strain. 2002. The immune system as a physiological indicator of marginal copper status? *Br. J. Nutr.* 87:393–403.

Bonilla, D. L., Y. Y. Fan, R. S. Chapkin, and D. N. McMurray. 2010. Transgenic mice enriched in omega-3 fatty acids are more susceptible to pulmonary tuberculosis: impaired resistance to tuberculosis in fat-1 mice. *J. Infect. Dis.* 201:399–408.

Brewer, G. J. 2009. The risks of copper toxicity contributing to cognitive decline in the aging population and to Alzheimer's disease. *J. Am. Coll. Nutr.* 28:238–242.

Byleveld, P. M., G. T. Pang, R. L. Clancy, and D. C. Roberts. 1999. Fish oil feeding delays influenza virus clearance and impairs production of interferon-gamma and virus-specific immunoglobulin A in the lungs of mice. *J. Nutr.* 129:328–335.

Byleveld, M., G. T. Pang, R. L. Clancy, and D. C. Roberts. 2000. Fish oil feeding enhances lymphocyte proliferation but impairs virus-specific T lymphocyte cytotoxicity in mice following challenge with influenza virus. *Clin. Exp. Immunol.* 119:287–292.

Calado, R. T. and N. S. Young. 2009. Telomere diseases. *New Engl. J. Med.* 361:2353–2365.

Calder, P. C. 2010. The 2008 ESPEN Sir David Cuthbertson Lecture: fatty acids and inflammation – from the membrane to the nucleus and from the laboratory bench to the clinic. *Clin. Nutr.* 29:5–12.

Candore, G., C. Caruso, E. Jirillo, T. Magrone, and S. Vasto. 2010. Low grade inflammation as a common pathogenetic denominator in age related diseases: novel drug targets for anti-ageing strategies and successful ageing achievement. *Curr. Pharm. Des.* 16:584–596.

Chang, H. R., A. G. Dulloo, I. R. Vladoianu, P. F. Piguet, D. Arsenijevic, L. Girardier, and J. C. Pechere. 1992. Fish oil decreases natural resistance of mice to infection with Salmonella typhimurium. *Metabolism* 41:1–2.

Chapkin, R. S., W. Kim, J. R. Lupton, and D. N. McMurray. 2009. Dietary docosahexaenoic and eicosapentaenoic acid: emerging mediators of inflammation. *Prostaglandins. Leukot. Essent. Fatty Acids.* 81:187–191.

Coombes, J. L. and F. Powrie. 2008. Dendritic cells in intestinal immune regulation. *Nat. Rev. Immunol.* 8:435–446.

Criqui, M. H. and B. L. Ringel. 1994. Does diet or alcohol explain the French Paradox? *Lancet.* 344: 1719–1723.

Das, H., A. Kumar, Z. Lin, W. D. Patino, P. M. Hwang, M. W. Feinberg, P. K. Majumder, and M. K. Jain. 2006. Kruppel-like factor 2 (KLF2) regulates proinflammatory activation of monocytes. *Proc. Natl Acad. Sci. USA* 103:6653–6658.

Davinelli, S., N. Sapere, M. Visentin, D. Zella, and G. Scapagnini. 2013. Enhancement of mitochondrial biogenesis with polyphenols: combined effects of resveratrol and equol in human endothelial cells. *Immun. Ageing* 10:28.

De la Fuente, M., S. Medina, I Baeza, and L. Jiménez. 2011. Improvement of leucocyte functions in mature and old mice after 15 and 30 weeks of diet supplementation with polyphenol-rich biscuits. *Eur. J. Nutr.* 50:563–573.

de Lorgeril, M. and P. Salen. 1999. Wine ethanol, platelets, and Mediterranean diet. *Lancet.* 353:1067.

Dorshkind, K. and E. Montecino-Rodriguez. 2007. Fetal B-cell lymphopoiesis and the emergence of B-1-cell potential. *Nat. Rev. Immunol.* 7:213–219.

Ekiz, C., L. Agaoglu, Z. Karakas, N. Gurel, and I. Yalcin. 2005. The effect of iron deficiency anemia on the function of the immune system. *Hematol. J.* 5:579–583.

Enck, P., K. Zimmermann, K. Rusch, A. Schwiertz, S. Klosterhalfen, and J. S. Frick. 2009. The effects of ageing on the colonic bacterial microflora in adults. *Z. Gastroenterol.* 47:653–658.

Ershler, W. B. and E. T. Keller. 2000. Age-associated increased interleukin-6 gene expression, late-life diseases, and frailty. *Annu. Rev. Med.* 51:245–270.

Fernandes, G. 2008. Progress in nutritional immunology. *Immunol. Res.* 40:244–261.

Fessler. J., A. Ficjan, C. Duftner, and C. Dejaco. 2013. The impact of aging on regulatory T-cells. *Front. Immunol.* 4:231.

Franceschi, C. 2007. Inflammaging as a major characteristic of old people: can it be prevented or cured? *Nutr. Rev.* 65:S173–S176.

Franceschi, C., M. Capri, D. Monti, S. Giunta, F. Olivieri, F. Sevini, M.P. Panourgia, L. Invidia, L. Celani, M. Scurti, E. Cevenini, G.C. Castellani, and S. Salvioli. 2007. Inflammaging and anti-inflammaging: a systemic perspective on aging and longevity emerged from studies in humans. *Mech. Ageing Dev.* 128:92–105.

Frasca, D. and B. B. Blomberg. 2009. Effects of aging on B cell function. *Curr. Opin. Immunol.* 21:425–430.

Freeman, G. J., J. M. Casasnovas, D. T. Umetsu, and R. H. De Kruyff. 2010. TIM genes: a family of cell surface phosphatidylserine receptors that regulate innate and adaptive immunity. *Immunol. Rev.* 235:172–189.

Fritsche, K. 2007. Important differences exist in the dose–response relationship between diet and immune cell fatty acids in humans and rodents. *Lipids.* 42:961–979.

Fritsche, K. L., L. M. Shahbazian, C. Feng, and J. N. Berg. 1997. Dietary fish oil reduces survival and impairs bacterial clearance in C3H/Hen mice challenged with Listeria monocytogenes. *Clin. Sci. (Lond.)* 92:95–101.

Galli, C. and P. C. Calder. 2009. Effects of fat and fatty acid intake on inflammatory and immune responses: a critical review. *Ann. Nutr. Metab.* 55:123–139.

Giacconi, R., M. Malavolta, L. Costarelli, F. Busco, R. Galeazzi, G. Bernardini, N. Gasparini, and E. Mocchegiani. 2012. Comparison of intracellular zinc signals in nonadherent lymphocytes from young-adult and elderly donors: role of zinc transporters (Zip family) and proinflammatory cytokines. *J. Nutr. Biochem.* 23:1256–1263.

Gill, H. S., Rutherfurd, K. J., Cross, M. L. and Gopal, P. K. 2001. Enhancement of immunity in the elderly by dietary supplementation with the probiotic *Bifidobacterium lactis* HN019. *Am. J. Clin. Nutr.* 74:833–839.

Girodon, F., P. Galan, A. L. Monget, M. C. Boutron-Ruault, P. Brunet-Lecomte, P. Preziosi, J. Arnaud, J. C. Manuguerra, and S. Herchberg. 1999. Impact of trace elements and vitamin supplementation on immunity and infections in institutionalized elderly patients: a randomized controlled trial. *MIN. VIT. AOX. geriatric network. Arch. Intern. Med.* 159:748–754.

Guigoz, Y., F. Rochat, G. Perruisseau-Carrier, I. Rochat, and E. Schiffrin. 2002. Effects of oligosaccharide on the faecal flora and non-specific immune system in elderly people. *Nutr. Res.* 22:13–25.

Guyatt, G. H., C. Patterson, M. Ali, J. Singer, M. Levine, I. Turpie, and R. Meyer. 1990. Diagnosis of iron-deficiency anemia in the elderly. *Am. J. Med.* 88:205–209.

Haase, H. and L. Rink. 2009. The immune system and the impact of zinc during aging. *Immun. Ageing* 6:9.

Hartmann, H. J., K. Felix, W. Nagel, and U. Weser. 1993. Intestinal administration of copper and its transient release into venous rat blood serum concomitantly with metallothionein. *Biometals* 6:115–118.

Harvey, L. J., K. Ashton, L. Hooper, A. Casgrain, and S. J. Fairweather-Tait. 2009. Methods of assessment of copper status in humans: a systematic review. *Am. J. Clin. Nutr.* 89:2009S–2024S.

Hatakka, K. and M. Saxelin. 2008. Probiotics in intestinal and non-intestinal infectious diseases-clinical evidence. *Curr. Pharm. Des.* 14:1351–1367.

Hazeldine, J. and J. M. Lord. 2013. The impact of ageing on natural killer cell function and potential consequences for health in older adults. *Ageing Res. Rev.* 12:1069–1078.

He, F., A. C. Ouwehand, E. Isolauri, M. Hosoda, Y. Benno, and S. Salminen. 2001. Differences in composition and mucosal adhesion of bifidobacteria isolated from healthy adults and healthy seniors. *Curr. Microbiol.* 43:351–354.

Hoang, B. X., G. Shaw, P. Pham, and S. A. Levine. 2010. Lactobacillus rhamnosus cell lysate in the management of resistant childhood atopic eczema. *Inflamm. Allergy. Drug. Targets* 9:192–196.

Holme, A. L. and S. Pervaiz. 2007. Resveratrol in cell fate decisions. *J. Bioenerg. Biomembr.* 39:59–63.

Hoursburg, C. R. Jr, M. O'Donnel, S. Chamblee, J. L. Moreland, J. Johnson, B. J. Marsh, M. Narita, L. S. Johnson, and C. F. von Reyn. 2010. Revisiting rates of reactivation tuberculosis: a population best approach. *Am. J. Respir. Crit. Care Med.* 182:420–425.

Huang, Z., A. H. Rose, and P. R. Hoffmann. 2012. The role of selenium in inflammation and immunity: from molecular mechanisms to therapeutic opportunities. *Antioxid. Redox Signal.* 16:705–743.

Hume, M. E. 2011. Historic perspective: prebiotics, probiotics, and other alternatives to antibiotics. *Poult. Sci.* 90:2663–2669.

Italian Multicentric Study on Centenarians. 1998. Laboratory parameters of Italian centenarians. *Arch. Gerontol. Geriatr.* 27:67–74.

Jenny, M., M. Klieber, D. Zaknun, S. Schroecksnadel, K. Kurz, M. Ledochowski, H. Schennach, and D. Fuchs. 2011. In vitro testing for anti-inflammatory properties of compounds employing peripheral blood mononuclear cells freshly isolated from healthy donors. *Inflamm. Res.* 60:127–135.

Jirillo, E., G. Candore, T. Magrone, and C. Caruso. 2008. A scientific approach to anti-ageing therapies: state of the art. *Curr. Pharm. Des.* 14:2637–2642.

Jordao, L., A. Lengeling, Y. Bordat, F. Boudou, B. Gicquel, O. Neyrolles, P. D. Becker, C. A. Guzman, G. Griffiths, and E. Anes. 2008. Effects of omega-3 and -6 fatty acids on *Mycobacterium tuberculosis* in macrophages and in mice. *Microbes Infect.* 10:1379–1386.

Kahmann, L., P. Uciechowski, S. Warmuth, M. Malavolta, E. Mocchegiani, and L. Rink. 2006. Effect of improved zinc status on T helper cell activation and TH1/TH2 ratio in healthy elderly individuals. *Biogerontology* 7:429–435.

Kalra, E. K. 2003. Nutraceutical: definition and introduction. *AAPS Pharm. Sci.* 5:E25.

Kang, Y. J., J. Chen, M. Otsuka, J. Mols, S. Ren, Y. Wang, and J. Han. 2008. Macrophage deletion of p38α partially impairs lipopolysaccharide induced cellular activation. *J. Immunol.* 180:5075–5082.

Kant, A. K. 2000. Consumption of energy-dense, nutrient-poor foods by adult Americans: nutritional and health implications. The third National Health and Nutrition Examination Survey, 1988–1994. *Am. J. Clin. Nutr.* 72:929–936.

Kau, A. L., P. P. Ahern, N. W. Griffin, A. L. Goodman, and J. I. Gordon. 2011. Human nutrition, the gut microbiome and the immune system. *Nature* 474:327–336.

Kawaguchi, K., T. Matsumoto, and Y. Kumazawa. 2011. Effects of antioxidant polyphenols on TNF-α-related diseases. *Curr. Top. Med. Chem.* 11:1767–1779.

Kim, W., N. A. Khan, D. N. McMurray, I. A. Prior, N. Wang, and R. S. Chapkin. 2010. Regulatory activity of polyunsaturated fatty acids in T-cell signaling. *Prog. Lipid Res.* 49:250–261.

Kogut, I., J. L. Scholz, M. P. Cancro, and J. C. Cambier. 2012. B cell maintenance and function in aging. *Semin. Immunol.* 24:342–349.

Kohli, P. and B. D. Levy. 2009. Resolvins and protectins: mediating solutions to inflammation. *Br. J. Pharmacol.* 158:960–971.

Koller, L. D., S. A. Mulhern, N. C. Frankel, M. G. Steven, and J. R. Williams. 1987. Immune dysfunction in rats fed a diet deficient in copper. *Am. J. Clin. Nutr.* 45:997–1006.

Lages, C. S., I. Suffia, P. A. Velilla, B. Huang, G. Warshaw, D. A. Hildeman, Y. Belkaid, and C. Chougnet. 2008. Functional regulatory T cells accumulate in aged hosts and promote chronic infectious disease reactivation. *J. Immunol.* 181:1835–1848.

Lagouge, M., C. Argmann, Z. Gerhart-Hines, H. Meziane, C. Lerin, F. Daussin, N. Messadeq, J. Milne, P. Lambert, P. Elliott, B. Geny, M. Laakso, P. Puigserver, and J. Auwerx. 2006. Resveratrol improves mitochondrial function and protects against metabolic disease by activating SIRT1 and PGC-1alpha. *Cell* 127:1109–1122.

Li, W. 2013. Phagocyte dysfunction, tissue aging and degeneration. *Ageing Res. Rev.* 12:1005–1012.

López-Lluch, G., P. M. Irusta, P. Navas, and R. de Cabo. 2008. Mitochondrial biogenesis and healthy aging. *Exp. Gerontol.* 43:813–819.

Lynch, H. E., G. L. Goldberg, A. Chidgey, M. R. Van den Brink, R. Boyd, and G. D. Sempowski. 2009. Thymic involution and immune reconstitution. *Trends Immunol.* 30:366–373.

Maassen, C. B. M. and E. Claassen. 2008. Strain-dependent effects of probiotic lactobacilli on EAE autoimmunity. *Vaccine* 26:2056–2057.

Magrone, T. and E. Jirillo. 2010. Polyphenols from red wine are potent modulators of innate and adaptive immune responsiveness. *Proc. Nutr. Soc.* 69:279–285.

Magrone, T. and E. Jirillo. 2011. Potential application of dietary polyphenols from red wine to attaining healthy ageing. *Curr. Top. Med. Chem.* 11:1780–1796.

Magrone, T. and E. Jirillo. 2013a. The interaction between gut microbiota and age-related changes in immune function and inflammation. *Immun. Ageing* 10:31.

Magrone, T. and E. Jirillo. 2013b. The interplay between the gut immune system and microbiota in health and disease: nutraceutical intervention for restoring intestinal homeostasis. *Curr. Pharm. Des.* 19:1329–1342.

Magrone, T., A. Tafaro, F. Jirillo, M. A. Panaro, P. Cuzzuol, A. C. Cuzzuol, V. Pugliese, L. Amati, E. Jirillo, and V. Covelli. 2007. Red wine consumption and prevention of atherosclerosis: an in vitro model using human peripheral blood mononuclear cells. *Curr. Pharm. Des.* 13:3718–3725.

Magrone, T., G. Candore, C. Caruso, E. Jirillo, and V. Covelli. 2008a. Polyphenols from red wine modulate immune responsiveness: biological and clinical significance. *Curr. Pharm. Des.* 14:2733–2748.

Magrone, T., A. Tafaro, F. Jirillo, L. Amati, E. Jirillo, and V. Covelli. 2008b. Elicitation of immune responsiveness against antigenic challenge in age-related diseases: effects of red wine polyphenols. *Curr. Pharm. Des.* 14:2749–2757.

Magrone, T., M. A. Panaro, E. Jirillo, and V. Covelli. 2008c. Molecular effects elicited in vitro by red wine on human healthy peripheral blood mononuclear cells: potential therapeutical application of polyphenols to diet-related chronic diseases. *Curr. Pharm. Des.* 14:2758–2766.

Magrone, T., G. Marzulli, and E. Jirillo. 2012. Immunopathogenesis of neurodegenerative diseases: current therapeutic models of neuroprotection with special reference to natural products. *Curr. Pharm. Des.* 18:34–42.

Magrone, T., F. Perez de Heredia, E. Jirillo, G. Morabito, A. Marcos, and M. Serafini. 2013. Functional foods and nutraceuticals as therapeutic tools for the treatment of diet-related diseases. *Can. J. Physiol. Pharmacol.* 91:387–396.

Magrone, T., V. Pugliese, S. Fontana, and E. Jirillo. 2014. Human Use Of Leucoselect® Phytosome® with special reference to inflammatory-allergic pathologies in frail elderly patients. *Curr. Pharm. Des.* 20:1011–1009.

Mañé, J., E. Pedrosa, V. Lorén, M.A. Gassull, J. Espadaler, J. Cuñé, S. Audivert, M.A. Bonachera, and E. Cabré. 2011. A mixture of *Lactobacillus plantarum* CECT 7315 and CECT 7316 enhances systemic immunity in elderly subjects. A dose–response, double-blind, placebo-controlled, randomized pilot trial. *Nutr. Hosp.* 26:228–235.

Mariani, E., S. Neri, L. Cattini, E. Mocchegiani, M. Malavolta, G. V. Dedoussis, S. Kanoni, L. Rink, J. Jajte, and A. Facchini. 2008. Effect of zinc supplementation on plasma IL-6 and MCP-1 production and NK cell function in healthy elderly: interactive influence of +647 MT1a and -174 IL-6 polymorphic alleles. *Exp. Gerontol.* 43:462–471.

Marzulli, G., T. Magrone, K. Kawaguchi, Y. Kumazawa, and E. Jirillo. 2012. Fermented grape marc (FGM): immunomodulating properties and its potential exploitation in the treatment of neurodegenerative diseases. *Curr. Pharm. Des.* 18:43–50.

Marzulli, G., T. Magrone, L. Vonghia, M. Kaneko, H. Takimoto, Y. Kumazawa, and E. Jirillo. 2014. Immunomodulating and anti-allergic effects of Negroamaro and Koshu *Vitis vinifera* fermented grape marc (FGM). *Curr. Pharm. Des.* 20:864–868.

McFarland, C. T., Y. Y. Fan, R. S. Chapkin, B. R. Weeks, and D. N. McMurray. 2008. Dietary polyunsaturated fatty acids modulate resistance to *Mycobacterium tuberculosis* in guinea pigs. *J. Nutr.* 138:2123–2128.

Meda, L., M. A. Cassatella, G. I. Szendrei, L. Otvos Jr, P. Baron, M. Villalba, D. Ferrari, and F. Rossi. 1995. Activation of microglial cells by beta-amyloid protein and interferon-gamma. *Nature* 374:647–650.

Meijerink, M. and J. M. Wells. 2010. Probiotic modulation of dendritic cells and T cell responses in the intestine. *Benef. Microbes* 1:317–326.

Merchant, A. T., G. C. Curhan, E. B. Rimm, W. C. Willett, and W. W. Fawzi. 2005. Intake of n-6 and n-3 fatty acids and fish and risk of community-acquired pneumonia in US men. *Am. J. Clin. Nutr.* 82:668–674.

Meydani, S. N., S. Endres, M. M. Woods, B. R. Goldin, C. Soo, A. Morrill-Labrode, C. A. Dinarello, and S. L. Gorbach. 1991. Oral (n-3) fatty acid supplementation suppresses cytokine production and lymphocyte proliferation: comparison between young and older women. *J. Nutr.* 121:547–555.

Meydani, S. N., A. H. Lichtenstein, S. Cornwall, M. Meydani, B. R. Goldin, H. Rasmussen, C. A. Dinarello, and E. J. Schaefer. 1993. Immunologic effects of national cholesterol education panel step-2 diets with and without fish-derived N-3 fatty acid enrichment. *J. Clin. Invest.* 92:105–113.

Mocchegiani, E., M. Muzzioli, C. Cipriano, and R. Giacconi. 1998. Zinc, T-cell pathways, aging: role of metallothioneins. *Mech. Ageing Dev.* 106:183–204.

Mocchegiani, E., M. Muzzioli, and R. Giacconi. 2000. Zinc and immunoresistance to infection in aging: new biological tools. *Trends Pharmacol. Sci.* 21:205–208.

Mocchegiani, E., M. Muzzioli, R. Giacconi, C. Cipriano, N. Gasparini, C. Franceschi, R. Gaetti, E. Cavalieri, and H. Suzuki. 2003. Metallothioneins/PARP-1/IL-6 interplay on natural killer cell activity in elderly: parallelism with nonagenarians and old infected humans. *Effect of zinc supply. Mech. Ageing Dev.* 124:459–468.

Mocchegiani, E., R. Giacconi, L. Costarelli, E. Muti, C. Cipriano, S. Tesei, S. Pierpaoli, C. Giuli, R. Papa, F. Marcellini, N. Gasparini, R. Pierandrei, F. Piacenza, E. Mariani, D. Monti, G. Dedoussis, S. Kanoni, G. Herbein, T. Fulop, L. Rink, J. Jajte, and M. Malavolta. 2008. Zinc deficiency and IL-6 -174G/C polymorphism in old people from different European countries: effect of zinc supplementation. *ZINCAGE study. Exp. Gerontol.* 43:433–444.

Mocchegiani, E., L. Costarelli, R. Giacconi, F. Piacenza, A. Basso, and M. Malavolta. 2012. Micronutrient (Zn, Cu, Fe)-gene interactions in ageing and inflammatory age-related diseases: implications for treatments. *Ageing Res. Rev.* 11:297–319.

Myles, I. A., N. M. Fontecilla, B. M. Janelsins, P. J. Vithayathil, J. A. Segre, and S. K. Datta. 2013. Parental dietary fat intake alters offspring microbiome and immunity. *J. Immunol.* 191:3200–3209.

Napoli, I. and H. Neumann. 2010. Protective effects of microglia in multiple sclerosis. *Exp. Neurol.* 225:24–28.

Nunes, C., E. Ferreira, V. Freitas, L. Almeida, R.M. Barbosa, and J. Laranjinha. 2013. Intestinal anti-inflammatory activity of red wine extract: unveiling the mechanisms in colonic epithelial cells. *Food. Funct.* 4:373–383.

Osaki, S. and D. A. Johnson. 1969. Mobilization of liver iron by ferroxidase (ceruloplasmin). *J. Biol. Chem.* 244:5757–5758.

Ou, B., M. Hampsch-Woodill, and R. L. Prior. 2001. Development and validation of an improved oxygen radical absorbance capacity assay using fluorescein as the fluorescent probe. *J. Agric. Food. Chem.* 49:4619–4626.

Pae, M., S. N. Meydani, and D. Wu. 2012. The role of nutrition in enhancing immunity in aging. *Aging. Dis.* 3:91–129.

Paul, K. P., M. Leichsenring, M. Pfisterer, E. Mayatepek, D. Wagner, M. Domann, H. G. Sonntag, and H. J. Bremer. 1997. Influence of n-6 and n-3 polyunsaturated fatty acids on the resistance to experimental tuberculosis. *Metabolism* 46:619–624.

Pearson, R., J. Fleetwood, S. Eaton, M. Crossley, and S. Bao. 2008. Krüppel-like transcription factors: a functional family. *Int. J. Biochem. Cell. Biol.* 40:1996–2001.

Pietersma, A., B. C. Tilly, M. Gaestel, N. de Jong, J. C. Lee, J. F. Koster, and W. Sluiter. 1997. p38 mitogen activated protein kinase regulates endothelial VCAM-1 expression at the post-transcriptional level. *Biochem. Biophys. Res. Commun.* 230:44–48.

Pompos, L. J. and K. L. Fritsche. 2002. Antigen-driven murine CD4+ T lymphocyte proliferation and interleukin-2 production are diminished by dietary (n-3) polyunsaturated fatty acids. *J. Nutr.* 132:3293–3300.

Potrykus, J., R. L. White, and S. L. Bearne. 2008. Proteomic investigation of amino acid catabolism in the indigenous gut anaerobe Fusobacterium varium. *Proteomics* 8:2691–2703.

Prasad, A., B. Bao, F. W. Beck, and F. H. Sarkar. 2006. Correction of interleukin-2 gene expression by in vitro zinc addition to mononuclear cells from zinc-deficient human subjects: a specific test for zinc deficiency in humans. *Transl. Res.* 148:325–333.

Rastall, R. A. and V. Maitin. 2002. Prebiotics and synbiotics: towards the next generation. *Curr. Opin. Biotechnol.* 13:490–496.

Rees, D., E. A. Miles, T. Banerjee, S. J. Wells, C. E. Roynette, K. W. Wahle, and P. C. Calder. 2006. Dose-related effects of eicosapentaenoic acid on innate immune function in healthy humans: a comparison of young and older men. *Am. J. Clin. Nutr.* 83:331–342.

Roberfroid, M., G. R. Gibson, L. Hoyles, A. L. McCartney, R. Rastall, I. Rowland, D. Wolvers, B. Watzl, H. Szajewska, B. Stahl, F. Guarner, F. Respondek, K. Whelan, V. Coxam, M. J. Davicco, L. Léotoing, Y. Wittrant, N. M. Delzenne, P. D. Cani, A. M. Neyrinck, and A. Meheust. 2010. Prebiotic effects: metabolic and health benefits. *Br. J. Nutr.* 104:S1–S63.

Rosen, G. M., S. Pou, C. L. Ramos, M. S. Cohen, and B. E. Britigan. 1995. Free radicals and phagocytic cells. *FASEB J.* 9:200–209.

Rubtsov, A. V., K. Rubtsova, A. Fischer, R. T. Meehan, J. Z. Gillis, J. W. Kappler, and P. Marrack. 2011. Toll-like receptor 7 (TLR7)-driven accumulation of a novel CD11c+ B-cell population is important for the development of autoimmunity. *Blood* 118:1305–1315.

Santos, P. C. and R. P. Falcão. 1990. Decreased lymphocyte subsets and K-cell activity in iron deficiency anemia. *Acta Haematol.* 84:118–121.

Scarpulla, R. C. 2008. Transcriptional paradigms in mammalian mitochondrial biogenesis and function. *Physiol. Rev.* 88:611–638.

Schmitt, V., L. Rink, and P. Uciechowski. 2013. The Th17/Treg balance is disturbed during aging. *Exp. Gerontol.* 48:1379–1386.

Schwerbrock, N. M., E. A. Karlsson, Q. Shi, P. A. Sheridan, and M. A. Beck. 2009. Fish oil-fed mice have impaired resistance to influenza infection. *J. Nutr.* 139:1588–1594.

Serhan, C. N., N. Chiang, and T. E. Van Dyke. 2008. Resolving inflammation: dual anti-inflammatory and pro-resolution lipid mediators. *Nat. Rev. Immunol.* 8:349–361.

Shaikh, S. R. and M. Edidin. 2006. Polyunsaturated fatty acids, membrane organization, T cells, and antigen presentation. *Am. J. Clin. Nutr.* 84:1277–1289.

Sijben, J. W. and P. C. Calder. 2007. Differential immunomodulation with long-chain n-3 PUFA in health and chronic disease. *Proc. Nutr. Soc.* 66:237–259.

Simone, R., A. Zicca, and D. Saverino. 2008. The frequency of regulatory $CD3^{+}CD8^{+}CD28^{-}$ CD25+ T lymphocytes in human peripheral blood increases with age. *J. Leukoc. Biol.* 84:1454–1461.

Smith, L. C. and R. Ratard. 2011. Clostridium difficile hospitalizations in Louisiana: a 10 year review. *J. La. State Med. Soc.* 163:192–195.

Solana, R., R. Tarazona, I. Gayoso, O. Lesur, G. Dupuis, and T. Fulop. 2012. Innate immunosenescence: effect of aging on cells and receptors of the innate immune system in humans. *Semin. Immunol.* 24:331–341.

Stadler, N., R. A. Lindner, and M. J. Davies. 2004. Direct detection and quantification of transition metal ions in human atherosclerotic plaques: evidence for the presence of elevated levels of iron and copper. *Arterioscler. Thromb. Vasc. Biol.* 24:949–954.

Stefenon, C. A., C. M. Bonesi, V. Marzarotto, D. Barnabé, F. R. Spinelli, V. Webber, and R. Vanderlinde. 2014. Phenolic composition and antioxidant activity in sparkling wines: modulation by the ageing on lees. *Food. Chem.* 145:292–299.

Tortorella, C., G. Piazzolla, F. Spaccavento, E. Jirillo, and S. Antonaci. 1999. Age-related effects of oxidative metabolism and cyclic AMP signaling on neutrophil apoptosis. *Mech. Ageing Dev.* 110:195–205.

Vallejo, A. N. 2005. CD28 extinction in human T cells: altered functions and the program of T-cell senescence. *Immunol. Rev.* 205:158–169.

Vitale, M., M. Della Chiesa, S. Carlomagno, D. Pende, M. Aricò, L. Moretta, and A. Moretta. 2005. NK-dependent DC maturation is mediated by TNFalpha and IFNgamma released upon engagement of the NKp30 triggering receptor. *Blood* 106:566–571.

Vulevic, J., A. Drakoularakou, P. Yaqoob, G. Tzortzis, and G. R. Gibson. 2008. Modulation of the fecal microflora profile and immune function by a novel transgalactooligosaccharide mixture (B-GOS) in healthy elderly volunteers. *Am. J. Clin. Nutr.* 88:1438–1446.

Wang. J. and K. Pantopoulos. 2011. Regulation of cellular iron metabolism. *Biochem. J.* 434:365–381.

Wapnir, R. A. 1998. Copper absorption and bioavailability. *Am. J. Clin. Nutr.* 67:1054S–1060S.

Wardwell, L., K. Chapman-Novakofski, S. Herrel, and J. Woods. 2008. Nutrient intake and immune function of elderly subjects. *J. Am. Diet Assoc.* 108:2005–2012.

Welch, K. D., C. A. Reilly, and S. D. Aust. 2002. The role of cysteine residues in the oxidation of ferritin. *Free Radic. Biol. Med.* 33:399–408.

Wolfe, K. L. and R. H. Liu. 2007. Cellular antioxidant activity (CAA) assay for assessing antioxidants, foods, and dietary supplements. *J. Agric. Food. Chem.* 55:8896–8907.

Wood, S. M., C. Beckham, A. Yosioka, H. Darban, and R. R. Watson. 2000. beta-Carotene and selenium supplementation enhances immune response in aged humans. *Integr. Med.* 2:85–92.

Xiuzhen, H., S. Tao, and L. Hongxiang. 2007. Dietary polyphenols and their biological significance. *Int. J. Mol. Sci.* 8:950–988.

Yan, F. and D. B. Polk. 2011. Probiotics and immune health. *Curr. Opin. Gastroenterol.* 27:496–501.

Zhang, P., W. Kim, L. Zhou, N. Wang, L. H. Ly, D. N. McMurray, and R. S. Chapkin. 2006. Dietary fish oil inhibits antigen-specific murine Th1 cell development by suppression of clonal expansion. *J. Nutr.* 136:2391–2398.

CHAPTER 6
Cardiovascular ageing

Carmen Brás Silva[1] and Delminda Neves[2]
[1] *Department of Physiology and Cardiothoracic Surgery, Faculty of Medicine, and Faculty of Nutrition and Food Sciences, University of Porto, Porto, Portugal*
[2] *Department of Experimental Biology, Faculty of Medicine, and Institute for Molecular and Cell Biology, University of Porto, Porto, Portugal*

6.1 Age-related cardiac changes

The most important determinant of cardiovascular health is a person's age. Since it delivers oxygenated blood to all tissues in the body, the health of the cardiovascular system is vital for the health of every tissue and longevity of the organism as a whole. Ageing results in a progressive functional and structural decline in multiple organs and, in particular, has profound effects on the heart and arterial system, leading to an increase in cardiovascular disease, including atherosclerosis, hypertension, heart failure, myocardial infarction and stroke (North & Sinclair, 2012).

6.1.1 Heart changes

There are a number of structural and functional changes in the heart with ageing and each of these changes can have significant implications for cardiovascular disease.

6.1.1.1 Structural changes

Concerning age-related structural changes of the aged heart, there is a significant increase in myocardial thickness as a direct consequence of individual increase in cardiomyocyte size. In addition, the heart changes its overall shape from elliptical to spheroid. These changes in thickness and shape have important implications for cardiac wall stress and overall cardiac efficiency (Strait & Lakatta, 2012). It appears, however, from the results of recent studies that there is no change in left ventricular (LV) mass with ageing in women, and a decease in LV mass can even be found in men (through the decrease in myocyte number). It seems thus that the increased wall thickness and changes in heart shape represent an asymmetric increase in the interventricular septum more than in the free wall, redistributing cardiac muscle in a way that does not increase total cardiac mass (Strait & Lakatta, 2012).

An increase in the amount (focal increases) and a change in the physical properties of collagen (purportedly owing to nonenzymatic crosslinking) also occur within the myocardium with ageing. The cardiac myocyte-to-collagen ratio in the older heart either remains constant or increases, however, because of the age-related increase in myocyte size (Lakatta & Levy, 2003).

Anti-Ageing Nutrients: Evidence-Based Prevention of Age-Associated Diseases, First Edition. Edited by Delminda Neves.

6.1.1.1.1 Changes in heart valves

Recent work has demonstrated age-related significant changes in heart valves composition and material properties (Stephens *et al.*, 2010, 2011). In normal hearts, aortic valve leaflet thickness is seen to increase with age. This change results in an increase in leaflet weight and overall coverage area. Histological characterization of the thickened leaflets demonstrates that it is associated with collagen deposition and degeneration, lipid accumulation and calcification (Kitzman & Edwards, 1990). Dilation of the aortic valve may also occur owing to the degeneration of collagen and deposition of lipids within the valve annulus. Leaflet thickening and valve dilation owing to ageing are associated with aortic valve sclerosis and severe aortic regurgitation, respectively (Collins *et al.*, 2014).

Additionally, it was shown in animal studies that pulmonary, mitral and aortic regurgitation became more frequent with age progression, but the severity remained unchanged. These functional changes were associated with degenerative myxoid thickening of the mitral and aortic valvular leaflets (Droogmans *et al.*, 2009).

Calcification of the valves is commonly associated with ageing and is the most frequent pathology seen in excised native valves (Butany *et al.*, 2005; Wu *et al.*, 2013). Vascular calcification can also lead to dysfunction of the heart valves, independently of their being native or bioprosthetic valves. In the valves, calcification of the leaflets can change the mechanical properties of the tissue and result in stenosis.

These valvular changes should be considered as part of the natural ageing process caused by hemodynamic and mechanical factors, and can be aggravated by several forms of stress, but the exact pathogenesis is not fully understood.

6.1.1.2 Functional changes

6.1.1.2.1 Cardiac systolic function

Despite a number of age-associated changes possibly limiting a person's functional capacity and promoting vascular stiffening, with consequent increased afterload, the overall resting systolic function of cardiac muscle does not change in healthy ageing. This does not signify that there is no change in components of cardiac systole. In fact, multiple changes occur in the mean shortening velocity and in the heart's interactions with the vasculature. The combined effects of these individual changes, however, balance each other and leave the net systolic function unaltered at rest (Strait & Lakatta, 2012).

The effects of ageing are most evident under exercise practice. An overall decrease in exercise tolerance is evident in the progressive decline in maximal oxygen uptake (VO_2 max), starting at age 20–30 years and falling by approximately 10% per decade (Fleg & Lakatta, 1988). This reduction in cardiac reserve is a result of multiple factors, including increased vascular afterload, arterial–ventricular load mismatching, reduced intrinsic myocardial contractility, impaired autonomic regulation and physical deconditioning (Strait & Lakatta, 2012).

6.1.1.2.2 Cardiac diastolic function

Despite maintenance of systolic function at rest, a noticeable number of changes in the diastolic phase of the cardiac cycle occur with ageing. In fact, the heart fills with blood more slowly in older vs younger healthy individuals, resulting in a lower proportion of total diastolic filling occurring during the passive, early diastolic phase (represented by the "E wave" on echocardiographic study of transmitral flow) owing mainly to an increase in the isovolumic relaxation time. As the bulk of ventricular filling shifts to later diastolic phase (in which an active diastolic filling occurs owing to atrial contraction represented by the "A wave") and there is significant atrial enlargement with ageing, the atrium contributes with a greater portion of the total end diastolic volume. This age-related change results in a decrease in the E/A ratio (Strait & Lakatta, 2012).

Normal exercise induces an increase in stroke volume and heart rate in order to increase overall cardiac output. This increased heart rate also increases the rate of isovolumic relaxation and produces a "suction" effect that helps fill the ventricle. However, these responses are diminished with ageing as a result of slowed relaxation, reduced β-adrenergic responsiveness, and alterations in the pattern of relaxation (Hees *et al.*, 2002; Spina *et al.*, 1998; Tan *et al.*, 2009). Surprisingly, while the rate of filling declines and is shifted to later in diastole, the end diastolic volume actually remains unchanged or increases somewhat with rest and low-level exercise, largely as a result of the slower heart rate (Tarasov *et al.*, 2009), which permits longer filling time and increase in the end systolic volume. Taken together, the reductions in early diastolic filling are partially compensated for by changes in adrenergic signaling that lower the maximal heart rate. However, the compensation mechanisms are not sufficient to maintain cardiac functional reserve when a subject is exposed to maximal exercise. In fact, a significant deficit is uncovered in the older population when the peak-filling rate at maximal exercise is compared between young and old individuals (Strait & Lakatta, 2012).

Interestingly, results from the Baltimore Longitudinal Study of Aging showed that increased visceral adiposity is associated with LV diastolic dysfunction and might explain some of the decline in LV diastolic function that accompanies ageing in healthy individuals. The phenomenon seems to be mediated by a metabolic pathway involving blood lipids and ectopic fat accumulation rather than adipokines (Canepa *et al.*, 2013).

6.1.1.2.3 Changes in cardiac conduction system and in heart rate

Ageing is associated with a generalized increase in elastic and collagenous tissue deposition in various organs. Additionally, ageing favors fat accumulation around the sinoatrial node, sometimes creating a partial or complete separation of the node from atrial tissue. A pronounced decline in the number of pacemaker cells and a variable degree of calcification on the left side of the cardiac skeleton also occurs with ageing. These conditions can impact the atrioventricular node, atrioventricular bifurcation and proximal left and right bundle branches, leading to significant risk of atrioventricular conduction block (North & Sinclair, 2012).

Heart rate modulation is also affected by age with a decrease in both rate variability and maximum heart rate (Antelmi *et al.*, 2004). Heart rate is influenced not only by the loss of cells in the sinoatrial node (responsible for controlling heart rate) but also by structural changes in the heart, including fibrosis and hypertrophy, which slow the propagation of electric impulse throughout the heart (North & Sinclair, 2012).

A number of other changes also occur in the cardiac conduction system that impact on the electrical properties of cardiac tissue in persons without evidence of cardiovascular disease. Such changes include a blunted respiratory sinus arrhythmia, a mild P–R interval prolongation, a leftward shift of the QRS axis, and increased prevalence, density and complexity of ectopic beats, both atrial and ventricular. Although these findings generally do not affect prognosis in clinically healthy older adults, other findings that become more prevalent with age, such as increased QRS voltage, Q waves, QT interval prolongation, and ST-T-wave abnormalities observed in the electrocardiogram, are generally associated with increased cardiovascular risk. Abnormalities such as left-bundle branch block or atrial fibrillation are strongly predictive of future cardiac morbidity and mortality among older adults, even if they are asymptomatic (Strait & Lakatta, 2012).

With ageing a number of cellular changes occur that slow the reactions controlling the beat of the heart as a whole (Lakatta & Sollott, 2002; Janczewski *et al.*, 2002). The action potential, transient increase in cytosolic Ca^{2+}, and rate of contraction of cardiomyocytes are all prolonged, which consequently prolongs systole and diastole of the heart, consistent with the lower maximal heart rate seen in older individuals during exercise (Strait & Lakatta, 2012).

6.1.1.2.4 Cardiac adrenergic responsiveness

Adrenergic signaling is a very important component of age-associated cardiovascular change. Conditions involving physical or psychological stress stimulate sympathetic modulation of this system. It is well known that the action of catecolamines is mediated by adrenergic receptors and that their effects on cardiovascular system include increased heart rate and myocardial contractility force and relaxation, increased cardiac output, reduced LV afterload and increased redistribution of blood to working muscles and skin to dissipate heat. However, with ageing, adrenergic responsiveness is altered and there is a reduction in the autonomic modulation of heart rate, LV contractility and arterial afterload related to the decline in the efficiency of post-synaptic β-adrenergic signaling (Strait & Lakatta, 2012).

In fact, both animal and human studies indicate a decline in heart rate, cardiac contractility, cardiac output and ejection fraction in response to β-adrenergic stimulation and exercise with ageing (Rinaldi *et al.*, 2006; Corbi *et al.*, 2012a, b). Part of the age-related decline in β-adrenergic responsiveness has been attributed to a general decrease in cardiac contractility. However, several observations indicate a crucial role of reduced β-adrenergic receptor density and some defects involving the adenylyl cyclase cascade beyond β-receptor levels (Ferrara *et al.*, 1995; Freedman *et al.*, 1995). In fact, the age-associated reduction in maximal heart rate during high levels of exercise correlates with a reduced β-adrenergic responsiveness to increased circulating levels of catecholamines (Corbi *et al.*, 2013). Ageing is associated with elevated neurohormonal activation, and characterized by elevated plasma catecholamine levels, owing to increased spillover from tissues (including the heart) and reduced plasma clearance (Ng *et al.*, 1993; Esler *et al.*, 1995). The "β-adrenergic desensitization" is, at least in part, due to the reduction of plasma membrane density of β-adrenergic receptors that are members of the G-protein-coupled receptor family, which act by coupling with guanine nucleotide binding proteins, as was described in the hearts of both senescent animals and elderly humans (White *et al.*, 1994, Xiao *et al.*, 1999). In addition to β-adrenergic receptor downregulation, the coupling of the β-adrenergic receptor to adenylyl cyclase via the Gs protein is altered, which leads to a reduction in the ability to increase cyclic adenosine monophosphate (cAMP) and to activate protein kinases. These modifications in adenylyl cyclase activity and ensuing responses are characteristic at molecular level of age-induced decrease in β-adrenoceptor responsiveness. An increase in Gαi subunit activity as well as the upregulation of G protein-coupled receptor kinases might also be possible additional mechanisms in "β-adrenergic desensitization" with ageing (Rengo *et al.*, 2012; Ferrara *et al.*, 2014).

6.1.1.3 Changes in cardioprotective and repair processes

Because of the many factors discussed earlier, the aged heart is placed under increasing levels of stress owing to its diminished functional reserve. Furthermore, increasing age is associated with the augmented occurrence of numerous disease processes (e.g. diabetes, hypertension) that interfere in heart function (Strait & Lakatta, 2012). The heart-protective systems that deal with such insult decline with age, resulting in a lower injury threshold. It is not yet clear if there are interventions that can be instituted in the elderly to delay or reverse these processes, but there are a number of promising candidates, such as physical conditioning, stem cells and ischemic preconditioning.

There is good evidence that regular aerobic exercise can provide improvements in peak oxygen consumption as well as increases in ventilatory threshold and submaximal endurance for older persons with heart failure (Fleg, 2002). Some researchers argue that the rate of cardiomyocyte turnover gradually decreases with ageing from 1% per year at 25 years to 0.45% per year at 75 years of age (Bergmann *et al.*, 2009). Indeed, there has been great interest in utilizing cardiac progenitor cells as a source of myocardial regeneration after injury or degenerative processes.

Ischemic preconditioning is the heart's endogenous capacity to resist ischemic damage and its effects includes suppression of ventricular arrhythmias and enhanced recovery of contractile function. This process is dependent on an initial, brief ischemic event, usually lasting less than 5 minutes. It appears to have both an early protective function lasting about 1 hour after preconditioning and also a late delayed action that returns around 24–96 hours later. Unfortunately, ageing results in decreased effectiveness of ischemic preconditioning and other protective pathways, which leads to a decreased injury threshold in the aged heart (Juhaszova *et al.*, 2005).

6.2 Age-related vascular changes

Rather than acting as simple conduits for blood flow, blood vessels are dynamic structures that adapt, repair, remodel and govern their structural and functional properties using complex signaling pathways in response to load, stress and age (Lakatta & Levy, 2003). In effect, the old aphorism "A man is as old as his arteries", as claimed by Thomas Sydenham (1624–1689), has been widely confirmed by epidemiological and observational studies establishing that cardiovascular diseases can be age-related in terms of their onset and progression (El Assar *et al.*, 2012). In addition, with ageing come a number of recognized physiological and morphological changes that alter vascular function and lead to subsequently increased risk of cardiovascular diseases, even in healthy asymptomatic individuals. Even though different adaptative mechanisms to protect blood vessels against mild stress have been described, the ageing process induces a progressive failure in most of them.

6.2.1 Central arterial changes

Arterial walls are composed of the intima (formed of endothelial cells and elastic lamina) and media (formed of smooth muscle, elastic and connective tissues) layers, and the cells that constitute arteries possess the ability to adapt function in response to injury, atherogenic factors and long-term modifications in hemodynamic conditions (Safar, 2010). Nevertheless, it has been demonstrated by both preclinical and clinical data that ageing is associated with alterations in the structural and functional properties of large arteries. Age-associated arterial changes in apparently healthy humans include luminal dilation, increase in arterial stiffness, intimal-medial thickening and endothelial dysfunction (Lakatta & Levy, 2003; Laurent, 2012; Collins *et al.*, 2014).

6.2.1.1 Arterial structural changes

6.2.1.1.1 Luminal dilatation

Cross-sectional studies show that elastic proximal arteries such as the central aorta and carotid artery dilate with age, leading to an increase in lumen diameter (Lakatta, 1993). Also, the difference in dilatation of the ascending aorta between systole and diastole decreases with age (Martin *et al.*, 2013).

Aortic root dilates modestly with age (approximating 6% between the fourth and eight decades). Similarly, the aortic knob diameter increases from 3.4 to 3.8 cm on average. Recent data suggest that, in individuals with hypertension (when aortic diameter is corrected for covariates), a relative decrease in effective aortic root diameter may contribute to increased load on the heart (Farasat *et al.*, 2008). In normal ageing, however, the aortic root dilatation provides an additional stimulus for LV hypertrophy because the larger volume of blood in the proximal aorta leads to a greater inertial load against which the senescent heart must pump (Strait & Lakatta, 2012).

6.2.1.1.2 Arterial stiffening and thickening

A positive correlation between increasing age and arterial stiffness has been demonstrated by measurements of pulse wave velocity (PWV), b-stiffness index, cardio-ankle vascular index and augmentation index (AI) (O'Rourke & Nichols, 2005; Choi *et al.*, 2013).

Collagen and elastin, normally stabilized by enzymatic crosslinking, provide the strength and elasticity, respectively, of the arterial wall. Age-related physiological changes are associated with a progressive decline in the elastic properties of the arterial wall (Aquaro *et al.*, 2013).

Vascular ageing begins in infancy, although it does not become apparent until middle age. The tunica media gradually stiffens owing to fracturing of elastin fibers and collagenous remodeling (O'Rourke *et al.*, 2010a). The mechanical principle of material fatigue predicts the fracture of the elastic lamella within the tunica media of the vessel after around 1 billion cycles, leading to 8% mean increase in vessel diameter per billion cycles as well, which occurs at approximately 40 years of age. In fact, following the loss of functional interlaminar elastic fibers, the elastic lamellae become further apart, and filled with proteoglycans and altered collagen – which goes from being thin, wavy fibers, to becoming thicker and more linear in arrangement with age (Martin *et al.*, 2013; Fritze *et al.*, 2012). Also, with increased age, a decreased quantity of smooth muscle cells (SMC) is found inside the tunica media, which are responsible for synthesizing elastin within the aorta. Moreover, although tropoelastin (a molecule responsible for forming the protein elastin) is expressed throughout life, its expression is decreased by 50% each decade, demonstrating a decrease in elastin regenerative potential with increasing age (Fritze *et al.*, 2012).

With ageing, the increase in collagen content, the nonenzymatic collagen crosslinking and the fraying of elastin fibrils that occurs in the medial layer reduce arterial distensibility and increase stiffness (Lakatta & Levy, 2003). The occurrence of irreversible nonenzymatic glycation-based crosslinking of collagen to form advanced glycation end-products (AGE) increases with age and is also associated with increased arterial stiffness in elderly people (Semba *et al.*, 2009). Furthermore, receptors for AGE are stimulated to produce a number of inflammatory and stress responses (Strait & Lakatta, 2012).

Aortic compliance is dependent on the ratio of collagen and elastin within the vascular wall. In normal tissue, the ratio of the two components is held relatively constant by a gradual production and degradation process. Collagen and elastin amounts are regulated by the collagenolytic and elastinolytic properties of catabolic matrix metalloproteinases (MMPs). These MMPs are regulated by multiple factors, including augmented gene expression, post-translational activation by the cleavage of pro-MMP protein, by MMP–MMP interactions and by plasmin, thrombin, and reactive oxygen species (ROS). Any alteration in the regulation of this process results in the overproduction of collagen within the artery as well as a reduction in the amount of functional elastin (Collins *et al.*, 2014). These changes result in a greatly stiffened arterial wall with thickened intima and media layers as well as a hypertrophy of SMC.

The increase in arterial wall thickness with age is mainly due to thickening of the media layer independent of atherosclerosis (Virmani *et al.*, 1991; Nagai *et al.*, 1998). This assumption is corroborated by ultrasound imaging cross-sectional studies that have shown that the intimal-medial layer thickens nearly 3-fold between the ages of 20 and 90 years in apparently healthy individuals (Lakatta & Levy, 2003).

6.2.1.1.3 Vascular calcification

Age has been previously identified as a nonmodifiable risk factor for atherosclerosis, but the influence that age has on disease progression is still uncertain (Collins *et al.*, 2014). In line with this, vascular calcification has been noted as a consequence of ageing for many decades. Growing evidence now suggests that vascular calcification, similar to bone remodeling, is an actively regulated process, dependent on both inductive and inhibitory influences (Bostrom *et al.*, 2011).

Although coronary and aortic calcium levels present correlation, and both are found to increase with increasing age, the calcium levels on their own may not affect athero-sclerotic wall burden. In a study of healthy elderly individuals undergoing magnetic resonance imaging, no significant association between atherosclerotic wall burden and aortic or coronary calcium levels, or progression of coronary calcium was found. This suggests that age may be a risk factor on its own pathway, and not dependent on vascular calcification, for atherosclerosis progression (Chen *et al.*, 2013).

6.2.1.1.4 Dimensional variation

The length of the aorta increases with increasing age (Hickson *et al.*, 2010). In particular, the ascending aorta considerably lengthens, which leads to widening of the aortic arch and an overall decrease in curvature (Sugawara *et al.*, 2008; Hickson *et al.*, 2010). This anatomical change in the arch is related to stiffening in the proximal aorta and induces an increase in LV mass (Redheuil *et al.*, 2011). The largest changes in diameter and stiffness occur in the ascending and abdominal aorta, respectively. Aortic stiffness is highest in the portions distal to the heart and decreases proximally, while average aortic diameter shows the inverse relationship. In fact, the diameter increase may function to counteract the increase in wall stiffness (Hickson *et al.*, 2010). A positive correlation between the wall volume of the descending thoracic aorta and age was also found (Chen *et al.*, 2013).

6.2.2 Peripheral arterial changes

In contrast to large vessels, changes in caliber and stiffness are less marked in the peripheral muscular arteries such as the brachial, radial and femoral arteries (Laurent, 2012; Benetos *et al.*, 1993; Boutouyrie *et al.*, 1992). The process of arterial ageing in specific circulation systems, such as cerebral and ocular, is discussed in other chapters of this book.

6.2.3 Arterial functional changes

6.2.3.1 Blood pressure

Arterial blood pressure is determined by the interplay of peripheral vascular resistance (PVR) and arterial stiffness. The concept of stiffness in this setting refers to time-varying cardiac elasticity throughout the cardiac cycle as a result of combined effects of active contractile and "passive" structural properties as well as the interaction of both. Systolic blood pressure (SBP), which is influenced by arterial stiffness, PVR and cardiac function, rises with age even in normotensive cohorts. In contrast, diastolic blood pressure (DBP), rises with increased PVR but is lowered by arterial stiffness, resulting in an increase in diastolic pressure until age 50 years, a leveling off between 50 and 60 years, then a decline after age 60 years (Tanaka *et al.*, 2000; O'Rourke & Nichols, 2005; Martin *et al.*, 2013). Thus, hypertension in the elderly is often characterized by isolated or predominant SBP elevation. Pulse pressure, the difference between SBP and DBP, is a useful clinical index of arterial stiffness and the pulsatile load on the arterial tree, and typically increases with ageing (Strait & Lakatta, 2012).

Central arterial stiffening occurs with ageing even in the absence of clinical hypertension (Vaitkevicius *et al.*, 1993). This condition can be demonstrated by AI determination. In fact, AI illustrates an important site of cardiac–vascular interaction. When the forward pulse wave reaches an area of impedance mismatch (vessel bifurcation or movement to a higher resistance vessel), a reflected wave that travels back up the arterial tree toward the central aorta is generated. This reflected wave is identified as a small notch, an inflection point, in the carotid and radial pulse waveforms, measured by arterial applanation tonometry (Strait & Lakatta, 2012). AI increases until about age 50 years, even in clinically healthy volunteers (Mitchell *et al.*, 2004). The clinical significance of these AI changes with age is that, in young subjects, the reflected wave typically arrives back at the proximal aorta in diastole and may assist in coronary artery diastolic filling. However, in older individuals, the reflected waves travel faster, thus arriving at the proximal aorta during late systole, thereby creating an increased load for the ventricle, a failure to augment DBP, and a potential compromise of coronary blood flow. Several studies in cohorts with cardiovascular disease have observed that higher AI is associated with adverse clinical outcomes (Williams & Lacy, 2010). A second method of arterial stiffness assessment, PWV, is a Doppler-based method that measures the speed with which an arterial pressure wave travels along the arterial tree, typically from the carotid region to the femoral artery. Multiple studies have shown that aortofemoral PWV increases with age, typically 2- to 3-fold across the adult lifespan (Strait & Lakatta, 2012). Furthermore, PWV has been shown in both clinically healthy cohorts and those with cardiovascular disease to be a predictor of future cardiovascular events, independently of blood pressure levels (Najjar *et al.*, 2008).

6.3 Changes in the interaction between heart and arterial system

It is not possible to describe hemodynamic changes associated with ageing without taking cardiac changes into account. In fact, there is a so-called cardiac–arterial coupling process that relies on crosstalk between cardiac function and the general circulation in the arterial tree. With increasing stiffening of the proximal thoracic aorta the reflected wave from the periphery back to the central circulation and the heart can no longer be accommodated. Instead this pulse wave energy will impact on the heart with increased pressure waves and augmentation during systole, leading to increased strain on the left ventricle. This continuous injury causes LV hypertrophy and a decreased perfusion pressure during diastole, leading to impaired blood flow in the coronary circulation. These two trends combined will increase the risk of morphological changes (LV hypertrophy) in combination with coronary ischemia, thus increasing the risk of coronary heart disease events. This is therefore a hemodynamic mechanism explaining some of the risk potential of arterial stiffness, as measured by increased PWV, for the development of coronary heart disease (Nilsson, 2014). It contributes to what has been called by O'Rourke, Safar and Dzau the "cardiovascular ageing continuum", which supports the independent association between chronological ageing and risk of cardiovascular disease (O'Rourke *et al.*, 2010b).

6.4 Endothelial dysfunction

A healthy endothelium maintains vascular tone and structure by regulating the balance between vasodilatation and vasoconstriction, growth inhibition and growth promotion, antithrombosis and prothrombosis, anti-inflammation and proinflammation, and also anti-oxidation and pro-oxidation. Ageing strongly contributes to endothelial dysfunction onset, as evidenced by the attenuation of endothelium-dependent vasodilatation observed in elderly subjects and animal models (Zeiher *et al.*, 1993; Safar *et al.*, 2001). Furthermore, age-related endothelial dysfunction leads to the pathogenesis, maintenance and development of atherosclerosis.

Several possible mechanisms by which advancing age impairs endothelial function are postulated. An imbalance between nitric oxide (NO) and ROS, related to oxidative stress, should be a key regulator of age-induced endothelial dysfunction. In fact, ageing activates nicotinamide adenine dinucleotide phosphate (NADPH) oxidase, xantine oxidase, cyclooxygenase and mitochondrial electron transport and inactivates the anti-oxidant system, including superoxide dismutase (SOD), glutathione peroxidase and catalase, leading to an increase in ROS production and a decrease in ROS degradation. First, ROS directly inhibit NO activity. In addition, ROS activate the PI3K/Ras/Akt/MAPK (phosphatidylinositol 3′ kinase/rat sarcoma/Akt/mitogen-activated protein kinase) pathway, related to redox transcription factors control, leading to redox-sensitive gene expression, which results in inhibition of endothelial NO synthase (eNOS) mRNA expression and reduced eNOS activity. Moreover, oxidation of tetrahydrobiopterin (BH4) by ROS induces eNOS uncoupling, which leads to a shift in eNOS activity that increases production of ROS rather than NO. In fact, under the oxidative stress conditions, BH4 predominantly promotes superoxide synthesis, leading further to peroxynitrite ($ONOO^-$) formation (Rodriguez-Crespo *et al.*, 1997; Kaufman, 1993).

Age-associated damage of the endothelium may not simply be a consequence of the endothelial cell malfunctioning, but also the result of impaired maintenance repair systems by endothelial progenitor cells (EPCs) (El Assar *et al.*, 2012; Williamson *et al.*, 2012). A deterioration of endogenous EPC function with age may culminate in a decreased capacity for neovascularization and/or reduced re-endothelinization of vascular lesions, facilitating the development, progression and clinical sequelae of cardiovascular disease (Williamson *et al.*, 2012). Hill *et al.* (2003) have shown that the number of EPCs is decreased in relation to the cumulative number of Framingham risk factors and that the number of EPCs is correlated with endothelial function measured by flow-mediated vasodilatation. In the early stage of endothelial dysfunction, impaired endothelial cells could be repaired by bone-marrow-derived EPCs. A decrease in the number of EPCs in bone marrow or inhibition of EPC mobilization may indeed contribute to progression of endothelial dysfunction. Additionally, Werner *et al.* (2005) suggest that the number of EPCs is a predictor of cardiovascular events. Several investigators have also shown a significant relationship between the number of EPCs and endothelial function in patients with cardiovascular diseases and even in normal subjects (Hill *et al.*, 2003; Umemura *et al.*, 2008). Multiple regression analysis has shown that age and hypertension are independent predictors of the number of EPCs. Experimental and clinical studies have clearly shown that excessive oxidative stress decreases the number of EPCs and impairs EPC function (Murasawa *et al.*, 2002; Ballard & Edelberg, 2007; Ballard, 2010). Under oxidative stress, age-associated decrease in NO bioavailability and decrease in the number of EPCs and EPC mobilization may form a vicious circle and lead to endothelial dysfunction (Higashi *et al.*, 2012).

After tissue injury, endothelial cells lose their ability to proliferate and migrate (Brandes *et al.*, 2005). Furthermore, endothelial barriers become porous and vascular SMC migrate into subendothelial spaces and deposit extracellular matrix proteins that result in intimal thickening (Strait & Lakata, 2012). Finally, the process of endothelial cell senescence itself may also play a critical role in endothelial dysfunction associated with ageing.

Telomere length in endothelial cells from human aortas and arteries shortens in an age-dependent fashion (Zhu *et al.*, 2011; Okuda *et al.*, 2000). Concomitantly with decreases in both NO production and eNOS activity in human umbilical vein endothelial cells (HUVEC) and human aortic endothelial cells (HAECs) (Sato *et al.*, 1993; Matsushita *et al.*, 2001). In agreement, several lines of evidence have shown that eNOS activity and NO production are decreased in senescent endothelial cells (Hayashi *et al.*, 2008; Farsetti *et al.*, 2009). Matsushita *et al.* (2001) demonstrated that shear stress-induced increase in NO production was diminished in senescent HAECs and that stable expression of telomerase reverse transcriptase (TERT) not only increased the chromosome telomeres length, but also restored decreased eNOS expression and NO production associated with ageing. In line with this, Minamino *et al.* (2002) reported that HAECs from human atherosclerotic lesions presented a phenotype of senescent cells and decrease in eNOS expression and eNOS activity. The introduction of TERT extended the life span and reversed endothelial functional alteration associated with senescence in HAECs. Interestingly, exogenous NO reduced HUVEC senescence and delayed age-dependent inhibition of telomerase activity, suggesting that telomerase inactivation precedes endothelial cell senescence and that NO prevents age-related downregulation of telomerase activity and delays endothelial cell senescence (Vasa *et al.*, 2000). Additionally, telomere lengths in white blood cells shorten in parallel with a decline in endothelial function in patients with various degrees of cardiovascular damage as well as in healthy subjects (Nakashima *et al.*, 2004). In brief, the process of endothelial dysfunction associated with ageing in relation to endothelial cell senescence is postulated to be as follows. Ageing activates NADPH oxidase, xantine oxidase, cyclooxygenase and mitochondrial electron transport and inactivate the anti-oxidant system, leading to an increase in ROS production and a decrease in ROS degradation. ROS induce the export of nuclear TERT into the cytosol through activation of Src-family kinases. Loss of nuclear TERT activity shortens telomere length, leading to a decrease in the endothelial cells lifespan, alteration in gene expression and a change from the phenotype of young cells to that of senescent cells. In addition, telomere shortening stimulates activation of p53, p21 and p16 proteins, which are triggers of cell senescence. The endogenous eNOS inhibitor asymmetrical dimethylarginine also accelerates endothelial cell senescence through an increase in production of ROS and inhibition of NO production. An imbalance between NO and ROS may be the initial step and may also play an important role in endothelial cell senescence, which results in endothelial dysfunction through various pathways (Higashi *et al.*, 2012).

6.5 Erectile dysfunction as an early signal of cardiovascular disease

Ageing constitutes an important risk factor for atherosclerosis even in healthy individuals (Michos *et al.*, 2009; Chen *et al.*, 2013). Owing to its systemic nature, atherosclerosis affects all vascular beds. However, the age-related loss of function does not manifest to the same extent in different vessels, and neither do the symptoms become evident at the same time in the organs. The manifestation of vascular impairment strongly depends on the vessel diameter. Supporting this, Montorsi *et al.* (2005) enunciated the "Artery Size Hypothesis" that states that small diameter arteries, such as those of the penis, manifest symptoms of dysfunction earlier, owing to the high percentage of lumen obstruction compared with larger vessels. In fact, among the vascular beds of the organism, the penile artery will be more narrowed by an equivalent amount of atherosclerotic plaque than coronary or carotid arteries, which present two or three times the diameter. The artery size hypothesis also demonstrated that erectile dysfunction (ED), defined as the inability to develop and maintain an erection for satisfactory sexual intercourse or activity, and systemic cardiovascular disease constitute two manifestations of the same disease, which was supported by the demonstration that ED is related to the clinical presentation and extent of coronary artery disease, and, that it manifests in patients before coronary artery disease by an average of 2–3 years (Montorsi *et al.*, 2006).

Currently, ED is considered an early manifestation of atherosclerosis and systemic cardiovascular disease, and every man who complains of ED should be considered at risk of cardiovascular disease by the clinicians until proven otherwise (Cheitlin, 2004; Jackson *et al.*, 2013). Interestingly, the structural modifications induced by nutritional patterns in erectile tissue seem to be more easily reversed than those observed in the heart, as demonstrated in rodents submitted to energy restriction (ER) after one year of regular consumption of a high-fat diet (Tomada *et al.*, 2013a). In line with this, it was reported that erectile function could be completely restored in patients by changing dietary habits, losing body weight or exercising (Esposito *et al.*, 2004), supporting the hypothesis that, despite loss of function manifesting earlier than in other organs, it is more responsive to external factors. Erectile dysfunction could be indeed considered a sentinel of vascular health, presenting when damage can still be reversed. In addition, the interventions available to improve erectile function may also ameliorate overall vascular health.

6.5.1 The erection mechanism

The penis is a highly vascularized organ. Two *corpora cavernosa* (CC) separated by an incomplete septum and constituted by erectile tissue extend along the length of the penis and fill with blood during erection, which significantly increases their volume. *Corpus cavernosum* presents a sponge-like texture, exhibiting a mesh of interconnected cavernous sinusoidal spaces, lined by endothelium and separated by trabeculae composed mainly of smooth muscle and connective tissue (collagen fibers and fibroblasts). Morphometric analysis after observation by transmission electron microscopy demonstrated that cavernous tissue in young men comprises 30% connective tissue and 50% SMC organized in long contractile fibers distributed within trabeculae. Ageing induces important modifications in cavernous tissue organization, leading to an inversion in the proportion of connective tissue relative to the SMC content (Tomada *et al.*, 2008).

The development of an erection is a complex event involving the integration of psychological, neurological, endocrine, vascular and local anatomic systems. In brief, sexual arousal is activated in higher cortical centers, which then stimulate the medial preoptic and paraventricular nuclei of the hypothalamus. These signals descend through an intricate neural network involving the parasympathetic nervous system and eventually activate terminations in the sacral area. The stimulus results in the inhibition of adrenergic tone and in the release of NO that is believed to originate from nerves and endothelial cells, synthesized by neuronal NO synthase (nNOS) and eNOS, respectively. It is thought that, while NO produced by nNOS only intervenes in the initiation of penile erection, NO generated by eNOS participates in the sustained erection required for normal sexual performance (Burnett *et al.*, 1996). However, it was recently reported that nNOS-derived NO is also produced throughout the erectile process (Hurt *et al.*, 2012). NO easily diffuses from nerves or endothelium to other cells, and subsequently, stimulates the enzyme guanylate cyclase in penile smooth muscle that converts guanosine triphosphate to cyclic guanosine monophosphate (cGMP). The increase in cGMP levels results in activation of protein kinase G and further decrease in intracellular calcium owing to promotion of its efflux, which triggers the relaxation of arterial and trabecular smooth muscle. Vasodilatation enhances arterial blood flow into the lacunar spaces of the penis, which increases intracavernous pressure by a veno-oclusion mechanism that consists of compression of the subtunical venules against the tunica albuginea and entrapment of the blood in CC. These coordinated actions establish the penis erection with adequate firmness for sexual activity (Ignarro *et al.*, 1990).

6.5.2 Contribution of ageing to erectile dysfunction onset

Both endothelium, which produces most of the NO in response to shear stress owing to increased blood flow to the CC, and SMCs, which support vasodilatation, play crucial roles in the erectile process. The erectile mechanism is thus particularly sensitive to endothelial structural and functional changes in sinusoidal small vessels of the penis (Kaya *et al.*, 2006). In fact, endothelium-dependent inability to induce vasodilatation – endothelial dysfunction – underlies the most prevalent form of ED, vasculogenic ED, which directly results from vascular disease of the penile arteries or failure of the corporal veno-occlusive or sinusoidal relax mechanisms (Shamloul & Ghanem, 2013). In line with this, age-associated ED is strongly associated with a decrease in bioavailability of NO, mainly through downregulation of eNOS activity (Garban *et al.*, 1995). Supporting this, an elegant study in 25-month-old rats demonstrated that treatment with cells transduced with adenovirus containing eNOS gene increased cGMP levels in penile tissue and improved erectile function (Bivalacqua *et al.*, 2007a). The contribution of endothelial dysfunction to ED onset is sufficiently relevant for these conditions to be considered equivalent by some authors (Goldstein, 2003; Guay, 2007).

Structural modifications in erectile tissue, such as those observed in the elderly (Tomada *et al.*, 2008, 2013b), also contribute to ED, which in part explains the age-related increase in the prevalence of this disorder. In fact, according to the Massachusetts Male Ageing Study, there is a global prevalence of 52% of any degree of ED in the male population, but while at 40 years approximately 40% of men are affected, the rate increases to nearly 70% in men aged 70 years (Feldman *et al.*, 1994). In addition, the prevalence of complete ED increases from 5 to 15% as age increases from 40 to 70 years. Corroborating this data, it was recently reported that age is the independent variable most strongly associated with ED (Ghalayini *et al.*, 2010). Nevertheless, the direct causes of age-dependent ED are poorly understood and likely to be multifactorial in origin. A European survey performed in 2005 demonstrated that, in addition to ageing, diabetes mellitus and hypertension are the most important risk factors for the development of ED (Ponholzer *et al.*, 2005). Corroborating these findings, the Global Online Sexuality Survey, an epidemiologic study based on validated questionnaires with applied age adjustment, reinforced diabetes mellitus, hypertension with and without antihypertensive treatment, coronary heart disease, obesity (defined by body mass index) and also psychological causes as serial risk factors for ED (Shaeer & Shaeer, 2013). Interestingly, alcohol consumption was not associated with higher prevalence of ED.

Analyzing together the conclusions of these important appraisals, it becomes clear that ED shares its chief risk factors with cardiovascular disease, which supports the common etiology of these disorders. In fact, this is generally accepted taking into account that endothelial dysfunction often precedes atherosclerosis formation, which is the basis of systemic cardiovascular disease (Lusis, 2000).

6.5.2.1 Age-related structural and molecular modifications of erectile tissue

The reasons why chronological ageing constitutes a main risk factor for ED and increases its severity remain to be completely elucidated, but unavoidable age-associated changes might contribute to the onset of this type of vascular disease. Ageing is strongly associated with an increase in oxidative stress (Stadtman, 1992; discussed in Chapter 1). In particular, an age-related increase in oxidative stress was demonstrated in the cavernous tissue of the rodent associated with a decrease in intracavernous pressure (Johnson *et al.*, 2011). The increase in cavernous oxidative stress strongly associates with fibrosis (Azadzoi *et al.*, 2005), which is aligned with our previous findings that demonstrated an increase in connective tissue proportion in erectile tissue of rodent and human origin throughout ageing (Cordeiro *et al.*, 2008; Tomada *et al.*, 2008, 2013a, b). However, the deleterious effects of oxidative stress are broader and affect erectile function in multiple ways (Jones *et al.*, 2002). First, oxidative stress favors superoxide anion formation, which is reported to have a direct vasoconstriction effect that potentially leads to ED (Katusic &

Vanhoutte, 1989). Second, it compromises NO bioavailability, in part because NO reacts with superoxide anion forming peroxynitrite, which directly decreases cGMP levels and impairs cavernosal smooth muscle relaxation, which is necessary to erectile function (Silva *et al.*, 2013). Third, oxidative stress is involved in formation of AGE (Baraibar *et al.*, 2012), which also induce oxidative stress (Higashi et al., 2009), constituting a deleterious vicious cycle that highly compromises normal erectile function. In fact, AGE upregulate the expression and activity of NADPH oxidase, an important source of vascular oxidative stress (Christ *et al.*, 2002) and decrease expression of enzymes involved in anti-oxidant systems, such as Mn-SOD (Su *et al.*, 2008). In addition, AGE directly reduce cellular NO bioavailability (Bucala *et al.*, 1992), which is negatively associated with the extent of endothelium-dependent vasodilatation (Sena *et al.*, 2012), by repression of mRNA expression coupled to downregulation of eNOS activity through modulation of phosphorylation of positive regulatory serine residues (Ser-1177) and negative regulatory threonine site (Thr-495) and uncoupling of the enzyme (Su *et al.*, 2008; Xu *et al.*, 2005). Furthermore, AGE are able to antagonize NO function by upregulating the expression of the vasoconstrictor endothelin-1 in endothelial cells (Quehenberger *et al.*, 2000). The increase in AGE adduct formation in tissues and serum is strongly associated with chronological ageing (Baraibar *et al.*, 2012; Jiaan *et al.*, 1995; Hipkiss, 2006; Schöneich, 2006). AGE formation progresses slowly along time and occurs predominantly on long-lived proteins, such as extracellular matrix proteins, which present a slow turnover. Over a person's lifespan the amount of AGE-modified tissue gradually increases, partly owing to the accumulation of AGE-modified proteins that resists to proteolytic degradation inside the cells, making it possible to estimate the "age" of any protein by its degree of AGE modification. Fourth, oxidative stress favors irreversible oxidation of proteins in parallel with glycation. Direct oxidation of proteins frequently results in carbonyl groups formation, also existing in AGE adducts. Similarly to AGE-modified compounds, oxidized proteins present abnormal conformations that result in the loss of native structure and catalytic activity, and are unable to exert their functions and to interact with target molecules, hence affecting the normal function of nonmodified proteins. Once formed, AGE adducts and carbonylated proteins accelerate the process of tissue deterioration. In fact, *in silico* approaches strongly suggest that carbonylated proteins and AGE are likely to be implicated in the molecular basis of ageing and age-associated diseases (Baraibar *et al.*, 2012).

The mechanisms by which AGE and oxidized proteins affect the *corpus cavernosum* and erectile function are complex (reviewed in Neves, 2013) and include modification of extracellular matrix characteristics and intercellular adhesion pattern, partly owing to increased collagen crosslinking, which favors its deposition in connective tissue (a hallmark of dysfunctional erectile tissue). Vascular wall thickening owing to AGE-modified collagen and decreased elasticity result in AGE modification of elastin, physically decreasing the extensibility of the erectile tissue and thus contributing to its dysfunction, as described earlier. AGE also leads to the trapping of macromolecules such as lipoproteins in the vessel wall owing to modifications in extracellular matrix proteins, which results in the accumulation of perivascular amorphous hyalinized material and favors atheroma formation (Knott *et al.*, 2003). In addition, subendothelial AGE adducts identified in atherosclerotic plaques (Harja *et al.*, 2008) are chemotactic for monocytes, which allows their migration through the endothelial monolayer and secretion of inflammatory molecules (Kirstein *et al.*, 1990). Monocyte-secreted products induce proliferation of

SMC, as demonstrated in a co-culture system with monocytes, endothelial cells and SMC that revealed synergistic effects of AGE on intercellular interactions implicated in the onset of atherosclerosis (Nam *et al.*, 2011). However, our studies indicate that the global content of SMCs density in human cavernous tissue significantly decreases with ageing (Tomada *et al.*, 2008, 2013b). Considering that smooth muscle fiber distribution in cavernous tissue of human origin is not restricted to the endothelium periphery, the age-associated fibrosis is apparently superimposed on the AGE-induced proliferative effects on SMCs. Nevertheless, returning to the previous observation of foam cells of muscle origin in erectile tissue of aged rats, the influence of age (and AGE) in atherosclerosis progression in the penis vessels seems relevant (Neves *et al.*, 2008).

The production and accumulation of AGE in cavernous tissue thus constitute a possible explanation for age-related increased ED risk. Supporting that, higher levels of AGE products, namely the fluorescent pentose-mediated protein crosslink pentosidine, have been detected in the CC of aged patients (Jiaan *et al.*, 1995).

Decrease in NO bioavailability in CC is affected by an increase in oxidative stress and by accumulation of AGE adducts. However, other molecular modifications that are associated with ageing also contribute to NO decay, such as an increase in the expression and activity of arginase, an enzyme that competes with NOS for the substrate L-arginine, and downregulation of nNOS activity, as demonstrated in experimental models of mouse and rabbit, respectively (Bivalacqua *et al.*, 2007b; Numao *et al.*, 2007). The physiological decay in angiogenic capability also contributes to the failure of NO production (Rivard *et al.*, 1999), considering that vascular endothelial growth factor (VEGF) induces NO synthesis through activation of eNOS (Gelinas *et al.*, 2002; Musicki *et al.*, 2005). VEGF is the main vascular growth factor in tissues and induces the proliferation and survival of endothelial cells *in vivo* (Ferrara & Davis-Smyth, 1997) after engagement of its specific tyrosine kinase receptor vascular endothelial growth factor receptor 2 (VEGFR2). In fact, most of the downstream effects normally attributed to VEGF result from VEGFR2 activation (Ferrara *et al.*, 2003). Expression of both VEGF and VEGFR2 decrease in the CC of the rodent and human (Neves *et al.*, 2006; Tomada *et al.*, 2010), and apparently are compensated for by other vascular growth factors such as angiopoietins, which crosstalk with VEGF in tissues (Cordeiro *et al.*, 2010; Neves *et al.*, 2010). The equilibrium among angiogenic factors contributes to vascular remodeling and repair, and their imbalance is associated with endothelium dysfunction, atherosclerosis and ED. In fact, local administration of the protein or gene of VEGF alone or in association with other angiogenic factors has been shown to restore erectile function in ED experimental models of hypercholesterolemia (Burchardt *et al.*, 2005; Ryu *et al.*, 2006).

During the ageing process, increased production of inflammatory cytokines and cell adhesion molecules such as E-selectin, intracellular adhesion molecule and vascular cell adhesion molecule was also found in rats (Tomada *et al.*, 2014), as well as a physiological decay in total testosterone levels. Low levels of testosterone, in particular, might contribute to the onset of ED (Feldman *et al.*, 2002), considering its important involvement in nearly every phase of male reproductive development and the erectile process, from pelvic ganglions to SMCs and endothelial cells of the CC. Testosterone engages androgen receptors on the target cell membrane and migrates to the nucleus, where it may exert genomic effects by upregulating expression of both androgen receptor and VEGF (Cai *et al.*, 2011). Androgens indeed modulate endothelial function and endothelial cell proliferation through VEGF action, and also play an important role in the development and maturation of EPCs, which as previously described, intervene in the repair of endothelial injury in vascular beds (Traish & Galoosian, 2013). It is also recognized that testosterone exhibits a direct vasodilatory action on the vascular smooth muscle (Jones *et al.*, 2003) owing to upregulation of cavernous NO synthesis (Reilly *et al.*, 1997). In line with this, hypogonadism leads to alterations in the erectile tissue equivalent to those observed in the elderly, such as reduction of SMC content in the penis coupled with an increase in connective tissue content and an increase in the caliber of vascular spaces (Tomada *et al.*, 2013b). Testosterone administration to hypogonadal men with ED strongly ameliorates erectile function by improving veno-occlusion (Yassin *et al.*, 2006).

6.6 Diet, nutrition and cardiovascular ageing

6.6.1 Obesity, energy restriction and cardiovascular ageing

Animal and human studies have shown that obesity adversely affects many of the risk factors for cardiovascular diseases and contributes to an increased rate of cardiovascular disease and reduced life expectancy (Everitt *et al.*, 2006; Fontana & Hu, 2014). Moreover, chronic overnutrition can cause cardiac insulin resistance, activation of the tissue renin–angiotensin–aldosterone system, mitochondrial uncoupling, impaired fatty acid metabolism, enhanced oxidative stress and endoplasmic reticulum stress in the heart. These conditions lead to structural and functional changes initially characterized by impaired diastolic relaxation, which can progress to heart failure (Mandavia *et al.*, 2012).

A 20–40% reduction in energy intake has been consistently shown to increase lifespan and to prevent the development of age-associated cardiovascular functional and structural changes in several model organisms (Haddad *et al.*, 1993; Taffet *et al.*, 1997; Guo *et al.*, 2002; Castello *et al.*, 2005; Seymour *et al.*, 2006; Mager *et al.*, 2006; Colman *et al.*, 2009; Fontana *et al.*, 2010). In particular, dietary restriction or ER has been shown to improve arterial flow-mediated vasodilatation (Dolinsky *et al.*, 2010; Rippe *et al.*, 2010) and to delay the development of atherosclerotic lesions in rodents (Guo *et al.*, 2002). Energy restriction significantly ameliorates LV diastolic function of the ageing heart and reduces arterial stiffness (Taffet *et al.*, 1997; Castello *et al.*, 2005; Seymour *et al.*, 2006; Dolinsky *et al.*, 2010). Moreover, long-term ER has been shown to improve autonomic function and, in particular, to increase the high-frequency component of the heart rate variability spectra, a marker for parasympathetic activity in rats (Mager *et al.*, 2006). Finally, long-term ER has a powerful effect in preventing/delaying the age-related increase in the severity of cardiomyopathy in rodents as well as in monkeys (Colman *et al.*, 2009; Fontana *et al.*, 2012).

There are a number of hypotheses regarding the mechanisms by which ER mediates its beneficial effects on ageing in lower organisms that could have relevance to slowing cardiovascular ageing in humans (discussed in Chapter 2). These include a decrease in chronic inflammation, a reduction in the levels of various hormones and growth factors, an increased resistance to oxidative stress, and an increase in anti-oxidant defense mechanisms (Fontana & Klein, 2007). The protection from free radical-induced tissue damage is conferred, at least in part, by the ER-mediated reduction in growth factor signaling. In the long-lived dwarf, growth hormone receptor-knockout, klotho transgenic and p66shc/ mice, the suppression of intracellular mitogenic signaling pathways increases the expression of ROS scavenging enzymes, such as catalase and SOD, thereby facilitating removal of these toxic oxygen species (Murakami, 2006). Also, human cells exposed to insulin-like growth factor 1 (IGF-1)-deficient human serum are more protected against oxidative DNA damage (Guevara-Aguirre *et al.*, 2011). In the heart of rats, these ER-dependent effects lead to a decrease in oxidative stress and an improved functional recovery after ischemia (Gredilla *et al.*, 2011; Colom *et al.*, 2007; Shinmura *et al.*, 2011). These effects as well as the reduced heart hypertrophy in ageing rats may be attributable to improvements in mitochondrial function (Niemann *et al.*, 2010). In fact, ER is a well-known intervention to delay the deterioration of mitochondrial respiratory function, the main source of ROS, by preserving enzymatic activities of the electron transport system and controlling proton leak (Ash & Merry, 2011). The protection against inflammation-mediated tissue damage and age-associated deterioration in immune function may also play an important role in preventing or delaying cardiovascular ageing, because it could lower the levels of inflammatory cytokines and oxidative stress involved in cardiovascular disease progression (Lee *et al.*, 2011). In fact, ER has been shown to lower the circulating levels of inflammatory cytokines [e.g. interleukin and tumor necrosis factor-alpha (TNF-α)] and to increase plasma adiponectin and cortisol concentration (Jolly, 2004; Fontana *et al.*, 2012). In addition, ER simultaneously affects multiple processes that are involved in cardiovascular ageing, including efficient removal of damaged proteins, oxidized lipids and lipoproteins, decreased protein glycation and collagen crosslinking, effects that suggest the involvement of autophagy (Cefalu *et al.*, 1995; Leeuwenburgh *et al.*, 1997; Sell *et al.*, 2003; Fontana *et al.*, 2012). Long-term ER in human volunteers, who call themselves CRONies (i.e. Calorie Restriction with Optimal Nutrition), causes profound reductions in several cardiometabolic risk factors for coronary heart disease, including lowering of total cholesterol, low-density-lipoprotein (LDL) cholesterol and triglycerides, and a large increase in high-density-lipoprotein (HDL) cholesterol concentrations. These individuals also present lower fasting glycemia, lower insulin resistance index, and considerably lower SBP and DBP levels (Fontana *et al.*, 2004; Fontana & Klein, 2007). Long-term ER in humans also has a powerful anti-inflammatory effect reflected by very low circulating levels of C-reactive protein and TNF-α. This decrease in systemic inflammation and other cardiometabolic markers is accompanied by a significantly lower thickness of the carotid artery intima-media thickness and by an improved LV diastolic function in the ER individuals compared with the age- and sex-matched control group (Fontana *et al.*, 2004; Meyer *et al.*, 2006). However, it is possible that some of the beneficial effects on the cardiometabolic risk factors are due not entirely to ER, but also to the high-quality diets consumed by the ER practioners. All of the CRONies have eliminated from their diets refined and processed foods containing salt, trans-fatty acids, dietary glyco-toxins and high-glycemic-index foods (e.g. refined carbohydrates, potato, white rice, sucrose- and fructose-enriched foods). They consume, instead, a wide variety of vegetables, low-glycemic-index fruit, nuts, low-fat dairy products, egg whites, wheat and soy proteins, fish and lean meat. Interestingly, men and women consuming energy-unrestricted strict vegan diets also have extremely low blood pressure, LDL cholesterol, triglycerides and fasting glucose concentrations, suggesting that the quality of the diet plays a major role in modulating blood pressure, lipid and glucose metabolism (Fontana *et al.*, 2007). Nevertheless, unlike in the CRONies, serum HDL-cholesterol and adiponectin concentrations were not significantly increased in these vegetarians and serum concentration of fasting insulin, TNF-α and triiodothyronine were higher than in age- and sex-matched individuals practicing ER. Short-term alternate-day fasting has also been shown to result in some beneficial cardiometabolic adaptations in obese individuals eating typical Western diets during the nonfasting days, including a reduction in body weight, blood pressure and serum cholesterol and triglycerides concentrations, but HDL-cholesterol, C-reactive protein and homocysteine concentrations did not change (Varady *et al.*, 2009; Bhutani *et al.*, 2010; Rizza *et al.*, 2013).

Recent studies have provided evidence for the role of the inactivation of growth hormone and IGF-I signaling pathways in the protective effects of ER on cellular resistance and ageing. In agreement with this, downregulation of the insulin/IGF-I pathway slows ageing and protects against several metabolic alterations that promote cardiovascular disease. However, the role of growth factors in modulating age-associated cardiovascular dysfunction has not been clearly defined (Fontana *et al.*, 2012).

Mechanisms that may underlie the beneficial effects of ER on vessel ageing include the preservation of extracellular matrix components within the vessel wall (Fornieri *et al.*, 1999), improvement of endothelial cell function through augmenting NO generation, reduction of sensitivity to oxidized LDL, reduction of oxidative stress by upregulating anti-oxidants and protection of mitochondria function (Yang *et al.*, 2004; Ungvari *et al.*, 2008; Shinmura, 2011; Dai *et al.*, 2012), and inhibition of inflammation (Csiszar *et al.*, 2009). Although ER may be inappropriate for many patients, drugs and dietary supplements that mimic ER effects without affecting nutritional balance may offer a wider therapeutic option (discussed in Chapter 2).

Sirtuins (Sirt 1–7) are a family of nicotinamide adenine dinucleotide (NAD^+)-dependent deacetylases and adenosine diphosphate–ribosyltransferases that may be partially responsible for the age-delaying effects of ER. Sirtuins have been reviewed in Chapter 2; therefore, only limited discussion is provided here. ER increases Sirt1 in some experimental models, leading to improved endothelial function (Rippe *et al.*, 2010; Zanetti *et al.*, 2010) while knocking down Sirt1 interferes with the ER-mediated anti-oxidant and anti-inflammatory vascular effects (Csiszar *et al.*, 2009). Similar to ER, over-expression of Sirt1 in the endothelium can improve vascular stiffness and attenuate the development of atherosclerosis, probably by activating eNOS, promoting NO production (Zhang *et al.*, 2008; Mattagajasingh *et al.*, 2007) and preventing endothelial cell senescence (Ota *et al.*, 2007). Indeed, Sirt1 deacetylation of eNOS may contribute to the atheroprotective effects of laminar stress (Chen *et al.*, 2010). Moreover, other sirtuin members, such as Sirt 3–5, may be protective in cardiovascular system as sensors of nutritional status, regulating the cellular response to stress, energy production, apoptosis and ROS production (Ahn *et al.*, 2008; Verdin *et al.*, 2010; Hafner *et al.*, 2010).

6.6.2 Diet patterns and cardiovascular ageing

Changes in lifestyle habits, such as diet and moderate exercise, can influence vascular repair mechanisms. Different studies have shown that a healthy diet and exercise induce a reduction of cell damage and endothelial dysfunction, both of which are factors responsible for reducing cardiovascular risk in the elderly (Yubero-Serrano *et al.*, 2011; Klonizakis *et al.*, 2012). The Mediterranean diet is a healthy diet that includes fish, vegetables, fruit, whole grains, legumes, olive oil and less red meat and dairy products, consumption of which has been associated with lower risk of cardiovascular disease (discussed in Chapter 11). In addition, several intervention studies have suggested that the consumption of flavonoid-rich foods such as tea, red wine (Dal-Ros *et al.*, 2012), cocoa and soya can improve endothelial function in patients with manifest cardiovascular disease (Zuchi *et al.*, 2010; Chiva-Blanch *et al.*, 2012). The Mediterranean diet significantly attenuates the postprandial inflammatory state, including nuclear factor kappa-light-chain-enhancer of activated B cells, MMP-9 and TNF-α (Cruz-Teno *et al.*, 2012; Scoditti *et al.*, 2012). In addition, consumption of a Mediterranean diet and exercise led to a greater decrease in blood pressure and a greater increase in the number of EPCs compared with the same diet without exercise (Fernandez *et al.*, 2012). The repair or prevention effects of Mediterranean diet in ageing have also been attributed to the presence of anti-oxidants, mainly contained in plant foods such as fruit, vegetables, whole grains, nuts and seeds (Marin *et al.*, 2013). Similarly, studies performed in elderly people have demonstrated that the consumption of a Mediterranean diet produces an increase in NO bioavailability, with a consequent improvement in endothelium-dependent endothelial function (Yubero-Serrano *et al.*, 2011). It is also associated with an improvement in endothelial regeneration capacity, producing an increased number of circulating EPCs and lower levels of endothelial cell microparticles compared with the consumption of a saturated fatty acid-rich diet and a low-fat and high-carbohydrate diet enriched with α-linoleic acid (Marin *et al.*, 2011, 2012; Fernandez *et al.*, 2012). An improvement in lifestyle habits is also positively correlated with telomere length. In fact, telomere length has been associated with nutritional status in both human and animal models. A healthy lifestyle, with a diet high in fruit and vegetables combined with exercise, the maintenance of low body mass and no smoking, is associated with longer telomeres (Mirabello *et al.*, 2009). Similarly, there is evidence to show the effect of the quality and quantity of dietary fat on telomere length, depending on the degree of oxidative stress that these diets produce. Therefore, the consumption of a saturated fatty acid-rich diet or a carbohydrate-rich diet induces telomere attrition, as a result of cell replication, which can be accelerated by the presence of increased oxidative stress (Marin *et al.*, 2011). However, the consumption of a Mediterranean-type diet (monounsaturated fat-rich diet), rich in virgin olive oil, improves this profile and leads to a reduction in the degree of oxidative stress (Yubero-Serrano *et al.*, 2011) and a decrease in the rate of telomere shortening (Marin *et al.*, 2012, 2013).

6.6.2.1 Contribution of dietary pattern to erectile dysfunction onset

In addition to chronological ageing, lifestyle and nutrition have also been increasingly recognized as central factors influencing erectile function. Exercise is the lifestyle factor most strongly correlated with erectile function through the increase in NO production owing to mechanical shear forces of blood flow (Meldrum *et al.*, 2010). Concerning nutritional habits, the Western diet pattern, which includes meat, poultry, dairy products and refined grains, and normally presents high contents of sucrose and saturated fat, has been adopted in industrialized countries in recent decades. The adoption of this diet pattern relates to an increase in obesity and cardiovascular disease prevalence. Supporting the contribution of the Western diet to cardiovascular disease and ED onset, La Favor *et al.* (2013) analyzed the endothelial-dependent and independent vasodilatation of coronary artery and erectile response to electric stimulus of rats treated for 4–12 weeks with a mimetic of Western diet (high sugar, high saturated fat and high level of omega-6 derived from linoleic acid). They did not find differences regarding body weight or composition; however, intracavernous pressure was significantly attenuated in response to electric stimulus following 8 or 12 weeks of Western diet. The authors of this study concluded that regular consumption of a Western diet (and not features secondary to diet) induced ED, and that this manifests before coronary artery endothelial dysfunction (on average

4 weeks). It was also demonstrated that the onset mechanism of ED induced by Western diet depends on the induction of NOS uncoupling, since it was reversed by sepiapterin treatment. It was previously demonstrated by Johnson *et al.* (2011) that sepiapterin augmented erectile function in 19-month-old rats, demonstrating that uncoupling of eNOS also underlies age-dependent ED. The isolated effect of diet fat content in erectile function outcomes has also been studied in experimental animal models fed with high-fat or hypercholesterolemic diets. All data clearly demonstrate that elevated fat content in diet induces structural and functional disturbances in erectile tissue that negatively affect erectile function. While treatment of Sprague–Dawley rats with a high-fat diet (45% of energy from lard) until 18 months of age induced an increase in cavernous connective tissue content and a decrease in eNOS phosphorylation at Ser1177 residue through the Akt-pathway compared with age-matched controls, chronological ageing did not modify eNOS expression and activation. These findings showed that long-term nutritional conditions override the influence of age in rat cavernous tissue (Tomada *et al.*, 2013a, 2014). Another study demonstrated that a diet consisting of 2% cholesterol and 10% lard for 6 months induced hyperplasia of the smooth muscle layer in cavernous tissue, which is typically associated with atherosclerotic processes, and reduced the number of nNOS-positive nerves and intracavernous pressure, despite the absence of differences in serum glucose and testosterone levels compared with the controls (Qiu *et al.*, 2011; Huang *et al.*, 2010). In line with these findings, it was shown that pigs fed with a diet containing 46% of energy from fat presented lower cGMP levels, increased eNOS uncoupling and production of thiobarbituric acid reactive substances (markers of oxidative stress) in the penis (Musicki *et al.*, 2008). Conversely, a study in aged rats demonstrated the beneficial effects of ER in erectile function (Maio *et al.*, 2012).

Concerning studies in humans, only a few studies have assessed the role of diet in ED onset. A case–control study exploring foods that were well represented or poorly represented in the diet of individuals with ED was carried out by Esposito *et al.* (2006). This study showed a negative correlation between ED prevalence and the intake of vegetables, fruit and nuts and a ratio of monounsaturated to saturated lipids typical of Mediterranean-style diet, in a cohort of 100 men with ED, but without diabetes or symptomatic cardiovascular diseases, compared with a group with an identical number of age- and disease-matched men without ED. In line with those findings, it was reported that high-protein, carbohydrate-reduced, low-fat and low-energy diet induced weight loss and promoted rapid improvement of endothelial and sexual function in obese diabetic men and sustained these beneficial effects for up to 1 year (Khoo *et al.*, 2011). Moreover, changes in diet pattern are often associated with loss of body weight, which independently ameliorates erectile function (Esposito *et al.*, 2004). However, the effect of weight loss has reduced impact in older men, as demonstrated in a cohort of 306 obese diabetic participants, aged 60 years on average (Wing *et al.*, 2010).

6.7 Nutritional intervention for cardiovascular disease prevention or amelioration

Several studies indicate that nutritional intervention could prevent or ameliorate not only overall cardiovascular diseases, but also in particular erectile dysfunction. Despite the high susceptibility of the cavernous tissue to loss of erectile capability as a result of nutritional habits, it seems to recover more easily after damage compared with myocardium (Tomada *et al.*, 2013a). The strategies to improve erectile function could be divided into nutritional pattern changes including reduction of high-fat and/or high-carbohydrates food, ER and ingestion of foodstuffs rich in anti-oxidants or other compounds proved to ameliorate erectile function, and, on the other hand, treatment with specific nutrients that intervene in molecular mechanisms involved in erectile function such as NO synthesis and AGE formation. Some of these nutrients are currently employed as co-adjuvants of drugs such as phosphodiesterase-5 (PDE5) inhibitors, which impede cGMP degradation in the SMC and are used as first-line treatment for ED. Lower doses of PDE5 inhibitors should thus be required, thus minimizing any side effects or complications of these medications.

6.7.1 Nutritional pattern modulation

AGE content in the Western diet, together with sugars and lipids, has significantly increased in the last 50 years, since they are naturally present in coffee, cola drinks and uncooked animal-derived products, and because cooking results in reactions between sugars and proteins leading to the formation of new AGE (Uribarri *et al.*, 2010). This could be deleterious to the health of the cardiovascular system, since exogenous AGE are believed to be absorbed after ingestion and are passed into the circulation. In fact, serum levels of AGE are strongly related to their consumption (Semba *et al.*, 2012), and may therefore contribute to cardiovascular diseases and ED onset. Thus, a low AGE intake could represent a strategy to avoid vascular disturbances, and despite it being difficult to maintain over the long term, the benefits in terms of the prevention of atherosclerosis and ED, even for healthy individuals, could be significant. This assumption is supported by a study that demonstrated a decrease in serum AGE levels in obese humans submitted to a short-term ER intervention (Gugliucci *et al.*, 2009). Decreasing the glycation burden prevents AGE accumulation, and the ensuing reduction in NO synthesis, increase in oxidative stress, inflammatory response and crosslinking with collagen fibers. Despite the fact that the exact contribution of the glycation-modified collagen in the cavernous connective tissue organization remains elusive, we believe that reduction of AGE adduct formation decreases the percentage of cavernous fibrous collagen deposed in connective tissue.

Beyond ER or dietary AGE reduction, some natural compounds available in food, most of them with anti-oxidant capability, could exert protective effects in the cardiovascular system. The main advantage is their accessibility and safety of their consumption. Some studies have employed entire foodstuffs, fruit juices, alcoholic beverages or mineral-rich natural water, and not isolated compounds, and indeed the global effect could be due to multiple mechanisms.

Polyphenols constitute a class of compounds that possess potent free radical-scavenging capacities and thus the consumption of food naturally rich in polyphenols by experimental animals and humans significantly inhibits oxidative stress, atherogenesis and atherosclerotic lesion development. Supporting the importance of mitigating oxidative stress in the preservation of erectile function, it was observed that lower levels of glutathione in the reduced state (GSH), an important intracellular anti-oxidant that also is an essential cofactor for NOS, strongly correlate with ED in men (Tagliabue *et al.*, 2005). In line with this, it was demonstrated that polyphenol-rich food improves erectile function in both arteriogenic ED and nonpathogenic conditions and prevents ischemia-induced fibrosis in the cavernous tissue (Azadzoi *et al.*, 2005). In fact, chronic administration of whole pomegranate juice or polyphenol extract to rabbits or rats caused significant increases in intracavernous blood flow and smooth muscle relaxation, possibly via increased NO bioavailability (Azadzoi *et al.*, 2005; Zhang *et al.*, 2011a; Ha *et al.*, 2012). Corroborating these findings, it was reported that pomegranate juice consumption improved erections in a cohort of 53 men with mild to moderate erectile dysfunction. However, the results in this study did not achieve statistical significance (Forest *et al.*, 2007). Several studies support the hypothesis that consumption of polyphenols of plant origin can not only induce NO formation in the endothelial cells, but also suppress activation of inducible NOS (iNOS), a isoform of NOS activated in inflammation and infection (Achike *et al.*, 2003). The inhibition of iNOS activity is particularly beneficial to erectile function, since iNOS-derived NO strongly contributes to the nitration of proteins, which causes damage in tissues and premature ageing (McCann *et al.*, 1998). Regular consumption of other beverages also naturally rich in polyphenols, such as red wine or green tea, also induces an apparent decrease in atherosclerotic progression in cavernous tissue in aged rats and activates selected mechanisms for the maintenance of cavernous tissue vascularization (Neves *et al.*, 2008, 2010; Mostafa *et al.*, 2013). Epidemiological studies agree with our findings in rats treated with red wine during 6 months, since alcoholic beverages, particularly those rich in anti-oxidants, ingested with moderation or infrequently may provide some protection against ED (Chew *et al.*, 2009).

Other foodstuffs also rich in anti-oxidants seem to favor NO synthesis and vasodilatation, such as cocoa, which in a dose of 821 mg of flavanols/day in acute or chronic administration induces potent flow-mediated vasodilatation in healthy individuals (Fisher *et al.*, 2003). Nonetheless, despite its promising effects, particularly in age-associated endothelial dysfunction (Fisher & Hollenberg, 2006), no studies exist regarding erectile function.

Ginseng is a natural product prepared from the roots of plants belonging to the genus *Panax* of the family Araliaceae. It may be included in small doses in energy drinks or tisanes and contains the active ingredients ginsenosides (also known as ginseng saponins or glycosylated steroidal saponins). More than 30 different ginsenosides have been isolated from the root of *Panax ginseng*. It has been employed in traditional Chinese medicine for more than 5000 years as a highly valued herb and has been applied to a variety of pathological conditions and illnesses, such as diabetes and ED. Recent evidence supports this belief, such as a study that demonstrated that extract of ginseng restored the anti-oxidant capability in several organs (kidney, liver, heart and lung) of aged rodents (Ramesh *et al.*, 2012), and another carried out in noninsulin-dependent diabetic rats that confirmed the anti-oxidant effect of 30 mg/kg oral administration of Korean red ginseng on the CC (Ryu *et al.*, 2005). Corroborating the efficacy of ginseng in preserving erectile function, another study demonstrated that ginsenosides induced *in vitro* nitric oxide-mediated relaxation and increase in cGMP in rabbit CC (Chen & Lee, 1995). The main conclusions of several clinical trials were reviewed by Moyad and Park (2012), who demonstrated that ginseng significantly improved erectile function in men compared with placebo, not so rapidly on average as PDE5 inhibitors do, but considering its favorable impact on libido and comparative cost saving and safety, ginseng presents its own set of advantages. In fact, to further ameliorate ED, ginsenosides present in ginseng may also provide some cardiovascular protection, apparently through NO-mediated mechanisms (Chen, 1996), as demonstrated in a small cohort of healthy, young patients who presented improved arterial stiffness as demonstrated by low radial AI after treatment with ginsenosides, but not ginseng polysaccharides (Jovanovski *et al.*, 2010).

Unexpectedly, Antep pistachio nuts, naturally rich in fat (although not in cholesterol), proteins, minerals (potassium, calcium and iron) and vitamins A and C, were also demonstrated to improve the International Index of Erectile Function (IIEF) and penile color Doppler ultrasound scores in ED patients, when 100 g was ingested for 3 weeks, without any associated side effects. Furthermore, the lipid parameters showed statistically significant improvements after this diet (Aldemir *et al.*, 2011). On the other hand, soy consumption could negatively affect erectile function, as demonstrated in rodents and in a diabetic patient (Pan *et al.*, 2008; Siepmann *et al.*, 2011). Owing to phytoestrogen effects, lower testosterone blood levels were found in rats and human after consumption of a soy protein-rich diet, as well as attenuated erectile parameters, including apomorphine-induced erections and intracavernous pressure in the rat.

6.7.2 Intervention of specific nutrients in cardiovascular disease protection

Beyond studies that analyze the effects of diet patterns or foods in endothelial function and cardiovascular disease progression, many other works have dissected the effect of isolated nutrients or non-nutrient dietary components. The nutrients that positively affect cardiovascular health belong to distinct classes and thus intervene in different pathways in cells.

6.7.2.1 Polyphenolic compounds

Dietary flavonoids constitute a large class of bioactive polyphenolic compounds commonly consumed in plant foods and beverages. According to the different patterns of this nucleus, they are categorized into six main subclasses: flavan-3-ols (e.g. catechin, epicatechin), flavonols (e.g. quercetin, myricetin, kaempferol), anthocyanidins (e.g. cyanidin, delphinidin), flavones (e.g. apigenin, diosmin), isoflavones (e.g. dadzein, genistein) and flavanones (e.g. naringenin, hesperetin). The bioavailability of flavonoids is generally low and may vary dramatically among different flavonoid classes as well as between individual compounds in a particular class. Isoflavones, flavonols, flavanones and flavan-3-ols may be absorbed sufficiently to exert possible cardio-protective effects *in vivo* (Lilamand *et al.*, 2014). Recent evidence supports the potential role of flavonoids in the reduction of cardiovascular diseases. In particular, flavonoid-rich food intake has been shown to improve endothelial function and peripheral blood pressure. In addition, the beneficial effect of flavonoids on arterial stiffness is becoming clear. Isoflavones (mainly found in soy products), anthocyanins (constituents of red and blue berries) and to a lesser extent cocoa flavanols have been shown to have a positive effect or to be associated with improved measures of vascular function, and in particular arterial stiffness assessed by PWV (Lilamand *et al.*, 2014).

The most studied polyphenols with vascular protective properties are curcumin, found in the Indian spice turmeric, epigallocatechin-3-gallate (EGCG), the most abundant polyphenol in green tea, resveratrol, a stilbene, available in grapes and red wine, and quercetin, present in capers, lovage, apples, onions and grapes.

Recent studies have focused on the development of ER mimetics to identify compounds that mimic the effects of ER by targeting cellular metabolic and stress response pathways without actually restricting energy intake. The polyphenol resveratrol was one the first compounds to be shown to mimic the cardiovascular protective effects of ER (Baur *et al.*, 2006; Barger *et al.*, 2008; Pearson *et al.*, 2008; Shinmura *et al.*, 2011), including induction of mitochondrial biogenesis (Csiszar *et al.*, 2009) and attenuation of mitochondrial oxidative stress (Ungvari *et al.*, 2009, 2010) in vascular endothelial cells and/or in cardiomyocytes (Dai *et al.*, 2012). Resveratrol also reduces endothelial cell apoptosis and increases aortic elasticity in aged rodents (Pearson *et al.*, 2008). The effects of resveratrol, in part, are attributed to its ability to upregulate and/or activate Sirt1, which deacetylates and activates peroxisome proliferator-activated receptor-gamma coactivator 1 alpha (PGC-1α) and other regulators of mitochondrial function (Lagouge *et al.*, 2006). In addition, resveratrol can also activate nuclear factor erythroid 2-related factor 2 in endothelial cells (Ungvari *et al.*, 2010), which may also contribute to its mitochondrial protective effects (discussed in Chapter 2).

AMP-activated protein kinase (AMPK) has emerged as a key nutrient sensor, acting as a master regulator of mitochondrial biogenesis, turnover, mitochondrial metabolism and mitochondrial anti-oxidant defenses (Quintero *et al.*, 2006). There is increasing evidence suggesting that AMPK upregulates Sirt1 activity (Canto *et al.*, 2009) and that AMPK activation may contribute to the cardioprotective effects of ER (Edwards *et al.*, 2010). Because polyphenols can activate AMPK (Zang *et al.*, 2006), this effect may contribute to the robust increases in cellular Sirt1 activity and other ER-like effects in vascular cells observed upon resveratrol treatment (Dai *et al.*, 2012).

Curcumin has been extensively studied and recently has been recognized as an anti-ageing nutrient (Lima *et al.*, 2011). Accumulating evidence suggests that it is a highly pleiotropic molecule that modulates abundant targets in cells, influencing numerous biochemical and molecular functions. Curcumin exhibits important anti-inflammatory properties and an inhibitory effect on AGE-dependent damage, apparently by direct trapping of methylglyoxal, intracellular levels of which were demonstrated to decrease in curcumin–treated endothelial cell lines in culture (Hu *et al.*, 2012; Kim *et al.*, 2011). Concerning SMC, it has been reported that curcumin inhibits migration and proliferation while promoting apoptosis (Chen & Huang, 1998).

Dietary supplementation with 0.2% curcumin for 4 weeks ameliorates age-related large elastic artery stiffening and vascular endothelial dysfunction through amelioration of oxidative stress and normalization of collagen I and AGE deposition, and restoration of NO bioavailability that lowers oxidative stress and improves vascular dysfunction in aged mice (Fleenor *et al.*, 2013). In line with this, it was recently reported that regular administration of water-soluble curcumin improved the erectile function in a rat model of diabetes, mainly owing to an upregulatory effect on expression of eNOS and nNOS, and repression of inflammatory genes and iNOS (Abdel Aziz *et al.*, 2012).

EGCG and quercetin share action mechanisms with curcumin, since all of them interact with the membranes of endothelial cells, restoring transmembrane potential and fluidity in the presence of AGE, apparently repressing the formation of atherosclerotic lesions (Margina *et al.*, 2013). Supporting these findings that reveal important interventions of polyphenols in cellular functions and potential protective effects in cavernous tissue, it was also demonstrated that resveratrol inhibits AGE-induced proliferation and collagen synthesis activity in vascular SMC, and that it also favors vasorelaxation response in the cavernous tissue of hypercholesterolemic rabbits (Mizutani *et al.*, 2000; Soner *et al.*, 2010) and diabetic rats when orally administrated alone in a dose of 5 mg/kg/day or in association with a PDE5 inhibitor (Yu *et al.*, 2013; Fukuhara *et al.*, 2011). In addition,

EGCG induces eNOS/cGMP activation, elicits dose-dependent vasodilatation in rat aortic rings (Lorenz *et al.*, 2004) and exerts significant cavernous anti-oxidant effects in rodents when orally administrated in a drinking solution in a dose of 7.6 mg/l (Mostafa *et al.*, 2013). Concerning quercetin, it was demonstrated that it presents an inhibitory effect on PDE5A activity, promotes relaxation of smooth muscle strips of guinea pig CC and increases intracavernous pressure and eNOS expression while improving anti-oxidative defenses in cavernous tissue of diabetic rats when intraperitoneally injected in a dose of 50 mg/kg (Lines & Ono, 2006; Hnatyszyn *et al.*, 2004; Zhang *et al.*, 2011b). No clinical trials were carried out to evaluate the effects of polyphenols administration on erectile function.

6.7.2.2 L-Carnitine and L-arginine

L-carnitine is the biologically active form of a small peptide available in red meat and dairy products, constituted by lysine and methionine and required for the transport of fatty acids from cytosol into mitochondria during the breakdown of lipids. Administration of L-carnitine to patients with ED seems promising, considering reports that demonstrate that oral administration of derivatives of L-carnitine significantly improved nocturnal penile tumescence and IIEF score, as well as other symptoms associated with male ageing (Cavallini *et al.*, 2004). When associated with niacin and L-arginine it was also demonstrated to ameliorate erectile dysfunction and satisfaction with sex life in a single-blind trial that included 54 ED patients (Gianfrilli *et al.*, 2012). Derivatives of L-carnitine have also been employed as adjuvants of PDE5 inhibitors, with very promising results for ED in diabetic patients (Gentile *et al.*, 2004). Association of L-carnitine with treatment was particularly beneficial for patients with ED refractory to PDE5 inhibitor monotherapy, since it frankly improved the endothelial function with clear amelioration of markers of inflammatory processes and vascular damage (Morano *et al.*, 2007).

The amino acid L-arginine is the raw material from which NO is synthesized by NOS. In the penis, L-arginine may be a substrate-limiting factor for NOS activity, particularly because the activity of arginase increases in aged cavernosal specimens, as shown in the rabbit (Numao *et al.*, 2007). Indeed, long-term oral administration of supraphysiological doses of L-arginine (2.25% dissolved in tap water) may upregulate penile NOS activity but not its expression, which improves erectile response in the ageing rat (Moody *et al.*, 1997). In human trials, two studies conducted 20 years ago demonstrated that high doses of orally administered L-arginine (5 g daily for 6 weeks) to compensate for its metabolization in the gut wall and liver significantly ameliorated ED (Zorgniotti & Lizza, 1994; Chen *et al.*, 1999). However, in the study of Chen *et al.* (1999), only one-third of the patients treated with L-arginine reported significant subjective improvement in sexual function without alteration of hemodynamics of the CC.

Oral supplementation with the amino acid L-citrulline, which is abundant in watermelon and present in free form in the human body, presents advantages compared with L-arginine, since it may be converted by the kidneys into L-arginine, escapes intestinal and liver metabolism and inhibits arginase activity (Morris, 2004). In fact, improved erectile function and penile tissue structure was demonstrated in rats that had been castrated or had acute arteriogenic ED, which were treated with 2% L-citrulline dissolved in drinking water for 4 weeks (Hotta *et al.*, 2013; Shiota *et al.*, 2013). Evidence of beneficial effects of L- citrulline was also reported in a human trial that showed that treatment with 1.5 g/day of L-citrulline divided into two doses during 1 month was able to restore normal erectile function in half of the ED patients enrolled in the study (Cormio *et al.*, 2011).

6.7.2.3 Fatty acids

The beneficial effects of Mediterranean diet are due in part to the abundance of omega-3 fatty acids, which directly ameliorate endothelial dysfunction, not only by promoting angiogenesis, EPC function and postnatal neovascularization, but also by increasing NO bioavailability in response to Akt kinase activation, as demonstrated in cultured human coronary artery endothelial cells treated with decosahexaenoic acid, one of the main omega-3 fatty acids (Stebbins *et al.*, 2008; Turgeon *et al.*, 2013). Supporting this finding, it was observed that dietary omega-3 fatty acid supplementation was accompanied by an increase in forearm blood flow in response to acetylcholine in aged patients (mean age of 73 years) with chronic heart failure (Morgan *et al.*, 2006). In addition, a recent randomized controlled trial in healthy middle-aged and older adults has shown that omega-3-polyunsaturated fatty acid supplementation lowered the concentration of serum pro-inflammatory cytokines (Kiecolt-Glaser *et al.*, 2012). Another study suggested that lower omega-6:omega-3 polyunsaturated fatty acid ratios can influence cell ageing, increasing telomere length (Kiecolt-Glaser *et al.*, 2013).

Alpha-lipoid acid could also be considered a promising strategy for ED treatment, since it prevents the formation of AGE-modified products in the presence of glucose, counteracts oxidative stress and blocks inflammatory responses induced by AGE in endothelial cells (Bierhaus *et al.*, 1997). In addition, an interesting study demonstrated that α-lipoic and γ-linolenic acids interact synergistically to improve NO-mediated neural and endothelium-dependent relaxation of CC in streptozotocin-induced diabetic rats, despite the absence of effect observed when each was employed alone (Keegan *et al.*, 2001).

6.7.2.4 Vitamins

Vitamin E is a blanket term for eight different nutrients – four different tocopherols and four different tocotrienols – with recognized anti-oxidant properties. Vegetables, fish, plant oils and in particular sunflower seeds are rich in vitamin E. Relevant to human, and specifically to elder, nutrition, most trials show that vitamin E derived from food, but not that from supplements, is inversely associated with mortality from coronary heart disease. For example, Kushi *et al.* (1996) as well as the Finnish trial (Knekt *et al.*, 1994) showed that modifying dietary habits to increase vitamin E intake may be worthwhile in preventing coronary heart disease.

Cherubini *et al.* (2001) suggested that maintaining proper vitamin E status is important to avoid increased risk of atherosclerosis with advanced age. Vitamin E is known to enhance endothelial function by increasing free radical trapping, which leads to an increase in circulating NO levels. Therefore, vitamin E directly improves NO-mediated arterial relaxation, as demonstrated in the rodent (Agarwal *et al.*, 2006; Keegan *et al.*, 1995). Owing to its impact on NO bioavailability, vitamin E was demonstrated to ameliorate ED when combined with a PDE5 inhibitor in an experimental model of streptozotocin-induced diabetic rats that presented an increase in intracavernous pressure and nNOS levels after treatment (De Young *et al.*, 2003). Anti-oxidant therapy with vitamin E also ameliorates age-associated ED, as demonstrated in 18-month-old aged rats treated with 80 IU of vitamin E/rat/day, revealing higher intracavernous pressure and penile NO_2/NO_3 levels, relating NO bioavailability, and lower levels of oxidative stress markers (Helmy & Senbel, 2012). In line with these findings, a study in a cohort of 89 men with ED who were low responders to PDE5 inhibitors demonstrated that treatment with 300 mg/day of α-tocophenol for at least 1 month increased the IIEF-5 score by an average of 3.3 points (Kondoh *et al.*, 2008).

Numerous studies in both experimental animals and humans show that tissue vitamin C (ascorbic acid) levels decline with age and do so in a gender-dependent manner, that is, men are more affected than women. This fact is apparently related to the incidence of mortality from stroke (Gale *et al.*, 1995, 2001), since it is highest in elders with the lowest ascorbic acid intake (<28 mg/day). Conversely, higher ascorbic acid intakes (>45 mg/day) are associated with lower mortality rate, regardless of social class or other dietary variables. Subjects in the upper two quintiles of ascorbic acid intake (>400 mg/day) of a study by Sahyoun *et al.* (1996), which enrolled 725 elderly men and women, had a lower incidence of overall mortality compared with the lowest two quintiles (<90 mg/day), largely owing to reduced mortality from heart disease. Vitamin C has been recently shown to restore proper flow-mediated vasodilatation in sedentary older men (Eskurza *et al.*, 2004). Ascorbic acid intake has also been shown to ameliorate endothelial dysfunction and hypertension in a number of clinical studies (Taddei *et al.*, 1998; Gokce *et al.*, 1999; Carr & Frei, 2000). The mechanisms by which ascorbic acid increases eNOS bioactivity and NO production have been thoroughly investigated and involve the maintenance of an intracellular reduced environment and of NOS cofactors, for example, tetrahydrobiopterin (Tomasian *et al.*, 2000; Heller *et al.*, 2001). In addition, vitamins C and E present synergistic effects after ingestion (Hamilton *et al.*, 2000).

The carotenoids are a group of red-, orange- and yellow-pigmented polyisoprenoid hydrocarbons synthesized by prokaryotes and higher plants, which concentrate in animal fat. Most of the carotenoids, such as carotene, are used in the formation of vitamin A in the body, whereas others, such as lycopene and lutein, show no vitamin A activity. The main sources of carotenoids that circulate in human plasma are fruit and vegetables: lycopene is the main tomato pigment whereas lutein is found in a number of vegetables (e.g. cabbage, corn, broccoli). Lycopene, lutein and other carotenoids can reduce vascular ageing. Their main anti-ageing action is as an ROS scavenger. Carotenoid anti-oxidant properties improve the atherosclerotic profile by augmentation of NO availability, reduction of plasma LDL and improved glucose tolerance and blood pressure control, which results in attenuation of the atherosclerotic process (Wolak & Paran, 2013). Anti-oxidants can potentially protect telomeric DNA from oxidative damage caused by extrinsic and intrinsic DNA damaging agents, so a diet lacking anti-oxidants leads to shorter telomeres, whereas consumption of an anti-oxidant-rich diet including vitamins C and E and β-carotene is associated with longer telomeres (Shen *et al.*, 2009; Marin *et al.*, 2012, 2013).

Vitamin B_9 (folic acid), abundant in leafy green vegetables, fruit, dried beans, peas, nuts and enriched bread or cereals, intervenes in the methylation of homocysteine (discussed in Chapter 3) and is also a cofactor in the normal production of NO. In addition, it helps to maintain eNOS in its coupled state (Moens *et al.*, 2008). Thus, novel evidence indicates that administration of folic acid improves erectile function and reduces intracavernosal oxidative stress in the diabetic rabbit, with reduced serum homocysteine levels (Shukla *et al.*, 2009). In line with this, a recent study conducted in diabetic patients treated with the PDE5 inihibitor tadalafil demonstrated that 5 mg of folic acid daily significantly increased the mean IIEF score (Hamidi Madani *et al.*, 2013).

Low plasma concentrations of vitamin B_6 (pyridoxine) have been associated with increased inflammatory status (Chiang *et al.*, 2005; Gori *et al.*, 2006). Given the important role played by inflammation in the onset and exacerbation of coronary heart disease, namely atherosclerosis, sufficient intake of vitamin B_6 might contribute to cardioprotection in the elderly (Visioli & Hagen, 2007).

Vitamin D levels are inversely associated with increased arterial stiffness in a normative ageing population, irrespective of traditional risk factor burden. Further research is needed to understand the mechanism of this association and to test the hypothesis that vitamin D supplementation can reduce arterial stiffness (Giallauria *et al.*, 2012).

Finally, a preventive role for vitamin K in vascular calcification has been proposed based on its role in activating matrix Gla protein, a calcification inhibitor that is expressed in vascular tissue. Although animal and *in vitro* data support this role of vitamin K, overall data from human studies are inconsistent (Shea & Holden, 2012).

6.7.2.5 Minerals

In animals exposed to short-term magnesium deficiency, the enzyme telomerase is downregulated in cells from all chambers of the heart as well as in aortic smooth muscle. In addition, this deficiency also induces oxidative DNA damage in cardiovascular tissues (Shah *et al.*, 2014). Taking these results into account, these authors recommend that water intake (e.g. tap water, well water, bottled water, beverages using tap/well/spring waters or desalinated water) in humans should contain at least 25–40 mg Mg^{2+}/l in order to prevent cardiovascular diseases and ameliorate the ageing process of body tissues and cells in humans (Shah *et al.*, 2014).

Dietary sodium restriction has also been found to improve arterial compliance. Gates *et al.* (2004) showed that sodium restriction rapidly improved the compliance of large elastic arteries in a population of older adults with stage 1 systolic hypertension.

6.7.2.6 Caffeine

Caffeine is a white crystalline xanthine alkaloid normally ingested in infusions prepared from seeds of the coffee plant and leaves of the tea bush. It was found that caffeine ingestion at doses of 10–20 mg/kg/day for 8 weeks positively impacted erectile function in streptozotocin-induced diabetic rats, increasing intracavernous pressure and upregulating cGMP synthesis (Yang *et al.*, 2008).

6.8 Conclusions

Cardiovascular diseases constitute a hallmark of the elderly population. Although this group of disorders is in part caused by age-related structural modifications and functional decay of the heart and vascular system, lifestyle also contributes to their progression. Nutritional intervention may indeed ameliorate or even prevent cardiovascular disease. Nutrients that possess anti-oxidant capability, mitigate AGE formation, activate NO synthesis or activate activity of Sirt1 or TERT can modulate the progression of ageing mechanisms and emerge as beneficial for elderly people. Future studies are, however, necessary to investigate the causal association between dietary pattern or specific nutrient consumption and cardiovascular function changes, in order to determine the adequate intake to obtain clinically significant modifications.

References

Abdel Aziz, M. T., T. Motawi, A. Rezq, T. Mostafa, H. H. Fouad, H. H. Ahmed, L. Rashed, D. Sabry, A. Senbel, A. Al-Malki, and R. El-Shafiey. 2012. Effects of a water-soluble curcumin protein conjugate vs. pure curcumin in a diabetic model of erectile dysfunction. *J. Sex. Med.* 9:1815–1833.

Achike, F. I. and C. Y. Kwan. 2003. Nitric oxide, human diseases and the herbal products that affect the nitric oxide signalling pathway. *Clin. Exp. Pharmacol. Physiol.* 30:605–615.

Agarwal, A., K. C. Nandipati, R. K. Sharma, C. D. Zippe, and R. Raina. 2006. Role of oxidative stress in the pathophysiological mechanism of erectile dysfunction. *J. Androl.* 27:335–347.

Ahn, B. H., H. S. Kim, S. Song, I. H. Lee, J. Liu, A. Vassilopoulos, C. X. Deng, and T. Finkel. 2008. A role for the mitochondrial deacetylase Sirt3 in regulating energy homeostasis. *Proc. Natl Acad. Sci. USA* 105:14447–14452.

Aldemir, M., E. Okulu, S. Neşelioğlu, O. Erel, and O. Kayıgil. 2011. Pistachio diet improves erectile function parameters and serum lipid profiles in patients with erectile dysfunction. *Int. J. Impot. Res.* 23:32–38.

Antelmi, I., R. S. de Paula, A. R. Shinzato, C. A. Peres, A. J. Mansur, and C. J. Grupi.2004. Influence of age, gender, body mass index, and functional capacity on heart rate variability in a cohort of subjects without heart disease. *Am. J. Cardiol.* 93:381–385.

Aquaro, G. D., A. Cagnolo, K. K. Tiwari, G. Todiere, S. Bevilacqua, G. Di Bella, L. Ait-Ali, P. Festa, M. Glauber, and M. Lombardi. 2013. Age-dependent changes in elastic properties of thoracic aorta evaluated by magnetic resonance in normal subjects. *Interact. Cardiovasc. Thorac. Surg.* 17:674–679.

Ash C. E. and B. J. Merry.2011. The molecular basis by which dietary restricted feeding reduces mitochondrial reactive oxygen species generation. *Mech. Ageing Dev.* 132:43–54.

Azadzoi, K. M., R. N. Schulman, M. Aviram, and M. B. Siroky. 2005. Oxidative stress in arteriogenic erectile dysfunction: prophylactic role of antioxidants. *J. Urol.* 174:386–393.

Ballard, V. L. 2010. Stem cells for heart failure in the aging heart. *Heart Fail. Rev.* 15:447–456.

Ballard, V. L. and J. M. Edelberg. 2007. Stem cells and the regeneration of the aging cardiovascular system. *Circ Res.* 100:1116–1127.

Baraibar, M. A., L. Liu, E. K. Ahmed, and B. Friguet. 2012. Protein oxidative damage at the crossroads of cellular senescence, aging and aging-related diseases. *Oxid. Med. Cell. Longev.* 919832.

Barger, J. L., T. Kayo, J. M. Vann, E. B. Arias, J. Wang, T. A. Hacker, Y. Wang, D. Raederstorff, J. D. Morrow, C. Leeuwenburgh, D. B. Allison, K. W. Saupe, G. D. Cartee, R. Weindruch, and T. A. Prolla. 2008. A low dose of dietary resveratrol partially mimics caloric restriction and retards aging parameters in mice. *PLoS One* 3:e2264.

Baur J. A., K. J. Pearson, N. L. Price, H. A. Jamieson, C. Lerin, A. Kalra, V. V. Prabhu, J. S. Allard, G. Lopez-Lluch, K. Lewis, P. J. Pistell, S. Poosala, K. G. Becker, O. Boss, D. Gwinn, M. Wang, S. Ramaswamy, K. W. Fishbein, R. G. Spencer, E. G. Lakatta, D. Le Couteur, R. J. Shaw, P. Navas, P. Puigserver, D. K. Ingram, R. de Cabo, and D. A. Sinclair. 2006. Resveratrol improves health and survival of mice on a high-calorie diet. *Nature* 444:337–342.

Benetos, A., S. Laurent, A. P. Hoeks, P. H. Boutouyrie, and M. E. Safar. 1993. Arterial alterations with aging and high blood pressure. A noninvasive study of carotid and femoral arteries. *Arterioscler. Thromb.* 13:90–97.

Bergmann, O., R. D. Bhardwaj, S. Bernard, S. Zdunek, F. Barnabe-Heider, S. Walsh, J. Zupicich, K. Alkass, B. A. Buchholz, H. Druid, S. Jovinge, and J. Frisen. 2009. Evidence for cardiomyocyte renewal in humans. *Science* 324:98–102.

Bhutani, S., M. C., Klempel, R. A. Berger, and K. A. Varady, 2010. Improvements in coronary heart disease risk indicators by alternate-day fasting involve adipose tissuemodulations. *Obesity (Silver Spring)* 18:2152–2159.

Bierhaus, A., S. Chevion, M. Chevion, M. Hofmann, P. Quehenberger, T. Illmer, T. Luther, E. Berentshtein, H. Tritschler, M. Müller, P. Wahl, R. Ziegler, and P. P. Nawroth. 1997. Advanced glycation end product-induced activation of NF-kappaB is suppressed by alpha-lipoic acid in cultured endothelial cells. *Diabetes* 46:1481–1490.

Bivalacqua T. J., W. Deng, M. Kendirci , M. F. Usta, C. Robinson, B. K. Taylor, S. N. Murthy, H. C. Champion, W. J. G. Hellstrom, and P. J. Kadowitz. 2007a. Mesenchymal stem cells alone or ex vivo gene modified with endothelial nitric oxide synthase reverse age-associated erectile dysfunction. *Am. J. Physiol.* 29:H1278–H1290.

Bivalacqua, T. J., A. L. Burnett, W. J. Hellstrom, and H. C. Champion. 2007b. Overexpression of arginase in the aged mouse penis impairs erectile function and decreases eNOS activity: influence of in vivo gene therapy of anti-arginase. *Am. J. Physiol.* 292:H1340–H1351.

Bostrom, K. I., M. Jumabay, A. Matveyenko, S. B. Nicholas, and Y. Yao. 2011. Activation of vascular bone morphogenetic protein signaling in diabetes mellitus. *Circul. Res.* 108:446–457.

Boutouyrie, P., S. Laurent, A. Benetos, X. J. Girerd, A. P. Hoeks, and M. E. Safar. 1992. Opposing effects of ageing on distal and proximal large arteries in hypertensives. *J. Hypertens. Suppl.* 10: S87–91.

Brandes, R.P., I. Fleming, and R. Busse. 2005. Endotheial aging. *Cardiovasc. Res.* 66(2):286–294.

Bucala, R., K. J. Tracey, and A. Cerami. 1991. Advanced glycosylation products quench nitric oxide and mediate defective endothelium-dependent vasodilatation in experimental diabetes. *J. Clin. Invest.* 87:432–438.

Burchardt, M., T. Burchardt, A. G. Anastasiadis, R. Buttyan, A. de la Taille, A. Shabsigh, J. Frank, and R. Shabsigh. 2005. Application of angiogenic factors for therapy of erectile dysfunction: protein and DNA transfer of VEGF 165 into the rat penis. *Urology* 66:665–670.

Burnett, A. L., R. J. Nelson, D. C. Calvin, J. X. Liu, G. E. Demas, S. L. Klein, L. J. Kriegsfeld , V. L. Dawson, T. M. Dawson, and S. H. Snyder. 1996. Nitric oxide-dependent penile erection in mice lacking neuronal nitric oxide synthase. *Mol. Med.* 2:288–296.

Butany, J., M. J. Collins, D. E. Demellawy, V. Nair, N. Israel, S. W. Leong, and M. A. Borger. 2005. Morphological and clinical findings in 247 surgically excised native aortic valves. *Can. J. Cardiol.* 21:747–755.

Cai, J., Y. Hong, C. Weng, C. Tan, J. Imperato-McGinley, and Y. S. Zhu. 2011. Androgen stimulates endothelial cell proliferation via an androgen receptor/VEGF/cyclin A-mediated mechanism. *Am. J. Physiol. Heart Circul. Physiol.* 300:H1210–1221.

Canepa, M., J. B. Strait, Y. Milaneschi, M. AlGhatrif, R. Ramachandran, S. Makrogiannis, M. Moni, M. David, C. Brunelli, E. G. Lakatta, and L. Ferrucci. 2013. The relationship between visceral adiposity and left ventricular diastolic function: results from the Baltimore Longitudinal Study of Aging. *Nutr. Metab. Cardiovasc. Dis.* 23:1263–1270.

Canto C., Z. Gerhart-Hines, J. N. Feige, M. Lagouge, L. Noriega, J. C. Milne, P. J. Elliott, P. Puigserver, and J. Auwerx. 2009. Ampk regulates energy expenditure by modulating nad+ metabolism and sirt1 activity. *Nature* 458:1056–1060.

Carr A. and B. Frei. 2000. The role of natural antioxidants in preserving the biological activity of endothelium-derived nitric oxide. *Free Radic. Biol. Med.*28:1806–1814.

Castello L., T. Froio, G. Cavallini, F. Biasi, A. Sapino, G. Leonarduzzi, E. Bergamini, G. Poli, and E. Chiarpotto. 2005. Calorie restriction protects against age-related rat aorta sclerosis. *FASEB J.* 19:1863–1865.

Cavallini, G., S. Caracciolo, G. Vitali, F. Modenini, and G. Biagiotti. 2004. Carnitine versus androgen administration in the treatment of sexual dysfunction, depressed mood, and fatigue associated with male aging. *Urology* 63:641–646.

Cefalu W. T., A. D. Bell-Farrow, Z. Q. Wang, W. E. Sonntag, M. X. Fu, J. W. Bayne, and S. R. Thorpe. 1995. Caloric restriction decreases age-dependent accumulation of the glycoxidation products, N epsilon-(carboxymethyl)lysine and pentosidine, in rat skin collagen. *J. Gerontol. A. Biol. Sci. Med. Sci.* 50:B337–B341.

Cheitlin, C. M. D. 2004. Erectile dysfunction: the earliest sign of generalized vascular disease? *J. Am. Coll. Cardiol.* 43:185–186.

Chen, H. W. and H. C. Huang. 1998. Effect of curcumin on cell cycle progression and apoptosis in vascular smooth muscle cells. *Br. J. Pharmacol.* 124:1029–1040.

Chen, J., Y. Wollman, T. Chernichovsky, A. Iaina, M. Sofer, and H. Matzkin. 1999. Effect of oral administration of high-dose nitric oxide donor L-arginine in men with organic erectile dysfunction: results of a double-blind, randomized, placebo-controlled study. *BJU Int.* 83:269–273.

Chen, M. A., M. Kawakubo, P. M. Colletti, D. Xu, L. Labree Dustin, R. Detrano, S. P. Azen, N. D. Wong, and X. Q. Zhao. 2013. Effect of age on aortic atherosclerosis. *J. Geriatr. Cardiol.* 10:135–140.

Chen, X. 1996. Cardiovascular protection by ginsenosides and their nitric oxide releasing action. *Clin. Exp. Pharmacol. Physiol.* 23:728–732.

Chen, X. and T. J. Lee. 1995. Ginsenosides-induced nitric oxide-mediated relaxation of the rabbit corpus cavernosum. *Br. J. Pharmacol.* 115:15–18.

Chen, Z., I. C. Peng, X. Cui, Y. S. Li, S. Chien, and J. Y. Shyy. 2010. Shear stress, SIRT1, and vascular homeostasis. *Proc. Natl Acad. Sci. USA* 107:10268–10273.

Cherubini A., G. Zuliani, F. Costantini, S. D. Pierdomenico, S. Volpato, A. Mezzetti, P. Mecocci, S. Pezzuto, M. Bregnocchi, R. Fellin, U. Senin, and the VASA Study Group. 2001. High vitamin E plasma levels and low low-density lipoprotein oxidation are associated with the absence of atherosclerosis in octogenarians. *J. Am. Geriatr. Soc.* 49:651–654.

Chew, K. K., A. Bremner, B. Stuckey, C. Earle, and K. Jamrozik. 2009. Alcohol consumption and male erectile dysfunction: an unfounded reputation for risk? *J. Sex. Med.* 6:1386–1394.

Chiang E. P., D. E. Smith, J. Selhub, G. Dallal, Y. C. Wang, and R. Roubenoff. 2005. Inflammation causes tissue-specific depletion of vitamin B_6. *Arthritis Res. Ther.* 7:R1254–1262.

Chiva-Blanch, G., M. Urpi-Sarda, E. Ros, S. Arranz, P. Valderas-Martinez, R. Casas, E. Sacanella, R. Llorach R. M. Lamuela-Raventos, C. Andres-Lacueva, and R. Estruch. 2012. Dealcoholized red wine decreases systolic and diastolic blood pressure and increases plasma nitric oxide: short communication. *Circul. Res.* 111:1065–1068.

Choi, S. Y., B. H. Oh, J. Bae Park, D. J. Choi, M. Y. Rhee, and S. Park. 2013. Age-associated increase in arterial stiffness measured according to the cardio-ankle vascular index without blood pressure changes in healthy adults. *J. Atheroscler. Thromb.* 20:911–923.

Christ, M., J. Bauersachs, C. Liebetrau, M. Heck, A. Günther, and M. Wehling. 2002. Glucose increases endothelial-dependent superoxide formation in coronary arteries by NAD(P)H oxidase activation: attenuation by the 3-hydroxy-3-methylglutaryl coenzyme A reductase inhibitor atorvastatin. *Diabetes* 51:2648–2652.

Collins, J. A., J. V. Munoz, T. R. Patel, M. Loukas, and R. S. Tubbs. 2014. The anatomy of the aging aorta. *Clin. Anat.* 27:463–466.

Colman R. J., R. M. Anderson, S. C. Johnson, E. K. Kastman, K. J. Kosmatka, T. M. Beasley, D. B. Allison, C. Cruzen, H. A. Simmons, J. W. Kemnitz, and R. Weindruch. 2009. Caloric restriction delays disease onset and mortality in rhesus monkeys. *Science*.325:201–204.

Colom B., J. Oliver, P. Roca, and F. J. Garcia-Palmer. 2007. Caloric restriction and gender modulate cardiac muscle mitochondrial H_2O_2 production and oxidative damage. *Cardiovasc. Res.* 74:456–465.

Corbi, G., V. Conti, G. Russomanno, G. Rengo, P. Vitulli, A. L. Ciccarelli, A. Filippelli, and N. Ferrara. 2012a. Is physical activity able to modify oxidative damage in cardiovascular aging? *Oxid. Med. Cell. Longev.* 2012:728547.

Corbi, G., V. Conti, G. Scapagnini, A. Filippelli, and N. Ferrara. 2012b. Role of sirtuins, calorie restriction and physical activity in aging. *Front. Biosci. (Elite Edn)* 4:768–778.

Corbi, G., V. Conti, G. Russomanno, G. Longobardi, G. Furgi, A. Filippelli, and N. Ferrara. 2013. Adrenergic signaling and oxidative stress: a role for sirtuins? *Front. Physiol.* 4:324.

Cordeiro, A. L., A. Figueiredo, F. Godinho, I. Martins, P. Vendeira, H. Almeida, and D. Neves. 2008. Ultrastructural characterization of corpus cavernosum of ageing, orchidectomy and diabetes rat experimental models. *Microsc. Microanal.* 14:S397–S398.

Cordeiro, A. L., A. Figueiredo, I. Tomada, H. Almeida, and D. Neves. 2010. Characterization of the expression of Ang1, Ang2 and Tie2 in the corpus cavernosum of the rat during aging. *Microsc. Microanal.* 16:1–11.

Cormio, L., M. De Siati , F. Lorusso, O. Selvaggio, L. Mirabella, F. Sanguedolce, and G. Carrieri. 2011. Oral L-citrulline supplementation improves erection hardness in men with mild erectile dysfunction. *Urology* 77:119–122.

Cruz-Teno, C., P. Perez-Martinez, J. Delgado-Lista, E. M. Yubero-Serrano, A. Garcia-Rios, C. Marin, P. Gomez, Y. Jimenez-Gomez, A. Camargo, F. Rodriguez-Cantalejo, M. M. Malagón, F. Pérez-Jiménez, H. M. Roche, and J. López-Miranda. 2012. Dietary fat modifies the postprandial inflammatory state in subjects with metabolic syndrome: the LIPGENE study. *Mol. Nutr. Food Res.* 56:854–865.

Csiszar, A., N. Labinskyy, R. Jimenez, J. T. Pinto, P. Ballabh, G. Losonczy, K. J. Pearson, R. de Cabo, and Z. Ungvari. 2009. Anti-oxidative and anti-inflammatory vasoprotective effects of caloric restriction in aging: role of circulating factors and SIRT1. *Mech. Ageing Dev.* 130:518–527.

Dai, D. F., P. S. Rabinovitch, and Z. Ungvari. 2012. Mitochondria and cardiovascular aging. *Circul. Res.* 110:1109–1124.

Dal-Ros, S., C. Bronner, C. Auger, and V. B. Schini-Kerth. 2012. Red wine polyphenols improve an established aging-related endothelial dysfunction in the mesenteric artery of middle-aged rats: Role of oxidative stress. *Biochem. Biophys. Res. Commun.* 419:381–387.

De Young, L., D. Yu, D. Freeman, and G. B. Brock. 2003. Effect of PDE5 inhibition combined with free oxygen radical scavenger therapy on erectile function in a diabetic animal model. *Int. J. Impot. Res.* 15:347–354.

Dolinsky V. W., J. S. Morton, T. Oka, I. Robillard-Frayne, M. Bagdan, G. D. Lopaschuk, C. Des Rosiers, K. Walsh, S. T. Davidge, and J. R. Dyck. 2010. Calorie restriction prevents hypertension and cardiac hypertrophy in the spontaneously hypertensive rat. *Hypertension* 56:412–421.

Droogmans, S., B. Roosens, B. Cosyns, S. Hernot, C. Weytjens, C. Degaillier, C. Garbar, V. Caveliers, M. Pipeleers-Marichal, P. R. Franken, A. Bossuyt, T. Lahoutte, D. Schoors, and G. Van Camp. 2009. Echocardiographic and histological assessment of age-related valvular changes in normal rats. *Ultrasound Med. Biol.* 35:558–565.

Edwards A. G., A. J. Donato, L. A. Lesniewski, R. A. Gioscia, D. R. Seals, and R. L. Moore. 2010. Life-long caloric restriction elicits pronounced protection of the aged myocardium: a role for ampk. *Mech Ageing Dev.* 131:739–742.

El Assar, M., J. Angulo, S. Vallejo, C. Peiro, C. F. Sanchez-Ferrer, and L. Rodriguez-Manas. 2012. Mechanisms involved in the aging-induced vascular dysfunction. *Front. Physiol.* 3:132.

Eskurza I., K. D. Monahan, J. A. Robinson, and D. R. Seals. 2004. Effect of acute and chronic ascorbic acid on flow-mediated dilatation with sedentary and physically active human ageing. *J. Physiol.* 556: 315–324.

Esler, M. D., A. G. Turner, D. M. Kaye, J. M. Thompson, B. A. Kingwell, M. Morris, G. W. Lambert, G. L. Jennings, H. S. Cox, and D. R. Seals. 1995. Aging effects on human sympathetic neuronal function. *Am. J. Physiol.* 268:R278–285.

Esposito, K., F. Giugliano, C. Di Palo, G. Giugliano, R. Marfella, F. D'Andrea, M. D'Armiento, and D. Giugliano. 2004. Effect of lifestyle changes on erectile dysfunction in obese men: a randomized controlled trial. *JAMA* 291:2978–2984.

Esposito, K., F. Giugliano , M. De Sio, D. Carleo, C. Di Palo, M. D'Armiento, and D. Giugliano. 2006. Dietary factors in erectile dysfunction. *Int. J. Impot. Res.* 18:370–374.

Everitt, A. V., S. N. Hilmer, J. C. Brand-Miller, H. A. Jamieson, A. S. Truswell, A. P. Sharma, R. S. Mason, B. J. Morris, and D. G. Le Couteur. 2006. Dietary approaches that delay age-related diseases. *Clin. Interv. Aging* 1:11–31.

Farasat, S. M., C. H. Morrell, A. Scuteri, C. T. Ting, F. C. Yin, H. A. Spurgeon, C. H. Chen, E. G. Lakatta, and S. S. Najjar. 2008. Pulse pressure is inversely related to aortic root diameter implications for the pathogenesis of systolic hypertension. *Hypertension* 51:196–202.

Farsetti, A., A. Grasselli, S. Bacchetti, C. Gaetano, and M. C. Capogrossi. 2009. The telomerase tale in vascular aging: regulation by estrogens and nitric oxide signaling. *J. Appl. Physiol. (1985)* 106:333–337.

Feldman, H. A., I. Goldstein, D. G. Hatzichristou, R. J. Krane, and J. B. McKinlay. 1994. Impotence and its medical and psychosocial correlates: results of the Massachusetts Male Aging Study. *J. Urol.* 151:54–61.

Feldman, H. A., C. Longcope, C. A. Derby, C. B. Johannes, A. B. Araujo, A. D. Coviello, W. J. Bremner, and J. B. McKinlay. 2002. Age trends in the level of serum testosterone and other hormones in middle-aged men: Longitudinal results from the Massachusetts male aging study. *J. Clin. Endocrinol. Metab.* 87:589–598.

Fernandez, J. M., D. Rosado-Alvarez, M. E. da Silva Grigoletto, O. A. Rangel-Zuniga, L. L. Landaeta-Diaz, J. Caballero-Villarraso, J. Lopez-Miranda, F. Perez-Jimenez, and F. Fuentes-Jimenez. 2012. Moderate-to-high-intensity training and a hypocaloric Mediterranean diet enhance endothelial progenitor cells and fitness in subjects with the metabolic syndrome. *Clin. Sci.* 123, 361–373.

Ferrara, N. and T. Davis-Smyth. 1997. The biology of vascular endothelial growth factor. *Endocr. Rev.* 18:4–25.

Ferrara, N., P. O'Gara, D. G. Wynne, L. A. Brown, F. del Monte, P. A. Poole-Wilson, and S. E. Harding. 1995. Decreased contractile responses to isoproterenol in isolated cardiac myocytes from aging guinea-pigs. *J. Mol. Cell. Cardiol.* 27:1141–1150.

Ferrara, N., H. P. Gerber, and J. L. Couter. 2003. The biology of VEGF and its receptors. *Nat. Med.* 9:669–676.

Ferrara, N., K. Komici, G. Corbi, G. Pagano, G. Furgi, C. Rengo, G. D. Femminella, D. Leosco, and D. Bonaduce. 2014. beta-adrenergic receptor responsiveness in aging heart and clinical implications. *Front. Physiol.* 4:396.

Fisher, N. D. and N. K. Hollenberg. 2006. Aging and vascular responses to flavanol-rich cocoa. J. Hypertens. 24:1575–1580.

Fisher, N. D., M. Hughes, M. Gerhard-Herman, and N. K. Hollenberg. 2003. Flavanol-rich cocoa induces nitric-oxide-dependent vasodilation in healthy humans. *J. Hypertens.* 21:2281–2286.

Fleenor, B. S., A. L. Sindler, N. K. Marvi, K. L. Howell, M. L. Zigler, M. Yoshizawa, and D. R. Seals. 2013. Curcumin ameliorates arterial dysfunction and oxidative stress with aging. *Exp. Gerontol.* 48:269–276.

Fleg, J. L. 2002. Can exercise conditioning be effective in older heart failure patients? *Heart Fail. Rev.* 7:99–103.

Fleg, J. L. and E. G. Lakatta. 1988. 'Role of muscle loss in the age-associated reduction in VO_2 max. *J Appl Physiol (1985)* 65(3):1147–1151.

Fontana, L. and F. B. Hu. 2014. Optimal body weight for health and longevity: bridging basic, clinical, and population research. *Aging Cell* 13:391–400.

Fontana L. and S. Klein. 2007. Aging, adiposity, and calorie restriction. *JAMA* 297:986 –994.

Fontana L., T. E. Meyer, S. Klein, and J. O. Holloszy. 2004. Long-term calorie restriction is highly effective in reducing the risk for atherosclerosis in humans. *Proc. Natl Acad. Sci. USA* 101:6659–6663.

Fontana L., D. T. Villareal, E. P. Weiss, S. B. Racette, K. Steger-May, K. Klein, J. O. Holloszy, and the Washington University School of Medicine CALERIE Group. 2007. Calorie restriction or exercise: effects on coronary disease risk factors. A randomized, controlled trial. *Am. J. Physiol. Endocrinol. Metab.* 293:E197–202.

Fontana L., L. Partridge, and V. D. Longo. 2010. Extending healthy life span – from yeast to humans. *Science* 328:321–326.

Fontana, L., M. Vinciguerra, and V. D. Longo. 2012. Growth factors, nutrient signaling, and cardiovascular aging. *Circul. Res.* 110:1139–1150.

Forest, C. P., H. Padma-Nathan, and H. R. Liker. 2007. Efficacy and safety of pomegranate juice on improvement of erectile dysfunction in male patients with mild to moderate erectile dysfunction: a randomized, placebo-controlled, double-blind, crossover study. *Int. J. Impot. Res.* 19:564–567.

Fornieri, C., F. Taparelli, D. Quaglino Jr, M. B. Contri, J. M. Davidson, S. Algeri, and I. P. Ronchetti. 1999. The effect of caloric restriction on the aortic tissue of aging rats. *Connect. Tissue Res.* 40:131–143.

Freedman, N. J., S. B. Liggett, D. E. Drachman, G. Pei, M. G. Caron, and R. J. Lefkowitz. 1995. Phosphorylation and desensitization of the human beta 1-adrenergic receptor. Involvement of G protein-coupled receptor kinases and cAMP-dependent protein kinase. *J. Biol. Chem.* 270:17953-17961.

Fritze, O., B. Romero, M. Schleicher, M. P. Jacob, D. Y. Oh, B. Starcher, K. Schenke-Layland, J. Bujan, and U. A. Stock. 2012. Age-related changes in the elastic tissue of the human aorta. *J. Vasc. Res.* 49:77–86.

Fukuhara, S., A. Tsujimura, H. Okuda, K. Yamamoto, T. Takao, Y. Miyagawa, N. Nonomura, and A. Okuyama. 2011. Vardenafil and resveratrol synergistically enhance the nitric oxide/cyclic guanosine monophosphate pathway in corpus cavernosal smooth muscle cells and its therapeutic potential for erectile dysfunction in the streptozotocin-induced diabetic rat: preliminary findings. *J. Sex. Med.* 8:1061–1071.

Gale, C. R., C. N. Martyn, P. D. Winter, and C. Cooper. 1995.Vitamin C and risk of death from stroke and coronary heart disease in cohort of elderly people. *BMJ* 310:1563–1566.

Gale C. R., H. E. Ashurst, H. J. Powers, and C. N. Martyn. 2001. Antioxidant vitamin status and carotid atherosclerosis in the elderly. *Am. J. Clin. Nutr.* 74:402–408.

Garban, H., D. Vernet, A. Freedman, J. Rajfer, and N. Gonzalez-Cadavid. 1995. Effect of aging on nitric oxide-mediated penile erection in rats. *Am. J. Physiol.* 268:H467–H475.

Gates, P. E., H. Tanaka, W. R. Hiatt, and D. R. Seals. 2004. Dietary sodium restriction rapidly improves large elastic artery compliance in older adults with systolic hypertension. *Hypertension* 44:35–41.

Gelinas, D. S., P. N. Bernatchez, S. Rollin, N. G. Bazan, and M. G. Sirois. 2002. Immediate and delayed VEGF-mediated NO synthesis in endothelial cells: role of PI3K, PKC and PLC pathways. *Br. J. Pharmacol.* 137:1021–1030.

Gentile, V., P. Vicini, G. Prigiotti, A. Koverech, and F. Di Silverio. 2004. Preliminary observations on the use of propionyl-L-carnitine in combination with sildenafil in patients with erectile dysfunction and diabetes. *Curr. Med. Res. Opin.* 20:1377–1384.

Ghalayini, I. F., M. A. Al-Ghazo, R. Al-Azab, I. Bani-Hani, Y. S. Matani, A. E. Barham, M. N. Harfeil, and Y. Haddad. 2010. Erectile dysfunction in a Mediterranean country: results of an epidemiological survey of a representative sample of men. *Int. J. Impot. Res.* 22:196–203.

Giallauria F., Y. Milaneschi, T. Tanaka, M. Maggio, M. Canepa, P. Elango, C. Vigorito, E. G. Lakatta, L. Ferrucci, and J. Strait. 2012. Arterial stiffness and vitamin D levels: the Baltimore longitudinal study of aging. *J. Clin. Endocrinol. Metab.* 97:3717–3723.

Gianfrilli, D., R. Lauretta, C. Di Dato, C. Graziadio, C. Pozza, J. De Larichaudy, E. Giannetta, A. M. Isidori, and A. Lenzi. 2012. Propionyl-L-carnitine, L-arginine and niacin in sexual medicine: a nutraceutical approach to erectile dysfunction. *Andrologia* 44:600–604.

Gokce N., J. F. Keaney Jr, B. Frei, M. Holbrook, M. Olesiak, B. J. Zachariah, C. Leeuwenburgh, J. W. Heinecke, and J. A. Vita. 1999. Long-term ascorbic acid administration reverses endothelial vasomotor dysfunction in patients with coronary artery disease. *Circulation* 99:3234–3240.

Goldstein. I. 2003. The association of ED (erectile dysfunction) with ED (endothelium dysfunction) in the *International Journal of Impotence Research: The Journal of Sexual Medicine. Int. J. Impot. Res.* 15:229–230.

Gori A. M., F. Sofi, A. M. Corsi, A. Gazzini, I. Sestini, F. Lauretani, S. Bandinelli, G. F. Gensini, L. Ferrucci, and R. Abbate. 2006. Predictors of vitamin B_6 and folate concentrations in older persons: the InCHIANTI study. *Clin. Chem.* 52:1318–1324.

Gredilla R., A. Sanz, M. Lopez-Torres, and G. Barja. 2001. Caloric restriction decreases mitochondrial free radical generation at complex i and lowers oxidative damage to mitochondrial DNA in the rat heart. *Faseb J.* 15:1589–1591.

Guay, A. T. 2007. ED2: erectile dysfunction = endothelial dysfunction. *Endocrinol. Metabol. Clin. N. Am.* 36:453–463.

Guevara-Aguirre J., P. Balasubramanian, M. Guevara-Aguirre, M. Wei, F. Madia, C. W. Cheng, D. Hwang, A. Martin-Montalvo, J. Saavedra, S. Ingles, de R. Cabo, P. Cohen, and V. D. Longo. 2011. Growth hormone receptor deficiency is associated with a major reduction in pro-aging signaling, cancer, and diabetes in humans. *Sci. Transl. Med.* 3:70ra13.

Gugliucci, A., K. Kotani, J. Taing, Y. Matsuoka, Y. Sano, M. Yoshimura, K. Egawa, C. Horikawa, Y. Kitagawa, Y. Kiso, S. Kimura, and N. Sakane. 2009. Short-term low calorie diet intervention reduces serum advanced glycation end products in healthy overweight or obese adults. *Ann. Nutr. Metab.* 54:197–201.

Guo Z., F. Mitchell-Raymundo, H. Yang, Y. Ikeno, J. Nelson, V. Diaz, A. Richardson, and R. Reddick. 2002. Dietary restriction reduces atherosclerosis and oxidative stress in the aorta of apolipoprotein E-deficient mice. *Mech. Ageing Dev.* 123:1121–1131.

Ha, U. S., J. S. Koh, H. S. Kim, J. C. Woo, S. J. Kim, H. Jang, B. I. Yoon, S. Y. Hwang, and S. W. Kim. 2012. Cyanidin-3-*O*-*β*-D-glucopyranoside concentrated materials from mulberry fruit have a potency to protect erectile function by minimizing oxidative stress in a rat model of diabetic erectile dysfunction. *Urol. Int.* 88:470–476.

Haddad F., P. W. Bodell, S. A. McCue, R. E. Herrick, and K. M. Baldwin. 1993. Food restriction-induced transformations in cardiac functional and biochemical properties in rats. *J. Appl. Physiol.* 74:606–612.

Hafner, A. V., J. Dai, A. P. Gomes, C. Y. Xiao, C. M. Palmeira, A. Rosenzweig, and D. A. Sinclair. 2010. Regulation of the mPTP by SIRT3-mediated deacetylation of CypD at lysine 166 suppresses age-related cardiac hypertrophy. *Aging (Albany NY)* 2:914–923.

Hamidi Madani, A., A. Asadolahzade, G. Mokhtari, R. Shahrokhi Damavand, A. Farzan, and S. Esmaeili. 2013. Assessment of the efficacy of combination therapy with folic acid and tadalafil for the management of erectile dysfunction in men with type 2 diabetes mellitus. *J. Sex. Med.*10:1146–1150.

Hamilton, I. M., W. S. Gilmore, I. F. Benzie, C. W. Mulholland, and J. J. Strain. 2000. Interactions between vitamins C and E in human subjects. *Br. J. Nutr.* 84:261–267.

Harja, E., D. X. Bu, B. I. Hudson, J. S. Chang, X. Shen, K. Hallam, A. Z. Kalea, Y. Lu, R. H. Rosario, S. Oruganti, Z. Nikolla, D. Belov, E. Lalla, R. Ramasamy, S. F. Yan, and A. M. Schmidt. 2008. Vascular and inflammatory stresses mediate atherosclerosis via RAGE and its ligands in apo$E^{-/-}$ mice. *J. Clin. Invest.* 118:183–194.

Hayashi, T., K. Yano, H. Matsui-Hirai, H. Yokoo, Y. Hattori, and A. Iguchi. 2008. Nitric oxide and endothelial cellular senescence. *Pharmacol. Ther.* 120:333–339.

Hees, P. S., J. L. Fleg, E. G. Lakatta, and E. P. Shapiro. 2002. Left ventricular remodeling with age in normal men versus women: novel insights using three-dimensional magnetic resonance imaging. *Am. J. Cardiol.* 90:1231–1236.

Heller R., A. Unbehaun, B. Schellenberg, B. Mayer, G. Werner-Felmayer, and E. R. Werner. 2001. L-Ascorbic acid potentiates endothelial nitric oxide synthesis via a chemical stabilization of tetrahydrobiopterin. *J. Biol. Chem.* 276:40–47.

Helmy, M. M. and A. M. Senbel. 2012. Evaluation of vitamin E in the treatment of erectile dysfunction in aged rats. *Life Sci.* 90:489–494.

Hickson, S. S., M. Butlin, M. Graves, V. Taviani, A. P. Avolio, C. M. McEniery, and I. B. Wilkinson. 2010. The relationship of age with regional aortic stiffness and diameter. *JACC Cardiovasc. Imag.* 3:1247–1255.

Higashi, Y., K. Noma, M. Yoshizumi, and Y. Kihara. 2009. Endothelial function and oxidative stress in cardiovascular diseases. *Circul. J.* 73:411–418.

Higashi, Y., Y. Kihara, and K. Noma. 2012. Endothelial dysfunction and hypertension in aging. *Hypertens. Res.* 35:1039–1047.

Hill, J. M., G. Zalos, J. P. Halcox, W. H. Schenke, M. A. Waclawiw, A. A. Quyyumi, and T. Finkel. 2003. Circulating endothelial progenitor cells, vascular function, and cardiovascular risk. *New Engl. J. Med.* 348:593–600.

Hipkiss, A. R. 2006. Accumulation of altered proteins and ageing: causes and effects. *Exp. Gerontol.* 41:464–473.

Hnatyszyn, O., V. Moscatelli, R. Rondina, M. Costa, C. Arranz, A. Balaszczuk, J. Coussio, and G. Ferraro. 2004. Flavonoids from Achyrocline satureioides with relaxant effects on the smooth muscle of guinea pig corpus cavernosum. *Phytomedicine* 11:366–369.

Hotta, Y., A. Shiota, T. Kataoka, M. Motonari, Y. Maeda, M. Morita, and K. Kimura. 2013. Oral L-citrulline supplementation improves erectile function and penile structure in castrated rats. *Int. J. Urol.* [Epub ahead of print]

Hu, T. Y., C. L. Liu, C. C. Chyau, and M. L. Hu. 2012. Trapping of methylglyoxal by curcumin in cell-free systems and in human umbilical vein endothelial cells. *J. Agric. Food Chem.* 60:8190–8196.

Huang, Y. C., H. Ning, A. W. Shindel, T. M. Fandel, G. Lin, A. M. Harraz, T. F. Lue, and C. S. Lin. 2010. The effect of intracavernous injection of adipose tissue-derived stem cells on hyperlipidemia-associated erectile dysfunction in a rat model. *J. Sex. Med.* 7:1391–1400.

Hurt, K. J., S. F. Sezen, G. F. Lagoda, B. Musicki, G. A. Rameau, S. H. Snyder, and A. L. Burnett. 2012. Cyclic AMP-dependent phosphorylation of neuronal nitric oxide synthase mediates penile erection. *Proc. Natl Acad. Sci. USA* 109:16624–16629.

Ignarro, L. J., P. A. Bush, G. M. Buga, K. S. Wood, J. M. Fukuto, and J. Rajfer. 1990. Nitric oxide and cyclic GMP formation upon electrical field stimulation cause relaxation of corpus cavernosum smooth muscle. *Biochem. Biophys. Res. Commun.* 31:843–850.

Jackson, G., A. Nehra, M. Miner, K. L. Billups, A. L. Burnett, J. Buvat, C. C. Carson, G. Cunningham, I. Goldstein, A. T. Guay, G. Hackett, R. A. Kloner, J. B. Kostis, P. Montorsi, M. Ramsey, R. Rosen, R. Sadovsky, A. D. Seftel, R. Shabsigh, C. Vlachopoulos, and F. C. Wu. 2013. The assessment of vascular risk in men with erectile dysfunction: the role of the cardiologist and general physician. *Int. J. Clin. Pract.* 67:1163–1172.

Janczewski, A. M., H. A. Spurgeon, and E. G. Lakatta. 2002. Action potential prolongation in cardiac myocytes of old rats is an adaptation to sustain youthful intracellular Ca^{2+} regulation. *J. Mol. Cell. Cardiol.* 34:641–648.

Jiaan D. B., A. D. Seftel, J. Fogarty, N. Hampel, W. Cruz, J. Pomerantz, M. Zuik, and V. M. Monnier. 1995: Age-related increase in an advanced glycation end product in penile tissue. *World J. Urol.* 13:369–375.

Johnson, J. M., T. J. Bivalacqua, G. A. Lagoda, A. L. Burnett, and B. Musicki. 2011. eNOS-uncoupling in age-related erectile dysfunction. *Int. J. Impot. Res.* 23:43–48.

Jolly C. A. 2004. Dietary restriction and immune function. *J. Nutr.* 134:1853–1856.

Jones, R. D., P. J. Pugh, T. H. Jones, and K. S. Channer. 2003. The vasodilatory action of testosterone: a potassium-channel opening or calcium antagonistic action? *Br. J. Pharmacol.* 138:733–744.

Jones, R. W., R. W. Rees, S. Minhas, D. Ralph, R. A. Persad, and J. Y. Jeremy. 2002. Oxygen free radicals and the penis. *Expert Opin. Pharmacother.* 3:889–897.

Jovanovski, E., A. Jenkins, A. G. Dias, V. Peeva, J. Sievenpiper, J. T. Arnason, D. Rahelic, R. G. Josse, and V. Vuksan. 2010. Effects of Korean red ginseng (*Panax ginseng* C. A. Mayer) and its isolated ginsenosides and polysaccharides on arterial stiffness in healthy individuals. *Am. J. Hypertens.* 23:469–472.

Juhaszova, M., C. Rabuel, D. B. Zorov, E. G. Lakatta, and S. J. Sollott. 2005. Protection in the aged heart: preventing the heart-break of old age? *Cardiovasc. Res.* 66:233–244.

Katusic, Z. S. and P. M. Vanhoutte. 1989. Superoxide anion is an endothelium-derived contracting factor. *Am. J. Physiol.* 257:H33–H37.

Kaufman, S. 1993. New tetrahydrobiopterin-dependent systems. *Annu. Rev. Nutr.* 13:261–286.

Kaya, C., Z. Uslu, and I. Karaman. 2006. Is endothelial function impaired in erectile dysfunction patients? *Int. J. Impot. Res.* 18:55–60.

Keegan, A., H. Walbank, M. A. Cotter, and N. E. Cameron. 1995. Chronic vitamin E treatment prevents defective endothelium-dependent relaxation in diabetic rat aorta. *Diabetologia* 38:1475–1478.

Keegan, A., M. A. Cotter, and N. E. Cameron. 2001. Corpus cavernosum dysfunction in diabetic rats: effects of combined alpha-lipoic acid and gamma-linolenic acid treatment. *Diabetes Metab. Res. Rev.* 17:380–386.

Khoo, J., C. Piantadosi, R. Duncan, S. G. Worthley, A. Jenkins, M. Noakes, M. I. Worthley, K. Lange, and G. A. Wittert. 2011. Comparing effects of a low-energy diet and a high-protein low-fat diet on sexual and endothelial function, urinary tract symptoms, and inflammation in obese diabetic men. *J. Sex. Med.* 8:2868–2675.

Kiecolt-Glaser, J. K., M. A. Belury, R. Andridge, W. B. Malarkey, B. S. Hwang, and R. Glaser. 2012. Omega-3 supplementation lowers inflammation in healthy middle-aged and older adults: a randomized controlled trial. *Brain Behav. Immun.* 26:988–995.

Kiecolt-Glaser, J. K., E. S. Epel, M. A. Belury, R. Andridge, J. Lin, R. Glaser, W. B. Malarkey, B. S. Hwang, and E. Blackburn. 2013. Omega-3 fatty acids, oxidative stress, and leukocyte telomere length: a randomized controlled trial. *Brain Behav. Immun.* 28:16–24.

Kim, D. C., W. Lee, and J. S. Bae. 2011. Vascular anti-inflammatory effects of curcumin on HMGB1-mediated responses in vitro. *Inflamm. Res.* 60:1161–1168.

Kirstein, M., J. Brett, S. Radoff, S. Ogawa, D. Stern, and H. Vlassara. 1990. Advanced protein glycosylation induces transendothelial human monocyte chemotaxis and secretion of platelet-derived growth factor: role in vascular disease of diabetes and aging. *Proc. Natl Acad. Sci. USA* 87:9010–9014.

Kitzman, D. W. and W. D. Edwards. 1990. Age-related changes in the anatomy of the normal human heart. *J. Gerontol.* 45:M33–39.

Klonizakis, M., A. Alkhatib, G. Middleton, and M. F. Smith. 2012. Mediterranean diet- and exercise-induced improvement in age-dependent vascular activity. *Clin. Sci.* 124, 579–575.

Knekt P., A. Reunanen, R. Jarvinen, R. Seppanen, M. Heliovaara, and A. Aromaa. 1994. Antioxidant vitamin intake and coronary mortality in a longitudinal population study. *Am. J. Epidemiol.* 139:1180–1189.

Knott, H. M., B. E. Brown, M. J. Davies, and R. T. Dean. 2003. Glycation and glycoxidation of low-density lipoproteins by glucose and low-molecular mass aldehydes. Formation of modified and oxidized particles. *Eur. J. Biochem.* 270:3572–3582.

Kondoh, N., Y. Higuchi, T. Maruyama, M. Nojima, S. Yamamoto, and H. Shima. 2008. Salvage therapy trial for erectile dysfunction using phosphodiesterase type 5 inhibitors and vitamin E: preliminary report. *Aging Male* 11:167–170.

Kushi L. H., A. R. Folsom, R. J. Prineas, P. J. Mink, Y. Wu, and R. M. Bostick. 1996. Dietary antioxidant vitamins and death from coronary heart disease in postmenopausal women. *New Engl. J. Med.* 334:1156–62.

La Favor, J. D., E. J. Anderson, R. C. Hickner, and C. J. Wingard. 2013. Erectile dysfunction precedes coronary artery endothelial dysfunction in rats fed a high-fat, high-sucrose, Western pattern diet. *J. Sex. Med.* 10:694–703.

Lagouge M., C. Argmann, Z. Gerhart-Hines, H. Meziane, C. Lerin, F. Daussin, N. Messadeq, J. Milne, P. Lambert, P. Elliott, B. Geny, M. Laakso, P. Puigserver, and J. Auwerx. 2006. Resveratrol improves mitochondrial function and protects against metabolic disease by activating sirt1 and pgc-1alpha. *Cell* 127:1109–1122.

Lakatta, E. G. 1993. Cardiovascular regulatory mechanisms in advanced age. *Physiol. Rev.* 73:413–467.

Lakatta, E. G. and D. Levy. 2003. Arterial and cardiac aging: major shareholders in cardiovascular disease enterprises: Part I: aging arteries: a "set up" for vascular disease. *Circulation* 107:139–146.

Lakatta, E. G. and S. J. Sollott. 2002. Perspectives on mammalian cardiovascular aging: humans to molecules. *Comp. Biochem. Physiol. A Mol. Integr. Physiol.* 132:699–721.

Laurent, S. 2012. Defining vascular aging and cardiovascular risk. *J. Hypertens.* 30 Suppl:S3–8.

Lee S., Y. Park, M. Y. Zuidema, M. Hannink, and C. Zhang. 2011. Effects of interventions on oxidative stress and inflammation of cardiovascular diseases. *World J. Cardiol.*3:18–24.

Leeuwenburgh C., P. Wagner, J. O. Holloszy, R. S. Sohal, and J. W. Heinecke. 1997. Caloric restriction attenuates dityrosine cross-linking of cardiac and skeletal muscle proteins in aging mice. *Arch. Biochem. Biophys.* 346:74–80.

Lilamand, M., E. Kelaiditi, S. Guyonnet, R. Antonelli Incalzi, A. Raynaud-Simon, B. Vellas, and M. Cesari. 2014. Flavonoids and arterial stiffness: promising perspectives. *Nutr. Metab. Cardiovasc. Dis.* 24:698–704.

Lima, C. F., C. Pereira-Wilson, and S. I. Rattan. 2011. Curcumin induces heme oxygenase-1 in normal human skin fibroblasts through redox signaling: relevance for anti-aging intervention. *Mol. Nutr. Food Res.* 55:430–442.

Lines, T. C. and M. Ono. 2006. FRS 1000, an extract of red onion peel, strongly inhibits phosphodiesterase 5A (PDE 5A). *Phytomedicine* 13:236–239.

Lorenz, M., S. Wessler, E. Follmann, W. Michaelis, T. Düsterhöft, G. Baumann, K. Stangl, and V. Stangl. 2004. A constituent of green tea, epigallocatechin-3-gallate, activates endothelial nitric oxide synthase by a phosphatidylinositol-3-OH-kinase-, cAMP-dependent protein kinase-, and Akt-dependent pathway and leads to endothelial-dependent vasorelaxation. *J. Biol. Chem.* 279:6190–6195.

Lusis, A. J. 2000. Atherosclerosis. *Nature* 407:233–241.

Mager D. E., R. Wan, M. Brown, A. Cheng, P. Wareski, D. R. Abernethy, and M. P. Mattson. 2006. Caloric restriction and intermittent fasting alter spectral measures of heart rate and blood pressure variability in rats. *FASEB J.* 20:631–637.

Maio, M. T., J. L. Hannan, M. Komolova, and M. A. Adams. 2012. Caloric restriction prevents visceral adipose tissue accumulation and maintains erectile function in aging rats. *J. Sex. Med.* 9:2273–2283.

Mandavia, C. H., L. Pulakat, V. DeMarco, and J. R. Sowers. 2012. Over-nutrition and metabolic cardiomyopathy. *Metabolism* 61:1205–1210.

Margina, D., D. Gradinaru, G. Manda, I. Neagoe, and M. Ilie. 2013. Membranar effects exerted in vitro by polyphenols – quercetin, epigallocatechin gallate and curcumin – on HUVEC and Jurkat cells, relevant for diabetes mellitus. *Food Chem. Toxicol.* 61:86–93.

Marin, C., R. Ramirez, J. Delgado-Lista, E. M. Yubero-Serrano, P. Perez-Martinez, J. Carracedo, A. Garcia-Rios, F. Rodriguez, F. M. Gutierrez-Mariscal, P. Gomez, F. Perez-Jimenez, and J. Lopez-Miranda. 2011. Mediterranean diet reduces endothelial damage and improves the regenerative capacity of endothelium. *Am. J. Clin. Nutr.* 93, 267–274.

Marin, C., J. Delgado-Lista, R. Ramirez, J. Carracedo, J. Caballero, P. Perez-Martinez, F. M., Gutierrez-Mariscal, A. Garcia-Rios, N. Delgado-Casado, C. Cruz-Teno, E. M. Yubero-Serrano, F. Tinahones, M. Malagon Mdel, F. Perez-Jimenez, and J. Lopez-Miranda. 2012. Mediterranean diet reduces senescence-associated stress in endothelial cells. *AGE* 34:1309–1316.

Marin, C., E. M. Yubero-Serrano, J. López-Miranda, and J. Pérez-Jiménez. 2013. Endothelial aging associated with oxidative stress can be modulated by a healthy mediterranean diet. *Int. J. Mol. Sci.* 14:8869–8889.

Martin, C., W. Sun, C. Primiano, R. McKay, and J. Elefteriades. 2013. Age-dependent ascending aorta mechanics assessed through multiphase CT. *Ann. Biomed. Eng.* 41:2565–2574.

Matsushita, H., E. Chang, A. J. Glassford, J. P. Cooke, C. P. Chiu, and P. S. Tsao, 2001. eNOS activity is reduced in senescent human endothelial cells: preservation by hTERT immortalization. *Circul. Res.* 89:793–798.

Mattagajasingh, I., C. S. Kim, A. Naqvi, T. Yamamori, T. A. Hoffman, S. B. Jung, J. DeRicco, K. Kasuno, and K. Irani. 2007. SIRT1 promotes endothelium-dependent vascular relaxation by activating endothelial nitric oxide synthase. *Proc. Natl Acad. Sci. USA* 104:14855–14860.

McCann, S. M., J. Licinio, M. L. Wong, W. H. Yu, S. Karanth, and V. Rettorri. 1998. The nitric oxide hypothesis of aging. *Exp. Gerontol.* 33:813–826.

Meldrum, D. R., J. C. Gambone, M. A. Morris, and L. J. Ignarro. 2010. A multifaceted approach to maximize erectile function and vascular health. *Fertil. Steril.* 94:2514–2520.

Meyer T. E., S. J. Kovacs, A. A. Ehsani, S. Klein, J. O. Holloszy, and L. Fontana. 2006. Long-term caloric restriction ameliorates the decline in diastolic function in humans. *J. Am. Coll. Cardiol.* 47:398–402.

Michos, E. D., K. M. Rice, M. Szklo, G. L. Burke, D. S. Siscovick, R. P. Tracy, R. G. Barr, J. A. Nettleton, P. Greenland , D. R. Jacobs Jr, and W. Post. 2009. Factors associated with low levels of subclinical vascular disease in older adults: multi-ethnic study of atherosclerosis. *Prev. Cardiol.* 12:72–79.

Minamino, T., H. Miyauchi, T. Yoshida, Y. Ishida, H. Yoshida, and I. Komuro. 2002. Endothelial cell senescence in human atherosclerosis: role of telomere in endothelial dysfunction. *Circulation* 105:1541–1544.

Mirabello, L., W. Y. Huang, J. Y. Wong, N. Chatterjee, D. Reding, E. D. Crawford, I. de Vivo, R. B. Hayes, and S. A. Savage. 2009. The association between leukocyte telomere length and cigarette smoking, dietary and physical variables, and risk of prostate cancer. *Aging Cell* 8:405–413.

Mitchell, G. F., H. Parise, E. J. Benjamin, M. G. Larson, M. J. Keyes, J. A. Vita, R. S Vasan, and D. Levy. 2004. Changes in arterial stiffness and wave reflection with advancing age in healthy men and women: the Framingham Heart Study. *Hypertension* 43:1239–1245.

Mizutani, K., K. Ikeda, and Y. Yamori. 2000. Resveratrol inhibits AGEs-induced proliferation and collagen synthesis activity in vascular smooth muscle cells from stroke-prone spontaneously hypertensive rats. *Biochem. Biophys. Res. Commun.* 274:61–67.

Moens, A. L., C. J. Vrints, M. J. Claeys, J. P. Timmermans, H. C. Champion, and D. A. Kass. 2008. Mechanisms and potential therapeutic targets for folic acid in cardiovascular disease. *Am. J. Physiol. Heart Circul. Physiol.* 294:H1971–H1977.

Montorsi, P., P. M. Ravagnani, S. Galli, F. Rotatori, A. Briganti, A. Salonia, P. Rigatti, and F. Montorsi. 2005. The artery size hypothesis: a macrovascular link between erectile dysfunction and coronary artery disease. *Am. J. Cardiol.* 96:19M–23M.

Montorsi, P., P. M. Ravagnani, S. Galli , F. Rotatori, F. Veglia, A. Briganti, A. Salonia, F. Dehò, P. Rigatti, F. Montorsi, and C. Fiorentini. 2006. Association between erectile dysfunction and coronary artery disease. Role of coronary clinical presentation and extent of coronary vessels involvement: the COBRA trial. *Eur. Heart J.* 27:2632–2639.

Moody, J. A., D. Vernet, S. Laidlaw, J. Rajfer, and N. F. Gonzalez-Cadavid. 1997. Effects of long-term oral administration of L-arginine on the rat erectile response. *J. Urol.* 158:942–947.

Morano, S., E. Mandosi, M. Fallarino, A. Gatti, C. Tiberti, M. Sensi, L. Gandini, B. Buchetti, L. Lenti, E. A. Jannini, and A. Lenzi. 2007. Antioxidant treatment associated with sildenafil reduces monocyte activation and markers of endothelial damage in patients with diabetic erectile dysfunction: a double-blind, placebo-controlled study. *Eur. Urol.* 52:1768–1774.

Morgan, D. R., L. J. Dixon, C. G. Hanratty, N. El-Sherbeeny, P. B. Hamilton, L. T. McGrath, W. J. Leahey, G. D. Johnston, and G. E. McVeigh. 2006. Effects of dietary omega-3 fatty acid supplementation on endothelium-dependent vasodilation in patients with chronic heart failure. *Am. J. Cardiol.* 97:547–551.

Morris, S. M. Jr. 2004. Enzymes of arginine metabolismo. *J. Nutr.* 134:2743S–2747S.

Mostafa, T., D. Sabry, A. M. Abdelaal, I. Mostafa, and M. Taymour. 2013. Cavernous antioxidant effect of green tea, epigallocatechin-3-gallate with/without sildenafil citrate intake in aged diabetic rats. *Andrologia* 45:272–277.

Moyad, M. A. and K. Park. 2012. What do most erectile dysfunction guidelines have in common? No evidence-based discussion or recommendation of heart-healthy lifestyle changes and/or *Panax ginseng*. *Asian J. Androl.* 14:830–841.

Murakami S. 2006. Stress resistance in long-lived mouse models. *Exp. Gerontol.* 41:1014–1019.

Murasawa, S., J. Llevadot, M. Silver, J. M. Isner, D. W. Losordo, and T. Asahara. 2002. Constitutive human telomerase reverse transcriptase expression enhances regenerative properties of endothelial progenitor cells. *Circulation* 106:1133–1139.

Musicki, B., M. F. Kramer, R. E. Becker, and A. L. Burnett. 2005. Age-related changes in phosphorylation of endothelial nitric oxide synthase in the rat penis. *J. Sex. Med.* 2:347–355.

Musicki, B., T. Liu, T. Strong, L. Jin, M. H. Laughlin, J. R. Turk, and A. L. Burnett. 2008. Low-fat diet and exercise preserve eNOS regulation and endothelial function in the penis of early atherosclerotic pigs: a molecular analysis. *J. Sex. Med.* 5:552–561.

Nagai, Y., E. J. Metter, C. J. Earley, M. K. Kemper, L. C. Becker, E. G. Lakatta, and J. L. Fleg. 1998. Increased carotid artery intimal-medial thickness in asymptomatic older subjects with exercise-induced myocardial ischemia. *Circulation* 98:1504–1509.

Najjar, S. S., A. Scuteri, V. Shetty, J. G. Wright, D. C. Muller, J. L. Fleg, H. P. Spurgeon, L. Ferrucci, and E. G. Lakatta. 2008. Pulse wave velocity is an independent predictor of the longitudinal increase in systolic blood pressure and of incident hypertension in the Baltimore Longitudinal Study of Aging. *J. Am. Coll. Cardiol.* 51:1377–1383.

Nakashima, H., R. Ozono, C. Suyama, T. Sueda, M. Kambe, and T. Oshima. 2004. Telomere attrition in white blood cell correlating with cardiovascular damage. *Hypertens. Res.* 27:319–325.

Nam, M. H., H. S. Lee, Y. Seomun, Y. Lee, and K. W. Lee. 2011. Monocyte-endothelium-smooth muscle cell interaction in co-culture: proliferation and cytokine productions in response to advanced glycation end products. *Biochim. Biophys. Acta* 1810:907–912.

Neves, D. 2013. Advanced glycation end-products: a common pathway in diabetes and age-related erectile dysfunction. *Free Rad. Res.* 47:49–69.

Neves D., J. Santos, N. Tomada, H. Almeida, and P. Vendeira. 2006. Ageing and orchidectomy modulate expression of VEGF receptors (Flt-1 and Flk-1) on corpus cavernosum of the rat. *Ann. NY Acad. Sci.* 1067:164–172.

Neves, D., M. Assunção, F. Marques, J. P. Andrade, and H. Almeida. 2008. Does regular consumption of green tea influence VEGF and its receptors expression in aged rat erectile tissue? Possible implications in vasculogenic erectile dysfunction progression. *AGE* 30:217–228.

Neves D., I. Tomada, M. Assunção, F. Marques, H. Almeida, and J. P. Andrade. 2010. Effects of chronic red wine consumption on the expression of vascular endothelial growth factor, angiopoietin 1, angiopoietin 2 and its receptors in rat erectile tissue. *J. Food Sci.* 75:H79–H86.

Ng, A. V., R. Callister, D. G. Johnson, and D. R. Seals. 1993. Age and gender influence muscle sympathetic nerve activity at rest in healthy humans. *Hypertension* 21:498–503.

Niemann B., Y. Chen, H. Issa, R. E. Silber, and S. Rohrbach. 2010. Caloric restriction delays cardiac ageing in rats: Role of mitochondria. *Cardiovasc. Res.* 88:267–276.

Nilsson, P. M. 2014. Hemodynamic aging as the consequence of structural changes associated with early vascular aging (EVA). *Aging Dis.* 5:109–113.

North, B. J. and D. A. Sinclair. 2012. The intersection between aging and cardiovascular disease. *Circul. Res.* 110:1097–1108.

Numao, N., H. Masuda, Y. Sakai, Y. Okada, K. Kinara, and H. Azuma. 2007. Roles of attenuated neuronal nitric-oxide synthase protein expression and accelerated arginase activity in impairing neurogenic relaxation of corpus cavernosum in aged rabbits. *BJU Int.* 99:1495–1499.

Okuda, K., M. Y. Khan, J. Skurnick, M. Kimura, H. Aviv, and A. Aviv. 2000. Telomere attrition of the human abdominal aorta: relationships with age and atherosclerosis. *Atherosclerosis* 152:391–398.

O'Rourke, M. F. and W. W. Nichols. 2005. Aortic diameter, aortic stiffness, and wave reflection increase with age and isolated systolic hypertension. *Hypertension* 45:652–658.

O'Rourke, M. F., A. Avolio, M. Safar, and W. Nichols. 2010a. Changes in the central arterial pressure pulse with aging. *J. Am. Coll. Cardiol.* 55:2183; author reply 84.

O'Rourke, M. F., M. E. Safar, and V. Dzau.2010b. The cardiovascular continuum extended: aging effects on the aorta and microvasculature. *Vasc. Med.* 15:461–468.

Ota, H., M. Akishita, M. Eto, K. Iijima, M. Kaneki, and Y. Ouchi. 2007. Sirt1 modulates premature senescence-like phenotype in human endothelial cells. *J. Mol. Cell Cardiol.* 43:571–579.

Pan, L., X. Xia, Y. Feng, C. Jiang, Y. Cui, and Y. Huang. 2008. Exposure of juvenile rats to the phytoestrogen daidzein impairs erectile function in a dose-related manner in adulthood. *J. Androl.* 29:55–62.

Pearson, K. J., J. A. Baur, K. N. Lewis, L. Peshkin, N. L. Price, N. Labinskyy, W. R. Swindell, D. Kamara, R. K. Minor, E. Perez, H. A. Jamieson, Y. Zhang, S. R. Dunn, K. Sharma, N. Pleshko, L. A. Woollett, A. Csiszar, Y. Ikeno, D. Le Couteur, P. J. Elliott, K. G. Becker, P. Navas, D. K. Ingram, N. S. Wolf, Z. Ungvari, D. Sinclair, and R. de Cabo. 2008. Resveratrol delays age-related deterioration and mimics transcriptional aspects of dietary restriction without extending life span. *Cell Metab.* 8:157–168.

Ponholzer, A., C. Temml, K. Mock, M. Marzlaekm, R. Obermayr, and S. Maderbacher. 2005. Prevalence and risk factors for erectile dysfunction in 2869 men using a validated questionnaire. *Eur. Urol.* 47:80–86.

Qiu, X., T. M. Fandel, G. Lin, Y. C. Huang, Y. T. Dai, T. F. Lue, and C. S. Lin. 2011. Cavernous smooth muscle hyperplasia in a rat model of hyperlipidaemia-associated erectile dysfunction. *BJU Int.* 108:1866–1872.

Quehenberger, P., A. Bierhaus, P. Fasching, C. Muellner, M. Klevesath, M. Hong, G. Stier, M. Sattler, E. Schleicher, W. Speiser, and P. P. Nawroth. 2000. Endothelin 1 transcription is controlled by nuclear factor-kappaB in AGE-stimulated cultured endothelial cells. *Diabetes* 49:1561–1570.

Quintero M., S. L. Colombo, A. Godfrey, and S. Moncada. 2006. Mitochondria as signaling organelles in the vascular endothelium. *Proc. Natl Acad. Sci. USA* 103:5379–5384.

Ramesh, T., S. W. Kim, S. Y. Hwang, S. H. Sohn, S. K. Yoo, and S. K. Kim. 2012. *Panax ginseng* reduces oxidative stress and restores antioxidant capacity in aged rats. *Nutr. Res.* 32:718–726.

Redheuil, A., W. C. Yu, E. Mousseaux, A. A. Harouni, N. Kachenoura, C. O. Wu, D. Bluemke, and J. A. Lima. 2011. Age-related changes in aortic arch geometry: relationship with proximal aortic function and left ventricular mass and remodeling. *J. Am. Coll. Cardiol.* 58:1262–1270.

Reilly C. M., P. Zamorano, V. S. Stopper, and T. M. Mills. 1997. Androgenic regulation of NO availability in rat penile erection. *J. Androl.* 18:110–115.

Rengo, G., P. Perrone-Filardi, G. D. Femminella, D. Liccardo, C. Zincarelli, C. de Lucia, G. Pagano, F. Marsico, A. Lymperopoulos, and D. Leosco. 2012. Targeting the beta-adrenergic receptor system through G-protein-coupled receptor kinase 2: a new paradigm for therapy and prognostic evaluation in heart failure: from bench to bedside. *Circul. Heart Fail.* 5:385–391.

Rinaldi, B., G. Corbi, S. Boccuti, W. Filippelli, G. Rengo, D. Leosco, F. Rossi, A. Filippelli, and N. Ferrara. 2006. Exercise training affects age-induced changes in SOD and heat shock protein expression in rat heart. *Exp. Gerontol.* 41:764–770.

Rippe, C., L. Lesniewski, M. Connell, T. LaRocca, A. Donato, and D. Seals. 2010. Short-term calorie restriction reverses vascular endothelial dysfunction in old mice by increasing nitric oxide and reducing oxidative stress. *Aging Cell* 9:304–312.

Rivard, A., J. E. Fabre, M. Silver, D. Chen, T. Murohara, M. Kearney, M. Magner, T. Asahara, and J. M. Isner. 1999. Age-dependent impairment of angiogenesis. *Circulation* 99:111–120.

Rizza, W., N. Veronese, and L. Fontana. 2013. What are the roles of calorie restriction and diet quality in promoting healthy longevity? *Ageing Res. Rev.* 13C:38–45.

Rodriguez-Crespo, I., P. Moenne-Loccoz, T. M. Loehr, and P. R. Ortiz de Montellano. 1997. Endothelial nitric oxide synthase: modulations of the distal heme site produced by progressive N-terminal deletions. *Biochemistry* 36:8530–8538.

Ryu, J. K., T. Lee, D. J. Kim, I. S. Park, S. M. Yoon, H. S. Lee, S. U. Song, and J. K. Suh. 2005. Free radical-scavenging activity of Korean red ginseng for erectile dysfunction in non-insulin-dependent diabetes mellitus rats. *Urology* 65:611–615.

Ryu, J. K., C. H. Cho, H. Y. Shin, S. U. Song, S. M. Oh, M. Lee, S. Piao, J. Y. Han, I. H. Kim, G. Y. Koh, and J. K. Suh. 2006. Combined angiopoietin-1 and vascular endothelial growth factor gene transfer restores cavernous angiogenesis and erectile function in a rat model of hypercholesterolemia. *Mol. Ther.* 13:705–715.

Safar, M. E. 2010. Arterial aging – hemodynamic changes and therapeutic options. *Nat. Rev. Cardiol.* 7:442–449.

Safar, M., P. Chamiot-Clerc, G. Dagher, and J. F. Renaud. 2001. Pulse pressure, endothelium function, and arterial stiffness in spontaneously hypertensive rats. *Hypertension* 38:1416–1421.

Sahyoun N. R., P. F. Jacques, and R. M. Russell. 1996. Carotenoids, vitamins C and E, and mortality in an elderly population. *Am. J. Epidemiol.* 144:501–11.

Sato, I., I. Morita, K. Kaji, M. Ikeda, M. Nagao, and S. Murota. 1993. Reduction of nitric oxide producing activity associated with in vitro aging in cultured human umbilical vein endothelial cell. *Biochem. Biophys. Res. Commun.* 195:1070–1076.

Schöneich C. 2006. Protein modification in aging: an update. *Exp. Gerontol.* 41:807–812.

Scoditti, E., N. Calabriso, M. Massaro, M. Pellegrino, C. Storelli, G. Martines, R. de Caterina, and M. A. Carluccio. 2012. Mediterranean diet polyphenols reduce inflammatory angiogenesis through MMP-9 and COX-2 inhibition in human vascular endothelial cells: A potentially protective mechanism in atherosclerotic vascular disease and cancer. *Arch. Biochem. Biophys.* 527:81–89.

Sell D. R., M. A. Lane, M. E. Obrenovich, J. A. Mattison, A. Handy, D. K. Ingram, R. G. Cutler, G. S. Roth, and V. M. Monnier. 2003. The effect of caloric restriction on glycation and glycoxidation in skin collagen of nonhuman primates. *J. Gerontol. A. Biol. Sci. Med. Sci.* 58:508–516.

Semba, R. D., S. S. Najjar, K. Sun, E. G. Lakatta, and L. Ferrucci. 2009. Serum carboxymethyl-lysine, an advanced glycation end product, is associated with increased aortic pulse wave velocity in adults. *Am. J. Hypertens.* 22:74–79.

Semba, R. D., A. Ang, S. Talegawkar, C. Crasto, M. Dalal, P. Jardack, M. G. Traber, L. Ferrucci, and L. Arab 2012. Dietary intake associated with serum versus urinary carboxymethyl-lysine, a major advanced glycation end product, in adults: the Energetics Study. *Eur. J. Clin. Nutr.* 66:3–9.

Sena, C. M., P. Matafome, J. Crisóstomo, L. Rodrigues, R. Fernandes, P. Pereira, and R. M. Seiça. 2012. Methylglyoxal promotes oxidative stress and endothelial dysfunction. *Pharmacol. Res.* 65:497–506.

Seymour E. M., R. V. Parikh, A. A. Singer, and S. F. Bolling. 2006. Moderate calorie restriction improves cardiac remodeling and diastolic dysfunction in the Dahl-SS rat. *J. Mol. Cell Cardiol.* 41:661–668.

Shaeer, O. and K. Shaeer. 2013. The Global Online Sexuality Survey (GOSS): the United States of America in 2011. Chapter I: erectile dysfunction among English-speakers. *J. Sex. Med.* 10:2904–2911.

Shah, N. C., G. J. Shah, Z. Li, X. C. Jiang, B. T. Altura, and B. M. Altura. 2014. Short-term magnesium deficiency downregulates telomerase, upregulates neutral sphingomyelinase and induces oxidative DNA damage in cardiovascular tissues: relevance to atherogenesis, cardiovascular diseases and aging. *Int. J. Clin. Exp. Med.* 7:497–514.

Shamloul, R. and H. Ghanem. 2013. Erectile dysfunction. *Lancet* 381:153–165.

Shea, M. K. and R. M. Holden, 2012. Vitamin K status and vascular calcification: evidence from observational and clinical studies. *Adv. Nutr.* 3:158–165.

Shen, J., M. D. Gammon, M. B. Terry, Q. Wang, P. Bradshaw, S. L. Teitelbaum, A. I. Neugut, and R. M. Santella. 2009. Telomere length, oxidative damage, antioxidants and breast cancer risk. *Int. J. Cancer* 124:1637–1643.

Shinmura, K. 2011. Cardiovascular protection afforded by caloric restriction: essential role of nitric oxide synthase. *Geriatr. Gerontol. Int.* 11:143–156.

Shinmura, K., K. Tamaki, M. Sano, N. Nakashima-Kamimura, A. M. Wolf, T. Amo, S. Ohta, Y. Katsumata, K. Fukuda, K. Ishiwata, M. Suematsu, and T. Adachi. 2011. Caloric restriction primes mitochondria for ischemic stress by deacetylating specific mitochondrial proteins of the electron transport chain. *Circul. Res.* 109:396–406.

Shiota, A., Y. Hotta, T. Kataoka, M. Morita, Y. Maeda, and K. Kimura. 2013. Oral L-citrulline supplementation improves erectile function in rats with acute arteriogenic erectile dysfunction. *J. Sex. Med.* 10:2423–2429.

Shukla, N., M. Hotston, R. Persad, G. D. Angelini, and J. Y. Jeremy. 2009. The administration of folic acid improves erectile function and reduces intracavernosal oxidative stress in the diabetic rabbit. *BJU Int.* 103:98–103.

Siepmann, T., J. Roofeh, F. W. Kiefer, and D. G. Edelson. 2011. Hypogonadism and erectile dysfunction associated with soy product consumption. *Nutrition* 27:859–862.

Silva, F. H., F. Z. Mónica, F. R. Báu, A. F. Brugnerotto, F. B. Priviero, H. A. Toque, and E. Antunes. 2013. Superoxide anion production by NADPH oxidase plays a major role in erectile dysfunction in middle-aged rats: prevention by antioxidant therapy. *J. Sex. Med.* 10:960–971.

Soner, B. C., N. Murat, O. Demir, H. Guven, A. Esen, and S. Gidener. 2010. Evaluation of vascular smooth muscle and corpus cavernosum on hypercholesterolemia. Is resveratrol promising on erectile dysfunction? *Int. J. Impot. Res.* 22:227–233.

Spina, R. J., M. J. Turner, and A. A. Ehsani. 1998. Beta-adrenergic-mediated improvement in left ventricular function by exercise training in older men. *Am. J. Physiol.* 274: H397–404.

Stadtman ER. 1992. Protein oxidation and aging. *Science* 257:1220–1224.

Stebbins, C. L., J. P. Stice, C. M. Hart, F. N. Mbai, and A. A. Knowlton. 2008. Effects of dietary decosahexaenoic acid (DHA) on eNOS in human coronary artery endothelial cells. *J. Cardiovasc. Pharmacol. Ther.* 13:261–268.

Stephens, E. H., N. de Jonge, M. P. McNeill, C. A. Durst, and K. J. Grande-Allen. 2010. Age-related changes in material behavior of porcine mitral and aortic valves and correlation to matrix composition. *Tissue Eng. Part A* 16:867–878.

Stephens, E. H., C. A. Durst, J. L. West, and K. J. Grande-Allen. 2011. Mitral valvular interstitial cell responses to substrate stiffness depend on age and anatomic region. *Acta Biomater.* 7:75–82.

Strait, J. B. and E. G. Lakatta. 2012. Aging-associated cardiovascular changes and their relationship to heart failure. *Heart Fail. Clin.* 8:143–164.

Su, J., P. A. Lucchesi, R. A. Gonzalez-Villalobos, D. I. Palen, B. M. Rezk, Y. Suzuki, H. A., Boulares, and K. Matrougui. 2008. Role of advanced glycation end products with oxidative stress in resistance artery dysfunction in type 2 diabetic mice. *Arterioscler. Thromb. Vasc. Biol.* 28:1432–1438.

Sugawara, J., K. Hayashi, T. Yokoi, and H. Tanaka. 2008. Age-associated elongation of the ascending aorta in adults. *JACC Cardiovasc. Imag.* 1:739–748.

Taddei, S., A. Virdis, L. Ghiadoni, A. Magagna, and A. Salvetti. 1998. Vitamin C improves endothelium-dependent vasodilation by restoring nitric oxide activity in essential hypertension. *Circulation* 97:2222–2229.

Taffet, G. E., T. T. Pham, and C. J. Hartley. 1997. The age-associated alterations in late diastolic function in mice are improved by caloric restriction. *J. Gerontol. A. Biol. Sci. Med. Sci.* 52:B285–B290.

Tagliabue, M., S. Pinach, C. Di Bisceglie, L. Brocato, M. Cassader, A. Bertagna, C. Manieri, and G. P. Pescarmona. 2005. Glutathione levels in patients with erectile dysfunction, with or without diabetes mellitus. *Int. J. Androl.* 28:156–162.

Tan, Y. T., F. Wenzelburger, E. Lee, G. Heatlie, F. Leyva, K. Patel, M. Frenneaux, and J. E. Sanderson, 2009. The pathophysiology of heart failure with normal ejection fraction: exercise echocardiography reveals complex abnormalities of both systolic and diastolic ventricular function involving torsion, untwist, and longitudinal motion. *J. Am. Coll. Cardiol.* 54:36–46.

Tanaka, H., F. A. Dinenno, K. D. Monahan, C. M. Clevenger, C. A. DeSouza, and D. R. Seals. 2000. Aging, habitual exercise, and dynamic arterial compliance. *Circulation* 102:11, 1270–1275.

Tarasov, K. V., S. Sanna, A. Scuteri, J. B., Strait, M. Orru, A. Parsa, P. I. Lin, A. Maschio, S. Lai, M. G. Piras, M. Masala, T. Tanaka, W. Post, J. R. O'Connell, D. Schlessinger, A. Cao, R. Nagaraja, B. D. Mitchell, G. R. Abecasis, A. R. Shuldiner, M. Uda, E. G. Lakatta, and S. S. Najjar. 2009. COL4A1 is associated with arterial stiffness by genome-wide association scan. *Circul. Cardiovasc. Genet.* 2:2, 151–158.

Tomada, I., D. Fernandes, J. T. Guimarães, H. Almeida, and D. Neves. 2013a. Energy restriction ameliorates Metabolic Syndrome-induced cavernous tissue structural modifications in aged rats. *AGE* 35:1721–1739.

Tomada, I., N. Tomada, H. Almeida, and D. Neves. 2013b. Androgen depletion in humans leads to cavernous tissue reorganization and upregulation of Sirt1–eNOS axis. *AGE* 35:35–47.

Tomada, I., R. Negrão, H. Almeida, and D. Neves. 2014. Long term high-fat consumption leads to down-regulation of Akt phosphorylation of eNOS at Ser1177 and upregulation of Sirtuin-1 expression in rat cavernous tissue. *AGE* 36:597–611.

Tomada, N., R. Oliveira, I. Tomada, P. Vendeira, and D. Neves. 2008. Comparative ultrastructural study of human corpus cavernosum during ageing. *Microsc. Microanal.* 14:S3152–3155.

Tomada, N., Tomada I., Vendeira P., Cruz F. and D. Neves. 2010. Characterization of VEGF and Angiopoietins expression in human corpus cavernosum during aging. *J. Sex. Med.* 7:1410–1418.

Tomasian, D., J. F. Keaney, and J. A. Vita. 2000. Antioxidants and the bioactivity of endothelium-derived nitric oxide. *Cardiovasc. Res.* 47:426–435.

Traish, A. M. and A. Galoosian. 2013. Androgens modulate endothelial function and endothelial progenitor cells in erectile physiology. *Korean J. Urol.* 54:721–731.

Turgeon, J., S. Dussault, F. Maingrette, J. Groleau, P. Haddad, G. Perez, and A. Rivard. 2013. Fish oil-enriched diet protects against ischemia by improving angiogenesis, endothelial progenitor cell function and postnatal neovascularization. *Atherosclerosis* 229:295–303.

Umemura, T., J. Soga, T. Hidaka, H. Takemoto, S. Nakamura, D. Jitsuiki, K. Nishioka, C. Goto, H. Teragawa, M. Yoshizumi, K. Chayama, and Y. Higashi. 2008. Aging and hypertension are independent risk factors for reduced number of circulating endothelial progenitor cells. *Am. J. Hypertens.* 21:1203–1209.

Ungvari, Z., C. Parrado-Fernandez, A. Csiszar, and de R. Cabo. 2008. Mechanisms underlying caloric restriction and lifespan regulation: implications for vascular aging. *Circul. Res.* 102:519–528.

Ungvari, Z., N. Labinskyy, P. Mukhopadhyay, J. T. Pinto, Z. Bagi, P. Ballabh, C. Zhang, P. Pacher, and A. Csiszar. 2009. Resveratrol attenuates mitochondrial oxidative stress in coronary arterial endothelial cells. *Am. J. Physiol. Heart Circul. Physiol.* 297:H1876–1881.

Ungvari, Z., G. Kaley, R. de Cabo, W. E. Sonntag, and A. Csiszar. 2010. Mechanisms of vascular aging: New perspectives. *J. Gerontol. A. Biol. Sci. Med. Sci.* 65:1028–1041.

Uribarri, J., S. Woodruff, S. Goodman, W. Cai, X. Chen, R. Pyzik, A. Yong, G. E. Striker, and H. Vlassara. 2010. Advanced glycation end products in foods and a practical guide to their reduction in the diet. *J Am. Diet. Assoc.* 110:911–916.e12.

Vaitkevicius, P. V., J. L. Fleg, J. H. Engel, F. C. O'Connor, J. G. Wright, L. E. Lakatta, F. C. Yin, and E. G. Lakatta. 1993. Effects of age and aerobic capacity on arterial stiffness in healthy adults. *Circulation* 88:1456–1462.

Varady, K. A., S. Bhutani, E. C. Church, and M. C. Klempel. 2009. Short-term modifiedalternate-day fasting: a novel dietary strategy for weight loss and cardioprotection in obese adults. *Am. J. Clin. Nutr.* 90:1138–1143.

Vasa, M., K. Breitschopf, A. M. Zeiher, and S. Dimmeler. 2000. Nitric oxide activates telomerase and delays endothelial cell senescence. *Circul. Res.* 87:540–542.

Verdin, E., M. D. Hirschey, L. W. Finley, annd M. C. Haigis. 2010. Sirtuin regulation of mitochondria: energy production, apoptosis, and signaling. *Trends Biochem. Sci.* 35:669–675.

Virmani, R., A. P. Avolio, W. J. Mergner, M. Robinowitz, E. E. Herderick, J. F. Cornhill, S. Y. Guo, T. H. Liu, D. Y. Ou, and M. O'Rourke. 1991. Effect of aging on aortic morphology in populations with high and low prevalence of hypertension and atherosclerosis. Comparison between occidental and Chinese communities. *Am. J. Pathol.* 139:1119–1129.

Visioli, F. and T. M. Hagen. 2007. Nutritional strategies for healthy cardiovascular aging: Focus on micronutrients. *Pharmacol. Res.* 55:199–206.

Werner, N., S. Kosiol, T. Schiegl, P. Ahlers, K. Walenta, A. Link, M. Bohm, and G. Nickenig. 2005. Circulating endothelial progenitor cells and cardiovascular outcomes. *New Engl. J. Med.* 353:999–1007.

White, M., R. Roden, W. Minobe, M. F. Khan, P. Larrabee, M. Wollmering, J. D. Port, F. Anderson, D. Campbell, A. M. Feldman, and M. R. Bristow. 1994. Age-related changes in beta-adrenergic neuroeffector systems in the human heart. *Circulation* 90:1225–1238.

Williams, B. and P. S. Lacy, 2010. Central haemodynamics and clinical outcomes: going beyond brachial blood pressure? *Eur. Heart J.* 31:1819–1822.

Williamson, K., S. E. Stringer, and M. Y. Alexander. 2012. Endothelial progenitor cells enter the aging arena. *Front. Physiol.* 3:30.

Wing, R. R., R. C. Rosen, J. L. Fava, J. Bahnson, F. Brancati, I. N. Gendrano III, A. Kitabchi, S. H. Schneider, and T. A. Wadden. 2010. Effects of weight loss intervention on erectile function in older men with type 2 diabetes in the Look AHEAD trial. *J. Sex. Med.* 7:156–165.

Wolak, T. and T. Paran. 2013. Can carotenoids attenuate vascular aging? *Vasc. Pharmacol.* 59:63–66.

Wu, M., C. Rementer, and C. M. Giachelli. 2013. Vascular calcification: an update on mechanisms and challenges in treatment. *Calcif. Tissue Int.* 93:365–373.

Xiao, R. P., H. Cheng, Y. Y. Zhou, M. Kuschel, and E. G. Lakatta. 1999. Recent advances in cardiac beta(2)-adrenergic signal transduction. *Circul. Res.* 85:1092–1100.

Xu, B., Y. Ji, K. Yao, Y. X. Cao, and A. Ferro. 2005. Inhibition of human endothelial cell nitric oxide synthesis by advanced glycation end-products but not glucose: relevance to diabetes. *Clin. Sci. (Lond.)* 10:439–446.

Yang, H., M. Shi, J. Story, A. Richardson, and Z. Guo. 2004. Food restriction attenuates age-related increase in the sensitivity of endothelial cells to oxidized lipids. *J. Gerontol. A. Biol. Sci. Med. Sci.* 59: 316–323.

Yang, R., J. Wang, Y. Chen, Z. Sun, R. Wang, and Y. Dai. 2008. Effect of caffeine on erectile function via up-regulating cavernous cyclic guanosine monophosphate in diabetic rats. *J. Androl.* 29:586–591.

Yassin, A. A., F. Saad, and A. Traish. 2006. Testosterone undecanoate restores erectile function in a subset of patients with venous leakage: a series of case reports. *J. Sex. Med.* 3:727–735.

Yu, W., Z. Wan, X. F. Qiu, Y. Chen, and Y. T. Dai. 2013. Resveratrol, an activator of SIRT1, restores erectile function in streptozotocin-induced diabetic rats. *Asian J. Androl.* 15:646–651.

Yubero-Serrano, E. M. A. Garcia-Rios, J. Delgado-Lista, N. Delgado-Casado, P. Perez-Martinez, F. Rodriguez-Cantalejo, F. Fuentes, C. Cruz-Teno, I. Tunez, I. Tasset-Cuevas, F. J. Tinahones, F. Perez-Jimenez, and J. Lopez-Miranda. 2011. Postprandial effects of the Mediterranean diet on oxidant and antioxidant status in elderly men and women. *J. Am. Geriatr. Soc.* 59:938–940.

Zanetti, M., G. Gortan Cappellari, I. Burekovic, R. Barazzoni, M. Stebel, and G. Guarnieri. 2010. Caloric restriction improves endothelial dysfunction during vascular aging: effects on nitric oxide synthase isoforms and oxidative stress in rat aorta. *Exp. Gerontol.* 45:848–855.

Zang M., S. Xu, K. A. Maitland-Toolan, A. Zuccollo, X. Hou, B. Jiang, M. Wierzbicki, T. J. Verbeuren, and R. A. Cohen. 2006. Polyphenols stimulate amp-activated protein kinase, lower lipids, and inhibit accelerated atherosclerosis in diabetic ldl receptor-deficient mice. *Diabetes* 55:2180–2191.

Zeiher, A. M., H. Drexler, B. Saurbier, and H. Just. 1993. Endothelium-mediated coronary blood flow modulation in humans. Effects of age, atherosclerosis, hypercholesterolemia, and hypertension. *J. Clin. Invest.* 92:652–662.

Zhang, Q. J., Z. Wang, H. Z. Chen, S. Zhou, W. Zheng, G. Liu, Y. S. Wei, H. Cai, D. P. Liu, and C. C. Liang. 2008. Endothelium-specific overexpression of class III deacetylase SIRT1 decreases atherosclerosis in apolipoprotein E-deficient mice. *Cardiovasc. Res.* 80:191–199.

Zhang, Q., Z. M. Radisavljevic, M. B. Siroky, and K. M. Azadzoi. 2011a. Dietary antioxidants improve arteriogenic erectile dysfunction. *Int. J. Androl.* 34:225–235.

Zhang, W., Y. Wang, Z. Yang, J. Qiu, J. Ma, Z. Zhao, and T. Bao. 2011b. Antioxidant treatment with quercetin ameliorates erectile dysfunction in streptozotocin-induced diabetic rats. *J. Biosci. Bioeng.* 112:215–218.

Zhu, H., M. Belcher, and P. van der Harst. 2011. Healthy aging and disease: role for telomere biology? *Clin. Sci. (Lond.)* 120:427–440.

Zorgniotti, A. W. and E. F. Lizza. 1994. Effect of large doses of the nitric oxide precursor, L-arginine, on erectile dysfunction. *Int. J. Impot. Res.* 6:33–35.

Zuchi, C., G. Ambrosio, T. F. Luscher, and U. Landmesser. 2010. Nutraceuticals in cardiovascular prevention: lessons from studies on endothelial function. *Cardiovasc. Ther.* 28:187–201.

CHAPTER 7

Bone and muscle ageing

Joana Carvalho[1], Elisa Marques[1] and Pedro Moreira[1,2]

[1] *Research Centre in Physical Activity, Health and Leisure, Faculty of Sport Science, University of Porto, Porto, Portugal*

[2] *Faculty of Nutrition and Food Sciences, University of Porto, Porto, Portugal*

7.1 Introduction

One of the most striking effects of age is the involuntary loss of muscle mass, strength and functional performance, and bone fragility. Both phenomena are associated with decreased metabolic rate and increased risk of falls/fracture, and frequently result in increased morbidity and loss of independence in the elderly.

Bone mass declines with advancing age, causing bone fragility, which leads to so-called "senile osteoporosis". This bone loss, which should not be understood as synonymous with resorptive removal of bone, as it also represents the failure of bone formation, is the net result of the amount of bone resorbed on the endosteal surfaces and the amount formed in the periosteal surface. Thus, age-related bone loss can be seen as a result of an alteration in bone turnover, which becomes progressively attenuated (Duque & Troen, 2008). It has been estimated that the number of hip fractures will double to 2.6 million by the year 2025, with a greater percentage increase in men than in women (Gullberg *et al.*, 1997). Decreasing the prevalence of osteoporotic fracture and public health burdens will certainly depend on modifying the regulation of bone biology and/or other mechanisms underlying bone loss and neuromuscular degenerations. Improving bone mineral density (BMD) through a significant decrease in the rate of bone loss is a common goal for people with low bone mass, particularly postmenopausal women and older adults.

Coupled with bone loss, ageing is strongly associated with muscle mass atrophy that, in turn, decreases quality of life and physical independence and increases disablement. A progressive loss of muscle mass occurs approximately after the fourth decade of life. This loss, which is greater in men as compared with women (Iannuzzi-Sucich *et al.*, 2002), has been estimated to be about 8% per decade until the age of 70 years, after which the loss increases to 15% per decade (Baumgartner *et al.*, 1995). Despite the great variability between individuals at any given age, most individuals aged over 70 years will possess about 80% of the muscle mass of those aged 20–30 years (Janssen *et al.*, 2000). The magnitude of this phenomenon, also termed sarcopenia, as a public health problem of significant dimensions, is well-established, being considered as a geriatric syndrome since 2010 (Cruz-Jentoft *et al.*, 2010).

This chapter describes how an integrated approach to the study of bone and muscle can be applied to increase our understanding of musculoskeletal ageing. The internal and

Anti-Ageing Nutrients: Evidence-Based Prevention of Age-Associated Diseases, First Edition. Edited by Delminda Neves.

external environments are discussed. The focus for the external environment is on nutrition and physical activity, two key modifiable factors identified as essential for bone heath and for the prevention of sarcopenia in later life.

7.1.1 Determinants of bone loss in ageing

The fundamental determinants of bone loss have been systematically studied across the spectrum of potential risk factors. In addition to age, the major factors that influence bone mass are genetics, lifestyle and menopausal status (NAMS, 2010).

It is well established that BMD is under a strong genetic control. Heredity plays a determining role in peak bone mass acquisition (i.e. the maximal BMD gained during the skeletal development and maturation phase), accounting for up to 80–90% of its variability (Duncan & Brown, 2010; Ralston & de Crombrugghe, 2006). The genetic component of osteoporosis is determined by an assembly of multiple genes with small individual effects; each gene is most likely responsible for less than 5% of the genetic variance in the general population (Kung & Huang, 2007). Both linkage (family-based linkage studies) and association (candidate-gene association studies) methods have been used to identify genetic susceptibility loci for osteoporosis (Duncan & Brown, 2010).

Several lifestyle factors associated with the risk of low BMD have been identified, including poor nutrition, insufficient physical activity, cigarette smoking and heavy alcohol consumption (NAMS, 2010; Kung & Huang, 2007). A balanced diet modulates bone development and the maintenance of bone health throughout life (Cashman, 2007). As older adults commonly have deficient diets, because of inadequate consumption of the recommended servings of dairy products, fruit, vegetables or whole grains, nutrition plays a crucial role in this population (Morley, 2001; Milaneschi *et al.*, 2010).

Being thin and/or having a body mass index less than 20 kg/m^2 are risk factors for low BMD (De Laet *et al.*, 2005). It is well established that body weight is related to BMD (Reid, 2010) and change in body weight is also a predictor of bone alterations (Shapses & Riedt, 2006). Body weight is largely made up of two components: fat mass and lean mass. Similarities between obesity and osteoporosis have been identified, suggesting some type of pathologic linkage (Cao, 2011; Rosen & Bouxsein, 2006), but obese individuals are thought to have a reduced risk of osteoporosis (Bacon *et al.*, 2004), potentially owing to increased skeletal loading and increased concentrations of certain hormones, such as oestradiol in women (Rosen & Bouxsein, 2006). In addition to the relationship with bone composition, obesity is associated with low-grade systemic inflammation, which is related to an increased risk of type 2 diabetes and cardiovascular disease (Fantuzzi, 2005), but also osteoporosis (Pfeilschifter *et al.*, 2002). Based on the current state of knowledge, it is thus unclear whether fat has beneficial effects on bone (Zhao *et al.*, 2008). Moreover, the relative contribution of fat mass and lean mass to the variation in BMD (Ho-Pham *et al.*, 2010) is currently highly contentious.

Regular exercise practice has been associated with increased BMD, by positively changing bone turnover in favour of bone formation. There is general agreement that weight-bearing and high-impact exercise provides a positive osteogenic stimulus (Kohrt *et al.*, 2004).

Chronic alcoholism leads to lower BMD and higher fracture risk owing to a combination of factors: (a) poor nutritional status of critical nutrients, particularly calcium, magnesium and zinc; (b) liver disease, abnormal vitamin D metabolites and parathyroid function; and (c) direct toxicity to osteoblasts (Ilich & Kerstetter, 2000). It is believed that cigarette smokers may have impaired calcium absorption (Krall & Dawson-Hughes, 1999) although the exact mechanisms by which smoking might adversely affect bone mass are unknown. Compared with nonsmokers, women smokers tend, on average, to lose bone more rapidly, have lower bone mass and reach menopause 2 years earlier (Kato *et al.*, 1998).

The increased rate of bone resorption immediately after menopause clearly indicates a hormonal influence on bone density in women. Clearly, loss of oestrogen leads to increased rate of remodelling and tilts the balance between bone resorption and formation in favour of the former (Frenkel *et al.*, 2010). Classical oestrogen receptors α and β or androgen receptors are present in chondrocytes, bone marrow stromal cells, osteoblasts and osteoclasts and their progenitors, indicating that the effects of sex steroids on bone result, at least in part, from direct activation (Frenkel *et al.*, 2010). Thus, it is now believed that loss of oestrogens and androgens stimulates both osteoclastogenesis and osteoblastogenesis, and that they have a critical role in osteocytes apoptosis (Manolagas *et al.*, 2002).

Finally, diverse medications (e.g. aromatase inhibitors, cytotoxic agents, excessive thyroxine doses, gonadotropin-releasing hormone agonists or analogues, heparin, immunosuppressives), disease states (e.g. celiac disease, Crohn's disease) and genetic disorders (e.g. hemochromatosis, hypophosphatasia, osteogenesis imperfect, thalassaemia) are associated with bone loss, being categorized as secondary causes of bone loss.

Despite the compelling evidence mostly extrapolated from cross-sectional studies, some studies have failed to demonstrate a clear influence of all the previously described risk factors. A recent systematic review (Papaioannou *et al.*, 2009) showed that advancing age, smoking and low weight/weight loss were consistent risk factors for bone loss in older men. Although less evidence was available, physical/functional limitations and prevalent fracture (after age 50), but not physical activity, alcohol consumption, calcium intake, muscle strength, family history of fracture or osteoporosis, or height or height loss, were also associated with low BMD/bone loss (Papaioannou *et al.*, 2009). Data from a 4-year longitudinal study on risk factors for change in BMD in older adults showed that risk factors consistently associated with bone loss include female sex, thinness and weight loss, while weight gain appears to protect against bone loss (Hannan *et al.*, 2000). In addition, data suggested that current oestrogen use might help to maintain bone in women, whereas current smoking was associated with bone loss in men. Surprisingly, bone loss was not affected by caffeine, physical activity, serum vitamin D or calcium intake (Hannan *et al.*, 2000).

7.1.2 Regulation of muscle atrophy in ageing

Sarcopenia increases with advanced adult age and is accelerated by poor nutrition, physical inactivity and comorbidities (Thomas, 2010). Other factors contributing to sarcopenia are genetics, hormones, neuromuscular dysfunction and trauma (Thomas, 2010).

In fact, despite its aetiology not being completely clear, a number of factors associated with ageing that contribute to the progress of sarcopenia have been identified. Among these factors, the loss of α-motoneurons (Clark & Fielding, 2012), an increase in inflammatory cytokines (Thomas, 2010), a decrease a physical activity (Evans & Cyr-Campbell, 1997), bedrest (Kortebein *et al.*, 2007) and humoral factors, such as hormone decrease, are prominent (Lamberts *et al.*, 1997).

A motor unit is made up of a single α-motoneuron and all the muscle fibres connected with it. If an α-motoneuron is lost, the muscle fibres will denervate and disappear. Neuron loss is a progressive and irreversible process that increases with age. Motoneuron death seems to be more evident in the larger motor units that typically are composed of faster muscle fibres that generate higher forces, meaning that, with age, atrophy rather affects type II fibres (Clark & Fielding, 2012).

Inflammation is also a key factor in the genesis of sarcopenia. Ageing itself may be considered as a form of stress, since it is associated with increased circulating levels of proinflammatory molecules such as tumour necrosis factor-α (TNF-α), interleukin-6 (IL-6), interleukin-1 (IL-1) and C-reactive protein (CRP) (Thomas, 2010). These age-related changes in immune function (discussed in Chapter 9) are associated with a progressive increase in glucocorticoid and catecholamine levels and decreased hormone levels (sexual and growth hormones) that may contribute to the development of sarcopenia. In addition to the age-related subclinical level of inflammation, an increase in certain catabolic factors or impaired anabolism, through a decrease in anabolic factors or reduced anabolic response (Thomas, 2010), is pivotal for skeletal system atrophy. Several anabolic factors such as growth hormone, androgens (testosterone), insulin and insulin-like growth factor-1 (IGF-1) play a prominent role in muscle grow, with the latter being central owing to its ability to control different muscular mechanisms such as cell proliferation and differentiation, myofibre growth and regeneration (Sakuma & Yamaguchi, 2012). Likewise, the age-dependent decline in testosterone and growth hormone, in combination with lower IGF-1 levels, contributes to the development of sarcopenia (Sakuma & Yamaguchi, 2012). In support of this evidence, a decrease of 24% in women and 37% in men, when individuals aged 20–32 years were compared with those aged 70–83 years, was observed in the number of satellite cells (a population of undifferentiated myogenic cells that play a important role in postnatal muscle growth) per muscle fibre, leading to a loss of regenerative function (Kadi & Ponsot, 2010). A final mechanism contributing to muscle loss in older men and women is the reported increase in the levels of myostatin in this population. Considering that myostatin is a negative regulator of muscle mass, an increase in circulating levels may lead to muscle atrophy.

Overall, the most recognizable cause of sarcopenia is disuse and inactivity. For example, older adults are particularly prone to losing muscle mass when confined to bed (Kortebein *et al.*, 2007). Although current evidence points to an early and transient rise in muscle protein breakdown contributing to this decline in muscle mass, the main factor seems to be a drop in muscle protein synthesis, in part owing to the amplification of anabolic resistance to amino acid provision (Marimuthu *et al.*, 2011). Furthermore, prolonged muscle disuse causes increased production of reactive oxygen species (ROS), including free radicals, and subsequent injury in inactive muscle fibres, as seen upon experimental immobilization of skeletal muscles (Powers *et al.*, 2012). With ageing a reduction in the cellular anti-oxidant defence mechanisms and an increase in the generation of free radicals owing to dysfunction in the mitochondrial respiratory chain result in an increase in the oxidative stress to which the cell is exposed (Barreiro *et al.*, 2006), leading to α-motoneuron atrophy and a reduced number and function of satellite cells (Howard *et al.*, 2007). In addition, protein degradation in skeletal muscle is stimulated by excessive oxidative stress (Powers *et al.*, 2007). Finally, the literature points out that apoptosis increases in skeletal muscle during normal ageing and thus may contribute to sarcopenia (Dirks & Leeuwenburgh, 2005; Leeuwenburgh, 2003).

It is likely that no single mechanism can explain muscle atrophy and dysfunction in the elderly and that all of the above factors contribute to some degree to the development of sarcopenia. The mechanisms that contribute to sarcopenia are complex, overlapping and interdependent.

Exercise (muscle contraction), in opposition to inactivity, causes the release of muscle growth factors (IGF and mechanogrowth factor) to stimulate satellite cells and protein synthesis. Since an adequate nutrient intake is also essential to maintain muscle mass (Morley *et al.*, 2010), an active life style and diet seem to be powerful protective factors against sarcopenia.

7.2 Osteoporosis and fragility fractures in the elderly

Osteoporosis is the most common skeletal disorder characterized by compromised bone strength, which becomes a serious health threat, especially for ageing postmenopausal women, by predisposing them to an increased risk of fracture (NIH Consensus Development Panel, 2001) that in turn is associated with substantial morbidity and mortality (Johnell & Kanis, 2005). To standardize values from different bone densitometry tests, results are reported as either a *Z*-score or a *T*-score, with both expressed as standard deviation (SD) units. The North American Menopause Society (NAMS) supports the World Health Organization and International Society for Clinical Densitometry definitions (Kanis, 1994) of osteoporosis in a postmenopausal woman or a man over age 50 as a BMD *T*-score ≤ -2.5 SD at the total hip, femoral neck or lumbar spine (at least two vertebral levels measured in the posterior–anterior projection, not the lateral projection). In addition to diagnosis through densitometry, osteoporosis can be diagnosed clinically (e.g. the presence of a fragility fracture), regardless of the *T*-score (Kanis, 2002).

Osteoporosis is categorized as either primary or secondary. Primary osteoporosis is usually due to bone loss that occurs with ageing. Secondary osteoporosis is a result of medications (e.g. glucocorticoids) or diseases (e.g. malabsorption) that adversely affect skeletal health (NAMS, 2010).

The clinical significance of osteoporosis lies in the fractures that occur. Many fracture types are associated with osteoporosis, but the hip, spine, forearm and shoulder are the most common sites of osteoporotic fragility fractures (Cooper *et al.*, 2011). Fractures of the neck and trochanteric regions of the femur are currently one of the most serious healthcare problems and source of morbidity and mortality for ageing populations (Marks *et al.*, 2003). Therefore, there is currently an urgent need to prevent the anticipated rise in hip fracture incidence observed in most countries and especially to investigate the underlying causes of this condition. The probability of sustaining osteoporotic fractures varies markedly in different regions of the world. In Europe, the highest risks ("very high risk") of hip fracture are seen in Norway, Iceland, Sweden and Denmark (with the USA also showing very high risk), whereas countries like Germany, Switzerland, Finland, Greece, The Netherlands, Hungary, Italy, the UK and Portugal have been described as "high risk" countries, defined as having a hip fracture probability that lies between 50 and 75% of that observed in Sweden (Kanis *et al.*, 2002).

BMD can be used to predict an individual's risk of an osteoporosis-related fracture and is the most commonly measured attribute compared with other qualities of bone. Qualities of bone other than BMD (including degree of mineralization, hydroxyapatite crystal size, collagen structure, heterogeneity of bone microstructure, connectivity of trabeculae and microdamage) are difficult or impossible to measure in clinical practice at this time. Although BMD is an important component of assessing fracture risk, other factors should also be considered. These include prior fracture, age, family history of osteoporotic fracture or long-term glucocorticoid therapy, among others, all of which should be taken into account in the assessment of fracture risk in patients (Miller, 2006; Kanis *et al.*, 2005).

Despite the contribution of a variety of risk factors, BMD is consistently identified as an important determinant of fracture risk, especially in women aged 65 and older (Johnell *et al.*, 2005; Kanis *et al.*, 2005). BMD and fracture risk are most closely related when BMD is used to predict the fracture risk at that same site. Risks for spine fracture and hip fracture increase 2.3- and 2.6-fold, respectively, for each decrease of 1 SD in age-adjusted BMD (Cummings *et al.*, 1993). Nevertheless, people with low BMD will not always develop fractures, but the probability of fractures is increased. There is a continuous relationship between fracture probability and BMD, that is, fracture probably increases progressively as bone density declines. Despite the obvious relationship between these two variables, only 15% of fractures occur in persons with osteoporosis (Siris *et al.*, 2001). In fact, risk factors for hip fracture are more strongly related to predictors of falls and factors that may modify the impact force of a fall (e.g. environmental hazards, postural instability, location of distance to impact, lower extremity muscle weakness/atrophy) than to low bone mass *per se* (Marks *et al.*, 2003).

History of fragility fracture is also a relevant risk factor for osteoporotic fractures. In fact, after the age of 40, a history of fragility fracture is associated with a 1.5- to 9.5-fold increased risk of future fracture, depending on the patient's age and the number and site of prior fractures (Klotzbuecher *et al.*, 2000). Also, as inactivity can lead to muscle weakness and atrophy, it is associated with an increased risk of fracture in elderly people (Marks *et al.*, 2003).

7.3 Nutritional mechanisms of age-related bone loss

Many nutrients and food components can potentially have a positive [calcium, copper, zinc, fluoride, magnesium, phosphorus, potassium, vitamin C, vitamin D, vitamin K, B vitamins, omega-3 polyunsaturated fatty acids (PUFA), protein, phyto-oestrogens, nondigestible oligosaccharides] or negative (excess of alcohol, caffeine, sodium, fluoride and phosphorus, excess/insufficient protein, and vitamin A) impact on bone health (Table 7.1). They may influence bone by various mechanisms, including alteration of bone structure, the rate of bone metabolism, the endocrine and/or paracrine system, and homeostasis of calcium and possibly of other bone-active minerals (Cashman, 2007).

We will briefly describe the potential effects of some key nutrients and their known mechanisms of actions by which they play a role in counteracting age-related bone loss or, conversely, in increasing the incidence of osteoporosis. The importance of calcium and vitamin D in promoting bone health is summarized in the next section.

It is now established that protein is both detrimental and beneficial to bone health, depending on a variety of factors, including the level of protein in the diet, the protein source, calcium intake, weight loss and the acid–base balance of the diet (Heaney & Layman, 2008). Protein intake affects bone in several ways: (a) it provides the structural matrix of bone; (b) it optimizes IGF-1 levels, and it is reported (c) to increase urinary

Table 7.1 Potential nutritional and dietary determinants of bone health (adapted from Cashman, 2007).

Nutritional adequacy for Protective factors	Potentially detrimental dietary factors
Calcium	Alcoholism
Copper	Excess caffeine
Zinc	Excess sodium
Fluoride	Excess fluoride
Magnesium	Excess/insufficient protein
Phosphorus	Excess phosphorus
Potassium	Excess vitamin A
Boron	
Vitamin C	
Vitamin D	
Vitamin K	
Folate, B6 and B12 vitamins	
n-3 and n-6/n-3 PUFA	
Protein	
Phytochemicals	

calcium excretion and (d) intestinal calcium absorption (Heaney & Layman, 2008). Interestingly, findings regarding the effect of protein on calcium balance and bone health are far from being focused (Kerstetter *et al.*, 1998, 2005; Hunt *et al.*, 2009), considering that increased calciuria does not necessarily translate to calcium loss, negative calcium balance and reduced bone mass (Bonjour, 2005). Overall, however, there is general agreement that moderate protein content diets (~1.0–1.5 g/kg/day) are associated with normal calcium metabolism and do not alter bone metabolism (Kerstetter *et al.*, 2003).

Although a depletion of phosphorus leads to impaired mineralization, there is more concern about the effects of high dietary phosphorus on bone, especially if combined with a low-calcium diet (Palacios, 2006). High phosphate levels in the blood reduce the formation of the active form of vitamin D3, 1-α,25-dihydroxyvitamin D3 [1,25 $(OH)_2D_3$] in the kidneys, reduce blood calcium and lead to increased parathyroid hormone (PTH) release by the parathyroid glands (Ilich & Kerstetter, 2000). In addition, the function of fluoride in bone health is also not clear, as it is indicated as both a positive and a negative modulator.

Despite the generalized analysis of the effect of each isolated nutrient on bone health, attention should also be given to the combined effect of multiple nutrients. For example, bone loss may be attributable, in part, to the mobilization of skeletal salts to balance the endogenous acid generated from acid-forming foods (Krieger *et al.*, 2004). By preserving calcium in bones, which might otherwise be mobilized to maintain normal pH, potassium-rich foods may help to prevent osteoporosis (Ilich & Kerstetter, 2000).

This relationship may explain the reported beneficial influence of fruit and vegetables on bone health (New, 2003; New *et al.*, 2000). The detrimental effect of dietary acidity on the skeleton is relatively small (Welch *et al.*, 2007), but a sustained small effect may have a large impact over time (New, 2003).

Cereal grains and meat, poultry, eggs, dairy and fish, are metabolized to acidic residues, whereas fruit, vegetables and nuts have an alkaline residue (containing the cations potassium, calcium and magnesium). Therefore the balance among intakes of these major dietary components will determine the net potential acid load of a diet (Remer & Manz, 1995). An excess acid load is buffered by bone and in the process calcium is released. Epidemiologic studies have observed that greater intakes of fruit and vegetables are associated with greater BMD (Chen *et al.*, 2006; New *et al.*, 2000), and an acidic environment leads to progressive bone loss (Macdonald *et al.*, 2005; Tucker *et al.*, 2001). Algorithms based on dietary intakes of key nutrients can be used to measure acid–base load, such as the dietary potential renal acid load, and to explore the association between dietary acidity and bone health (Macdonald *et al.*, 2005).

It is suggested that metabolic acidosis stimulates mineral dissolution and subsequently cell-mediated bone resorption. Acidosis suppresses the activity of bone-forming cells, osteoblasts, decreasing gene expression of specific matrix proteins and alkaline phosphatase activity (Cao & Nielsen, 2010). There is a concomitant acid stimulation of prostaglandin production by osteoblasts, which, acting in a paracrine manner, increases synthesis of the osteoblastic receptor activator of nuclear factor κ-B ligand (RANKL). The acid induction of RANKL then stimulates osteoclastic activity and the recruitment of new osteoclasts to promote bone resorption and buffering of the proton load (Krieger *et al.*, 2003). Both the regulation of RANKL and acid-induced calcium efflux from bone are mediated by prostaglandins (Krieger *et al.*, 2004).

Several other micronutrients with essential roles in bone health may also have inadequate content in the diets of the elderly. They are vitamins K, C and A, magnesium, boron and other trace minerals. Less research has been conducted on these micronutrients compared with calcium, phosphorus and vitamin D, but they nevertheless are essential for bone health. Indeed, magnesium plays an important role in calcium and bone metabolism. It has a direct effect on bone quality by decreasing hydroxyapatite crystal size, thereby preventing larger, more perfect mineral crystals that result in brittle bone (Palacios, 2006). Deficiency of this mineral could affect bone growth, osteoblastic and osteoclastic activity, osteopenia and bone fragility, and alter calcium metabolism (Rude *et al.*, 2009), resulting in hypocalcaemia, vitamin D abnormalities and neuromuscular hyperexcitability.

Finally, the negative influence of caffeine on bone health has been supported in previous studies (Massey & Whiting, 1993; Harris & Dawson-Hughes, 1994) but not consistently (Heaney, 2002). Caffeine is negatively correlated with intestinal calcium absorption with the net result being a more negative calcium balance, particularly when dietary calcium is inadequate (Rapuri *et al.*, 2001; Harris & Dawson-Hughes, 1994; Massey & Whiting, 1993).

7.4 Calcium and vitamin D and the ageing skeleton: Efficacy in the treatment of osteoporosis

Physiological alterations associated with the ageing process may make the elderly population most susceptible to vitamin D deficiency and its consequences. Age-induced skin changes reduce the amount of 7-dehydrocholesterol, the precursor of cholecalciferol (vitamin D3), as well as its rate of conversion (Tuohimaa, 2009). Absorption of dietary vitamin D is also reduced in older individuals (Christakos *et al.*, 2011). The ageing adult also has a reduction in the quantity and activity of the renal 1-α-hydroxylase, which affects the production of the most active metabolite of vitamin D, 1,25 $(OH)_2D_3$ (Tuohimaa, 2009), which plays a vital role in promoting intestinal calcium absorption. Regulation of calcium absorption is one of the most important functions attributed to vitamin D in the development and maintenance of skeleton mass. In addition, advanced age is associated with diminished renal and hepatic conversion of vitamin D precursors, decreased renal response to PTH and increased resistance of intestinal mucosal cells to the active form of vitamin D (Lanham-New, 2008).

Other conditions, further to physiological changes in vitamin D metabolism, affect the vitamin D status in older individuals. Sunlight deprivation for a variety of reasons, the increased use of medications that potentially interfere with vitamin D metabolism and the greater likelihood of medical conditions (e.g. renal disease, severe hepatic disease and malabsorption) that can also interfere with vitamin D metabolism all contribute to a greater prevalence of vitamin D deficiency in older adults (Tuohimaa, 2009; Ilich & Kerstetter, 2000).

Extensive clinical and animal studies support the concept that vitamin D deficiency and altered vitamin D metabolism contribute to bone loss, hip fractures, osteomalacia and reduced muscular function (Lips & van Schoor, 2011), which may increase risk of falling. There is extensive evidence that 1,25 $(OH)_2D_3$ stimulates both bone formation and resorption; however, the mechanisms of such actions remain unclear. As osteoblastic cells contain the vitamin D receptor, the actions of 1,25 $(OH)_2D_3$ on bone formation probably result from a direct stimulatory action further to that induced by steroid hormones on the osteoblast differentiation and osteoblastic synthetic functions (Song *et al.*, 2011). Moreover, 1,25 $(OH)_2D_3$ also stimulates calcium transport across the intestinal cells by inducing the production of a calcium-binding protein. Hence, vitamin D is critical for effective calcium absorption (Christakos *et al.*, 2011), but is less important at high calcium loads.

Despite these observations, vitamin D supplementation alone does not appear to reduce the incidence of hip or vertebral fractures, but the use of vitamin D in combination with calcium has been shown to be effective in reducing the risk of vertebral and nonvertebral fractures, including hip fractures (Avenell *et al.*, 2009).

Frequently, older adults are unable to obtain adequate amounts of calcium from the diet (Gennari, 2001). Thus, to smooth out fluctuations in calcium concentration, bone resorption is increased to regenerate the calcium supply, and bone reformation at the same site is also increased when the dietary intake of calcium increases (Cashman, 2002). In ageing, the ability of the kidney and gut to maintain extracellular calcium homeostasis also declines and the reasons for this are complex (Peacock, 2010). The consequences of these defects are that skeletal bone resorption rises and, together with the deficient bone regeneration associated with ageing, the outcome is osteoporosis (Hwang & Putney, 2011).

The flow of calcium into and out of the bone, gut, and kidney is regulated by a variety of mechanisms, only partly understood, which involve the principal hormonal regulator of calcium homeostasis, the vitamin D–PTH system (Peacock, 2010). Critical abnormalities in calcium homeostasis resulting in age-related osteoporosis involve all three main organs of calcium homeostasis, as summarized in Fig. 7.1.

On the supply side there is a reduction in gut calcium absorption (Need *et al.*, 1998; Morris *et al.*, 1991; Devine *et al.*, 1993), involving intrinsic gut wall defects and

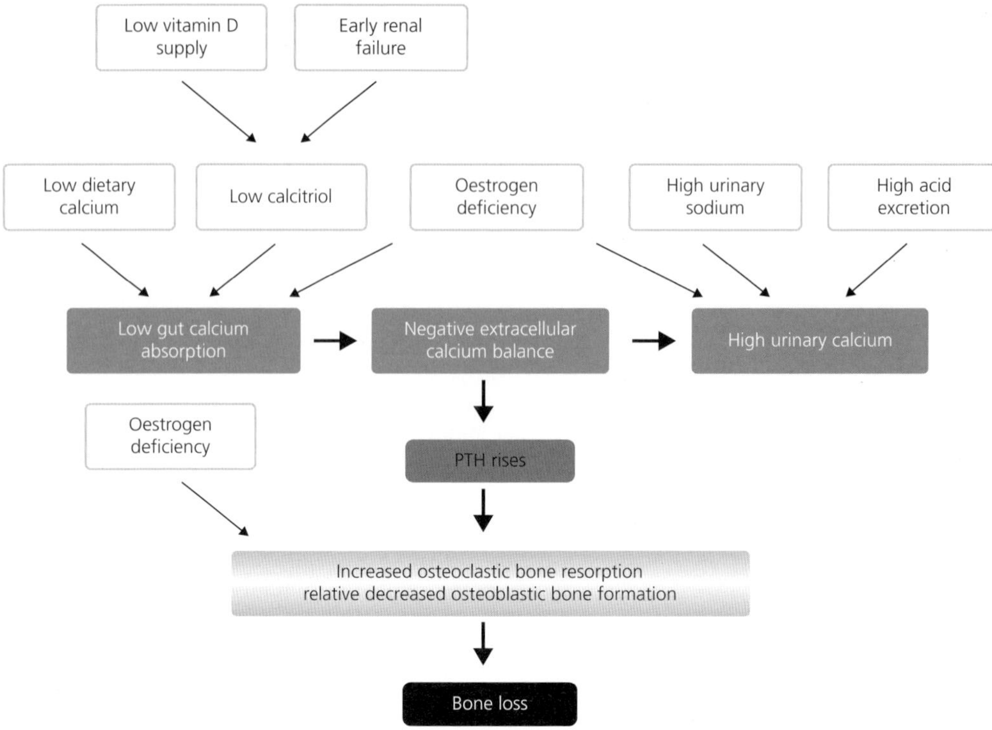

Figure 7.1 Schematic model of the disordered mechanisms of calcium homeostasis linked to age-related bone loss. PTH, Parathyroid hormone.

abnormalities in vitamin D and oestrogen status. On the demand side there is an increase in renal calcium excretion that, in women, occurs at menopause and persists during old age (Cashman, 2002) owing to oestrogen deficiency and other determinants of renal calcium excretion such as salt and acid–base balance.

As calcium serves as an indirect regulator of skeletal remodelling, a large number of epidemiological studies have examined the effect of dietary calcium and calcium supplements on fracture rates and BMD. Most of them found that calcium supplementation increases BMD and is linked to decreased risk of vertebral and hip fractures (Shea *et al.*, 2004; Jackson *et al.*, 2006, 2011). Accordingly, calcium seems to function as an antiresorptive agent. It does not antagonize PTH action on bone, as do oestrogen, the selective oestrogen receptor modulators and the bisphosphonates, but reduces remodelling by directly reducing PTH secretion (Heaney & Weaver, 2005).

Taken together, these findings demonstrate that calcium and vitamin D are necessary for normal skeletal homeostasis and are considered the first step in osteoporosis treatment.

7.5 Skeletal muscle age-related contributory mechanisms

In the strong relationship between muscle mass and function, the latter is the pivotal predictor of hospital admission, falls, fractures, gait disorders and mortality (Mitchell *et al.*, 2012). There is now evidence to suggest that dynapenia (which represents the lack of muscle strength and power – dyna refers to "power, strength, or force" and penia refers to "poverty") is an important factor in compromising autonomy, well-being and quality of life in old age (Clark & Manini, 2008). This concept stresses the idea of muscle quality, that is, the force generated per capacity per unit cross-sectional area.

Recent longitudinal data have advocated that, in addition to muscle atrophy, there are numerous other factors that lead to dynapenia (Clark & Manini, 2008). These embrace altered muscle energetics, changes in tendon insertion with increased collagenation, leading to a transformed angle of pennation, altered nerve motor unit input to muscle, changing muscle coordination, and decreased blood flow owing to reduced nitric oxide release in the capillary bed of the muscle. Fat infiltration into muscle (myosteatosis) is also associated with decreased strength and an increase in the prevalence of disability (Delmonico *et al.*, 2009). Generally, the deterioration in muscle performance is affected by both neurological and myogenic adaptations.

Neurological adaptations may involve changes in supraspinal drive generated from the cortex, with impaired ability of the nervous system to fully activate skeletal muscle voluntarily, which could result in suboptimal motor unit discharge rates (Clark & Taylor, 2011). Deficits in voluntary agonist activation and/or increased antagonistic coactivation muscles (Klass *et al.*, 2007) can contribute to older adults muscle weakness, as well as substantial morphometric changes in the motor cortex that affect maximal spinal cord output and muscle coordination (synergism).

Ageing also affects motor cortical properties at the system level (Kamen *et al.*, 1995). Studies have reported that older subjects exhibit ~35–40% lower maximal motor unit firing rates compared with young individuals. Additionally, there is probably a rearrangement in the motor unit pool. For example, the significant enlargement of the motor unit action potential in aged humans (Edstrom *et al.*, 2007) suggests that nerve sprouting and reinnervation of "orphaned" muscle fibres may provide an adaptive mechanism to maintain muscle mass despite substantial motor unit loss. The fact that older muscle displays an increase in fibre-type grouping compared with young muscle is also consistent with a denervation–reinnervation model (Edstrom *et al.*, 2007). Collectively, these changes in motor unit discharge properties seem to contribute to the decreased skeletal muscle functionality.

Concerning the potential contributory mechanisms of dynapenia, age-related muscle atrophy is undoubtedly considered to be a main factor. Loss of muscle mass in aged humans is well documented (Lee *et al.*, 2001). The excretion of urinary creatinine, reflecting muscle creatinine content and total muscle mass, decreases by nearly 50% between the ages of 20 and 90 years (Pahor *et al.*, 2009). Also, previous ultrasonography and computed tomography reports have shown that the quadriceps muscle cross-sectional area is smaller in elderly subjects when compared with younger counterparts (Frontera *et al.*, 2000). Decreased muscle density and increased concentrations of collagen and fat in muscle are also associated with age-related deterioration in muscle performance. Over the past decade, numerous studies have reported that ageing increases the adipocyte content between muscle groups (intermuscular adipose tissue) and between muscle fascicles (intramuscular adipose tissue; Delmonico *et al.*, 2009; Goodpaster *et al.*, 2000), suggesting that greater muscle fat content is associated with decreased muscle strength.

In addition to muscle size and anatomic structure, aged muscle appears to differ in other compositional manners. For instance, the concentration of myosin, the most important motor protein, is reduced in fibre types I and IIA from old subjects expressing different myosin heavy chain isoforms (D'Antona *et al.*, 2003). This may suggest that old muscle fibres have fewer cross-bridges per muscle fibre area (Frontera *et al.*, 2012) and therefore a lower capacity to generate force per area of contractile tissue. On the other hand, immobilization, common in this age group further reduces the concentration of myosin in human single fibres. Thus the combination of ageing and disuse may have serious deleterious effects on muscle function (D'Antona *et al.*, 2003).

Another pathway playing a consistent role in dynapenia relies on specific age-related changes on muscle geometry (the angles and lengths of its fibres or fascicles) that strongly influences its force production characteristics (Narici *et al.*, 2003; Thom *et al.*, 2007). The length of each fascicle will determine the number of sarcomeres in series and therefore the maximum velocity with which it contracts. Pennation allows more fibres to act in parallel and, with hypertrophy, the angle of pennation increases, contributing to loss of shortening velocity as well as force generation.

Moreover, studies with human single fibres show that ageing is associated with changes in fibre elasticity in both type I and IIA fibres (Ochala *et al.*, 2007). This increase in stiffness may be due to an increase in the number and proportion of actin–myosin cross-bridges in a low force state or alterations in the compliance of structures in series in muscle fibres.

Other studies suggest that the age-related mitochondria dysfunction seems to play a key role in muscle function decline, as the mitochondria are the main producers of both cellular energy and free radicals. Alterations in mitochondria have been noted in ageing, including decreased total volume, increased oxidative damage that results in augmentation of oxidative stress, decline in mitochondrial DNA (mtDNA), downregulation in some enzyme activities and alterations in mitochondrial respiratory chain (discussed in Chapter 1; Joseph *et al.*, 2012).

Finally, although there is no agreement in the literature, numerous studies describe a reduction of the muscular capillarization with advancing age. This compromised vascular responsiveness exposes aged muscles to potential hypoxia and free radical stress, and could compromise nutrient delivery (Mitchell *et al.*, 2012).

Concluding, dynapenic individuals could have fewer functioning motor units, which will theoretically affect muscle strength once a critical threshold is reached, particularly if collateral reinnervation does not occur or is incomplete. Similarly, it is plausible that the muscle system's ability to optimally produce force is impaired in dynapenic individuals, with this deficit in the intrinsic force-generating capacity of muscle (force/unit area) caused by potential changes in the excitation–contraction coupling process (Delbono, 2011; Russ *et al.*, 2011). Muscle ageing is characterized by a decline in functional performance and restriction of adaptability, owing to progressive loss of muscle tissue coupled with a decrease in strength and force output.

Regardless of these underlying conditions, since dynapenia is undoubtedly strictly connected with an increased risk in older adults of mobility limitations (Manini *et al.*, 2007), implying exercise intolerance, inability to manage daily activity and mortality (Takata *et al.*, 2012), the preservation of muscle function with advancing age is of high clinical and functional significance. Ideally, a multifaceted approach should involve adequate nutritional support and implementation of exercise training to stimulate muscle hypertrophy and function.

A number of reports have clearly demonstrated that elderly men and women, even up to 90 years of age, maintain their ability to increase their muscle mass, strength and power (reviewed in Liu & Latham, 2009). Presumably, this improvement is due to several factors including alterations in muscle morphology, muscle/connective tissue biomechanics and increase in neural activation, motor skill coordination and psychological drive (Candow *et al.*, 2012).

7.6 The role of nutrition in preventing ageing skeletal muscle atrophy

The diets of elderly people define to a large extent their health, and particularly the potential for counteracting the possible physiological aetiological factors of sarcopenia. In this section, dietary protein, PUFA and other bioactive nutritional components that have been shown to have a protective effect on muscle metabolism, inflammation and antioxidant status will be addressed.

7.6.1 Protein

Proteins are continuously broken down and resynthesized, and skeletal muscle may account for approximately one-quarter of the total body protein turnover (Waterlow, 1984). When the levels of protein intake are insufficient, turnover of tissue protein is diminished while the opposite may occur with increased intake. However, in the elderly, the amount of protein turned over decreases in relation to young adults (Young *et al.*, 1975).

Net protein balance in the skeletal muscle is the result of protein synthesis and protein breakdown. When muscle protein breakdown (MPB) exceeds the rate of muscle protein synthesis (MPS), net protein balance is negative, while the opposite corresponds to positive balance; balance is achieved when MPB equals MPS (Tang & Phillips, 2009). The installation of sarcopenia may be the consequence of an elevated basal-fasted rate of MPB and/or reduced basal MPS (Breen & Phillips, 2011). Nevertheless, MPB may also contribute to restore the functionality of proteins by allowing impaired proteins to be removed and recycled into new muscle proteins (Churchward-Venne *et al.*, 2012). MPS is more responsive than MPB to diet-induced changes in healthy subjects, making it the main target to stimulate muscle protein balance and eventual protein accretion (Churchward-Venne *et al.*, 2012).

Considerable discussion exists over the quantity of protein intake needed for optimal health in older adults, particularly when addressing it in the light of energy requirements (Millward *et al.*, 1997). Gersovitz *et al.* (1982) provided older adults with diets containing 0.8 g egg protein/kg/day, and concluded that this amount was not sufficient for most of the subjects. Campbell *et al.* (2001) also suggested that 0.8 g protein/kg/day may not be adequate to completely meet the requirements of virtually all older people. In a study to assess dietary protein intake and changes in lean mass in community-dwelling older adults, subjects in the highest quintile of protein intake (1.2 ± 0.4 g protein/kg body weight/day) lost about 40% less lean mass than did those in the lowest quintile of protein intake (0.8 ± 0.3 g protein/kg body weight/day; Houston *et al.*, 2008). According to some authors, the recommend intake for the prevention of sarcopenia is 0.8–1.2 g high-quality protein/kg body weight/day (Volkert, 2011), or even higher doses, such as 1.6 g protein/kg body weight/day (Evans, 2004).

Moreover, Paddon-Jones and Rasmussen (2009) emphasized that MPS was reduced in older adults when the ingested protein was less than about 20 g per meal, and a value of 25–30 g of high-quality protein per meal was advised to maximize the anabolic response. Therefore, promoting the distribution of protein intake in approximately equal parts through breakfast, lunch and dinner may be also an important determinant of protein efficacy (Tieland *et al.*, 2012).

7.6.2 PUFA and inflammation

Although biochemical processes underlying the roles of pro-inflammatory cytokines in skeletal muscle remain to be established (Podbregar *et al.*, 2013), increased circulation levels of cytokines such as IL-6, in addition to CRP and TNF-α receptor II, may has deleterious effects on protein synthetic rates (Toth *et al.*, 2005; Lang *et al.*, 2002).

However, these inflammatory processes may be reduced by long-chain omega-3 PUFA, such as eicosapentaenoic acid (EPA) and docosahexaenoic acid (DHA), which are found in foods, particularly fatty fish, and supplements (Villani *et al.*, 2013; Calder, 2013).

The effects of omega-3 PUFA intake on MPS and the respective metabolic intracellular signalling pathways in the elderly are not fully understood. In a randomized controlled trial designed to evaluate the effects of omega-3 PUFA on the rate of MPS in older adults, 8 weeks of daily supplementation with 1.86 g EPA plus 1.50 g DHA had no effect on the basal rate of MPS, but amplified the hyper-aminoacidaemia–hyperinsulinaemia-stimulated increase in the rate of MPS, which may be important to counteract the anabolic resistance associated with ageing (Smith *et al.*, 2011). Furthermore, the intake of oily fish was associated with an increase in grip strength in community-dwelling older adults, which raised the hypothesis of an anti-inflammatory effect of omega-3 PUFA and a possible role of these nutrients in the prevention of sarcopenia (Robinson *et al.*, 2008).

α-Linolenic acid (ALA) is the major plant-based omega-3 PUFA and its effects may also occur through its conversion to EPA and DHA, when dietary intake of marine PUFA is low (Galli & Calder, 2009; Anderson & Ma, 2009). Although the precise efficacy of metabolic conversion of ALA to EPA and/or to DHA is an unresolved question, it is accepted that, owing the low conversion from dietary ALA, desired tissue levels of EPA and DHA could be better achieved through consumption of these two nutrients (Harris *et al.*, 2009). Since long-chain PUFA synthesis occurs mainly in the liver, it is possible that natural changes in physiological state occurring with ageing, or any additional pathologic conditions that may exist, affect the availability of these nutrients in cells from different tissues (Galli & Calder, 2009). However, particularly in older adults, considering the antithrombotic properties of omega-3 PUFA, special attention should be given to the risks of potential severe adverse effects after high doses ingestion, such as bleeding (Villani *et al.*, 2013) or a slight rise in LDL cholesterol (Eslick *et al.*, 2009).

In a review of Calder (2013) addressing the consumption of fish oil supplements by healthy adults and its impact on inflammatory processes, it was indicated that an EPA plus DHA intake higher than 2 g/day seemed to be required to obtain anti-inflammatory actions. The existence of Dietary Reference Intakes for EPA + DHA is still a matter for discussion, but consumption levels for an adult of up to 500 mg/day do not appear to raise safety concerns (Harris *et al.*, 2009). Furthermore, Villani *et al.* (2013) performed a systematic review on fish oil administration in older adults, and concluded that the potential for adverse effects related to omega-3 supplementation seemed mild to moderate at worst and was seen as unlikely to be of clinical impact. However, data are limited to establish definitive conclusions about the safety of these nutrients.

7.6.3 Anti-oxidants and oxidative stress

Hiona and Christiaan Leeuwenburgh (2008) reviewed the potential mechanisms by which mtDNA mutations related to ageing that favour mitochondrial dysfunction may impact the skeletal muscle and concluded that mtDNA mutations may contribute to sarcopenia. According to the mitochondrial "vicious circle" hypothesis that is associated with the free radical theory of ageing, chronic ROS production and oxidative stress can favour mtDNA mutations, which in turn may lead to an increased mitochondrial ROS production, promoting a "vicious circle" of oxidative damage that may lead to muscle cell death (Hiona & Leeuwenburgh, 2008), which in turn may contribute to sarcopenia (Marzetti *et al.*, 2012).

The presence of elevated levels of pro-inflammatory cytokines that may occur with ageing also contributes to an increase in the oxidative stress in skeletal muscle (Arthur & Cooley, 2012). Thus counteracting oxidative stress by exposure to anti-oxidants may be an important strategy to prevent sarcopenia (Semba *et al.*, 2007).

Although is debatable whether oxidative stress is the first event responsible for the loss of muscle mass and muscle strength in the elderly, anti-oxidants are considered by the International Working Group on Sarcopenia as promising biomarkers of this condition (Cesari *et al.*, 2012).

The primary and auxiliary extra- and intracellular anti-oxidant protection systems include nutritive anti-oxidants (e.g. vitamin C, vitamin E, carotenoids, conjugated dienoic isomers of linoleic acid, carnosine, anserine and histidine), non-nutritive anti-oxidants (e.g. natural and synthetic phenols, and furanones/furfurals), enzymes (e.g. glutathione peroxidase/transferase or glutathione disulphide reductase that catalyse anti-oxidants regeneration), transition metal (e.g. iron, copper) binders and exporters (glutathione-conjugate transporter; Bonorden & Pariza, 1994).

Although an adequate intake of anti-oxidants may be considered as an important strategy to prevent sarcopenia (Volkert, 2011), in the study of Chaput *et al.* (2007), there were no significant differences in anti-oxidant intakes between the group of elderly subjects with sarcopenia and the nonsarcopenic group; however, in that study (Chaput *et al.*, 2007), the intake of anti-oxidant nutrients in older adults with sarcopenia reached fewer of the Recommended Dietary Allowances than in the group of subjects without sarcopenia.

Nutritional approaches that have been proposed to prevent oxidative stress or benefit muscle protein metabolism by anti-oxidants include the mediation effects of resveratrol (Ryan *et al.*, 2010b) vitamin E, vitamin C (Ryan *et al.*, 2010a), carotenoids (Semba *et al.*, 2003), vitamin A (Marzani *et al.*, 2008), dehydroepiandrosterone, ornithine, cysteine, *N*-acetylcysteine, carnitine, epigallocatechin gallate (Bonetto *et al.*, 2009) zinc and selenium (Marzani *et al.*, 2008).

Considering that oxidative stress may favour the initiation of sarcopenia (Marzetti *et al.*, 2012; Martin *et al.*, 2007; Arthur & Cooley, 2012), future research should clarify specific protein targets for oxidative damage (Baraibar *et al.*, 2013) and the mechanistic pathways by which anti-oxidants in foods or supplements may decrease oxidative stress. Future randomized controlled trials using single or several anti-oxidants, in supplements or food preparations, should also be tested for efficacy to reduce oxidative stress in the muscle, and promote net protein balance in older adults.

7.6.4 Vitamin D

Vitamin D metabolites may affect muscle mass and function through indirect mechanisms such as the hypophosphataemia (Schubert & DeLuca, 2010) or the secondary hyperparathyroidism of vitamin D deficiency (Rejnmark, 2011; Baczynski *et al.*, 1985). Direct effects may also occur through the 1,25 $(OH)_2D_3$ receptor in muscle tissue (Bischoff *et al.*, 2001; Janssen *et al.*, 2002). In addition, a relationship between lower 25-hydroxyvitamin D (25-OHD) (and higher PTH levels) and risk of sarcopenia was reported in older men and women (Visser *et al.*, 2003; Janssen *et al.*, 2002; for a review of mechanisms of how vitamin D affect muscle cell metabolism see Boland *et al.*, 1995; and for clinical and laboratory studies that have examined the role of vitamin D in skeletal muscle see Ceglia & Harris, 2013).

In a systematic review evaluating the effects of exposure to vitamin D on muscle function, Rejnmark (2011) identified 16 randomized controlled trials, and all except one of the studies were performed in subjects above 50 years of age; in seven studies, vitamin D supplementation showed positive effects on muscle strength (Rejnmark, 2011; Stockton *et al.*, 2011). Another systematic review and meta-analysis by Muir and Montero-Odasso (2011), which assessed the efficacy of vitamin D supplementation on muscle strength in elderly subjects aged over 60 years, showed that all studies with ingested doses of 800–1000 IU per day reported beneficial effects on muscle strength.

Vitamin D deficiency, defined by serum 25-OHD concentrations less than 15 ng/ml, in persons older than 60 years, was also demonstrated in the Third National Health and Nutrition Survey to associate with frailty (Wilhelm-Leen *et al.*, 2010). Furthermore, low vitamin D nutritional status is a risk factor for falls in the elderly (Faulkner *et al.*, 2006; Snijder *et al.*, 2006), and its supplementation was indicated as an important strategy to reduce the risk of falls among ambulatory or institutionalized older individuals (Bischoff-Ferrari *et al.*, 2004). However, evidence on whether vitamin D supplementation affects muscle mass is scarce (Ceglia & Harris, 2013).

Although vitamin D functions include an important role for muscle health (Janssen *et al.*, 2002; Schott & Wills, 1976), an inadequate vitamin D nutritional status is frequently seen in older adults. In a study with older adults from 11 European countries, 36% of men and 47% of women had appointed concentrations less than 12 ng/ml in wintertime, this being the lowest mean concentration found in Southern European countries (van der Wielen *et al.*, 1995). Serum vitamin D levels may vary widely between subjects from different countries (Lips, 2007) and variations in vitamin D status seem to be related to contrasts in nutritional intake, sunlight exposure and clinical, therapeutic, sociodemographic and environmental factors (Sakuma & Yamaguchi, 2012; National Research Council, 2011).

The Recommended Dietary Allowance in healthy adults under 70 years is 600 IU/day, and in older adults over 70 years it is 800 IU/day (National Research Council, 2011), which may require supplementation (Boucher, 2012). However, some research also indicates that too much vitamin D may be harmful (National Research Council, 2011; Bernstein & Munoz, 2012) and further research is needed to determine optimal vitamin D nutritional status in the elderly for the prevention of sarcopenia.

7.6.5 Food and dietary patterns

The eating habits of older adults are influenced by several factors, including food preferences that have been established throughout life, physiological changes associated with ageing, socioeconomic conditions, transportation, being institutionalized or not, and living with a spouse or alone. Food insecurity and hunger are issues of concern for many older adults, particularly for those living alone, having low socioeconomic status or from minority ethnic groups (Kuczmarski & Weddle, 2005; Bernstein & Munoz, 2012).

Energy needs decline with increasing age, and increased physical activity or exercise may be important to counteract this trend. Furthermore, with higher energy intake by those with increased energy needs, it is easier to provide the amount of food necessary to meet the nutritional recommendations, particularly for micronutrients (Schlenker, 1992).

The modern Western-type diet is rich in animal products and scarce in fruit and vegetables (Adeva & Souto, 2011), which results in a net acid production, in contrast with diets abundant in potassium that possess an alkalinizing effect (Cordain *et al.*, 2005; Adeva & Souto, 2011). In addition protein, an adequate potassium intake and alkaline diets may favour lean tissue mass in older adults (Dawson-Hughes *et al.*, 2008), while acidosis (Adeva & Souto, 2011) can amplify the decrease in muscle mass. This is also particularly important considering that the normal decrease in kidney function associated with age may also favour acidosis (Adeva & Souto, 2011).

In addition to being important for potassium intake, consumption of fruit and vegetables is negatively associated with inflammation in older adults (Semba *et al.*, 2007) and ensuring an adequate intake of these foods is also important to achieve adequate ingestion of anti-oxidants, namely carotenoids (Doria *et al.*, 2012), polyphenols, tocopherols, ascorbate and selenium (Buonocore *et al.*, 2011).

Many of the components previously reported as beneficial to inflammation and redox status, particularly omega-3 PUFA and dietary anti-oxidants, are natural constituents of the Mediterranean diet, a cultural paradigm for healthy eating, considering its high content of vegetables, legumes, fruit, nuts, seeds, whole grain cereals, olive oil, fish and herbal infusions, with moderate amounts of wine (Bach-Faig *et al.*, 2011). Therefore, nutritional strategies are needed to limit muscle wasting and to counteract muscle mass and function decline. When examining associations between grip strength and empirically healthy dietary patterns such as the prudent dietary pattern – generally characterized by high consumption of vegetables, fruit, fatty fish and whole grains and a low consumption of white bread, chips, sugar and full-fat dairy products (Bhupathiraju & Tucker, 2011; Robinson *et al.*, 2008) – grip strength was positively related to prudent diet score in community-dwelling older men and women (Robinson *et al.*, 2008).

Looking for nutrients and foods using a whole dietary pattern approach may present numerous advantages over a "single nutrient approach", considering the high number of interactions and synergies that may occur between food components, and future studies should also address this multidimensional perspective of intake.

7.7 Resistance exercise and nutrition: Effective treatment strategy to counteract age-related muscle wasting and bone loss

Progressive resistance exercise (RE) training is a potent, nonpharmacological, efficacious therapy for the impairment of muscle quantity and quality in older adults. Several studies and systematic reviews have shown that, even in the elderly, RE increases muscle mass, muscle power and muscle strength (Liu & Latham, 2009; Latham *et al.*, 2004). Overwhelming evidence from randomized controlled trials and/or observational studies suggests that older adults can substantially increase their strength and muscular power after RE (Chodzko-Zajko *et al.*, 2009). Strong evidence also demonstrates that increases in muscle quality are similar between older and younger adults (Chodzko-Zajko *et al.*, 2009).

Muscle accretion from RE may be regulated by an increase in the activation of the mTOR muscle protein synthetic pathway (Fujita *et al.*, 2007), satellite cell activation and proliferation (Verdijk *et al.*, 2009a) and anabolic hormone production (Smilios *et al.*, 2007) and a decrease in catabolic cytokine activity (Cornish & Chilibeck, 2009).

Additionally, evidence from both animal and human studies indicates that exercise in general, and mechanical signals in particular, are both anabolic and anticatabolic to bone tissue and benefit both bone quantity and quality (Rubin *et al.*, 2008). Loading derives from forces applied to a bone, either from a muscle pulling on an origin or insertion region, or from external forces acting on a bone across a joint or from the outside world (e.g. the ground; Pearson & Lieberman, 2004). Strong evidence also suggests that high-intensity RE training preserves or improves BMD relative to sedentary controls (Ryan *et al.*, 2004; Marques *et al.*, 2012). Mechanical loading forces become less effective in eliciting an osteogenic effect with increasing age, suggesting a progressive loss of bone sensitivity to chemical and physical signals (Rubin *et al.*, 1992).

There is a growing body of evidence suggesting that nutritional interventions, when applied in conjunction with RE, may further augment the increase in muscle mass and strength (Candow *et al.*, 2012). There are several ways in which nutrition contributes to intensification of musculoskeletal health, particularly by: (a) providing bone-forming minerals; (b) assuring nutritional balance for calcium-phosphate homeostasis; and (c) supplying of energy, amino acids and nutrients involved in anti-inflammatory and proteic anabolic responses.

Although research indicates that creatine monohydrate, essential fatty acids and vitamin D may all have beneficial effects, high-quality protein intake (such as those from milk or whole egg protein) is appointed as an important factor to enhance the anabolic effect of RE on muscle. The resulting increase in the delivery of essential amino acids (EAA) after high-intensity RE may favour hiperaminoacidaemia and MPS to a greater extent than eating protein without exercise (for a review see Phillips *et al.*, 2009). This improved anabolic response when RE was combined with EEA or high-quality protein intake was observed in middle aged (Robinson *et al.*, 2013) and older adults (Symons *et al.*, 2011; Drummond *et al.*, 2008).

7.7.1 Protein and resistance exercise

The required dose of protein to maximally stimulate MPS in older adults following RE generates strong debate and controversy. In the study by Welle and Thornton (1998), contributions of high-quality protein intake in the meals corresponding to 7, 14 and 28% of total energy intake were described as equally effective in increasing MPS in older adults after RE. When considering the absolute intake of high-quality protein, 20 g of protein after exercise was suggested to be sufficient to maximally stimulate MPS in young men (Moore *et al.*, 2009). However, older adults may respond to higher intakes of protein (e.g. 40 g of high quality protein) after RE (Yang *et al.*, 2012), suggesting that an attenuated anabolic response in older adults may be compensated for if an adequate amount of EEA or high-quality protein intake is provided (Drummond *et al.*, 2012).

The ability of amino acids to act as a trigger element for the initiation of protein synthesis is not universal, and leucine has been suggested to have the most marked anabolic characteristics of all nutrients (Wilkinson *et al.*, 2013; Atherton *et al.*, 2010). A dose effect has also been described, and increasing leucine above a certain level was hypothesised to be fundamental in stimulating MPS in elderly subjects (reviewed in Breen and Philips, 2011).

In fact, older adults showed less anabolic sensitivity and responsiveness of MPS to EAA than younger adults (Cuthbertson *et al.*, 2005), and a high proportion of leucine may also be required in the elderly for optimal stimulation of MPS (Katsanos *et al.*, 2006). In this context, the metabolic efficacy of proteins will depend on its content of EAA, particularly leucine, and its bioavailability, particularly degree of digestibility and rate of absorption, in order to rapidly increase aminoacidaemia (Breen & Phillips, 2011).

The existence of a "window of opportunity" to amplify MPS with protein intake, particularly shortly after RE, is controversial (Breen & Phillips, 2011). In older adults, the study of Dideriksen *et al.* (2011), for example, showed that MPS did not differ when high-quality protein was fed immediately before or after heavy RE, while in the study of Jordan *et al.* (2010), when protein (from a chocolate milk beverage) was consumed immediately after exercise rather than before, nitrogen balance was more positive. Nevertheless, although conflicting results exist, recommendations for protein intake include the consumption of high-quality protein in doses of 20 g or more, or in doses between 30–40 g of protein, close in time to the RE session, and at intervals throughout the day after RE (Breen & Phillips, 2011). Drummond *et al.* (2012) accepted as possible the hypothesis that a dose of 40 g of high-quality protein (approximately 20 g of EAA) should be given early after exercise in order to amplify muscle hypertrophy and strength after RE, although providing such an amount of protein may not be an easy task in the elderly considering the protein content in usual foods (Tieland *et al.*, 2012).

Future research is needed to clarify in older adults the importance of the quality and quantity of dietary protein, and the exact amounts of leucine and other EAA intake, considering the effects of shorter and longer periods of consumption that improve muscle strength, maximize lean mass maintenance (Breen & Phillips, 2011) and increase the magnitude or duration of MPS under the conditions of RE (Churchward-Venne *et al.*, 2012). The questions of whether these potential benefits and others vary according to the amount (Verdijk *et al.*, 2009b) and timing of protein consumption also need to be addressed.

In a review of Churchward-Venne *et al.* (2012), the main factors emphasized in the modulation of the magnitude (and eventually the duration) of MPS with RE included the consumption and timing of protein and EAA intake, and the dietary source of the protein (such as egg albumin, soy, beef, whey, or casein; Moore *et al.*, 2009; Tang *et al.*, 2009; Robinson *et al.*, 2013), and differences in MPS can also be found between proteins that exhibit high quality levels (Tang *et al.*, 2009; Churchward-Venne *et al.*, 2012). Accordingly, whey protein was described as more effective than casein in stimulating muscle protein accretion (Pennings *et al.*, 2011), and this difference may be related to different digestion and absorption kinetics, and amino acid composition (Pennings *et al.*, 2012), which may impact the bioavailability and bioefficacy of proteins. Since postprandial MPS may also depend on postprandial plasma amino acid levels (Bohé *et al.*, 2003), the physical food form in which these nutrients are delivered is also hypothesized to have implications for anabolic processes, and amino acid concentrations may be higher in protein meals in liquid form than in solid form (Conley *et al.*, 2011). Different methods of food preparation or processing may also modify postprandial protein digestion and absorption, and Pennings *et al.* (2013) showed that minced meat originated more rapid protein digestion and absorption than beef steak in the elderly, despite the absence of a significant postprandial muscle protein synthetic response. The preparation of texture-modified foods is an important issue in older adults, particularly when dental problems (such as tooth loss) reduce chewing capacity, which in turn may decrease meat protein utilization for protein synthesis (Remond *et al.*, 2007). In summary, MPS following resistance exercise may be increased after high-quality protein intake, although more research is needed to determine the exact required doses of EAA and protein to maximally stimulate anabolic response in the older adults.

Another important nutritional condition to be considered during exercise and recovery is glycogen availability, since an increased rate of net protein degradation may occur if a state of low muscle glycogen content is observed (Blomstrand & Saltin, 1999). Even supposing that carbohydrate alone after RE may improve net protein balance (Borsheim *et al.*, 2004), consuming protein and carbohydrate together is also described as being more important to attenuate indices of protein breakdown (Aragon & Schoenfeld, 2013; Borsheim *et al.*, 2004) or to increase the stimulus for MPS, compared with the ingestion of carbohydrate alone (Howarth *et al.*, 2009). Nevertheless, the higher exercise-induced protein accretion after concurrent ingestion of protein and carbohydrates vs protein alone was not found by all researchers (Staples *et al.*, 2011).

7.8 Concluding remarks

Despite the existence of evidence clearly demonstrating that regular exercise can minimize the physiological effects of an otherwise sedentary lifestyle by limiting the development and progression of chronic disease and disabling conditions, only a limited number of older adults are physically active. Several physical activity guidelines for older adults have been published and frequently updated showing the types and amounts of physical activity recommended. Evidence is accumulating that dietary amino acid supplementation may also improve muscle protein balance in older adults. Muscle and bone should be considered together as a functional unit, and a combined exercise and nutritional guideline for older adults is needed to provide the best possible information, supporting older adults to make informed choices related to nutrition and physical activity. Nonetheless, older adults should optimize both nutrition and exercise as both are important modifiable factors that increase muscle strength and mass, and contribute to the maintenance of bone mass and the prevention and treatment of osteoporosis.

References

Adeva, M. M. and G. Souto. 2011. Diet-induced metabolic acidosis. *Clin. Nutr.* 30:416–421.

Anderson, B. M. and D. W. Ma. 2009. Are all n-3 polyunsaturated fatty acids created equal? *Lipids Health Dis.* 8:33.

Aragon, A. A. and B. J. Schoenfeld. 2013. Nutrient timing revisited: is there a post-exercise anabolic window? *J. Int. Soc. Sports Nutr.* 10.

Arthur, S. T. and I. D. Cooley. 2012. The effect of physiological stimuli on sarcopenia; impact of Notch and Wnt signaling on impaired aged skeletal muscle repair. *Int. J. Biol. Sci.* 8:731–760.

Atherton, P. J., K. Smith, T. Etheridge, D. Rankin, and M. J. Rennie. 2010. Distinct anabolic signalling responses to amino acids in C2C12 skeletal muscle cells. *Amino Acids* 38:1533–1539.

Avenell, A., W. J. Gillespie, L. D. Gillespie, and D. O'Connell. 2009. Vitamin D and vitamin D analogues for preventing fractures associated with involutional and post-menopausal osteoporosis. *Cochrane Database Syst. Rev.* 15:CD000227.

Bach-Faig, A., E. M. Berry, D. Lairon, J. Reguant, A. Trichopoulou, S. Dernini, F. X. Medina, M. Battino, R. Belahsen, G. Miranda, and L. Serra-Majem. 2011. Mediterranean diet pyramid today. Science and cultural updates. *Public Health Nutr.* 14:2274–2284.

Bacon, L., J. S. Stern, N. L. Keim, and M. D. Van Loan. 2004. Low bone mass in premenopausal chronic dieting obese women. *Eur. J. Clin. Nutr.* 58:966–971.

Baczynski, R., S. G. Massry, M. Magott, S. el-Belbessi, R. Kohan, and N. Brautbar. 1985. Effect of parathyroid hormone on energy metabolism of skeletal muscle. *Kidney Int.* 28:722–727.

Baraibar, M. A., M. Gueugneau, S. Duguez, G. Butler-Browne, D. Bechet, and B. Friguet. 2013. Expression and modification proteomics during skeletal muscle ageing. *Biogerontology* 14(3):339–352.

Barreiro, E., C. Coronell, B. Lavina, A. Ramirez-Sarmiento, M. Orozco-Levi, and J. Gea. 2006. Aging, sex differences, and oxidative stress in human respiratory and limb muscles. *Free Radic. Biol. Med.* 41:797–809.

Baumgartner, R. N., P. M. Stauber, D. McHugh, K. M. Koehler, and P. J. Garry. 1995. Cross-sectional age differences in body composition in persons 60+ years of age. *J. Gerontol. A. Biol. Sci. Med. Sci.* 50: M307–316.

Bernstein, M. and N. Munoz. 2012. Position of the Academy of Nutrition and Dietetics: food and nutrition for older adults: promoting health and wellness. *J. Acad. Nutr. Diet.* 112:1255–1277.

Bhupathiraju, S. N. and K. L. Tucker. 2011. Coronary heart disease prevention: nutrients, foods, and dietary patterns. *Clin. Chim. Acta* 412:1493–1514.

Bischoff, H. A., M. Borchers, F. Gudat, U. Duermueller, R. Theiler, H. B. Stahelin, and W. Dick. 2001. In situ detection of 1,25-dihydroxyvitamin D3 receptor in human skeletal muscle tissue. *Histochem. J.* 33:19–24.

Bischoff-Ferrari, H. A., B. Dawson-Hughes, W. C. Willett, H. B. Staehelin, M. G. Bazemore, R. Y. Zee, and J. B. Wong. 2004. Effect of vitamin D on falls: a meta-analysis. *JAMA* 291:1999–2006.

Blomstrand, E. and B. Saltin. 1999. Effect of muscle glycogen on glucose, lactate and amino acid metabolism during exercise and recovery in human subjects. *J. Physiol.* 514 (Pt 1):293–302.

Bohé, J., A. Low, R. R. Wolfe, and M. J. Rennie. 2003. Human muscle protein synthesis is modulated by extracellular, not intramuscular amino acid availability: a dose–response study. *J. Physiol.* 552: 315–324.

Boland, R., A. R. de Boland, M. J. Marinissen, G. Santillan, G. Vazquez, and S. Zanello. 1995. Avian muscle cells as targets for the secosteroid hormone 1,25-dihydroxy-vitamin D3. *Mol. Cell. Endocrinol.* 114:1–8.

Bonetto, A., F. Penna, M. Muscaritoli, V. G. Minero, F. Rossi Fanelli, F. M. Baccino, and P. Costelli. 2009. Are antioxidants useful for treating skeletal muscle atrophy? *Free Radic. Biol. Med.* 47:906–916.

Bonjour, J. P. 2005. Dietary protein: an essential nutrient for bone health. *J. Am. Coll. Nutr.* 24:526S–536S.

Bonorden, W. R. and M. W. Pariza. 1994. Antioxidant nutrients and protection from free radicals. *In*: Kotsonis, F., M. Mackey, and J. Hjelle (eds) *Nutritional Toxicology*. New York: Raven Press, pp. 19–48.

Borsheim, E., M. G. Cree, K. D. Tipton, T. A. Elliott, A. Aarsland, and R. R. Wolfe. 2004. Effect of carbohydrate intake on net muscle protein synthesis during recovery from resistance exercise. *J. Appl. Physiol.* 96:674–678.

Boucher, B. J. 2012. The problems of vitamin d insufficiency in older people. *Aging Dis.* 3:313–329.

Breen, L. and S. M. Phillips. 2011. Skeletal muscle protein metabolism in the elderly: Interventions to counteract the "anabolic resistance" of ageing. *Nutr. Metab. (Lond.)* 8.

Buonocore, D., S. Rucci, M. Vandoni, M. Negro, and F. Marzatico. 2011. Oxidative system in aged skeletal muscle. *Muscles Ligaments Tendons J.* 1:85–90.

Calder, P. C. 2013. Omega-3 polyunsaturated fatty acids and inflammatory processes: nutrition or pharmacology? *Br. J. Clin. Pharmacol.* 75:645–662.

Campbell, W. W., T. A. Trappe, R. R. Wolfe, and W. J. Evans. 2001. The recommended dietary allowance for protein may not be adequate for older people to maintain skeletal muscle. *J. Gerontol. A. Biol. Sci. Med. Sci.* 56:M373–M380.

Candow, D. G., S. C. Forbes, J. P. Little, S. M. Cornish, C. Pinkoski, and P. D. Chilibeck. 2012. Effect of nutritional interventions and resistance exercise on aging muscle mass and strength. *Biogerontology* 13:345–358.

Cao, J. J. 2011. Effects of obesity on bone metabolism. *J. Orthop. Surg. Res.* 6:30.

Cao, J. J. and F. H. Nielsen. 2010. Acid diet (high-meat protein) effects on calcium metabolism and bone health. *Curr. Opin. Clin. Nutr. Metab. Care* 13:698–702.

Cashman, K. D. 2002. Calcium intake, calcium bioavailability and bone health. *Br. J. Nutr.* 87 Suppl 2:S169–177.

Cashman, K. D. 2007. Diet, nutrition, and bone health. *J. Nutr.* 137:2507S–2512S.

Ceglia, L. and S. S. Harris. 2013. Vitamin D and its role in skeletal muscle. *Calcif. Tissue Int.* 92:151–162.

Cesari, M., R. A. Fielding, M. Pahor, B. Goodpaster, M. Hellerstein, G. A. Van Kan, S. D. Anker, S. Rutkove, J. W. Vrijbloed, M. Isaac, Y. Rolland, C. M'Rini, M. Aubertin-Leheudre, J. M. Cedarbaum, M. Zamboni, C. C. Sieber, D. Laurent, W. J. Evans, R. Roubenoff, J. E. Morley, and B. Vellas. 2012. Biomarkers of sarcopenia in clinical trials – recommendations from the International Working Group on Sarcopenia. *J. Cachexia Sarcopenia Muscle* 3:181–190.

Chaput, J. P., C. Lord, M. Cloutier, M. Aubertin Leheudre, E. D. Goulet, S. Rousseau, A. Khalil, and I. J. Dionne. 2007. Relationship between antioxidant intakes and class I sarcopenia in elderly men and women. *J. Nutr. Health Aging* 11:363–369.

Chen, Y. M., S. C. Ho, and J. L. Woo. 2006. Greater fruit and vegetable intake is associated with increased bone mass among postmenopausal Chinese women. *Br. J. Nutr.* 96:745–751.

Chodzko-Zajko, W. J., D. N. Proctor, M. A. Fiatarone Singh, C. T. Minson, C. R. Nigg, G. J. Salem, and J. S. Skinner. 2009. American College of Sports Medicine position stand. Exercise and physical activity for older adults. *Med. Sci. Sports Exerc.* 41:1510–1530.

Christakos, S., P. Dhawan, A. Porta, L. J. Mady, and T. Seth. 2011. Vitamin D and intestinal calcium absorption. *Mol. Cell. Endocrinol.* 347:25–29.

Churchward-Venne, T. A., N. A. Burd, and S. M. Phillips. 2012. Nutritional regulation of muscle protein synthesis with resistance exercise: strategies to enhance anabolism. *Nutr. Metab. (Lond.)* 9:40.

Clark, B. C. and T. M. Manini. 2008. Sarcopenia =/= dynapenia. *J. Gerontol. A. Biol. Sci. Med. Sci.* 63: 829–834.

Clark, B. C. and J. L. Taylor. 2011. Age-related changes in motor cortical properties and voluntary activation of skeletal muscle. *Curr. Aging Sci.* 4:192–199.

Clark, D. J. and R. A. Fielding. 2012. Neuromuscular contributions to age-related weakness. *J. Gerontol. A. Biol. Sci. Med. Sci.* 67:41–47.

Conley, T. B., J. W. Apolzan, H. J. Leidy, K. A. Greaves, E. Lim, and W. W. Campbell. 2011. Effect of food form on postprandial plasma amino acid concentrations in older adults. *Br. J. Nutr.* 106:203–207.

Cooper, C., Z. A. Cole, C. R. Holroyd, S. C. Earl, N. C. Harvey, E. M. Dennison, L. J. Melton, S. R. Cummings, and J. A. Kanis. 2011. Secular trends in the incidence of hip and other osteoporotic fractures. *Osteoporos. Int.* 22:1277–1288.

Cordain, L., S. B. Eaton, A. Sebastian, N. Mann, S. Lindeberg, B. A. Watkins, J. H. O'Keefe, and J. Brand-Miller. 2005. Origins and evolution of the Western diet: health implications for the 21st century. *Am. J. Clin. Nutr.* 81:341–354.

Cornish, S. M. and P. D. Chilibeck. 2009. Alpha-linolenic acid supplementation and resistance training in older adults. *Appl. Physiol. Nutr. Metab.* 34:49–59.

Cruz-Jentoft, A. J., F. Landi, E. Topinkova, and J. P. Michel. 2010. Understanding sarcopenia as a geriatric syndrome. *Curr. Opin. Clin. Nutr. Metab. Care* 13:1–7.

Cummings, S. R., D. M. Black, M. C. Nevitt, W. Browner, J. Cauley, K. Ensrud, H. K. Genant, L. Palermo, J. Scott, and T. M. Vogt. 1993. Bone density at various sites for prediction of hip fractures. The Study of Osteoporotic Fractures Research Group. *Lancet* 341:72–75.

Cuthbertson, D., K. Smith, J. Babraj, G. Leese, T. Waddell, P. Atherton, H. Wackerhage, P. M. Taylor, and M. J. Rennie. 2005. Anabolic signaling deficits underlie amino acid resistance of wasting, aging muscle. *FASEB J.* 19:422–424.

D'Antona, G., M. A. Pellegrino, R. Adami, R. Rossi, C. N. Carlizzi, M. Canepari, B. Saltin, and R. Bottinelli. 2003. The effect of ageing and immobilization on structure and function of human skeletal muscle fibres. *J. Physiol.* 552:499–511.

Dawson-Hughes, B., S. S. Harris, and L. Ceglia. 2008. Alkaline diets favor lean tissue mass in older adults. *Am. J. Clin. Nutr.* 87:662–665.

De Laet, C., J. A. Kanis, A. Oden, H. Johanson, O. Johnell, P. Delmas, J. A. Eisman, H. Kroger, S. Fujiwara, P. Garnero, E. V. McCloskey, D. Mellstrom, L. J. Melton, 3rd, P. J. Meunier, H. A. Pols, J. Reeve, A. Silman, and A. Tenenhouse. 2005. Body mass index as a predictor of fracture risk: a meta-analysis. *Osteoporos. Int.* 16:1330–1338.

Delbono, O. 2011. Expression and regulation of excitation–contraction coupling proteins in aging skeletal muscle. *Curr. Aging Sci.* 4:248–259.

Delmonico, M. J., T. B. Harris, M. Visser, S. W. Park, M. B. Conroy, P. Velasquez-Mieyer, R. Boudreau, T. M. Manini, M. Nevitt, A. B. Newman, and B. H. Goodpaster. 2009. Longitudinal study of muscle strength, quality, and adipose tissue infiltration. *Am. J. Clin. Nutr.* 90:1579–1585.

Devine, A., R. L. Prince, D. A. Kerr, I. M. Dick, R. A. Criddle, G. N. Kent, R. I. Price, and P. G. Webb. 1993. Correlates of intestinal calcium absorption in women 10 years past the menopause. *Calcif. Tissue Int.* 52:358–360.

Dideriksen, K. J., S. Reitelseder, S. G. Petersen, M. Hjort, I. C. Helmark, M. Kjaer, and L. Holm. 2011. Stimulation of muscle protein synthesis by whey and caseinate ingestion after resistance exercise in elderly individuals. *Scand. J. Med. Sci. Sports* 21:e372–e383.

Dirks, A. J. and C. Leeuwenburgh. 2005. The role of apoptosis in age-related skeletal muscle atrophy. *Sports Med.* 35:473–483.

Doria, E., D. Buonocore, A. Focarelli, and F. Marzatico. 2012. Relationship between human aging muscle and oxidative system pathway. *Oxid. Med. Cell. Longev.* 2012:830257.

Drummond, M. J., H. C. Dreyer, B. Pennings, C. S. Fry, S. Dhanani, E. L. Dillon, M. Sheffield-Moore, E. Volpi, and B. B. Rasmussen. 2008. Skeletal muscle protein anabolic response to resistance exercise and essential amino acids is delayed with aging. *J. Appl. Physiol.* 104:1452–1461.

Drummond, M. J., R. L. Marcus, and P. C. Lastayo. 2012. Targeting anabolic impairment in response to resistance exercise in older adults with mobility impairments: potential mechanisms and rehabilitation approaches. *J. Aging Res.* 2012:486930.

Duncan, E. L. and M. A. Brown. 2010. Genetic determinants of bone density and fracture risk – state of the art and future directions. *J. Clin. Endocrinol. Metab.* 95:2576–2587.

Duque, G. and B. R. Troen. 2008. Understanding the mechanisms of senile osteoporosis: new facts for a major geriatric syndrome. *J. Am. Geriatr. Soc.* 56:935–941.

Edstrom, E., M. Altun, E. Bergman, H. Johnson, S. Kullberg, V. Ramirez-Leon, and B. Ulfhake. 2007. Factors contributing to neuromuscular impairment and sarcopenia during aging. *Physiol. Behav.* 92:129–135.

Eslick, G. D., P. R. Howe, C. Smith, R. Priest, and A. Bensoussan. 2009. Benefits of fish oil supplementation in hyperlipidemia: a systematic review and meta-analysis. *Int. J. Cardiol.* 136:4–16.

Evans, W. J. 2004. Protein nutrition, exercise and aging. *J. Am. Coll. Nutr.* 23:601S–609S.

Evans, W. J. and D. Cyr-Campbell. 1997. Nutrition, exercise, and healthy aging. *J. Am. Diet. Assoc.* 97:632–638.

Fantuzzi, G. 2005. Adipose tissue, adipokines, and inflammation. *J. Allergy Clin. Immunol.* 115:911–919; quiz 920.

Faulkner, K. A., J. A. Cauley, J. M. Zmuda, D. P. Landsittel, A. B. Newman, S. A. Studenski, M. S. Redfern, K. E. Ensrud, H. A. Fink, N. E. Lane, and M. C. Nevitt. 2006. Higher 1,25-dihydroxyvitamin D3 concentrations associated with lower fall rates in older community-dwelling women. *Osteoporos. Int.* 17: 1318–1328.

Frenkel, B., A. Hong, S. K. Baniwal, G. A. Coetzee, C. Ohlsson, O. Khalid, and Y. Gabet. 2010. Regulation of adult bone turnover by sex steroids. *J. Cell. Physiol.* 224:305–310.

Frontera, W. R., V. A. Hughes, R. A. Fielding, M. A. Fiatarone, W. J. Evans, and R. Roubenoff. 2000. Aging of skeletal muscle: a 12-yr longitudinal study. *J. Appl. Physiol. (1985)* 88:1321–1326.

Frontera, W. R., A. R. Zayas, and N. Rodriguez. 2012. Aging of human muscle: understanding sarcopenia at the single muscle cell level. *Phys. Med. Rehabil. Clin. N. Am.* 23:201–207, xiii.

Fujita, S., T. Abe, M. J. Drummond, J. G. Cadenas, H. C. Dreyer, Y. Sato, E. Volpi, and B. B. Rasmussen. 2007. Blood flow restriction during low-intensity resistance exercise increases S6K1 phosphorylation and muscle protein synthesis. *J. Appl. Physiol. (1985)* 103:903–910.

Galli, C. and P. C. Calder. 2009. Effects of fat and fatty acid intake on inflammatory and immune responses: a critical review. *Ann. Nutr. Metab.* 55:123–139.

Gennari, C. 2001. Calcium and vitamin D nutrition and bone disease of the elderly. *Public Health Nutr.* 4:547–559.

Gersovitz, M., K. Motil, H. N. Munro, N. S. Scrimshaw, and V. R. Young. 1982. Human protein requirements: assessment of the adequacy of the current Recommended Dietary Allowance for dietary protein in elderly men and women. *Am. J. Clin. Nutr.* 35:6–14.

Goodpaster, B. H., D. E. Kelley, F. L. Thaete, J. He, and R. Ross. 2000. Skeletal muscle attenuation determined by computed tomography is associated with skeletal muscle lipid content. *J. Appl. Physiol. (1985)* 89:104–110.

Gullberg, B., O. Johnell, and J. A. Kanis. 1997. World-wide projections for hip fracture. *Osteoporos. Int.* 7:407–413.

Hannan, M. T., D. T. Felson, B. Dawson-Hughes, K. L. Tucker, L. A. Cupples, P. W. Wilson, and D. P. Kiel. 2000. Risk factors for longitudinal bone loss in elderly men and women: the Framingham Osteoporosis Study. *J. Bone Miner. Res.* 15:710–720.

Harris, S. S. and B. Dawson-Hughes. 1994. Caffeine and bone loss in healthy postmenopausal women. *Am. J. Clin. Nutr.* 60:573–578.

Harris, W. S., D. Mozaffarian, M. Lefevre, C. D. Toner, J. Colombo, S. C. Cunnane, J. M. Holden, D. M. Klurfeld, M. C. Morris, and J. Whelan. 2009. Towards establishing dietary reference intakes for eicosapentaenoic and docosahexaenoic acids. *J. Nutr.* 139:804S–819S.

Heaney, R. P. 2002. Effects of caffeine on bone and the calcium economy. *Food Chem. Toxicol.* 40:1263–1270.

Heaney, R. P. and D. K. Layman. 2008. Amount and type of protein influences bone health. *Am. J. Clin. Nutr.* 87:1567S–1570S.

Heaney, R. P. and C. M. Weaver. 2005. Newer perspectives on calcium nutrition and bone quality. *J. Am. Coll. Nutr.* 24:574S–581S.

Hiona, A. and C. Leeuwenburgh. 2008. The role of mitochondrial DNA mutations in aging and sarcopenia: implications for the mitochondrial vicious cycle theory of aging. *Exp. Gerontol.* 43:24–33.

Ho-Pham, L. T., N. D. Nguyen, T. Q. Lai, and T. V. Nguyen. 2010. Contributions of lean mass and fat mass to bone mineral density: a study in postmenopausal women. *BMC Musculoskelet. Disord.* 11:59.

Houston, D. K., B. J. Nicklas, J. Ding, T. B. Harris, F. A. Tylavsky, A. B. Newman, J. S. Lee, N. R. Sahyoun, M. Visser, and S. B. Kritchevsky. 2008. Dietary protein intake is associated with lean mass change in older, community-dwelling adults: the Health, Aging, and Body Composition (Health ABC) Study. *Am. J. Clin. Nutr.* 87:150–155.

Howard, C., L. Ferrucci, K. Sun, L. P. Fried, J. Walston, R. Varadhan, J. M. Guralnik, and R. D. Semba. 2007. Oxidative protein damage is associated with poor grip strength among older women living in the community. *J. Appl. Physiol. (1985)* 103:17–20.

Howarth, K. R., N. A. Moreau, S. M. Phillips, and M. J. Gibala. 2009. Coingestion of protein with carbohydrate during recovery from endurance exercise stimulates skeletal muscle protein synthesis in humans. *J. Appl. Physiol.* 106:1394–1402.

Hunt, J. R., L. K. Johnson, and Z. K. Fariba Roughead. 2009. Dietary protein and calcium interact to influence calcium retention: a controlled feeding study. *Am. J. Clin. Nutr.* 89:1357–1365.

Hwang, S. Y. and J. W. Putney, Jr. 2011. Calcium signaling in osteoclasts. *Biochim. Biophys. Acta* 1813: 979–983.

Iannuzzi-Sucich, M., K. M. Prestwood, and A. M. Kenny. 2002. Prevalence of sarcopenia and predictors of skeletal muscle mass in healthy, older men and women. *J. Gerontol. A. Biol. Sci. Med. Sci.* 57:M772–777.

Ilich, J. Z. and J. E. Kerstetter. 2000. Nutrition in bone health revisited: a story beyond calcium. *J. Am. Coll. Nutr.* 19:715–737.

Jackson, R. D., A. Z. LaCroix, M. Gass, R. B. Wallace, J. Robbins, C. E. Lewis, T. Bassford, S. A. Beresford, H. R. Black, P. Blanchette, D. E. Bonds, R. L. Brunner, R. G. Brzyski, B. Caan, J. A. Cauley, R. T. Chlebowski, S. R. Cummings, I. Granek, J. Hays, G. Heiss, S. L. Hendrix, B. V. Howard, J. Hsia, F. A. Hubbell, K. C. Johnson, H. Judd, J. M. Kotchen, L. H. Kuller, R. D. Langer, N. L. Lasser, M. C. Limacher, S. Ludlam, J. E. Manson, K. L. Margolis, J. McGowan, J. K. Ockene, M. J. O'Sullivan, L. Phillips, R. L. Prentice, G. E. Sarto, M. L. Stefanick, L. Van Horn, J. Wactawski-Wende, E. Whitlock, G. L. Anderson, A. R. Assaf, and D. Barad. 2006. Calcium plus vitamin D supplementation and the risk of fractures. *New Engl. J. Med.* 354:669–683.

Jackson, R. D., N. C. Wright, T. J. Beck, D. Sherrill, J. A. Cauley, C. E. Lewis, A. Z. LaCroix, M. S. LeBoff, S. Going, T. Bassford, and Z. Chen. 2011. Calcium plus vitamin D supplementation has limited effects on femoral geometric strength in older postmenopausal women: the Women's Health Initiative. *Calcif. Tissue Int.* 88:198–208.

Janssen, H. C., M. M. Samson, and H. J. Verhaar. 2002. Vitamin D deficiency, muscle function, and falls in elderly people. *Am. J. Clin. Nutr.* 75:611–615.

Janssen, I., S. B. Heymsfield, Z. M. Wang, and R. Ross. 2000. Skeletal muscle mass and distribution in 468 men and women aged 18–88 yr. *J. Appl. Physiol.* 89:81–88.

Johnell, O. and J. Kanis. 2005. Epidemiology of osteoporotic fractures. *Osteoporos. Int.* 16 Suppl 2:S3–7.

Johnell, O., J. A. Kanis, A. Oden, H. Johansson, C. De Laet, P. Delmas, J. A. Eisman, S. Fujiwara, H. Kroger, D. Mellstrom, P. J. Meunier, L. J. Melton, 3rd, T. O'Neill, H. Pols, J. Reeve, A. Silman, and A. Tenenhouse. 2005. Predictive value of BMD for hip and other fractures. *J. Bone Miner. Res.* 20:1185–1194.

Jordan, L. Y., E. L. Melanson, C. L. Melby, M. S. Hickey, and B. F. Miller. 2010. Nitrogen balance in older individuals in energy balance depends on timing of protein intake. *J. Gerontol. A. Biol. Sci. Med. Sci.* 65:1068–1076.

Joseph, A. M., P. J. Adhihetty, T. W. Buford, S. E. Wohlgemuth, H. A. Lees, L. M. Nguyen, J. M. Aranda, B. D. Sandesara, M. Pahor, T. M. Manini, E. Marzetti, and C. Leeuwenburgh. 2012. The impact of aging on mitochondrial function and biogenesis pathways in skeletal muscle of sedentary high- and low-functioning elderly individuals. *Aging Cell* 11:801–809.

Kadi, F. and E. Ponsot. 2010. The biology of satellite cells and telomeres in human skeletal muscle: effects of aging and physical activity. *Scand. J. Med. Sci. Sports* 20:39–48.

Kamen, G., S. V. Sison, C. C. Du, and C. Patten. 1995. Motor unit discharge behavior in older adults during maximal-effort contractions. *J. Appl. Physiol. (1985)* 79:1908–1913.

Kanis, J. A. 1994. Assessment of fracture risk and its application to screening for postmenopausal osteoporosis: synopsis of a WHO report. WHO Study Group. *Osteoporos. Int.* 4:368–381.

Kanis, J. A. 2002. Diagnosis of osteoporosis and assessment of fracture risk. *Lancet* 359:1929–1936.

Kanis, J. A., O. Johnell, C. De Laet, B. Jonsson, A. Oden, and A. K. Ogelsby. 2002. International variations in hip fracture probabilities: implications for risk assessment. *J. Bone Miner. Res.* 17:1237–1244.

Kanis, J. A., F. Borgstrom, C. De Laet, H. Johansson, O. Johnell, B. Jonsson, A. Oden, N. Zethraeus, B. Pfleger, and N. Khaltaev. 2005. Assessment of fracture risk. *Osteoporos. Int.* 16:581–589.

Kato, I., P. Toniolo, A. Akhmedkhanov, K. L. Koenig, R. Shore, and A. Zeleniuch-Jacquotte. 1998. Prospective study of factors influencing the onset of natural menopause. *J. Clin. Epidemiol.* 51: 1271–1276.

Katsanos, C. S., H. Kobayashi, M. Sheffield-Moore, A. Aarsland, and R. R. Wolfe. 2006. A high proportion of leucine is required for optimal stimulation of the rate of muscle protein synthesis by essential amino acids in the elderly. *Am. J. Physiol. Endocrinol. Metab.* 291:E381–E387.

Kerstetter, J. E., K. O. O'Brien, and K. L. Insogna. 1998. Dietary protein affects intestinal calcium absorption. *Am. J. Clin. Nutr.* 68:859–865.

Kerstetter, J. E., K. O. O'Brien, and K. L. Insogna. 2003. Dietary protein, calcium metabolism, and skeletal homeostasis revisited. *Am. J. Clin. Nutr.* 78:584S–592S.

Kerstetter, J. E., K. O. O'Brien, D. M. Caseria, D. E. Wall, and K. L. Insogna. 2005. The impact of dietary protein on calcium absorption and kinetic measures of bone turnover in women. *J. Clin. Endocrinol. Metab.* 90:26–31.

Klass, M., S. Baudry, and J. Duchateau. 2007. Voluntary activation during maximal contraction with advancing age: a brief review. *Eur. J. Appl. Physiol.* 100:543–551.

Klotzbuecher, C. M., P. D. Ross, P. B. Landsman, T. A. Abbott, 3rd, and M. Berger. 2000. Patients with prior fractures have an increased risk of future fractures: a summary of the literature and statistical synthesis. *J. Bone Miner. Res.* 15:721–739.

Kohrt, W. M., S. A. Bloomfield, K. D. Little, M. E. Nelson, and V. R. Yingling. 2004. American College of Sports Medicine Position Stand: physical activity and bone health. *Med. Sci. Sports Exerc.* 36:1985–1996.

Kortebein, P., A. Ferrando, J. Lombeida, R. Wolfe, and W. J. Evans. 2007. Effect of 10 days of bed rest on skeletal muscle in healthy older adults. *JAMA* 297:1772–1774.

Krall, E. A. and B. Dawson-Hughes. 1999. Smoking increases bone loss and decreases intestinal calcium absorption. *J. Bone Miner. Res.* 14:215–220.

Krieger, N. S., D. A. Bushinsky, and K. K. Frick. 2003. Cellular mechanisms of bone resorption induced by metabolic acidosis. *Semin. Dial.* 16:463–466.

Krieger, N. S., K. K. Frick, and D. A. Bushinsky. 2004. Mechanism of acid-induced bone resorption. *Curr. Opin. Nephrol. Hypertens.* 13:423–436.

Kuczmarski, M. F. and D. O. Weddle. 2005. Position paper of the American Dietetic Association: nutrition across the spectrum of aging. *J. Am. Diet. Assoc.* 105:616–633.

Kung, A. W. and Q. Y. Huang. 2007. Genetic and environmental determinants of osteoporosis. *J. Musculoskelet. Neuronal. Interact.* 7:26–32.

Lamberts, S. W., A. W. van den Beld, and A. J. van der Lely. 1997. The endocrinology of aging. *Science* 278:419–424.

Lang, C. H., R. A. Frost, A. C. Nairn, D. A. MacLean, and T. C. Vary. 2002. TNF-alpha impairs heart and skeletal muscle protein synthesis by altering translation initiation. *Am. J. Physiol. Endocrinol. Metab.* 282:E336–347.

Lanham-New, S. A. 2008. Importance of calcium, vitamin D and vitamin K for osteoporosis prevention and treatment. *Proc. Nutr. Soc.* 67:163–176.

Latham, N. K., D. A. Bennett, C. M. Stretton, and C. S. Anderson. 2004. Systematic review of progressive resistance strength training in older adults. *J. Gerontol. A. Biol. Sci. Med. Sci.* 59:48–61.

Lee, R. C., Z. M. Wang, and S. B. Heymsfield. 2001. Skeletal muscle mass and aging: regional and whole-body measurement methods. *Can. J. Appl. Physiol.* 26:102–122.

Leeuwenburgh, C. 2003. Role of apoptosis in sarcopenia. *J. Gerontol. A. Biol. Sci. Med. Sci.* 58:999–1001.

Lips, P. 2007. Vitamin D status and nutrition in Europe and Asia. *J. Steroid. Biochem. Mol. Biol.* 103:620–625.

Lips, P. and N. M. van Schoor. 2011. The effect of vitamin D on bone and osteoporosis. *Best Pract. Res. Clin. Endocrinol. Metab.* 25:585–591.

Liu, C. J. and N. K. Latham. 2009. Progressive resistance strength training for improving physical function in older adults. *Cochrane Database Syst. Rev.* 8:CD002759.

Macdonald, H. M., S. A. New, W. D. Fraser, M. K. Campbell, and D. M. Reid. 2005. Low dietary potassium intakes and high dietary estimates of net endogenous acid production are associated with low bone mineral density in premenopausal women and increased markers of bone resorption in postmenopausal women. *Am. J. Clin. Nutr.* 81:923–933.

Manini, T. M., M. Visser, S. Won-Park, K. V. Patel, E. S. Strotmeyer, H. Chen, B. Goodpaster, N. De Rekeneire, A. B. Newman, E. M. Simonsick, S. B. Kritchevsky, K. Ryder, A. V. Schwartz, and T. B. Harris. 2007. Knee extension strength cutpoints for maintaining mobility. *J. Am. Geriatr. Soc.* 55: 451–457.

Manolagas, S. C., S. Kousteni, and R. L. Jilka. 2002. Sex steroids and bone. *Recent Prog. Horm. Res.* 57:385–409.

Marimuthu, K., A. J. Murton, and P. L. Greenhaff. 2011. Mechanisms regulating muscle mass during disuse atrophy and rehabilitation in humans. *J. Appl. Physiol. (1985)* 110:555–560.

Marks, R., J. P. Allegrante, C. Ronald MacKenzie, and J. M. Lane. 2003. Hip fractures among the elderly: causes, consequences and control. *Ageing Res. Rev.* 2:57–93.

Marques, E. A., J. Mota, and J. Carvalho. 2012. Exercise effects on bone mineral density in older adults: a meta-analysis of randomized controlled trials. *Age* 34:1493–1515.

Martin, C., H. Dubouchaud, L. Mosoni, J. M. Chardigny, A. Oudot, E. Fontaine, C. Vergely, C. Keriel, L. Rochette, X. Leverve, and L. Demaison. 2007. Abnormalities of mitochondrial functioning can partly explain the metabolic disorders encountered in sarcopenic gastrocnemius. *Aging Cell* 6:165–177.

Marzani, B., M. Balage, A. Venien, T. Astruc, I. Papet, D. Dardevet, and L. Mosoni. 2008. Antioxidant supplementation restores defective leucine stimulation of protein synthesis in skeletal muscle from old rats. *J. Nutr.* 138:2205–2211.

Marzetti, E., R. Calvani, R. Bernabei, and C. Leeuwenburgh. 2012. Apoptosis in skeletal myocytes: a potential target for interventions against sarcopenia and physical frailty – a mini-review. *Gerontology* 58:99–106.

Massey, L. K. and S. J. Whiting. 1993. Caffeine, urinary calcium, calcium metabolism and bone. *J. Nutr.* 123:1611–1614.

Milaneschi, Y., T. Tanaka, and L. Ferrucci. 2010. Nutritional determinants of mobility. *Curr. Opin. Clin. Nutr. Metab. Care* 13:625–629.

Miller, P. D. 2006. Guidelines for the diagnosis of osteoporosis: T-scores vs fractures. *Rev. Endocr. Metab. Disord.* 7:75–89.

Millward, D. J., A. Fereday, N. Gibson, and P. J. Pacy. 1997. Aging, protein requirements, and protein turnover. *Am. J. Clin. Nutr.* 66:774–786.

Mitchell, W. K., J. Williams, P. Atherton, M. Larvin, J. Lund, and M. Narici. 2012. Sarcopenia, dynapenia, and the impact of advancing age on human skeletal muscle size and strength; a quantitative review. *Front. Physiol.* 3:260.

Moore, D. R., M. J. Robinson, J. L. Fry, J. E. Tang, E. I. Glover, S. B. Wilkinson, T. Prior, M. A. Tarnopolsky, and S. M. Phillips. 2009. Ingested protein dose response of muscle and albumin protein synthesis after resistance exercise in young men. *Am. J. Clin. Nutr.* 89:161–168.

Morley, J. E. 2001. Decreased food intake with aging. *J. Gerontol. A. Biol. Sci. Med. Sci.* 56(spec. no. 2): 81–88.

Morley, J. E., J. M. Argiles, W. J. Evans, S. Bhasin, D. Cella, N. E. Deutz, W. Doehner, K. C. Fearon, L. Ferrucci, M. K. Hellerstein, K. Kalantar-Zadeh, H. Lochs, N. MacDonald, K. Mulligan, M. Muscaritoli, P. Ponikowski, M. E. Posthauer, F. Rossi Fanelli, M. Schambelan, A. M. Schols, M. W. Schuster, and S. D. Anker. 2010. Nutritional recommendations for the management of sarcopenia. *J. Am. Med. Dir. Assoc.* 11:391–396.

Morris, H. A., A. G. Need, M. Horowitz, P. D. O'Loughlin, and B. E. Nordin. 1991. Calcium absorption in normal and osteoporotic postmenopausal women. *Calcif. Tissue Int.* 49:240–243.

Muir, S. W. and M. Montero-Odasso. 2011. Effect of vitamin D supplementation on muscle strength, gait and balance in older adults: a systematic review and meta-analysis. *J. Am. Geriatr. Soc.* 59:2291–2300.

NAMS. 2010. Management of osteoporosis in postmenopausal women: 2010 position statement of The North American Menopause Society. *Menopause* 17:25–54.

Narici, M. V., C. N. Maganaris, N. D. Reeves, and P. Capodaglio. 2003. Effect of aging on human muscle architecture. *J. Appl. Physiol. (1985)* 95:2229–2234.

National Research Council. 2011. *Dietary Reference Intakes for Calcium and Vitamin D*. Washington, DC: The National Academies Press.

Need, A. G., H. A. Morris, M. Horowitz, E. Scopacasa, and B. E. Nordin. 1998. Intestinal calcium absorption in men with spinal osteoporosis. *Clin. Endocrinol. (Oxf.)* 48:163–168.

New, S. A. 2003. Intake of fruit and vegetables: implications for bone health. *Proc. Nutr. Soc.* 62:889–899.

New, S. A., S. P. Robins, M. K. Campbell, J. C. Martin, M. J. Garton, C. Bolton-Smith, D. A. Grubb, S. J. Lee, and D. M. Reid. 2000. Dietary influences on bone mass and bone metabolism: further evidence of a positive link between fruit and vegetable consumption and bone health? *Am. J. Clin. Nutr.* 71: 142–151.

NIH Consensus Development Panel. 2001. Osteoporosis prevention, diagnosis, and therapy. *JAMA* 285:785–795.

Ochala, J., W. R. Frontera, D. J. Dorer, J. Van Hoecke, and L. S. Krivickas. 2007. Single skeletal muscle fiber elastic and contractile characteristics in young and older men. *J. Gerontol. A. Biol. Sci. Med. Sci.* 62:375–381.

Paddon-Jones, D. and B. B. Rasmussen. 2009. Dietary protein recommendations and the prevention of sarcopenia. *Curr. Opin. Clin. Nutr. Metab. Care* 12:86–90.

Pahor, M., T. Manini, and M. Cesari. 2009. Sarcopenia: clinical evaluation, biological markers and other evaluation tools. *J. Nutr. Health Aging* 13:724–728.

Palacios, C. 2006. The role of nutrients in bone health, from A to Z. *Crit. Rev. Food Sci. Nutr.* 46:621–628.

Papaioannou, A., C. C. Kennedy, A. Cranney, G. Hawker, J. P. Brown, S. M. Kaiser, W. D. Leslie, C. J. O'Brien, A. M. Sawka, A. Khan, K. Siminoski, G. Tarulli, D. Webster, J. McGowan, and J. D. Adachi. 2009. Risk factors for low BMD in healthy men age 50 years or older: a systematic review. *Osteoporos. Int.* 20:507–518.

Peacock, M. 2010. Calcium metabolism in health and disease. *Clin. J. Am. Soc. Nephrol.* 5 Suppl 1:S23–30.

Pearson, O. M. and D. E. Lieberman. 2004. The aging of Wolff's "law": ontogeny and responses to mechanical loading in cortical bone. *Am. J. Phys. Anthropol.* Suppl 39:63–99.

Pennings, B., Y. Boirie, J. M. G. Senden, A. P. Gijsen, H. Kuipers, and L. J. C. van Loon. 2011. Whey protein stimulates postprandial muscle protein accretion more effectively than do casein and casein hydrolysate in older men. *Am. J. Clin. Nutr.* 93:997–1005.

Pennings, B., B. Groen, A. de Lange, A. P. Gijsen, A. H. Zorenc, J. M. G. Senden, and L. J. C. van Loon. 2012. Amino acid absorption and subsequent muscle protein accretion following graded intakes of whey protein in elderly men. *Am. J. Physiol. Endocrinol. Metab.* 302:E992–E999.

Pennings, B., B. B. Groen, J. W. van Dijk, A. de Lange, A. Kiskini, M. Kuklinski, J. M. Senden, and L. J. van Loon. 2013. Minced beef is more rapidly digested and absorbed than beef steak, resulting in greater postprandial protein retention in older men. *Am. J. Clin. Nutr.* 98:121–128.

Pfeilschifter, J., R. Koditz, M. Pfohl, and H. Schatz. 2002. Changes in proinflammatory cytokine activity after menopause. *Endocr. Rev.* 23:90–119.

Phillips, S. M., J. E. Tang, and D. R. Moore. 2009. The role of milk- and soy-based protein in support of muscle protein synthesis and muscle protein accretion in young and elderly persons. *J. Am. Coll. Nutr.* 28:343–354.

Podbregar, M., M. Lainscak, O. Prelovsek, and T. Mars. 2013. Cytokine response of cultured skeletal muscle cells stimulated with proinflammatory factors depends on differentiation stage. *Sci. Wld J.* 2013:617170.

Powers, S. K., A. N. Kavazis, and J. M. McClung. 2007. Oxidative stress and disuse muscle atrophy. *J. Appl. Physiol. (1985)* 102:2389–2397.

Powers, S. K., M. P. Wiggs, J. A. Duarte, A. M. Zergeroglu, and H. A. Demirel. 2012. Mitochondrial signaling contributes to disuse muscle atrophy. *Am. J. Physiol. Endocrinol. Metab.* 303:E31–39.

Ralston, S. H. and B. de Crombrugghe. 2006. Genetic regulation of bone mass and susceptibility to osteoporosis. *Genes. Dev.* 20:2492–2506.

Rapuri, P. B., J. C. Gallagher, H. K. Kinyamu, and K. L. Ryschon. 2001. Caffeine intake increases the rate of bone loss in elderly women and interacts with vitamin D receptor genotypes. *Am. J. Clin. Nutr.* 74:694–700.

Reid, I. R. 2010. Fat and bone. *Arch. Biochem. Biophys.* 503:20–27.

Rejnmark, L. 2011. Effects of vitamin d on muscle function and performance: a review of evidence from randomized controlled trials. *Ther. Adv. Chronic. Dis.* 2:25–37.

Remer, T. and F. Manz. 1995. Potential renal acid load of foods and its influence on urine pH. *J. Am. Diet. Assoc.* 95:791–797.

Remond, D., M. Machebeuf, C. Yven, C. Buffiere, L. Mioche, L. Mosoni, and P. Patureau Mirand. 2007. Postprandial whole-body protein metabolism after a meat meal is influenced by chewing efficiency in elderly subjects. *Am. J. Clin. Nutr.* 85:1286–1292.

Robinson, S. M., K. A. Jameson, S. F. Batelaan, H. J. Martin, H. E. Syddall, E. M. Dennison, C. Cooper, and A. A. Sayer. 2008. Diet and its relationship with grip strength in community–dwelling older men and women: the Hertfordshire cohort study. *J. Am. Geriatr. Soc.* 56:84–90.

Robinson, M. J., N. A. Burd, L. Breen, T. Rerecich, Y. F. Yang, A. J. Hector, S. K. Baker, and S. M. Phillips. 2013. Dose-dependent responses of myofibrillar protein synthesis with beef ingestion are enhanced with resistance exercise in middle-aged men. *Appl. Physiol. Nutr. Metab.* 38:120–125.

Rosen, C. J. and M. L. Bouxsein. 2006. Mechanisms of disease: is osteoporosis the obesity of bone? *Nat. Clin. Pract. Rheumatol.* 2:35–43.

Rubin, C., J. Rubin, and S. Judex. 2008. Exercise and the prevention of osteoporosis. *In*: C. J. Rosen (ed.) *Primer on the Metabolic Bone Diseases and Disorders of Mineral Metabolism*, 7th edn. Washington, DC: American Society for Bone Mineral Research, pp. 227–233.

Rubin, C. T., S. D. Bain, and K. J. McLeod. 1992. Suppression of the osteogenic response in the aging skeleton. *Calcif. Tissue Int.* 50:306–313.

Rude, R. K., F. R. Singer, and H. E. Gruber. 2009. Skeletal and hormonal effects of magnesium deficiency. *J. Am. Coll. Nutr.* 28:131–141.

Russ, D. W., J. S. Grandy, K. Toma, and C. W. Ward. 2011. Ageing, but not yet senescent, rats exhibit reduced muscle quality and sarcoplasmic reticulum function. *Acta Physiol.* 201:391–403.

Ryan, A. S., F. M. Ivey, D. E. Hurlbut, G. F. Martel, J. T. Lemmer, J. D. Sorkin, E. J. Metter, J. L. Fleg, and B. F. Hurley. 2004. Regional bone mineral density after resistive training in young and older men and women. *Scand. J. Med. Sci. Sports* 14:16–23.

Ryan, M. J., H. J. Dudash, M. Docherty, K. B. Geronilla, B. A. Baker, G. G. Haff, R. G. Cutlip, and S. E. Alway. 2010a. Vitamin E and C supplementation reduces oxidative stress, improves antioxidant enzymes and positive muscle work in chronically loaded muscles of aged rats. *Exp. Gerontol.* 45:882–895.

Ryan, M. J., J. R. Jackson, Y. Hao, C. L. Williamson, E. R. Dabkowski, J. M. Hollander, and S. E. Alway. 2010b. Suppression of oxidative stress by resveratrol after isometric contractions in gastrocnemius muscles of aged mice. *J. Gerontol. A. Biol. Sci. Med. Sci.* 65:815–831.

Sakuma, K. and A. Yamaguchi. 2012. Sarcopenia and age-related endocrine function. *Int. J. Endocrinol.* 2012:127362.

Schlenker, E. D. 1992. Nutrition for aging and the aged. *In*: S. R. Williams and B. S. Worthington-Roberts (eds) *Nutrition through the Life Cycle*. St Louis, MO: Mosby -Year Book, pp. 344–383.

Schott, G. D. and M. R. Wills. 1976. Muscle weakness in osteomalacia. *Lancet* 1:626–629.

Schubert, L. and H. F. DeLuca. 2010. Hypophosphatemia is responsible for skeletal muscle weakness of vitamin D deficiency. *Arch. Biochem. Biophys.* 500:157–161.

Semba, R. D., C. Blaum, J. M. Guralnik, D. T. Moncrief, M. O. Ricks, and L. P. Fried. 2003. Carotenoid and vitamin E status are associated with indicators of sarcopenia among older women living in the community. *Aging Clin. Exp. Res.* 15:482–487.

Semba, R. D., R. Varadhan, B. Bartali, L. Ferrucci, M. O. Ricks, C. Blaum, and L. P. Fried. 2007. Low serum carotenoids and development of severe walking disability among older women living in the community: the women's health and aging study I. *Age Ageing* 36:62–67.

Shapses, S. A. and C. S. Riedt. 2006. Bone, body weight, and weight reduction: what are the concerns? *J. Nutr.* 136:1453–1456.

Shea, B., G. Wells, A. Cranney, N. Zytaruk, V. Robinson, L. Griffith, C. Hamel, Z. Ortiz, J. Peterson, J. Adachi, P. Tugwell, and G. Guyatt. 2004. Calcium supplementation on bone loss in postmenopausal women. *Cochrane Database Syst. Rev.*:CD004526.

Siris, E. S., P. D. Miller, E. Barrett-Connor, K. G. Faulkner, L. E. Wehren, T. A. Abbott, M. L. Berger, A. C. Santora, and L. M. Sherwood. 2001. Identification and fracture outcomes of undiagnosed low bone mineral density in postmenopausal women: results from the National Osteoporosis Risk Assessment. *JAMA* 286:2815–2822.

Smilios, I., T. Pilianidis, M. Karamouzis, A. Parlavantzas, and S. P. Tokmakidis. 2007. Hormonal responses after a strength endurance resistance exercise protocol in young and elderly males. *Int. J. Sports Med.* 28:401–406.

Smith, G. I., P. Atherton, D. N. Reeds, B. S. Mohammed, D. Rankin, M. J. Rennie, and B. Mittendorfer. 2011. Dietary omega-3 fatty acid supplementation increases the rate of muscle protein synthesis in older adults: a randomized controlled trial. *Am. J. Clin. Nutr.* 93:402–412.

Snijder, M. B., N. M. van Schoor, S. M. Pluijm, R. M. van Dam, M. Visser, and P. Lips. 2006. Vitamin D status in relation to one-year risk of recurrent falling in older men and women. *J. Clin. Endocrinol. Metab.* 91:2980–2985.

Song, L., X. Zhang, and Y. Zhou. 2011. A synergetic role of 1,25-dihydroxyvitamin D(3) in 17beta-estradial induced-proliferation and differentiation of osteoblastic MC3T3-E1 cells. *Eur. J. Pharmacol.* 659: 273–280.

Staples, A. W., N. A. Burd, D. W. D. West, K. D. Currie, P. J. Atherton, D. R. Moore, M. J. Rennie, M. J. Macdonald, S. K. Baker, and S. M. Phillips. 2011. Carbohydrate does not augment exercise-induced protein accretion versus protein alone. *Med. Sci. Sports Exerc.* 43:1154–1161.

Stockton, K. A., K. Mengersen, J. D. Paratz, D. Kandiah, and K. L. Bennell. 2011. Effect of vitamin D supplementation on muscle strength: a systematic review and meta-analysis. *Osteoporos. Int.* 22:859–871.

Symons, T. B., M. Sheffield-Moore, M. M. Mamerow, R. R. Wolfe, and D. Paddon-Jones. 2011. The anabolic response to resistance exercise and a protein-rich meal is not diminished by age. *J. Nutr. Health Aging* 15:376–381.

Takata, Y., T. Ansai, I. Soh, S. Awano, Y. Yoshitake, Y. Kimura, I. Nakamichi, K. Goto, R. Fujisawa, K. Sonoki, A. Yoshida, K. Toyoshima, and T. Nishihara. 2012. Physical fitness and 6.5-year mortality in an 85-year-old community-dwelling population. *Arch. Gerontol. Geriatr.* 54:28–33.

Tang, J. E. and S. M. Phillips. 2009. Maximizing muscle protein anabolism: the role of protein quality. *Curr. Opin. Clin. Nutr. Metab. Care* 12:66–71.

Tang, J. E., D. R. Moore, G. W. Kujbida, M. A. Tarnopolsky, and S. M. Phillips. 2009. Ingestion of whey hydrolysate, casein, or soy protein isolate: effects on mixed muscle protein synthesis at rest and following resistance exercise in young men. *J. Appl. Physiol.* 107:987–992.

Thom, J. M., C. I. Morse, K. M. Birch, and M. V. Narici. 2007. Influence of muscle architecture on the torque and power-velocity characteristics of young and elderly men. *Eur. J. Appl. Physiol.* 100:613–619.

Thomas, D. R. 2010. Sarcopenia. *Clin. Geriatr. Med.* 26:331–346.

Tieland, M., K. Borgonjen-Van den Berg, L. C. Loon, and L. P. G. M. Groot. 2012. Dietary protein intake in community-dwelling, frail, and institutionalized elderly people: scope for improvement. *Eur. J. Nutr.* 51:173–179.

Toth, M. J., D. E. Matthews, R. P. Tracy, and M. J. Previs. 2005. Age-related differences in skeletal muscle protein synthesis: relation to markers of immune activation. *Am. J. Physiol. Endocrinol. Metab.* 288: E883–891.

Tucker, K. L., M. T. Hannan, and D. P. Kiel. 2001. The acid–base hypothesis: diet and bone in the Framingham Osteoporosis Study. *Eur. J. Nutr.* 40:231–237.

Tuohimaa, P. 2009. Vitamin D and aging. *J. Steroid Biochem. Mol. Biol.* 114:78–84.

van der Wielen, R. P., M. R. Lowik, H. van den Berg, L. C. de Groot, J. Haller, O. Moreiras, and W. A. van Staveren. 1995. Serum vitamin D concentrations among elderly people in Europe. *Lancet* 346:207–210.

Verdijk, L. B., B. G. Gleeson, R. A. Jonkers, K. Meijer, H. H. Savelberg, P. Dendale, and L. J. van Loon. 2009a. Skeletal muscle hypertrophy following resistance training is accompanied by a fiber type-specific increase in satellite cell content in elderly men. *J. Gerontol. A. Biol. Sci. Med. Sci.* 64:332–339.

Verdijk, L. B., R. A. Jonkers, B. G. Gleeson, M. Beelen, K. Meijer, H. H. Savelberg, W. K. Wodzig, P. Dendale, and L. J. van Loon. 2009b. Protein supplementation before and after exercise does not further augment skeletal muscle hypertrophy after resistance training in elderly men. *Am. J. Clin. Nutr.* 89:608–616.

Villani, A. M., M. Crotty, L. G. Cleland, M. J. James, R. J. Fraser, L. Cobiac, and M. D. Miller. 2013. Fish oil administration in older adults: is there potential for adverse events? A systematic review of the literature. *BMC Geriatr.* 13:41.

Visser, M., D. J. Deeg, and P. Lips. 2003. Low vitamin D and high parathyroid hormone levels as determinants of loss of muscle strength and muscle mass (sarcopenia): the Longitudinal Aging Study Amsterdam. *J. Clin. Endocrinol. Metab.* 88:5766–5772.

Volkert, D. 2011. The role of nutrition in the prevention of sarcopenia. *Wien. Med. Wochenschr.* 161: 409–415.

Waterlow, J. C. 1984. Protein turnover with special reference to man. *Q. J. Exp. Physiol.* 69:409–438.

Welch, A. A., S. A. Bingham, J. Reeve, and K. T. Khaw. 2007. More acidic dietary acid–base load is associated with reduced calcaneal broadband ultrasound attenuation in women but not in men: results from the EPIC-Norfolk cohort study. *Am. J. Clin. Nutr.* 85:1134–1141.

Welle, S. and C. A. Thornton. 1998. High-protein meals do not enhance myofibrillar synthesis after resistance exercise in 62- to 75-yr-old men and women. *Am. J. Physiol.* 274(4 Pt 1):E677–683.

Wilhelm-Leen, E. R., Y. N. Hall, I. H. Deboer, and G. M. Chertow. 2010. Vitamin D deficiency and frailty in older Americans. *J. Intern. Med.* 268:171–180.

Wilkinson, D. J., T. Hossain, D. S. Hill, B. E. Phillips, H. Crossland, J. Williams, P. Loughna, T. A. Churchward-Venne, L. Breen, S. M. Phillips, T. Etheridge, J. A. Rathmacher, K. Smith, N. J. Szewczyk, and P. J. Atherton. 2013. Effects of leucine and its metabolite β-hydroxy-β-methylbutyrate on human skeletal muscle protein metabolism. *J. Physiol.* 591(Pt 11):2911–2923.

Yang, Y., L. Breen, N. A. Burd, A. J. Hector, T. A. Churchward-Venne, A. R. Josse, M. A. Tarnopolsky, and S. M. Phillips. 2012. Resistance exercise enhances myofibrillar protein synthesis with graded intakes of whey protein in older men. *Br. J. Nutr.* 108:1780–1788.

Young, V. R., W. P. Steffee, P. B. Pencharz, J. C. Winterer, and N. S. Scrimshaw. 1975. Total human body protein synthesis in relation to protein requirements at various ages. *Nature* 253:192–194.

Zhao, L. J., H. Jiang, C. J. Papasian, D. Maulik, B. Drees, J. Hamilton, and H. W. Deng. 2008. Correlation of obesity and osteoporosis: effect of fat mass on the determination of osteoporosis. *J. Bone Miner. Res.* 23:17–29.

CHAPTER 8

Nutrition and the ageing eye

Ângela Carneiro

Department of Ophthalmology of Hospital de São João and Department of sense organs, Faculty of Medicine, University of Porto, Porto, Portugal

8.1 The ageing eye

The human eye is a complex organ with multiple layers and components that detect light and convert it in a set of electrochemical impulses that are transmitted to the brain. In a very simplified approach, the human eye has a fibrous outer coat (comprising the opaque posterior sclera and the transparent anterior cornea), an intermediate vascular tunic (composed by the choroid, ciliary body and iris) and a thin sheet covering the inner posterior surface of the eyeball, the retina. Additionally to the cornea, the aqueous humor, lens and vitreous body, collectively termed ocular media, serve to focus an image on the retina by transmitting and refracting the light (Gray *et al.*, 2005).

Below we will describe the anatomy, function and changes with ageing of two components of the human eye more affected by ageing and oxidative stress and with more data available from laboratory, animal and clinical studies: the lens and the retina.

8.1.1 The lens

The lens exerts a simple function in the eye: it serves as an optical element that, with the cornea, brings light rays to a precise focus on retinal photoreceptors. This function can be preserved only as long as the lens is transparent. The lens is an encapsulated organ without blood vessels or nerves. The anterior hemisphere of the lens is covered by a single layer of epithelial cells containing a full complement of subcellular organelles. At the lens equator, the epithelial cells elongate and differentiate to become fiber cells. When completely differentiated they possess no organelles but are filled with structural proteins known as crystallins (Tasman *et al.*, 2001). The high density and special arrangement of the crystallins produce a uniform refractive index within the lens, with the required transparency to achieve its function.

The shape of the crystalline lens, in histological sections, changes with age from a reniform configuration in infants to oval in adults (Spencer, 1985). The lens increases in weight from approximately 90 mg at birth to 190 mg at the age of 40 years and 240 mg at the age of 80 years (Grossniklaus *et al.*, 2013). The lens also suffers an age-related change in color: from almost complete transparency at birth to a yellow-brown color later in life.

Many investigators have shown that the human lens hardens over time, leading to the hypothesis that presbyopia occurs when the lens becomes too hard to change shape in response to ciliary muscle contraction. Supporting that, studies using a variety of methods have shown that a marked increase in lens stiffness begins in the third to

Anti-Ageing Nutrients: Evidence-Based Prevention of Age-Associated Diseases, First Edition. Edited by Delminda Neves.

fifth decades of life, which is roughly the age at which loss of accommodation becomes noticeable in the early stages of presbyopia (Heys *et al.*, 2004; Petrash, 2013).

Lens fiber cells, owing to the absence of organelles, are no longer able to synthesize proteins. As a consequence, lens proteins, particularly those located in the nucleus, are among the oldest proteins in the human body. With age there is a progressive accumulation of damaged proteins inside the fibers, leading to a progressive loss of transparency of the lens. The progressive accumulations of damaged crystallins and the aggregation of proteins leads to light scattering, lens opacification and the development of cataracts (Boscia *et al.*, 2000).

8.1.2 The retina

The retina is a sensory multilayered tissue covering the internal surface of eyeball from the optic nerve to the ora serrata. It consists of a pigmented epithelial layer and a complex sensorial layer (Guyer, 1999). Retinal anatomy is highly organized with vascular and avascular components strictly segregated owing to the presence of blood–retinal barriers. The blood–retinal barriers, inner and outer, are fundamental for the integrity of structure and optimization of function in the retina (Cunha-Vaz, 2004). The outer retina, which includes the photoreceptors and the retinal pigment epithelium (RPE), adjacent to Bruch's membrane and the choriocapillaris, is the region of the retina more susceptible to changes with ageing and thus more predisposed to develop degenerative age-associated diseases. The RPE is a polarized epithelium consisting of a monolayer of cuboid-shaped cells, that in the macular area are tall, narrow and highly uniform in size and shape (Friedman & Ts'o, 1968). Interdigitation of the apical processes of the RPE with the outer segments of the cones and rods is important for some RPE-related functions such as regeneration of visual pigments, transport of fluids and ions, formation and maintenance of interphotoreceptor matrix and phagocytosis of the outer segments (de Jong, 2006). The total number of RPE cells diminishes with age. In addition, macular RPE cells become narrower and increase in height (Friedman & Ts'o, 1968; Feeney-Burns *et al.*, 1990). In each RPE cell there is a progressive accumulation of lipofuscin, a hallmark of ageing cells (discussed in Chapter 1), throughout life. In people over 80 years of age, the debris can occupy more than one-fifth of the total volume of the cell (Feeney-Burns *et al.*, 1984). The major component of lipofuscin in the retina cells is *N*-retinylidene-*N*-retinylethanolamine, a retinoid product of the visual cycle that interferes with the function of RPE cells, addressing their apoptosis when in excess (Coleman *et al.*, 2008; Sparrow & Boulton, 2005). Age-related changes also include loss of basal interdigitations and irregularity in shape. In aged retina, the cells become separated from their basal membrane by membranous debris and abnormal secretory products, with subsequent deposition of collagen and fibronectin and later formation of insoluble basal laminar deposits (Tabandeh *et al.*, 2006).

Bruch's membrane is a thin acellular and well-delineated membrane constituted by five layers. From internal to external the layers are: (a) the basement membrane of the RPE; (b) the inner collagenous zone; (c) the elastic tissue layer; (d) the outer collagenous zone; and (e) the basement membrane of the choriocapillaris. It is composed of elements from the retina and choroid, but it is an integral part of the choroid (Tasman *et al.*, 2001). Owing to its specific location and properties, this structure is thought to be a vital limiting layer for metabolic transport between the RPE cells and the choriocapillaris (Huang *et al.*, 2007). With the advancement of age, both the thickness and complexity of Bruch's membrane increase, primarily owing to extracellular matrix remodeling and accumulation of amorphous material in this region (Ramrattan *et al.*, 1994). The lipid concentration within Bruch's membrane increases during life and consequently the fluid permeability and nutrient transport across the membrane decrease (Starita *et al.*, 1996). Bruch's membrane calcifies and doubles in thickness between the ages of 10 and 90 years (Ramrattan *et al.*, 1994). There is a linear thickening owing to deposits of collagen, lipids and debris. In normal conditions Bruch's membrane acts as an intercellular matrix regulator of adjacent RPE and choriocapillaris cell survival. Its diminished function results in apoptosis of these cells, in part owing to incorrect cell adhesion (Gilmore, 2005). On the other hand, extracellular deposits around Bruch's membrane lead to chronic inflammation, invasion by dendritic cells and the release of inflammatory cytokines, angiogenic factors and immune complexes (Penfold *et al.*, 1997; Guymer *et al.*, 2004).

The choriocapillaris consists of a continuous layer of fenestrated endothelial cells surrounded by a basement membrane. The fenestrations, 60–80 nm in diameter, are abundant and seem to play an important role in permitting the passage of glucose and vitamin A to the RPE and retina. The choriocapillaris supplies oxygen and nutrients to cells adjacent to the Bruch's membrane and to those localized in the outer third of the retina, except in the macula, where it supplies the entire retina (Tasman *et al.*, 2001). The peculiar structure of the choroidal vascular tree in the macula provides this area with the highest rate of blood flow of any tissue in the body (Gass, 1997). With ageing, the lumina of the choriocapillaris and the choroidal thickness become reduced by half (Ramrattan *et al.*, 1994; Margolis & Spaide, 2009). There is clinical data using optical coherence tomography, indicating an inverse relationship between age and choroidal volume (Barteselli *et al.*, 2012).

8.2 Nutrients in the structure and physiology of the healthy human eye

The eye is directly exposed to light and therefore is damaged by its own function. The eye responds to visible light but is vulnerable to it owing to its internal structure and intrinsic metabolism. The importance of micronutrients in the structure and physiology of the healthy human eye is supported by evidence coming from a variety of sources: laboratory, biochemical, animal and clinical studies.

8.2.1 Vitamins

Vitamin A is fundamental to the formation of rhodopsin, the visual pigment found in the disk membranes of rods and cones in the retina. Rhodopsin comprises a transmembrane protein (opsin) covalently bound to retinal (the aldehyde form of vitamin A). When one photon of light converts 11-*cis* retinal to all-*trans* retinal, the generation of the visual signal is initiated (Hargrave & McDowell, 1992). Vitamin A has activities in the retina and in the epithelial cells of the eye surface and its deficiency induces the gradual progression from xerophthalmia and night blindness to keratomalacia. According to the World Health Organization vitamin A deficiency is one of the world's leading causes of blindness (Resnikoff *et al.*, 2004).

Carotenoids are identified in almost all eye structures with the exception of cornea, sclera and vitreous. Lutein and zeaxanthin, light-absorbing yellow carotenoids, are concentrated in the inner layers of the macula. They are fundamental for photopic vision and their concentrations in blood strongly correlate with dietary intake (Lien & Hammond,

2011; Hammond *et al.*, 1997). Both improve the visibility of targets by absorbing scattered light and reduce glare disability (Stringham & Hammond, 2007).

Vitamin C (ascorbic acid) is usually considered the most effective anti-oxidant in the human plasma. In the retina vitamin C presents a concentration 10 times higher than in the plasma and its importance in the protection of the lens against oxidative stress and cataract development is well documented (Friedman & Zeidel, 1999; Ravindran *et al.*, 2011; Tan *et al.*, 2008).

Vitamin E (α-tocopherol) is found in the RPE and rod outer segments, with higher concentrations outside the macula (Friedrichson *et al.*, 1995). It is transparent to visible light and plays an important role as an effective anti-oxidant under high oxygen pressures such as the conditions maintained in the outer retina (Wang & Quinn, 1999).

8.2.2 Polyunsaturated fatty acids

The omega-3 long-chain polyunsaturated fatty acids eicosapentaenoic acid (EPA) and docosahexaenoic acid (DHA) are important in the structure and metabolism of the photoreceptors (PR). DHA is the primary fatty acid found in high concentrations in the structural phospholipids of the PR outer segment disk membrane, with higher concentrations in the retina than in any other tissue of the human body (Lien & Hammond, 2011; Anderson *et al.*, 1974). EPA is present in the blood but, owing to its rapid metabolism resulting in the synthesis of DHA, it is poorly integrated in the tissues (Stone *et al.*, 1979).

8.2.3 Zinc

Zinc levels are high in ocular tissues particularly in the cornea and retina. Zinc is the most abundant trace metal in the retina, located in the inner nuclear, RPE and PR layers. Zinc ions in photoreceptors might play a role in the phototransduction cascade and in rhodopsin regeneration (Ugarte & Osborne, 2014; Ugarte *et al.*, 2013).

8.3 The human eye and the oxidative stress

The production of free radicals is a enduring phenomenon in living cells associated with cellular aerobic metabolism and oxidoreduction reactions (Halliwell, 1997). The human eye is exposed to light and its main function is to convert the incident light into a change in membrane potential at the outer segments of the photoreceptors. The regeneration of the visual pigment, rhodopsin, the constant disk shedding at the interface between RPE and rods and cones, and the efficient recycling of phospholipids and other structural components of the photoreceptors' outer segments, are only some of the activities requiring high metabolic rates. Consequently, the retina is the most metabolically active tissue within the human body, which results in increased formation of free radicals (SanGiovanni & Chew, 2005). Moreover, the human eye, and the retina in particular, is particularly exposed to the production of free radicals owing to a combination of the following factors: (a) it is highly vascularized, which results in high oxygen tension in rods and cones; (b) at the fovea, light-induced stress can be particularly dangerous owing to the increased cellular density and metabolism; (c) rods and cones are rich in unsaturated fatty acids such as DHA, which is highly susceptible to oxidation; (d) other photosensitizing compounds form within the retina; and (e) the tissue is regularly exposed to extremely high rates of cumulative radiation (Sickel, 1972; Lien & Hammond, 2011).

Owing to the pro-oxidative environment, singlet oxygen free radicals can be generated in the retina and these free radicals will extract hydrogen atoms from molecules with available double bounds, such as DHA. In the sequence of the free radical attack, DHA becomes a lipid hydroperoxide, which can create additional free radicals in a self-perpetuating chain reaction, resulting in lipid peroxidation (Lien & Hammond, 2011). Lipid peroxides cross-link with proteins, nucleic acids and other cellular components, adversely affecting cell structure and function (Offord *et al.*, 2000).

The continuous penetration of sunlight in the eye during the visual process is also responsible for the production of superoxide anion, hydrogen peroxide, hydroxyl radical and other oxygen reactive molecular species in the aqueous humor and lens (Kisic *et al.*, 2012). Oxidation can damage lens proteins, lens fiber membranes and lipids, leading to the formation of molecular aggregates with high molecular weight (Tan *et al.*, 2008). These aggregates cause light scattering and lens opacities, features characteristic of cataract (Kisic *et al.*, 2012).

8.4 The anti-oxidant systems in the eye

The balance between the production and catabolism of oxidant molecules by cells and tissues is fundamental to the maintenance of the biologic integrity of the tissues. In the eye, an anti-oxidant system with multiple components intervenes from the aqueous humor to the retina.

Among the enzymatic anti-oxidant defenses of the eye lens, superoxide dismutase, catalase and glutathione peroxidase are the three primary enzymes (Manikandan *et al.*, 2010a; Thiagarajan & Manikandan, 2013). In addition, glutathione reductase, glucose-6-phosphate dehydrogenase and cytosolic glutathione-*S*-transferase are also known anti-oxidants of eye lens (Thiagarajan & Manikandan, 2013; Manikandan *et al.*, 2010b). The nonenzymatic anti-oxidants include, reduced glutathione, ascorbate, carotene, glutathione, pyruvate and α-tocopherol (Harding, 1991; Thiagarajan & Manikandan, 2013).

The high concentration of ascorbate in the aqueous humor is important for scavenging of hydroxyl and superoxide anion radicals and to act as a filter to prevent the deep penetration of UV light within the lens, thus protecting the lens tissue from photo-induced damage (Kannan *et al.*, 2001). Accordingly, diurnal animals present ascorbic acid concentrations in some ocular tissues 20–70 times higher than those circulating in the plasma. These high concentrations in the aqueous humor is sustained by continuous active transport from plasma through the blood–aqueous barrier (Kisic *et al.*, 2012). In the lens, ascorbic acid prevents cation pumps damage induced by UV radiation and reduces photoperoxidation in the membranes (Garland, 1991). However, vitamin C has not only anti-oxidant but also pro-oxidant properties, and its direction of work depends on its own concentration, oxygen and the presence of metal ions, especially iron, lead and copper (Kisic *et al.*, 2012; Cekic, 1998). Some authors believe that ascorbate can even contribute to protein modifications, when acting as prooxidant and participating in reactions that generate reactive radicals. These reactions assume a particular importance when cells lose their ability to eliminate metals, making them permanently available for reaction, and/or when cells lose their ability to maintain vitamin C in a reduced form. During ageing of the lens the concentration of copper and iron increases, although it is lower in noncataract lenses (Balaji *et al.*, 1992; Garner *et al.*, 2000).

The retina possesses an anti-oxidant system with several components: vitamins C and E and also the carotenoids lutein and zeaxanthin. Vitamins C and E cooperatively reduce epoxide adducts within the retina and participate in its protection from blue light-induced damage (Sparrow *et al.*, 2003). The carotenoids are concentrated in the plexiform area of the macula, but the spatial distributions of lutein and zeaxanthin differ, with zeaxanthin dominating the central foveal region and lutein dominating the periphery. This differentiated distribution makes zeaxanthin a more effective anti-oxidant in the area where the risk of oxidative damage is higher (Handelman *et al.*, 1988). Additionally, carotenoids are found in the outer segments of rods and probably of cones, where the concentration of DHA is highest, which are the most susceptible areas to lipid oxidation (Sommerburg *et al.*, 1999). In fact, lutein is a powerful anti-oxidant, which can return singlet oxygen to the ground state and remove the resultant energy as heat, resulting in its autoregeneration (Lien & Hammond, 2011; Stahl & Sies, 2002). Compared with α-tocopherol, lutein is a much more efficient quencher of singlet oxygen (Fukuzawa *et al.*, 1998).

8.5 How can diet interfere with the ocular anti-oxidant system?

The dietary intake of vitamins, carotenoids, essential fatty acids and other oligoelements in developed countries is usually sufficient to supply the needs of a healthy person. Table 8.1 summarizes the reference daily intakes based on recommended dietary allowances and adequate intakes) and enumerates the main sources in the diet of some micronutrients that can interfere with ocular structure and function. While the recommended dietary allowance is the average daily dietary intake level sufficient to meet the nutrient requirements of nearly all (97–98%) healthy individuals, adequate intake is believed to cover the needs of all healthy individuals.

Other nutrients such as DHA, EPA, lutein and zeaxanthin are fundamental for ocular structure and function. Humans can synthesize saturated fatty acids *de novo* through the fatty acid synthase system. However, they do not possess the enzyme systems necessary to insert double bonds at the n-3 or n-6 positions, and dietary sources of these fatty acids are essential (Innis, 1991). The major dietary sources of the 18 carbon fatty acids α-linolenic acid (ALA; C18:3 n-3) and linoleic acid (LA; C18:2 n-6)

Table 8.1 Dietary reference intakes in the population older than 50 years.

	Vitamin A (μg/day)	Vitamin C (mg/day)	Vitamin E (mg/day)	Selenium (μg/day)	Zinc (mg/day)
Male	900	90	15	55	11
Female	700	75	15	55	8
Sources	Fish, fish oil, liver, milk, dairy products, vegetables	Fruit, vegetables, liver, meat, fish	Grains, olive oil, fruit, oily fish, vegetables	Mushrooms, seafood, olive oil, fish, cereals, meat, eggs	Seafood, liver, fish, cheese, eggs, dairy products

Adapted from Food and Nutrition Board, Institute of Medicine, National Academies data.

are vegetable oils. The biologically active EPA, DHA and arachidonic acid are more unsaturated and present longer chains. Diets rich in fish, meat and eggs will provide these fatty acids, but they can also be synthesized from ALA and LA (Lien & Hammond, 2011; Ugarte *et al.*, 2013).

On the other hand, lutein and zeaxanthin are carotenoids, which are not synthesized by humans. They are found in high concentrations in green leafy vegetables and their conversion to vitamin A is not possible. Lutein is found in fruit and spices. Zeaxanthin is found in vegetables such as lettuce, broccoli and spinach.

A balanced nutritional pattern may ensure the maximum effectiveness of the defensive systems, considering that different types of diet provide different amounts of nutrients. The Mediterranean diet has been indicated to have some distinctive components.

A clear definition of "Mediterranean diet" is difficult. It is predominantly characterized by high consumption of vegetables, grains and cereals, fruit and nuts, low consumption of meat and meat products, increased consumption of fish relative to Western diets, moderate consumption of milk and dairy products, the use of olive oil with a high monounsaturated/saturated fat ratio for cooking, and low to moderate red wine consumption (Rees *et al.*, 2013; Estruch *et al.*, 2013). A 2013 Cochrane review included 11 random controlled trials in which the intervention consisted of the full Mediterranean diet or at least two of the characteristics defined earlier (Rees *et al.*, 2013). Control groups had no intervention. They concluded that there is limited evidence to date, but the Mediterranean diet may reduce some cardiovascular risk factors (total cholesterol levels, LDL cholesterol levels). However, regarding the eye, no studies to date have demonstrated beneficial effects of the Mediterranean diet on the prevalence of eye diseases.

8.6 Nutritional intervention in age-associated eye diseases

8.6.1 Cataract

Cataract is, by definition, the opacification of the crystalline lens. According to a 2012 World Health Organization report it is estimated that 39 million people are blind worldwide and that cataract is the main cause, affecting almost 18 million people (Petrash, 2013; Rao *et al.*, 2011). The incidence of cataract is known to increase with age and the burden disproportionately affects low- and middle-income countries. Cataract is essentially an aggregation disease involving the crystalline proteins that accumulate to high concentrations in fiber cells. The fiber cells, the major cell type that constitutes the lens, are thus endowed with high concentrations of proteins that are not replenished and remain *in situ* for the lifetime of the tissue. Lens cells experience decades of exposure to ultraviolet light and chemical insult, stresses that are known to destabilize protein structure, function and interactions with other molecules. Additionally, the supply and activity of enzymes that usually search for and destroy damaged proteins are also limited (Petrash, 2013), and strongly decline with ageing (discussed in Chapter 1).

Cataract in humans is clearly a multifactorial and progressive process in which independent events occurring over time can culminate in a loss of transparency of the lens. Experimental studies using animal models demonstrated that nutritional supplementation with vitamin C or glutathione, the two major hydrophilic anti-oxidants inside the lens, prevents cataract development (Taylor & Hobbs, 2001). Additionally, vitamin E and the carotenoids lutein and zeaxanthin, lipophilic anti-oxidants, in animal models slow cataractogenesis (Taylor & Hobbs, 2001; Bernstein *et al.*, 2001).

In line with these findings, numerous observational epidemiological studies have found inverse relationships between levels of dietary micronutrients and the development of age-related cataract (Kuzniarz *et al.*, 2001; Tan *et al.*, 2008; Mares-Perlman *et al.*, 2000; Jacques *et al.*, 2001; Ravindran *et al.*, 2011; Christen *et al.*, 2008; Pastor-Valero, 2013). Some clinical trials have tested whether the intake of selected anti-oxidant micronutrients or vitamins affects cataract development (Chang *et al.*, 2011; Christen *et al.*, 2003, 2004, 2010a, b; AREDS Research Group, 2001a; Mares-Perlman *et al.*, 2000; Leske *et al.*, 1995). The results of some relevant studies are presented and discussed later.

8.6.1.1 The blue mountains eye study

The Blue Mountains Eye Study is a population-based cohort study of vision, common eye and systemic conditions in a population aged 49 years or older, living in a defined region of Australia. At baseline (1992–94) 3654 persons participated and surviving participants were invited to attend follow-up examinations after 5 and 10 years. At each examination, lens photography was performed and patients responded a questionnaire focused on nutritional habits, including a 145-item semiquantitative food-frequency questionnaire. Intake of anti-oxidants, including β-carotene, zinc and vitamins A, C and E, was assessed. Higher intakes of vitamin C or the above-median intake of combined anti-oxidants (vitamins C and E, β-carotene and zinc) had long-term protective associations against the development of nuclear cataract (Tan *et al.*, 2008). Anti-oxidant intake was not associated with incident cortical or posterior subcapsular cataract (Tan *et al.*, 2008).

8.6.1.2 The beaver dam eye study

The Beaver Dam Eye Study is a population-based prospective study that enrolled 4926 participants aged 43–86 years at the baseline, designed to investigate the association of use of vitamins, minerals and nonvitamin/nonmineral supplements (herbal, amino acids or other supplements not approved by the Food and Drug Administration) with the development of age-related macular degeneration (AMD) (discussed further later) and cataract. The cohort was re-examined at 5, 10 and 15 years with lens photographs, and all medications and supplements taken by the participant were brought to each examination with duration of use and dose indicated. Compared with nonusers, the 5-year risk for any cataract was 60% lower among persons who, at follow-up, reported the use of multivitamins or any supplement containing vitamin C or E for more than 10 years. Taking multivitamins for more than 10 years lowered the risk for nuclear and cortical cataracts but not for posterior subcapsular cataracts (Mares-Perlman *et al.*, 2000). However, at 15 years of follow-up, there was no evidence of any significant association between supplement use and posterior subcapsular or nuclear cataract. Patients who used multivitamins and single supplements or combinations containing vitamins A and D and zinc appeared to have decreased odds of incident cortical cataract (Klein *et al.*, 2008).

8.6.1.3 The India age-related eye disease study

A population-based study was conducted in two centers in the north and south India to examine the prevalence and risk factors for cataract and specifically to investigate correlation between vitamin C intake and cataract in 5638 people aged 60 years or over. Participants were interviewed and invited to describe their diet assessed by 24 h period, and plasma vitamin C was measured. Lens opacities were graded according to the Lens Opacities Classification System III in lens digital photographs. The study found a strong inverse association between plasma vitamin C levels and cataract; however, a vitamin C-depleted population was considered in this study (Ravindran *et al.*, 2011).

8.6.1.4 The Spanish segment of European eye study (EUREYE)

The EUREYE is a multicenter population-based cross-sectional study aimed primarily at estimating the prevalence of AMD and contributing factors for the disease, including diet, in an elderly population. This study analyzed data from the Spanish segment of the EUREYE, collected between February 2000 and November 2001 in 599 patients at least 65 years of age. Energy-adjusted intake of fruit and vegetables and anti-oxidant vitamins was estimated using a semiquantitative food-frequency questionnaire. Plasma concentrations of vitamin C, carotenoids and α-tocopherol were determined. Analyzed data demonstrated that high daily intakes of fruit and vegetables and vitamins C and E were associated with a significant decrease in the prevalence of cataract or cataract surgery (Pastor-Valero, 2013).

8.6.1.5 The physicians' health study

The Physicians' Health Study is a randomized, double-masked, placebo-controlled trial primarily aimed at evaluating the effects of aspirin and high levels of vitamins E (400 IU) and C (500 mg) and β-carotene (50 mg on alternate days) on cardiovascular disease and cancer. Secondary analysis includes ocular end-points of AMD and age-related cataract in male US physicians registered with the American Medical association, 50 years or older, based on self-report with confirmation using medical records. For the vitamins E and C, 11,545 male physicians were followed and treated for 8 years, and for β-carotene, 22,071 male physicians were followed for a mean of 12 years. No statistically significant differences among treated and placebo groups in the incidence of cataract were observed (Christen *et al.*, 2003; Ugarte & Osborne, 2014).

8.6.1.6 The women's health study

The Women's Health Study is a randomized, double-masked, placebo-controlled trial, performed at Brigham and Women's Hospital and Harvard Medical School, aiming to investigate the effects of β-carotene (50 mg in alternate days), vitamin E (600 IU) and aspirin on the primary prevention of cancer and cardiovascular disease. The enrolled participants were 39,876 female health professionals 45 years or older, and the main ocular outcomes measured were visually significant cataract and cataract extraction. These outcomes were obtained with self-reports and confirmed by medical records. After an average follow-up of 2.1 years, the randomization for the β-carotene arm was stopped, without demonstration of statistically significant benefit for the development of cataract. Concerning vitamin C, after a mean follow-up of 9.7 years, no significant difference between vitamin C and placebo groups was demonstrated either for the development of cataracts or for the need for cataract surgery (Christen *et al.*, 2004, 2008).

8.6.1.7 The age-related eye disease study (AREDS)

The AREDS is a randomized clinical trial that evaluated the effect of high doses of anti-oxidant vitamins (500 mg vitamin C, 400 IU vitamin E), β-carotene (15 mg) and zinc (80 mg) on the incidence and progression of AMD and cataracts. A total of 4757 participants, followed in 11 eye care centers specializing in retinal diseases in the USA, were enrolled in AREDS from 1992 to 1998. The mean follow-up was 6.3 years in 4629 AREDS participants, comprising both men and women aged 55–80 years. No effect of high doses of anti-oxidants on progression of the three types of cataract (nuclear, cortical and posterior subcapsular) or the incidence of cataract surgery was observed (AREDS Research Group, 2001a).

8.6.1.8 The age-related eye disease study 2 (AREDS2)

The AREDS2 is a double-masked clinical trial that enrolled 4203 participants, aged 50–85 years, previously identified as being at risk of progression to advanced AMD in 82 centers in the USA. The participants were randomly assigned to receive daily placebo, lutein/zeaxanthin (10 mg/2 mg), omega-3 long-chain polynsaturated acids (1 g) or a combination of both to evaluate the effects on progression to advanced AMD. A secondary outcome was to evaluate the effects of lutein/zeaxanthin on the subsequent need for cataract surgery. The daily supplementation with lutein/zeaxanthin did not show a significant overall effect on rates of cataract surgery or vision loss (Chew *et al.*, 2013b).

The randomized clinical trials and observational studies have focused only on individual anti-oxidants such as vitamins C and E and various carotenoids, and have reported inconsistent results. A recent Cochrane review concluded that there is no evidence from randomized clinical trials that supplements of β-carotene or vitamin C or E prevent or even slow the progression of age-related cataract (Mathew *et al.*, 2012). However, the recent concept of total anti-oxidant capacity (TAC) aims to measure the capacity from all dietary anti-oxidants in a single estimate by taking into account synergistic effects among compounds.

The recent questionnaire-based nutrition survey within the prospective Swedish Mammography Cohort study, which included 30,607 women (aged 49–83 years) observed for cataract incidence for a mean period of 7.7 years, aimed to investigate the association between the TAC of the diet and the incidence of age-related cataract. The main contributors to dietary TAC in the study population were fruit and vegetables (44.3%), whole grains (17.0%) and coffee (15.1%). A total of 4309 incident cases of age-related cataracts were identified during the 7.7 years of follow-up, the risk being apparently inversely associated with dietary TAC (Rautiainen *et al.*, 2014). However, this data needs to be confirmed in larger epidemiological studies.

8.6.2 Age-related macular degeneration

According to the data of the World Health Organization from 2002, AMD is the third leading cause of blindness worldwide, after cataract and glaucoma, and the first in industrialized countries (Resnikoff *et al.*, 2004). The prevalence of AMD increases sharply with age and differences in prevalence rates among studies are mainly due to the use of different classification criteria and differences in age distribution. Indeed, only studies using the International Classification and Grading System for the diagnosis and classification of AMD are comparable (Bird *et al.*, 1995). The prevalence of AMD appears to be similar in Caucasian populations from the USA, Australia and European countries, despite major geographical and lifestyle differences. In a meta-analysis performed in 2004 by Friedman *et al.*, the prevalence rates for the late forms of the disease increased from less than 0.5% in subjects aged 50–60 years to 12–16% in people of at least 80 years. For early AMD, an increase from about 1.5% in Caucasians aged 40–49 years to more than 25% in those aged 80 years or more was reported (Friedman *et al.*, 2004).

With increasing age, the outer retina suffers alterations in cells and increased formation of extracellular deposits. Basal laminar deposits, composed of basement membrane proteins, including long-spaced collagen located between the RPE and basement membranes, are considered the precursors of AMD, emerging around the age of 40 years (Sarks *et al.*, 2007). In addition, basal linear deposits, consisting of granular, vesicular or membranous lipid-rich material located externally to the basement membrane of the RPE, represent a specific marker of the disease (Curcio & Millican, 1999). These two types of deposits can only be found in pathological specimens and not by clinical evaluation. The combination of the deposits with secondary changes in the RPE results in the formation of drusen. Drusen are localized deposits of extracellular material (a core of glycoproteins, fragments of RPE cells, crystallins, apolipoproteins B and E, amyloid P and β, and complement factors) lying between the basement membrane of the RPE and the inner collagen layer of Bruch's membrane (Ding *et al.*, 2009; Crabb *et al.*, 2002; Wang *et al.*, 2009). Drusen change in size, shape, color, distribution and consistency with the passing of years (Gass, 1967). Small drusen (Figure 8.1) are defined as being less than 63 μm in diameter (Bird *et al.*, 1995), and are visible in ophthalmoscopy when their diameter exceeds 25 μm, as dots ranging in color from white to yellow. The presence of small, hard drusen alone is not sufficient to diagnose early AMD, because these deposits are ubiquitous and not age dependent (Klein *et al.*, 1997). On the other hand, soft drusen (Figure 8.2) are larger and associated with pigment epithelial detachment and diffuse abnormal Bruch's membrane alterations. Soft drusen have tendency to cluster and merge, and when they become larger than 125 μm, the greater the area that they cover, the higher the risk of progression to late AMD becomes (Bressler *et al.*, 1994; Sarks *et al.*, 1999; Gass, 1973). RPE degeneration and nongeographic atrophy of the RPE are characterized by pigment mottling and stippled hypopigmentation associated with thinning of the neurosensory retina (Bressler *et al.*, 1989). These findings are characteristic of early AMD and usually not associated with relevant visual loss.

Conversely, late AMD is characterized by visual loss owing to geographic atrophy (GA) of the RPE (dry AMD) and/or the development of choroidal neovascularization (wet AMD). Geographic atrophy (Figure 8.3) is clinically characterized by roughly oval areas of hypopigmentation, a consequence of RPE loss, allowing increased exposure of the underlying choroidal vessels. Loss of RPE cells leads to gradual degeneration of

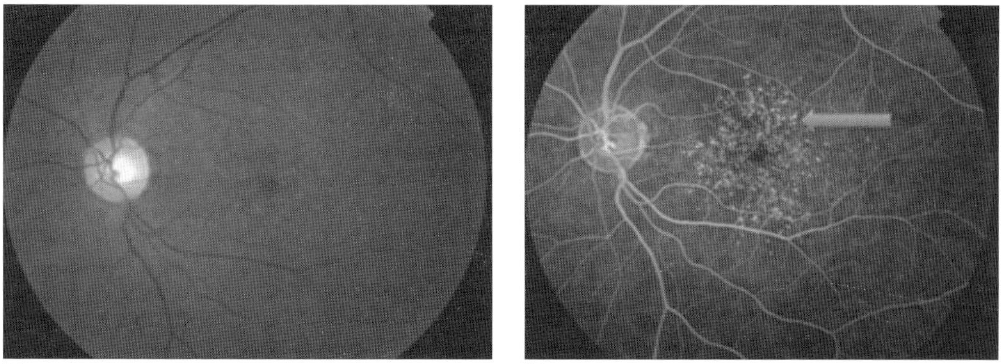

(a) (b)

Figure 8.1 Small hard drusen (arrow) in fundus photograph (a) and fluorescein angiography (b).

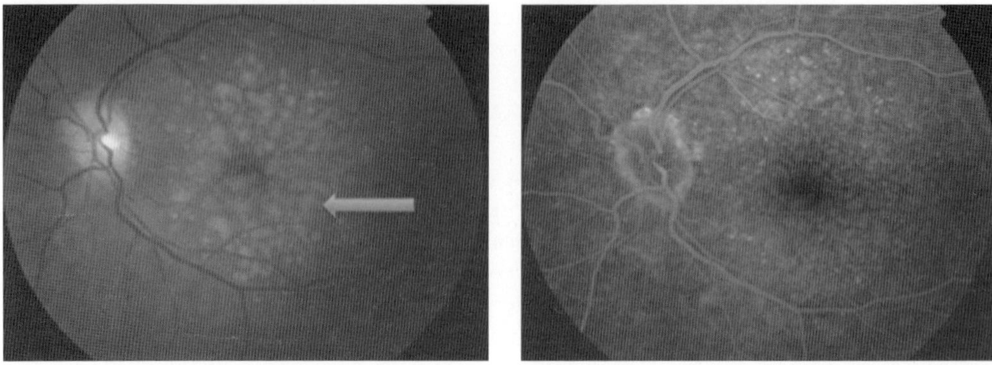

(a) (b)

Figure 8.2 Soft large drusen (arrow) on fundus photograph (a) and fluorescein angiography (b).

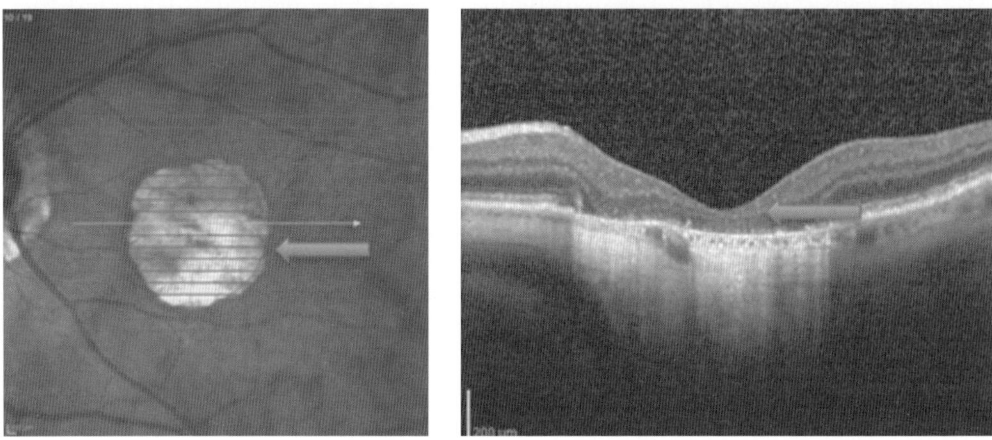

(a) (b)

Figure 8.3 Geographic atrophy in infrared fundus image (a) and optical coherence tomography (b). Note an oval area of retinal pigment epithelium loss (arrow) associated with thinning of the neurosensorial retina (arrow) on the optical coherence tomography.

photoreceptors and thinning of the retina that may extend to the outer plexiform and inner nuclear layers (Ding *et al.*, 2009; de Jong, 2006). In neovascular AMD, also known as wet or exudative AMD (Figure 8.4), early choroidal neovascularization occurs under the RPE and eventually breaks through, enteing the space between the photoreceptors and RPE cells and growing laterally in the subretinal space (Grossniklaus & Green, 2004).

AMD is a complex disease occurring in older people, caused by the combination of genetic predisposition and environmental factors. The genetic component of the disease has been elucidated from family, twin and sibling studies (Smith & Mitchell, 1998; Luo *et al.*, 2008). Many of these studies suggest that the genes involved in AMD lie on chromosomes 1 (1q25–31) and 10 (10q26) (Fisher *et al.*, 2005). The identification of persistent single changes, substitutions or variants of a single base with a frequency of greater than 1% in at least one population, that is, single nucleotide polymorphisms (SNPs), has shown tremendous progress in the elucidation of the genetics of AMD. Among the studied SNPs, the best available markers of AMD risk are in complement factor H (gene

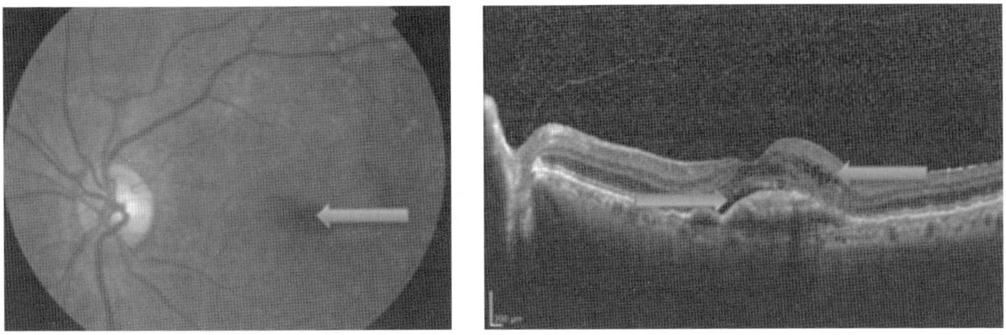

(a) (b)

Figure 8.4 Neovascular AMD. Note a subfoveal lesion of choroidal neovascularization with blood (arrow) in color fundus photograph (a); and retinal pigment epithelium detachment associated to subretinal (left arrow) and intraretinal fluid (right arrow) in the optical coherence tomography (b). (Color version of the figure is available in the online version.)

localized in 1q23–32), in age-related maculopathy sensitivity 2 (ARMS2) and high-temperature required factor A-1 (HTRA1) (genes located on 10q26). SNPs in these genes capture a substantial fraction of AMD risk and permit the identification of individuals at high risk of developing this disease (Thakkinstian *et al.*, 2006; Fritsche *et al.*, 2008; Launay *et al.*, 2008).

Smoking is the most recognized environmental risk factor for AMD (Jager *et al.*, 2008). Most of the studies found that the risk of late AMD is multiplied by 2.5–4.5 in current smokers and a clear dose-dependent relationship was observed (Khan *et al.*, 2006; Chakravarthy *et al.*, 2007; Tan *et al.*, 2007; Mitchell *et al.*, 2002). In contrast, associations with early AMD, with smoking or other lifestyle conditions, are weaker in the vast majority of published studies (Khan *et al.*, 2006; Chakravarthy *et al.*, 2007; Tan *et al.*, 2007; Klein *et al.*, 2002).

The exact pathogenesis of AMD is unknown, although oxidative stress is considered to comprise an important role in the mechanisms that lead to the onset of the disease. The role of nutrition and nutritional supplements has been raised by a number of observational and randomized clinical trials. Three main types of nutritional factors have been investigated for their potential protection against eye age-associated diseases: antioxidants (mainly vitamins C and E and zinc), the carotenoids lutein and zeaxanthin, and omega-3 polynsaturated fatty acids. The results of the most important clinical trials concerning nutritional effects on AMD are presented and discussed later.

8.6.2.1 AREDS

As described earlier, AREDS is a randomized, double-masked, placebo-controlled clinical trial designed to evaluate the effect of vitamins C (500 mg) and E (400 IU), and β-carotene (15 mg), with or without zinc (80 mg) and copper (2 mg) as an adjuvant of zinc, on progression of AMD and cataract. The 4757 AREDS participants, aged 55–80 years, were followed for a mean period of 6.3 years. At the beginning of the study, 1117 of those enrolled had few if any drusen (Category 1), 1063 had extensive small drusen, pigment abnormalities or at least one intermediate size drusen (Category 2); 1621 had extensive intermediate drusen, GA not involving the center of the macula, or at least one large drusen (Category 3); and 956 had advanced AMD or visual acuity less than 20/32 owing to AMD in one eye (Category 4). The results from AREDS demonstrated that treatment with zinc alone or in combination with anti-oxidants reduced the risk of progression to advanced AMD in participants in Categories 3 and 4. The risk reduction at 5 years for those taking anti-oxidants plus zinc was 25%, when compared with placebo group. The treatment effect appeared to persist following five additional years of follow-up after the clinical trial was stopped (Chew *et al.*, 2013a). During the study, 407 participants without GA at baseline developed at least moderate GA (>360 μm) not necessarily involving the center of the macula. No significant difference among treatments with anti-oxidants, zinc or anti-oxidants plus zinc on AMD progression during the AREDS was reported (AREDS Research Group, 2001b).

8.6.2.2 AREDS2

As described earlier, the AREDS2 is a multicenter, randomized, double-masked, placebo-controlled clinical trial, phase 3 study, conducted in 2006–2012, which enrolled 4203 participants, aged 50–85 years, at risk for progression to advanced AMD with bilateral large drusen or large drusen in one eye and advanced AMD in the other eye. The participants were assigned randomly to placebo, lutein (10 mg)/zeaxanthin (2 mg), omega-3 fatty acids (DHA 350 mg and EPA 650 mg), or a combination of lutein/zeaxanthin and omega-3 fatty acids. In addition, all of the participants were administered either the original AREDS formulation or some modification of the AREDS formulation (either elimination of β-carotene, lowering of the zinc, or a combination of the two; Chew *et al.*, 2012). Addition of lutein + zeaxanthin, DHA + EPA, or both to the AREDS formulation in primary analyses did not further reduce the risk of progression to advanced AMD (AREDS Research Group, 2013). More lung cancers were noted in the β-carotene vs no β-carotene group, mostly in former smokers (AREDS Research Group, 2013). In the analyses that used the entire population (>4000) to conduct the analysis of the main effects, that is, evaluating all those assigned to lutein/zeaxanthin (2123) vs those not assigned lutein/zeaxanthin (2080), there was an additional 10% reduction in the risk of progression to advanced AMD in patients assigned to lutein/zeaxanthin vs those not assigned. When analyses were restricted to those with lowest dietary intake of lutein/zeaxanthin, there was a further reduction in the risk of advanced AMD in those patients in the lowest quintile of dietary intake of carotenoids (Chew *et al.*, 2014). In brief, the totality of evidence on beneficial and adverse effects from AREDS2 and other studies suggests that lutein/zeaxanthin could be more appropriate than β-carotene in the AREDS-type supplements, particularly for former or current smokers. Supporting that, studies based on plasma levels also found a correlation between high levels of lutein/zeaxanthin in the plasma and low risk of AMD, for example the Pathologies Oculaires Liées à l'Age (POLA Study) and Gale and coworkers (Delcourt *et al.*, 2006; Gale *et al.*, 2003; Aslam *et al.*, 2013). On the other hand, most large-scale epidemiologic observational studies, such as the Eye Disease Case–Control Study (USA), agree with the findings of beneficial effects of dietary intake of carotenoids (Seddon *et al.*, 1994).

Various studies have demonstrated an increase in macular pigment with carotenoid intake (Weigert *et al.*, 2011; Koh *et al.*, 2004; Aslam *et al.*, 2013), but some results from epidemiological studies have been contradictory, for example the Rotterdam study showed a decreased risk for AMD in subjects with high dietary intakes of β-carotene, vitamins C and E and zinc (van Leeuwen *et al.*, 2005), while the Physicians' Health Study failed to show any marked benefits for vitamin C or E (Christen *et al.*, 1999).

Interestingly, data from the USA differ from those from Europe, which could be explained by differences in nutritional patterns or supplement intake. For example, in the USA the majority of the participants in AREDS study used vitamin supplements in addition to the supplementation tested in the study (AREDS Research Group, 2001a). The mean baseline plasma vitamin C concentration was 62 μmol/l in AREDS-enrolled patients, whereas it was 31.6 μmol/l in men and 40.5 μmol/l in women participating in the POLA Study, performed in France (AREDS Research Group, 2001a; Birlouez-Aragon *et al.*, 2001). The values of the POLA study were quite similar to those of the EUREYE Study performed in seven European countries (Fletcher *et al.*, 2008).

Regarding the effect of intake of omega-3 fatty long-chain polyunsaturated acids in preventing or slowing the progression of AMD, a Cochrane database review published in 2012, in accordance with AREDS2 results concluded that there is currently no evidence to support increasing levels of omega-3 fatty acids in the diet for the explicit purpose of preventing or slowing the progression of AMD (Lawrenson & Evans, 2012). The systematic review of prospective studies of dietary intake found no evidence that diets high in anti-oxidant vitamins prevent AMD (Evans & Lawrenson, 2012; Chong *et al.*, 2007).

8.7 Nutrigenomics

Nutrigenomics is a novel field of research focused on the interactions between genetic variability and nutritional factors, and represents a new challenge in accounting for interindividual variations in disease susceptibility and potential responses to nutritional supplementation (anti-oxidants, minerals) (Delcourt, 2007). AREDS Caucasian patients with category 3 disease in one eye and category 1–4 disease in the other eye at enrollment were evaluated for known AMD genetic risk markers and treatment category. Over an average of 10.1 years, individuals with one or two complement factor H (CFH) risk alleles derived maximum benefit from anti-oxidants alone. In these patients, the addition of zinc negated the benefits of anti-oxidants. On the other hand, patients with ARMS2 risk alleles derived maximum benefit from zinc-containing regimens, with a deleterious response to anti-oxidant supplementation. These results demonstrate that individuals homozygous for CFH and ARMS2 risk alleles derive no benefit from any category of AREDS treatment. On the other hand, patients with no CFH risk alleles and with one or two ARMS2 risk alleles derive maximum benefit from zinc-only supplementation (Awh *et al.*, 2013). These findings need to be confirmed in larger clinical trials, but these recommendations may lead to an improvement of outcomes through genotype-directed therapy (Awh *et al.*, 2013).

8.8 Conclusions

The eye, an organ particularly exposed to light, is probably the ideal model in which to study the biological effects of oxidative stress. Moreover, the eye's accessibility to study and the development of new noninvasive techniques allow the possibility of easily following pathologies related to ageing and oxidative stress.

Several laboratory and animal studies have suggested that micronutrient supplementation could be useful in slowing the development and progression of cataract and AMD.

Additionally, nutritional intervention in these diseases has been extensively evaluated with observational studies. Despite some contradictory findings, results from observational studies have provided the rational for interventional studies.

Concerning cataract, the data from randomized clinical trials have mostly failed to demonstrate beneficial effects of nutritional supplements for the either the prevention or the treatment of this disease. Regarding AMD, the AREDS study demonstrated that the AREDS formulation that included vitamins C and E, β-carotene and zinc reduced the progression to advanced AMD by 25% over 5 years in persons with bilateral large drusen or in persons with large drusen in one eye and advanced AMD in the fellow eye. This is one of the few nutritional supplements known to have beneficial effects in any eye disease. However, other nutrients, such as omega-3 fatty acids, failed to demonstrate any beneficial effect and the results of lutein/zeaxanthin supplementation need to be further investigated.

New evidence related to genetic information may also be relevant to evaluating different patterns of response and explaining differences found among individuals. The pathogenesis of these two age-related pathologies is not yet completely understood, considering that the progression of the diseases is slow, and that randomized multicenter clinical trials in these entities are long, expensive and difficult to perform and analyze. However, even a modest protective effect on the progression of these diseases would have a significant impact on patient welfare and on the burden related to cataract and AMD.

References

AREDS Research Group. 2001a. A randomized, placebo-controlled, clinical trial of high-dose supplementation with vitamins C and E and beta carotene for age-related cataract and vision loss: AREDS report no. 9. *Arch. Ophthalmol.* 119:1439–1452.

AREDS Research Group. 2001b. A randomized, placebo-controlled, clinical trial of high-dose supplementation with vitamins C and E, beta carotene, and zinc for age-related macular degeneration and vision loss: AREDS report no. 8. *Arch. Ophthalmol.* 119:1417–1436.

AREDS Research Group. 2013. Lutein+zeaxanthin and omega-3 fatty acids for age-related macular degeneration: the Age-related Eye Disease Study 2 (AREDS2) randomized clinical trial. *JAMA* 309:2005–2015.

Anderson, R. E., R. M. Benolken, P. A. Dudley, D. J. Landis and T. G. Wheeler. 1974. Proceedings: polyunsaturated fatty acids of photoreceptor membranes. Exp. *Eye Res.* 18:205–213.

Aslam, T., C. Delcourt, R. Silva, F. G. Holz, A. Leys, A. Garcia Layana and E. Souied. 2013. Micronutrients in age-related macular degeneration. *Ophthalmologica* 229:75–79.

Awh, C. C., A. M. Lane, S. Hawken, B. Zanke and I. K. Kim. 2013. CFH and ARMS2 genetic polymorphisms predict response to antioxidants and zinc in patients with age-related macular degeneration. *Ophthalmology* 120:2317–2323.

Balaji, M., K. Sasikala and T. Ravindran. 1992. Copper levels in human mixed, nuclear brunescence, and posterior subcapsular cataract. *Br. J. Ophthalmol.* 76:668–669.

Barteselli, G., J. Chhablani, S. El-Emam, H. Wang, J. Chuang, I. Kozak, L. Cheng, D. U. Bartsch and W. R. Freeman. 2012. Choroidal volume variations with age, axial length, and sex in healthy subjects: a three-dimensional analysis. *Ophthalmology* 119:2572–2578.

Bernstein, P. S., F. Khachik, L. S. Carvalho, G. J. Muir, D. Y. Zhao and N. B. Katz. 2001. Identification and quantitation of carotenoids and their metabolites in the tissues of the human eye. *Exp. Eye Res.* 72:215–223.

Bird, A. C., N. M. Bressler, S. B. Bressler, I. H. Chisholm, G. Coscas, M. D. Davis, P. T. De Jong, C. C. Klaver, B. E. Klein, R. Klein *et al.* 1995. An international classification and grading system for age-related maculopathy and age-related macular degeneration. *The International ARM Epidemiological Study Group. Surv. Ophthalmol.* 39:367–374.

Birlouez-Aragon, I., C. Delcourt, F. Tessier and L. Papoz. 2001. Associations of age, smoking habits and diabetes with plasma vitamin C of elderly of the POLA study. *Int. J. Vitam. Nutr. Res.* 71:53–59.

Boscia, F., I. Grattagliano, G. Vendemiale, T. Micelli-Ferrari and E. Altomare. 2000. Protein oxidation and lens opacity in humans. *Invest. Ophthalmol. Vis. Sci.* 41:2461–2465.

Bressler, N. M., S. B. Bressler, S. K. West, S. L. Fine and H. R. Taylor. 1989. The grading and prevalence of macular degeneration in Chesapeake Bay watermen. *Arch. Ophthalmol.* 107:847–852.

Bressler, N. M., J. C. Silva, S. B. Bressler, S. L. Fine and W. R. Green. 1994. Clinicopathologic correlation of drusen and retinal pigment epithelial abnormalities in age-related macular degeneration. *Retina* 14:130–142.

Cekic, O. 1998. Effect of cigarette smoking on copper, lead, and cadmium accumulation in human lens. *Br. J. Ophthalmol.* 82:186–188.

Chakravarthy, U., C. Augood, G. C. Bentham, P. T. De Jong, M. Rahu, J. Seland, G. Soubrane, L. Tomazzoli, F. Topouzis, J. R. Vingerling, J. Vioque, I. S. Young and A. E. Fletcher. 2007. Cigarette smoking and age-related macular degeneration in the EUREYE Study. *Ophthalmology* 114:1157–1163.

Chang, J. R., E. Koo, E. Agron, J. Hallak, T. Clemons, D. Azar, R. D. Sperduto, F. L. Ferris, 3rd and E. Y. Chew. 2011. Risk factors associated with incident cataracts and cataract surgery in the Age-related Eye Disease Study (AREDS): AREDS report number 32. *Ophthalmology* 118:2113–2119.

Chew, E. Y., T. Clemons, J. P. Sangiovanni, R. Danis, A. Domalpally, W. Mcbee, R. Sperduto and F. L. Ferris. 2012. The Age-related Eye Disease Study 2 (AREDS2): study design and baseline characteristics (AREDS2 report number 1). *Ophthalmology* 119:2282–2289.

Chew, E. Y., T. E. Clemons, E. Agron, R. D. Sperduto, J. P. Sangiovanni, N. Kurinij and M. D. Davis. 2013a. Long-term effects of vitamins C and E, beta-carotene, and zinc on age-related macular degeneration: AREDS report no. 35. *Ophthalmology* 120:1604–1611 e1604.

Chew, E. Y., J. P. Sangiovanni, F. L. Ferris, W. T. Wong, E. Agron, T. E. Clemons, R. Sperduto, R. Danis, S. R. Chandra, B. A. Blodi, A. Domalpally, M. J. Elman, A. N. Antoszyk, A. J. Ruby, D. Orth, S. B. Bressler, G. E. Fish, G. B. Hubbard, M. L. Klein, T. R. Friberg, P. J. Rosenfeld, C. A. Toth and P. Bernstein. 2013b. Lutein/zeaxanthin for the treatment of age-related cataract: AREDS2 randomized trial report no. 4. *JAMA Ophthalmol.* 131:843–850.

Chew, E. Y., T. E. Clemons, J. P. Sangiovanni, R. P. Danis, F. L. Ferris, 3rd, M. J. Elman, A. N. Antoszyk, A. J. Ruby, D. Orth, S. B. Bressler, G. E. Fish, G. B. Hubbard, M. L. Klein, S. R. Chandra, B. A. Blodi, A. Domalpally, T. Friberg, W. T. Wong, P. J. Rosenfeld, E. Agron, C. A. Toth, P. S. Bernstein and R. D. Sperduto. 2014. Secondary analyses of the effects of lutein/zeaxanthin on age-related macular degeneration progression: AREDS2 report no. 3. *JAMA Ophthalmol.* 132:142–149.

Chong, E. W., T. Y. Wong, A. J. Kreis, J. A. Simpson and R. H. Guymer. 2007. Dietary antioxidants and primary prevention of age related macular degeneration: systematic review and meta-analysis. *BMJ* 335:755.

Christen, W. G., U. A. Ajani, R. J. Glynn, J. E. Manson, D. A. Schaumberg, E. C. Chew, J. E. Buring and C. H. Hennekens. 1999. Prospective cohort study of antioxidant vitamin supplement use and the risk of age-related maculopathy. *Am. J. Epidemiol.* 149:476–484.

Christen, W. G., J. E. Manson, R. J. Glynn, J. M. Gaziano, R. D. Sperduto, J. E. Buring and C. H. Hennekens. 2003. A randomized trial of beta carotene and age-related cataract in US physicians. *Arch. Ophthalmol.* 121:372–378.

Christen, W., R. Glynn, R. Sperduto, E. Chew and J. Buring. 2004. Age-related cataract in a randomized trial of beta-carotene in women. *Ophthalmic Epidemiol.* 11:401–412.

Christen, W. G., S. Liu, R. J. Glynn, J. M. Gaziano and J. E. Buring. 2008. Dietary carotenoids, vitamins C and E, and risk of cataract in women: a prospective study. *Arch. Ophthalmol.* 126:102–109.

Christen, W. G., R. J. Glynn, E. Y. Chew and J. E. Buring. 2010a. Vitamin E and age-related macular degeneration in a randomized trial of women. *Ophthalmology* 117:1163–1168.

Christen, W. G., R. J. Glynn, H. D. Sesso, T. Kurth, J. Macfadyen, V. Bubes, J. E. Buring, J. E. Manson and J. M. Gaziano. 2010b. Age-related cataract in a randomized trial of vitamins E and C in men. *Arch. Ophthalmol.* 128:1397–1405.

Coleman, H. R., C. C. Chan, F. L. Ferris, 3rd and E. Y. Chew. 2008. Age-related macular degeneration. *Lancet* 372:1835–1845.

Crabb, J. W., M. Miyagi, X. Gu, K. Shadrach, K. A. West, H. Sakaguchi, M. Kamei, A. Hasan, L. Yan, M. E. Rayborn, R. G. Salomon and J. G. Hollyfield. 2002. Drusen proteome analysis: an approach to the etiology of age-related macular degeneration. *Proc Natl Acad Sci USA* 99:14682–14687.

Cunha-Vaz, J. G. 2004. The blood–retinal barriers system. Basic concepts and clinical evaluation. *Exp. Eye Res.* 78:715–721.

Curcio, C. A. and C. L. Millican. 1999. Basal linear deposit and large drusen are specific for early age-related maculopathy. *Arch. Ophthalmol.* 117:329–339.

De Jong, P. T. 2006. Age-related macular degeneration. *New Engl. J. Med.* 355:1474–1485.

Delcourt, C. 2007. Application of nutrigenomics in eye health. *Forum Nutr.* 60:168–175.

Delcourt, C., I. Carriere, M. Delage, P. Barberger-Gateau and W. Schalch. 2006. Plasma lutein and zeaxanthin and other carotenoids as modifiable risk factors for age-related maculopathy and cataract: the POLA Study. *Invest. Ophthalmol. Vis. Sci.* 47:2329–2335.

Ding, X., M. Patel and C. C. Chan. 2009. Molecular pathology of age-related macular degeneration. *Prog. Retin Eye Res.* 28:1–18.

Estruch, R., E. Ros, J. Salas-Salvado, M. I. Covas, D. Corella, F. Aros, E. Gomez-Gracia, V. Ruiz-Gutierrez, M. Fiol, J. Lapetra, R. M. Lamuela-Raventos, L. Serra-Majem, X. Pinto, J. Basora, M. A. Munoz, J. V. Sorli, J. A. Martinez and M. A. Martinez-Gonzalez. 2013. Primary prevention of cardiovascular disease with a Mediterranean diet. *N. Engl. J. Med.* 368:1279–1290.

Evans, J. R. and J. G. Lawrenson. 2012. Antioxidant vitamin and mineral supplements for slowing the progression of age-related macular degeneration. *Cochrane Database Syst. Rev.* 11:CD000254.

Feeney-Burns, L., E. S. Hilderbrand and S. Eldridge. 1984. Aging human RPE: morphometric analysis of macular, equatorial, and peripheral cells. *Invest. Ophthalmol. Vis. Sci.* 25:195–200.

Feeney-Burns, L., R. P. Burns and C. L. Gao. 1990. Age-related macular changes in humans over 90 years old. *Am. J. Ophthalmol.* 109:265–278.

Fisher, S. A., G. R. Abecasis, B. M. Yashar, S. Zareparsi, A. Swaroop, S. K. Iyengar, B. E. Klein, R. Klein, K. E. Lee, J. Majewski, D. W. Schultz, M. L. Klein, J. M. Seddon, S. L. Santangelo, D. E. Weeks, Y. P. Conley, T. S. Mah, S. Schmidt, J. L. Haines, M. A. Pericak-Vance, M. B. Gorin, H. L. Schulz, F. Pardi, C. M. Lewis and B. H. Weber. 2005. Meta-analysis of genome scans of age-related macular degeneration. *Hum. Mol. Genet.* 14:2257–2264.

Fletcher, A. E., G. C. Bentham, M. Agnew, I. S. Young, C. Augood, U. Chakravarthy, P. T. De Jong, M. Rahu, J. Seland, G. Soubrane, L. Tomazzoli, F. Topouzis, J. R. Vingerling and J. Vioque. 2008. Sunlight exposure, antioxidants, and age-related macular degeneration. *Arch. Ophthalmol.* 126:1396–1403.

Friedman, D. S., B. J. O'Colmain, B. Munoz, S. C. Tomany, C. Mccarty, P. T. De Jong, B. Nemesure, P. Mitchell and J. Kempen. 2004. Prevalence of age-related macular degeneration in the United States. *Arch. Ophthalmol.* 122:564–572.

Friedman, E. and M. O. Ts'o. 1968. The retinal pigment epithelium. II. Histologic changes associated with age. *Arch. Ophthalmol.* 79:315–320.

Friedman, P. A. and M. L. Zeidel. 1999. Victory at C. *Nat Med.* 5:620–621.

Friedrichson, T., H. L. Kalbach, P. Buck and F. J. Van Kuijk. 1995. Vitamin E in macular and peripheral tissues of the human eye. *Curr. Eye Res.* 14:693–701.

Fritsche, L. G., T. Loenhardt, A. Janssen, S. A. Fisher, A. Rivera, C. N. Keilhauer and B. H. Weber. 2008. Age-related macular degeneration is associated with an unstable ARMS2 (LOC387715) mRNA. *Nat. Genet.* 40:892–896.

Fukuzawa, K., Y. Inokami, A. Tokumura, J. Terao and A. Suzuki. 1998. Rate constants for quenching singlet oxygen and activities for inhibiting lipid peroxidation of carotenoids and alpha-tocopherol in liposomes. *Lipids* 33:751–756.

Gale, C. R., N. F. Hall, D. I. Phillips and C. N. Martyn. 2003. Lutein and zeaxanthin status and risk of age-related macular degeneration. *Invest. Ophthalmol. Vis. Sci.* 44:2461–2465.

Garland, D. L. 1991. Ascorbic acid and the eye. *Am. J. Clin. Nutr.* 54:1198S–1202S.

Garner, B., M. J. Davies and R. J. Truscott. 2000. Formation of hydroxyl radicals in the human lens is related to the severity of nuclear cataract. *Exp. Eye Res.* 70:81–88.

Gass, J. D. 1967. Pathogenesis of disciform detachment of the neuroepithelium. *Am. J. Ophthalmol.* 63:Suppl 1–139.

Gass, J. D. 1973. Drusen and disciform macular detachment and degeneration. *Arch. Ophthalmol.* 90:206–217.

Gass, J. D. M. 1997. *Stereoscopic Atlas of Macular Diseases: Diagnosis and Treatment.* St Louis, MO: Mosby.

Gilmore, A. P. 2005. Anoikis. *Cell Death Differ.* 12 Suppl 2:1473–1477.

Gray, H., S. Standring, H. Ellis and B. K. B. Berkovitz. 2005. *Gray's Anatomy: the Anatomical Basis of Clinical Practice.* Edinburgh: Elsevier Churchill Livingstone.

Grossniklaus, H. E. and W. R. Green. 2004. Choroidal neovascularization. *Am. J. Ophthalmol.* 137:496–503.

Grossniklaus, H. E., J. M. Nickerson, H. F. Edelhauser, L. A. Bergman and L. Berglin. 2013. Anatomic alterations in aging and age-related diseases of the eye. *Invest. Ophthalmol. Vis. Sci.* 54:ORSF23–27.

Guyer, D. R. 1999. *Retina, Vitreous, Macula*. Philadelphia, PA: Saunders.

Guymer, R. H., A. C. Bird and G. S. Hageman. 2004. Cytoarchitecture of choroidal capillary endothelial cells. *Invest Ophthalmol. Vis. Sci.* 45:1660–1666.

Halliwell, B. 1997. Antioxidants and human disease: a general introduction. *Nutr. Rev.* 55:S44–49; discussion S49–52.

Hammond, B. R., Jr, E. J. Johnson, R. M. Russell, N. I. Krinsky, K. J. Yeum, R. B. Edwards and D. M. Snodderly. 1997. Dietary modification of human macular pigment density. *Invest. Ophthalmol. Vis. Sci.* 38:1795–1801.

Handelman, G. J., E. A. Dratz, C. C. Reay and J. G. Van Kuijk. 1988. Carotenoids in the human macula and whole retina. *Invest. Ophthalmol. Vis. Sci.* 29:850–855.

Harding, J. 1991. *Cataract: Biochemistry, Epidemiology, and Pharmacology*. London: Chapman and Hall.

Hargrave, P. A. and J. H. Mcdowell. 1992. Rhodopsin and phototransduction: a model system for G protein-linked receptors. *FASEB J.* 6:2323–2331.

Heys, K. R., S. L. Cram and R. J. Truscott. 2004. Massive increase in the stiffness of the human lens nucleus with age: the basis for presbyopia? *Mol. Vis.* 10:956–963.

Huang, J. D., J. B. Presley, M. F. Chimento, C. A. Curcio and M. Johnson. 2007. Age-related changes in human macular Bruch's membrane as seen by quick-freeze/deep-etch. *Exp. Eye Res.* 85:202–218.

Innis, S. M. 1991. Essential fatty acids in growth and development. *Prog. Lipid Res.* 30:39–103.

Jacques, P. F., L. T. Chylack, Jr, S. E. Hankinson, P. M. Khu, G. Rogers, J. Friend, W. Tung, J. K. Wolfe, N. Padhye, W. C. Willett and A. Taylor. 2001. Long-term nutrient intake and early age-related nuclear lens opacities. *Arch. Ophthalmol.* 119:1009–1019.

Jager, R. D., W. F. Mieler and J. W. Miller. 2008. Age-related macular degeneration. *New Engl. J. Med.* 358:2606–2617.

Kannan, R., A. Stolz, Q. Ji, P. D. Prasad and V. Ganapathy. 2001. Vitamin C transport in human lens epithelial cells: evidence for the presence of SVCT2. *Exp. Eye Res.* 73:159–165.

Khan, J. C., D. A. Thurlby, H. Shahid, D. G. Clayton, J. R. Yates, M. Bradley, A. T. Moore and A. C. Bird. 2006. Smoking and age related macular degeneration: the number of pack years of cigarette smoking is a major determinant of risk for both geographic atrophy and choroidal neovascularisation. *Br. J. Ophthalmol.* 90:75–80.

Kisic, B., D. Miric, L. Zoric, A. Ilic and I. Dragojevic. 2012. Antioxidant capacity of lenses with age-related cataract. *Oxid. Med. Cell Longev.* 2012:467130.

Klein, R., B. E. Klein, S. C. Jensen and S. M. Meuer. 1997. The five-year incidence and progression of age-related maculopathy: the Beaver Dam Eye Study. *Ophthalmology* 104:7–21.

Klein, R., B. E. Klein, S. C. Tomany and S. E. Moss. 2002. Ten-year incidence of age-related maculopathy and smoking and drinking: the Beaver Dam Eye Study. *Am. J. Epidemiol.* 156:589–598.

Klein, B. E., M. D. Knudtson, K. E. Lee, J. O. Reinke, L. G. Danforth, A. M. Wealti, E. Moore and R. Klein. 2008. Supplements and age-related eye conditions the beaver dam eye study. *Ophthalmology* 115: 1203–1208.

Koh, H. H., I. J. Murray, D. Nolan, D. Carden, J. Feather and S. Beatty. 2004. Plasma and macular responses to lutein supplement in subjects with and without age-related maculopathy: a pilot study. *Exp. Eye Res.* 79:21–27.

Kuzniarz, M., P. Mitchell, R. G. Cumming and V. M. Flood. 2001. Use of vitamin supplements and cataract: the Blue Mountains Eye Study. *Am. J. Ophthalmol.* 132:19–26.

Launay, S., E. Maubert, N. Lebeurrier, A. Tennstaedt, M. Campioni, F. Docagne, C. Gabriel, L. Dauphinot, M. C. Potier, M. Ehrmann, A. Baldi and D. Vivien. 2008. HtrA1-dependent proteolysis of TGF-beta controls both neuronal maturation and developmental survival. *Cell Death Differ.* 15:1408–1416.

Lawrenson, J. G. and J. R. Evans. 2012. Omega 3 fatty acids for preventing or slowing the progression of age-related macular degeneration. *Cochrane Database Syst. Rev.* 11:CD010015.

Leske, M. C., S. Y. Wu, L. Hyman, R. Sperduto, B. Underwood, L. T. Chylack, R. C. Milton, S. Srivastava and N. Ansari. 1995. Biochemical factors in the lens opacities. Case–control study. The Lens Opacities Case–Control Study Group. *Arch. Ophthalmol.* 113:1113–1119.

Lien, E. L. and B. R. Hammond. 2011. Nutritional influences on visual development and function. *Prog. Retin Eye Res.* 30:188–203.

Luo, L., J. Harmon, X. Yang, H. Chen, S. Patel, G. Mineau, Z. Yang, R. Constantine, J. Buehler, Y. Kaminoh, X. Ma, T. Y. Wong, M. Zhang and K. Zhang. 2008. Familial aggregation of age-related macular degeneration in the Utah population. *Vision Res.* 48:494–500.

Manikandan, R., R. Thiagarajan, S. Beulaja, G. Sudhandiran and M. Arumugam. 2010a. Curcumin prevents free radical-mediated cataractogenesis through modulations in lens calcium. *Free Radic. Biol. Med.* 48:483–492.

Manikandan, R., R. Thiagarajan, S. Beulaja, G. Sudhandiran and M. Arumugam. 2010b. Effect of curcumin on selenite-induced cataractogenesis in Wistar rat pups. *Curr. Eye Res.* 35:122–129.

Mares-Perlman, J. A., B. J. Lyle, R. Klein, A. I. Fisher, W. E. Brady, G. M. Vandenlangenberg, J. N. Trabulsi and M. Palta. 2000. Vitamin supplement use and incident cataracts in a population-based study. *Arch. Ophthalmol.* 118:1556–1563.

Margolis, R. and R. F. Spaide. 2009. A pilot study of enhanced depth imaging optical coherence tomography of the choroid in normal eyes. *Am. J. Ophthalmol.* 147:811–815.

Mathew, M. C., A. M. Ervin, J. Tao and R. M. Davis. 2012. Antioxidant vitamin supplementation for preventing and slowing the progression of age-related cataract. *Cochrane Database Syst. Rev.* 6:CD004567.

Mitchell, P., J. J. Wang, W. Smith and S. R. Leeder. 2002. Smoking and the 5-year incidence of age-related maculopathy: the Blue Mountains Eye Study. *Arch. Ophthalmol.* 120:1357–1363.

Offord, E., G. Van Poppel and R. Tyrrell. 2000. Markers of oxidative damage and antioxidant protection: current status and relevance to disease. *Free. Radic. Res.* 33:S5–S19.

Pastor-Valero, M. 2013. Fruit and vegetable intake and vitamins C and E are associated with a reduced prevalence of cataract in a Spanish Mediterranean population. *BMC Ophthalmol.* 13:52.

Penfold, P. L., S. C. Liew, M. C. Madigan and J. M. Provis. 1997. Modulation of major histocompatibility complex class II expression in retinas with age-related macular degeneration. *Invest. Ophthalmol. Vis. Sci.* 38:2125–2133.

Petrash, J. M. 2013. Aging and age-related diseases of the ocular lens and vitreous body. *Invest. Ophthalmol. Vis. Sci.* 54:ORSF54–59.

Ramrattan, R. S., T. L. Van Der Schaft, C. M. Mooy, W. C. De Bruijn, P. G. Mulder and P. T. De Jong. 1994. Morphometric analysis of Bruch's membrane, the choriocapillaris, and the choroid in aging. *Invest. Ophthalmol. Vis. Sci.* 35:2857–2864.

Rao, G. N., R. Khanna and A. Payal. 2011. The global burden of cataract. *Curr. Opin. Ophthalmol.* 22:4–9.

Rautiainen, S., B. E. Lindblad, R. Morgenstern and A. Wolk. 2014. Total antioxidant capacity of the diet and risk of age-related cataract: a population-based prospective cohort of women. *JAMA Ophthalmol.* 132:247–252.

Ravindran, R. D., P. Vashist, S. K. Gupta, I. S. Young, G. Maraini, M. Camparini, R. Jayanthi, N. John, K. E. Fitzpatrick, U. Chakravarthy, T. D. Ravilla and A. E. Fletcher. 2011. Inverse association of vitamin C with cataract in older people in India. *Ophthalmology* 118:1958–1965; e1952.

Rees, K., L. Hartley, N. Flowers, A. Clarke, L. Hooper, M. Thorogood and S. Stranges. 2013. "Mediterranean" dietary pattern for the primary prevention of cardiovascular disease. *Cochrane Database Syst. Rev.* 8: CD009825.

Resnikoff, S., D. Pascolini, D. Etya'ale, I. Kocur, R. Pararajasegaram, G. P. Pokharel and S. P. Mariotti. 2004. Global data on visual impairment in the year 2002. *Bull. World Health Organ* 82:844–851.

Sangiovanni, J. P. and E. Y. Chew. 2005. The role of omega-3 long-chain polyunsaturated fatty acids in health and disease of the retina. *Prog. Retin Eye Res.* 24:87–138.

Sarks, S. H., J. J. Arnold, M. C. Killingsworth and J. P. Sarks. 1999. Early drusen formation in the normal and aging eye and their relation to age related maculopathy: a clinicopathological study. *Br. J. Ophthalmol.* 83:358–368.

Sarks, S., S. Cherepanoff, M. Killingsworth and J. Sarks. 2007. Relationship of basal laminar deposit and membranous debris to the clinical presentation of early age-related macular degeneration. *Invest. Ophthalmol. Vis. Sci.* 48:968–977.

Seddon, J. M., U. A. Ajani, R. D. Sperduto, R. Hiller, N. Blair, T. C. Burton, M. D. Farber, E. S. Gragoudas, J. Haller, D. T. Miller *et al.* 1994. Dietary carotenoids, vitamins A, C, and E, and advanced age-related macular degeneration. Eye Disease Case–Control Study Group. *JAMA* 272:1413–1420.

Sickel, W. 1972. Electrical and metabolic manifestations of receptor and higher-order neuron activity in vertebrate retina. *Adv. Exp. Med. Biol.* 24:101–118.

Smith, W. and P. Mitchell. 1998. Family history and age-related maculopathy: the Blue Mountains Eye Study. *Aust. NZ J. Ophthalmol.* 26:203–206.

Sommerburg, O. G., W. G. Siems, J. S. Hurst, J. W. Lewis, D. S. Kliger and F. J. Van Kuijk. 1999. Lutein and zeaxanthin are associated with photoreceptors in the human retina. *Curr. Eye Res.* 19:491–495.

Sparrow, J. R. and M. Boulton. 2005. RPE lipofuscin and its role in retinal pathobiology. *Exp. Eye Res.* 80:595–606.

Sparrow, J. R., H. R. Vollmer-Snarr, J. Zhou, Y. P. Jang, S. Jockusch, Y. Itagaki and K. Nakanishi. 2003. A2E-epoxides damage DNA in retinal pigment epithelial cells. Vitamin E and other antioxidants inhibit A2E-epoxide formation. *J. Biol. Chem.* 278:18207–18213.

Spencer, W. H. 1985. *Ophthalmic Pathology: an Atlas and Textbook.* Philadelphia, PA: W. B. Saunders.

Stahl, W. and H. Sies. 2002. Carotenoids and protection against solar UV radiation. *Skin Pharmacol. Appl. Skin Physiol.* 15:291–296.

Starita, C., A. A. Hussain, S. Pagliarini and J. Marshall. 1996. Hydrodynamics of ageing Bruch's membrane: implications for macular disease. *Exp. Eye Res.* 62:565–572.

Stone, W. L., C. C. Farnsworth and E. A. Dratz. 1979. A reinvestigation of the fatty acid content of bovine, rat and frog retinal rod outer segments. *Exp. Eye Res.* 28:387–397.

Stringham, J. M. and B. R. Hammond, Jr. 2007. The glare hypothesis of macular pigment function. *Optom. Vis. Sci.* 84:859–864.

Tabandeh, H., S. Dubovy and W. R. Green. 2006. Bilateral midperipheral large drusen and retinal pigment epithelial detachments associated with multifocal areas of choroidal neovascularization: a histopathologic study. *Retina* 26:1063–1069.

Tan, A. G., P. Mitchell, V. M. Flood, G. Burlutsky, E. Rochtchina, R. G. Cumming and J. J. Wang. 2008. Antioxidant nutrient intake and the long-term incidence of age-related cataract: the Blue Mountains Eye Study. *Am. J. Clin. Nutr.* 87:1899–1905.

Tan, J. S., P. Mitchell, A. Kifley, V. Flood, W. Smith and J. J. Wang. 2007. Smoking and the long-term incidence of age-related macular degeneration: the Blue Mountains Eye Study. *Arch. Ophthalmol.* 125:1089–1095.

Tasman, W., E. A. Jaeger and Wills Eye Hospital (Philadelphia, PA). 2001. *The Wills Eye Hospital Atlas of Clinical Ophthalmology*. Philadelphia, PA: Lippincott Williams & Wilkins.

Taylor, A. and M. Hobbs. 2001. 2001 assessment of nutritional influences on risk for cataract. *Nutrition* 17:845–857.

Thakkinstian, A., P. Han, M. Mcevoy, W. Smith, J. Hoh, K. Magnusson, K. Zhang and J. Attia. 2006. Systematic review and meta-analysis of the association between complement factor H Y402H polymorphisms and age-related macular degeneration. *Hum. Mol. Genet.* 15:2784–2790.

Thiagarajan, R. and R. Manikandan. 2013. Antioxidants and cataract. *Free Radic. Res.* 47:337–345.

Ugarte, M. and N. N. Osborne. 2014. Recent advances in the understanding of the role of zinc in ocular tissues. *Metallomics* 6:189–200.

Ugarte, M., N. N. Osborne, L. A. Brown and P. N. Bishop. 2013. Iron, zinc, and copper in retinal physiology and disease. *Surv. Ophthalmol.* 58:585–609.

Van Leeuwen, R., S. Boekhoorn, J. R. Vingerling, J. C. Witteman, C. C. Klaver, A. Hofman and P. T. De Jong. 2005. Dietary intake of antioxidants and risk of age-related macular degeneration. *JAMA* 294:3101–3107.

Wang, J., K. Ohno-Matsui, T. Yoshida, N. Shimada, S. Ichinose, T. Sato, M. Mochizuki and I. Morita. 2009. Amyloid-beta up-regulates complement factor B in retinal pigment epithelial cells through cytokines released from recruited macrophages/microglia: another mechanism of complement activation in age-related macular degeneration. *J. Cell. Physiol.* 220:119–128.

Wang, X. and P. J. Quinn. 1999. Vitamin E and its function in membranes. *Prog. Lipid Res.* 38:309–336.

Weigert, G., S. Kaya, B. Pemp, S. Sacu, M. Lasta, R. M. Werkmeister, N. Dragostinoff, C. Simader, G. Garhofer, U. Schmidt-Erfurth and L. Schmetterer. 2011. Effects of lutein supplementation on macular pigment optical density and visual acuity in patients with age-related macular degeneration. *Invest. Ophthalmol. Vis. Sci.* 52:8174–8178.

CHAPTER 9

Beauty from the inside: Nutrition and skin ageing

Alessandra Marini and Jean Krutmann
IUF - Leibniz Research Institute for Environmental Medicine, Heinrich-Heine-University Düsseldorf, Düsseldorf, Germany

9.1 Introduction

The relationship between nutrition and the effect on skin ageing has become an interesting topic that is exciting researchers, clinicians and the general population worldwide (reviewed in Krutmann & Humbert, 2011; Preedy, 2012). Increase in life expectancy has emerged as a new preoccupation for industrial countries and for nutritional science, and one of the challenges is to offer new strategies to improve the quality of human life (Piccardi & Manissier, 2009). Skin functions and healthy appearance depend on a sufficient supply of essential nutrients. In this context, nutritional supplements are used to optimize diet and to improve quality of life. In addition to the traditional use of topical skin care, nutritional supplements have emerged as a new strategy to improve skin beauty. Many attempts have been made to improve skin health and beauty by changing or by supplementing the diet (Burton, 1989). Vitamins, including carotenoids and tocopherols, flavonoids, minerals, fatty acids and a variety of plant extracts have been reported to possess potent anti-oxidant properties and have been widely used in the skin care industry in an attempt to prolong youthful skin appearance. Intervention studies indicate that it is possible to manipulate and to delay skin ageing and to improve skin condition through supplementation with selected nutritional supplements.

Skin ageing results from two independent distinct factors, the effects of which can be clearly distinguished at a clinical, histological and molecular level: intrinsic (genetic, endocrinologic) and extrinsic (environmental) factors. The general ageing process, which is a genetically determined loss of cell function and occurs by passing time alone, is called the intrinsic skin ageing process, whereas the skin ageing process induced by environmental factors, mainly chronic sun exposure and ultraviolet (UV) irradiation but also smoking and pollution, is called the extrinsic skin ageing process (Vierkötter & Krutmann, 2012). Kligmann coined the term "photoageing" to describe the modifications that occur in skin after years of exposure to UV radiation (Kligmann & Kligmann, 1986). In sun-exposed skin, the ageing process is accompanied by enhanced cumulative oxidative damage; as a consequence, collagen fibrils become disorganized and their synthesis decreases, while skin levels of type I and III collagen precursors and cross-links are reduced and an abnormal quantity of elastin-containing material accumulates in tissue

Anti-Ageing Nutrients: Evidence-Based Prevention of Age-Associated Diseases, First Edition. Edited by Delminda Neves.

(Morganti, 2012). Photooxidative stress is involved in processes of photoageing and photocarcinogenesis, and plays a major role in the pathogenesis of photodermatoses (Krutmann, 2000). The prevention of oxidative damage to cells and tissue and the repair of UV-dependent damage may be supported by molecules that are capable of inducing suitable repair systems: the anti-oxidants. They act as scavengers of reactive oxygen species generated in primary or secondary reactions following UV irradiation. Naturally human skin has endogenous enzymatic and nonenzymatic anti-oxidants. However, with ongoing ageing and environmental influences, the body's endogenous anti-oxidative defenses attenuate and the production of reactive oxygen species increases (discussed in Chapter 1; Wu *et al.*, 2012). Moreover, changes in personal lifestyles over the years have led to a significant increase in sunlight exposure and this had led to a surge in the incidence of skin cancer and photoageing.

Prevention of skin ageing is of constantly increasing importance to the general population; therefore in recent years, the concept of photoprotection has gained attention as the mainstay of skin protective strategies and a viable approach to reducing the occurrence of skin cancer and photoageing. Based on their structural features, promising candidates for endogenous photoprotection in humans are found among the anti-oxidant micronutrients, including carotenoids, tocopherols, flavonoids and other polyphenols, as well as vitamins C and E, essential omega-3-fatty acids, some proteins and lactobacilli (Sies & Stahl, 2004), which have been described as agents capable of promoting skin health and beauty. It has already been shown that nutrition-based anti-skin-ageing strategies are most effective if they are directed against extrinsic skin ageing (Marini, 2011; Krutmann, 2011). Human studies have underlined the possibility of preventing or at least minimizing photoageing by external use of efficient sunscreens or by the internal use of nutraceuticals (reviewed in Krutmann & Humbert, 2011; Morganti, 2012). Photoprotection obtained from nutrients is well documented. The most frequent damage induced by UV exposure is sunburn, and evidence of sunburn prevention by nutritional supplementation has been widely reported.

The modern idea of sun-protecting products is to combine a "passive" protection with a UV filter and an "active" protection with an anti-oxidant. Modern sunscreen products therefore frequently combine UV filters with one or more biologically active molecules that provide photoprotection through a mechanism that is not based on the absorption or reflection of UV rays and thus are completely different from UV filters (Krutmann & Yarosh, 2006). Rona and Berardesca (2008) suggested that a complete approach to dermocosmetic conditions could involve the correct association of a topical treatment with an oral one on the basis of their synergy (Rona & Berardesca, 2008). The development of novel active compounds for skin photoprotection is a highly innovative and dynamic field (Krutmann & Yarosh, 2006). The group of molecules being used as active compounds, with diverse target points for photoprotection, is heterogeneous and constantly growing. There is an increasing number of products marketed in the European Community as foods containing concentrated sources of nutrients and presented for supplementing the intake of those nutrients from the normal diet. According to the European Directive 2002/46/EC, "food supplements means foodstuffs the purpose of which is to supplement the normal diet and which are concentrated sources of nutrients or other substances with a nutritional or physiological effect, alone or in combination, marketed in dose form, namely forms such as capsules, pastilles, tablets, pills and other similar forms, sachets of powder, ampoules of liquids, drop dispensing bottles, and other similar forms of liquids and powders designed to be taken in measured small unit quantities" (Karajiannis & Fish, 2011). Today, nutritional supplements with cosmetic aims have a broad spectrum of ingredients, including four principal categories: carotenoids, vitamins, polyunsaturated fatty acids (PUFAs) and others (Morganti, 2012). Different names are used to identify these supplements, such as endocosmetics and nutricosmeceuticals (Rona & Berardesca, 2008). The objective of this work is to review the most interesting anti-oxidants and their properties, which have drawn attention for their unique anti-ageing effects, and particularly the photoprotective effects of nutrients. Table 9.1 summarizes the most important nutrients and their major sources.

Table 9.1 The most important nutrients and their major sources.

	Nutrients		Major sources	References
Vitamins	Vitamin C		Fresh fruit and vegetables, e.g. citrus fruit, kiwi, blackcurrant, tomatoes, rosehip, guava, chilli pepper oand parsley	Schagen *et al.* (2012)
	Vitamin E		Vegetables, oils, seeds, nuts, corn, soy, whole wheat flour, margarine, some types of meat and dairy products	Wu *et al.* (2012)
	Carotenoids	β-Carotene	Fresh fruit and vegetables, e.g. carrots, pumpkin, sweet potatoes, mangos and papaya	Stahl (2011a)
		Lycopene	All tomato products, watermelon, guava, rosehips, and pink grapefruit	Stahl (2011a)
		Astaxanthin	Microalgae, yeast, salmon, trout, krill, shrimp, crayfish and crustacean	Schagen *et al.* (2012)
		Retinol	Liver, milk, egg yolk, cheese and fatty fish	Schagen *et al.* (2012)
	Vitamin D		Animal-based foods, e.g. fatty fish and egg yolk. Some products like milk, cereals and margarine can be enriched with vitamin D	Schagen *et al.* (2012)
Polyphenols and flavonoids			Fruit, vegetables, cereals, chocolate, dry legumes and plant-derived beverages such as fruit juices, tea, coffee and red wine	Schagen *et al.* (2012)
Poly unsaturated fatty acids			Fish and shellfish, flaxseed, hemp oil, soya oil, canola oil, chia seeds, pumpkin seeds, sunflower seeds, leafy vegetables, walnuts, sesame seeds, avocados, salmon and albacore tuna	Schagen *et al.* (2012)
Pre- and probiotics	Prebiotics		Soybeans, inulin sources (such as Jerusalem artichoke and chicory root), raw oats, unrefined wheat, unrefined barley and yacon	Marini & Krutmann (2012)
	Probiotics		Live yoghurts, fermented dairy drinks, cheese, fromage frais and fruit juices	Marini & Krutmann (2012)

9.2 Vitamins

9.2.1 Vitamin C (L-ascorbic acid)

L-Ascorbic acid, also called vitamin C, is the most widely known vitamin and an essential micronutrient, required for multiple biological functions. Vitamin C is included in nutraceutical supplements to reduce skin photodamage, rebalance free radical-mediated pathologic processes and prevent photoageing (Morganti, 2012).

Vitamin C is not naturally synthesized by the human body and therefore an adequate dietary intake is required and essential for a healthy human diet. The richest natural sources are fresh fruit and vegetables, such as citrus fruit, kiwi, blackcurrant, tomatoes, rosehips, guava, chilli pepper and parsley (Schagen *et al.*, 2012).

Vitamin C plays an important role in skin biology, contributing to the formation of an efficient skin barrier and fibroblast proliferation and therefore essential for the maintenance of normal connective tissue as well as for wound healing (Marini, 2012). By stimulating collagen synthesis it improves the elasticity of the skin, thereby reducing wrinkles (Duarte & Almeida, 2012). The most commonly described cutaneous manifestations accompanying vitamin C deficiency are attributed to impaired collagen synthesis (Schagen *et al.*, 2012). Enlargement and keratosis of hair follicles and damaged hair have been described (Schagen *et al.*, 2012). Additionally, vitamin C deficiency is known to cause scurvy, a disease with symptoms such as capillary/vascular fragility, skin lesions, gum bleeding, ease of developing bruises and slow wound healing (Krutmann, 2000).

Ascorbic acid is considered to be one of the most powerful and least toxic natural anti-oxidants; it can scavenge deleterious free radicals that contribute to the process of skin ageing. Therefore it is used in cosmetic and dermatological products (Humbert *et al.*, 2012).

Topically Vitamin C is used in various cosmetic products, for example, for lightening skin dyspigmentation and in anti-ageing and sun-protection formulations. It is efficient in protecting against UVB radiation. It reduces the sunburn reaction and prevents the formation of thymine dimers, thus preventing DNA damage (Placzek *et al.*, 2005). Placzek *et al.* (2005) observed in a long-term study the effects of a combination of ascorbic acid and vitamin E administered orally to human volunteers on UVB-induced epidermal damage. The major direct DNA damage induced by UV exposure is the release of cyclobutane pyrimidine dimers (thymine dimers and 6–4 photoproducts; Piccardi & Manissier, 2009). Placzek *et al.* (2005) showed that oral administration of vitamins C (2 mg/day) and E (1000 IU/day) for 3 months had a protective effect against UV-induced thymine dimers. In line with this, Morganti *et al.* (2002) compared in an 8 week study topical and systemic anti-oxidants treatment, which both seemed to be good photoprotectants.

Furthermore, the ability of vitamin C to suppress skin pigmentation via the inhibition of tyrosinase activity in melanocytes makes it a useful whitening agent (Duarte & Almeida, 2012). However, the use of vitamin C in cosmetic products is difficult as its reducing capacity decays very rapidly and there seem to be many products in which the desired effects are not measurable (Wang *et al.*, 2011). Ascorbic acid is an unstable compound in aqueous solution; thus its oral administration could represent an alternative to topical application, benefiting from increased stability and less dependence on the vehicle (Duarte & Almeida, 2012).

9.2.2 Vitamin E (tocopherol)

The term "vitamin E" is a generic description for all tocopherol and tocotrienol derivatives (Traber & Sies, 1996). This group of compounds is highly lipophilic, and thus operative in membranes or lipoproteins. Their most important anti-oxidant function appears to be the inhibition of lipid peroxidation, scavenging lipid peroxyl radicals to yield lipid hydroperoxides and a tocopheroxyl radical (Brigelius-Flohe & Traber, 1999; Liebler, 1993). Vitamin E stabilizes cell membranes and protects tissues that are more sensitive to oxidation, such as the skin. Moreover, it helps in the preservation of other molecules, such as vitamin A, and prevents the oxidation of some hormones (Cassano, 2012). Natural sources of vitamin E include vegetables, oils, seeds, nuts, corn, soy, whole wheat flour, margarine, types sorts of meat and dairy products (Wu *et al.*, 2012). The intake of natural vitamin E products helps prevent collagen cross-linking and lipid peroxidation, which are both linked to ageing of the skin (Schagen *et al.*, 2012).

Vitamin E has been used in the healing of wounds of skin and photoprotection against sunburn, photocarcinogenesis, photoimmunoinhibition and changes in the dermal immunostimulation (Baumann, 2009). Many clinical trials have demonstrated the effects of tocopherol. The data seem to be controversial, but in 2001, Boelsma *et al.* (2001) reviewed the effects of vitamins, including carotenoids and fatty acid supplements, in optimizing skin condition and preventing skin diseases, and concluded that nutritional factors show potential beneficial actions on the skin and that high doses of oral vitamin E may affect the response to UVB in humans.

α-Tocopherol is the predominant isoform of vitamin E in humans and animals. It removes free radical intermediates and prevents oxidation reactions (Wu *et al.*, 2012). However, tocotrienol have been shown to have higher anti-oxidant, anticancer and neuroprotective properties. Yamada *et al.* (2008) observed that dietary tocotrienols protect the skin against damage produced by UVB in hairless mice.

Oral combination treatments of vitamins C and E increase the photoprotective effects compared with monotherapies. In a study with 12 volunteers, vitamin C was supplemented at 500 mg/day over a period of 8 weeks, and the erythemal response following UV-exposure was followed (McArdle *et al.*, 2002). Supplementation with only vitamin C had no effect on "sunburn threshold" or minimal erythemal dose (MED). In a study investigating the cooperative activity of both compounds vitamin E and vitamin C against UV-induced erythema (Fuchs & Kern, 1998), four treatment groups were followed over a period of 50 days. *RRR*-α-tocopherol and ascorbate were supplemented as single components at dose levels of 2 and 3 g/day, respectively. With the combination, 2 g/day of α-tocopherol plus 3 g/day of ascorbate were administered; controls remained without treatment. After treatment with the combination of both vitamins the MED was significantly increased from about 100 mJ/cm^2 before to about 180 mJ/m^2 after supplementation. Treatment with the single compounds provided only moderate protection, which was not statistically significant.

Short-term intervention with high doses of vitamins E and C provides some protection. When vitamin E was ingested at 1000 IU together with 2 g ascorbic acid/day over a period of 8 days, a minor increase in MED was determined (Eberlein-König & Placzek, 1998). Furthermore, vitamins E and C prevent phototoxic damage like UV-dependent erythema, the formation of sunburn cells, lipid peroxidation and DNA damage, as shown in several studies (Fuchs, 1998; McVean & Liebler, 1999). Cesarini *et al.* (2003) demonstrated that

α-tocopherol together with β-carotene, lycopene and selenium significantly reduced lipoperoxide levels, UV-induced erythema and sunburn cells. Therefore the experts recommend that the synergetic interplay of several anti-oxidants should be taken into consideration.

9.2.3 Vitamin B_6

Vitamin B_6 is a water-soluble vitamin and is part of the vitamin B complex group. Three forms of the vitamin are known, pyridoxine, pyridoxal and pyridoxamine. All three forms are precursors of an activated compound known as pyridoxal phosphate. This active form is a cofactor in many reactions of amino acid metabolism, including transamination, deamination and decarboxylation (Kato, 2012). Vitamin B_6 is obtained from various dietary sources (cereals, meat, fish, poultry, soy and some fruit such as bananas and avocado; Kato, 2012).

Vitamin B_6 was discovered as an antidermatitis factor. Additionally, it has been reported to have a strong anti-oxidant effect like a singlet oxygen quencher (Bilski *et al.*, 2000) and to prevent lipid peroxidation (Kannan & Jain, 2004). Therefore, vitamin B_6 is believed to be essential for skin development and maintenance.

The discovery of potential functions of vitamin B_6 as an anti-oxidant awakened interest in its protective roles. Recent growing evidence, however, has suggested that excessive doses can cause phototoxicity and adverse effects (Kato, 2012).

Kitazawa *et al.* (2005) examined the protective effects of an anti-oxidant derived from serine and vitamin B_6 on skin photoageing in hairless mice and they indicated the combination to be promising for the prevention of chronic skin photoageing. On the other hand, Lu *et al.* examined the effect of low dietary vitamin B_6 levels on UVB-induced skin tumorigenesis in hairless mice and found an exacerbation, suggesting that an interaction between vitamin B_6 and UV-radiation might be responsible for higher levels of carcinogenic processes in skin (Lu *et al.*, 2008). Wondrak *et al.* (2004) reported that vitamin B_6 has a strong cytotoxic effect after UV-irradiation in the cell culture system of human skin fibroblasts. Further research is essential to understand the mechanism of phototoxicity of vitamin B_6 and to define its use in the clinical practice.

9.2.4 Carotenoids

The carotenoids are examples of dietary constituents with beneficial effects on skin health. Carotenoids are vitamin A derivates such as β-carotene, astaxanthin, lycopene and retinol, which are all highly effective anti-oxidants and able to neutralize singlet oxygen and peroxyradicals. These compounds have been documented to possess photoprotective properties (Marini, 2011; Krutmann & Yarosh, 2006) and represent a class of lipophilic secondary plant components, and are among the most widespread natural colorants, with β-carotene as the most frequently applied endogenous sun protectant. Fruit and vegetables provide most of the carotenoids in the human diet with a mean daily intake of about 5 mg total carotenoids per day, as measured in Germany (Pelz *et al.*, 1998). Based on epidemiological observations, fruit and vegetables that are rich sources of carotenoids are thought to provide health benefits by decreasing the risk of various diseases (Stahl, 2011a). β-Carotene (from 15 to 180 mg/day) and lycopene (up to 10 mg/day), two efficient singlet oxygen quenchers, have been shown to prevent sunburn in humans (Köpcke & Krutmann, 2008; Stahl *et al.*, 2001; Sies & Stahl, 2004; Stahl, 2011a). Among the carotenoids, lycopene is the most efficient singlet oxygen quencher. When skin is exposed to UV light stress, more skin lycopene is destroyed compared with β-carotene, suggesting that lycopene has a role in mitigating oxidative damage (Ribaya-Mercado *et al.*, 1995). All tomato products are the major source of lycopene for the human organism. Further sources are watermelon, guava, rosehips and pink grapefruit.

Carrots, pumpkin, sweet potatoes, mangos and papaya are some examples of β-carotene-containing fruit and vegetables. Upon dietary supplementation, β-carotene can be further enriched in the skin, in which it is already a major carotenoid (Alaluf *et al.*, 2002). β-Carotene is an endogenous photoprotector, and its efficacy has been demonstrated in various trials (Sies & Stahl, 2004; Köpcke & Krutmann, 2008). In an intervention study with β-carotene it was shown that protection against UV-induced erythema can be achieved (Stahl *et al.*, 2000). The efficacy of β-carotene in systemic photoprotection depends on the duration of treatment and on the dose.

A number of recent studies in humans have shown that oral uptake of mixed carotenoids also has photoprotective effects. In healthy volunteers, a 12-week oral administration of at least a total of 12 mg of carotenoids per day results in a reduction of UV-induced erythema for more than 7 weeks (Stahl *et al.*, 2000). Similar effects have been described in volunteers receiving a lycopene-rich diet (Stahl & Sies, 2002). In order to investigate whether a diet rich in carotenoids is useful for photoprotection, tomato paste was selected as a dietary source containing high levels of lycopene (Gärtner *et al.*, 1997). To improve absorption, olive oil was co-ingested with the paste (20 g/day), providing 16 mg lycopene per day. Dietary intervention was performed over a period of 10 weeks, after which increased lycopene levels in serum and skin were determined. After 10 weeks of intervention, erythema formation was significantly lower in the group consuming the tomato paste compared with control (Stahl *et al.*, 2001), but no significant protection was found at week 4 of treatment. The data show that protection against UV-induced erythema can be achieved by a modulation of the diet. A combination of lycopene (6 mg), vitamin C (60 mg) and soy isoflavones (50 mg) has been shown to maintain skin density and improve skin firmness, microrelief, hydration and tone in postmenopausal women (Dréno, 2003).

In addition to the traditional carotenoids, other emerging ingredients are gaining in popularity. Astaxanthin is found in microalgae, yeast, salmon, trout, krill, shrimp, crayfish and crustacean (Schagen *et al.*, 2012). It prevents UVA-induced alterations in cellular superoxide dismutase activity (Lyons & O'Brien, 2002). Camera *et al.* (2009) showed in cultured human dermal fibroblasts significant photoprotection from a combination of astaxanthin, canthaxanthin and β-carotene (Camera *et al.*, 2009). The uptake of astaxanthin by fibroblasts was higher than that of canthaxanthin and β-carotene, which led to the assumption that the effect of astaxanthin toward photooxidative changes was stronger than that of the other substances. In addition, Suganuma *et al.* (2010) showed that astaxanthin could interfere with UVA-induced matrix-metalloproteinase (MMP)-1 and skin fibroblast elastase/neutral endopeptidase expression.

Retinol is a fat-soluble unsaturated isoprenoid essential for the growth, differentiation and maintenance of epithelial tissues. Natural retinol and retinol ester are contained in liver, milk, egg yolk, cheese and fatty fish. Topical retinoid inhibits the UV-induced, MMP-mediated breakdown of collagen and protects against UV-induced decreases in procollagen expression (Fisher *et al.*, 1997, 2000). Oral treatment with retinol or retinal derivatives has not been yet proposed as a possible anti-ageing treatment. It should be noted that the large CARET trial (the Beta-Carotene and Retinol Efficacy Trial) reported the lung cancer-promoting effects of 25,000 IU retinyl palmitate combined with 30 mg

β-carotene intake (Omenn *et al.*, 1996). Thus, the belief that chemical quenching of free radicals by natural compounds exerts always beneficial effects has been challenged and it is important to consider that the systemic increase of anti-oxidants by dietary supplementation may also lead to adverse effects.

9.2.5 Vitamin D

Vitamin D is a group of fat-soluble secosteroids responsible for enhancing intestinal absorption of calcium, iron, magnesium, phosphate and zinc. In humans, the most important compounds in this group are vitamin D3 (also known as cholecalciferol) and vitamin D2 (ergocalciferol). Vitamin D acts as a pro-hormone and the human body can synthesize it itself through sun exposure, therefore, the skin is the major source of vitamin D. Smaller amounts of vitamin D2 and D3 come from the dietary intake of animal-based foods such as fatty fish or egg yolk. Some products like milk, cereals and margarine can be enriched with vitamin D (Schagen *et al.*, 2012).

Numerous functions of the skin are regulated by vitamin D, such as inhibition of cell proliferation, stimulation of cell differentiation, including formation of the permeability barrier, promotion of innate immunity, regulation of the hair follicle cycle, and suppression of tumor formation (Bikle, 2012). Several *in vitro* and *in vivo* studies have documented the protective effect of 1-α,25-dihydroxyvitamin D3 against UVB-induced skin damage and carcinogenesis (De Haes *et al.*, 2005; Dixon *et al.*, 2005). It should be mentioned that the long-term intakes of vitamin D above the upper recommended intake levels can result in adverse health effects (Schagen *et al.*, 2012).

9.3 Polyphenols and flavonoids

Because of their anti-oxidant properties and the increasing studies showing their probable role in the prevention of various diseases associated with oxidative stress, polyphenols have drawn the attention of the anti-ageing researchers over the last decade. Polyphenols can be divided into many different functional groups such as phenolic acids, flavonoids, stilbenes and lignans (Manach *et al.*, 2004). Polyphenols are mostly found in fruit, vegetables, cereals, chocolate, dry legumes and plant-derived beverages such as fruit juices, tea, coffee and red wine (Schagen *et al.*, 2012).

Polyphenols such as green tea polyphenols, grape seed proanthocyanidins, resveratrol, silymarin and genistein, combined with sunscreen protection, have the ability to protect the skin from the adverse effects of UV radiation (Nichols & Katiyar, 2010).

Flavonoids comprise a group of secondary plant pigments that are used in cosmetics and dermatology. In addition to anti-oxidant properties, they exhibit other biological activities that probably contribute to their cutaneous effects. Flavonoids and flavonoid-rich products can protect skin against UV-induced damage at the molecular and cellular level and may also improve overall skin quality. Regular intake confers significant photoprotection and helps maintain skin health by improving skin structure and function (Stahl, 2011b). Among the flavonoids that have received attention for their photoprotective qualities, green tea has recently gained prominence for the health benefits observed in some, although not all, epidemiological studies. Green tea is made from unfermented leaves of the plant *Camellia sinensis*. Green tea polyphenols (GTP) act as potent anti-oxidants and offer protection against UVB-induced stress (Wu *et al.*, 2012). Treatment of cultured cells with EGCG (epigallocatechin gallate), a major polyphenolic constituent of green tea, directly inhibits the baseline expression of MMPs, such as MMP-2, MMP-9 and neutrophil elastase, even in the absence of UV exposure (Stahl & Mukhtar, 2006). Oral administration of green tea to mice as a sole source of liquid remarkably inhibited UV-induced expression of MMPs in mouse skin, suggesting that GTP has a potential anti-photoageing effect (Vayalil & Mittal, 2004). Treatment with EGCG diminishes UVA-induced skin damage (roughness and sagginess) and protects against the loss of dermal collagen in hairless mouse skin, and also blocks the UV-induced increase of collagenase mRNA level and the promoter-binding activities of activator protein 1 (AP-1) and nuclear factor κ-light chain enhancer of activated B cells in cultured human epidermal fibroblasts (Kim & Hwang, 2001).

Polyphenols provided by the ingestion of high-flavanol cocoa (326 mg/day) reduced UV-induced erythema (Heinrich *et al.*, 2006). *Polypodium leucomotos* (7.5 mg/kg body weight), a tropical fern plant used traditionally in Central America for the treatment of anti-inflammatory disorders, has also been shown to counteract the erythematogenic effect of UV exposure (Middelkamp-Hup *et al.*, 2004).

Phlorizin, a type of flavonoid belongs to the group of dihydrochalcones, and it can be found in the bark of pear (*Pyrus communis*), apple, cherry and other fruit trees. It has been used for over 150 years but its anti-ageing effects have only been reported recently (Schagen *et al.*, 2012).

Other polyphenols have been described to have potent anti-oxidant properties. Among them silymarin, genistein, and the nonflavonoids resveratrol and curcumi, have been demonstrated to have beneficial effects on skin ageing parameters.

Silymarin is a naturally polyphenolic flavonoid isolated from the milk thistle plant (*Silybum marianum* L. Gaertn), and is a mixture of several flavonolignans, including silybin, silibinin, silidianin, silychristin and isosylibin (Wagner *et al.*, 1974). The anti-oxidant effects of silymarin in mouse models have been established, and silybin is the main constituent responsible for these effects (Wagner *et al.*, 1974). Silymarin is effective against burn-induced oxidative damage and morphological alterations in rat skin (Toklu *et al.*, 2007).

Genistein and daidzein are isoflavones that have anti-oxidative and photoprotective effects (Wu *et al.*, 2012). Soybeans are a rich source of isoflavones, but these can also be found in *Ginkgo biloba* extract, Greek oregano and Greek sage. Genistein preserves cutaneous cell proliferation and repair mechanisms, and exerts photoprotective effects against acute UVB irradiation-induced damage on reconstituted skin (Moore *et al.*, 2006).

Resveratrol (*trans*-3,4 ,5-trihydroxystilbene), is a polyphenolic phytoalexin found largely in the skin and seeds of grapes, nuts, fruit and red wine. It has been the subject of intense interest in recent years owing to its range of unique anti-ageing properties (discussed in Chapter 2; Schagen *et al.*, 2012). Resveratrol is a potent anti-oxidant with anti-inflammatory and antiproliferative properties (Tsai *et al.*, 1999). Moreover, it has been suggested to protect skin from UV-induced photodamage and photoageing (Baumann, 2009). Resveratrol imparts its protective effects against multiple UVB exposure via modulations in the cki–cyclin–cdk network (cyclin kinase inhibitors, cyclins and cyclin-dependent kinases) and MAPK (mitogen-activated protein kinase) pathway (Reagan-Shaw *et al.*, 2004).

Curcumin is a dietary pigment from the plant *Curcuma longa* and has been shown to protect against the deleterious effects of injury on skin by attenuating oxidative stress and suppressing inflammation (reviewed in Heng, 2010).

9.4 Polyunsaturated fatty acids

PUFAs are categorized into omega-3, omega-6 and omega-9 families (Morganti, 2012). Omega-3 PUFAs are derived from linolenic acid, and omega-6 are derived from linoleic acid (Schagen *et al.*, 2012). They are present in multiple food sources, such as fish and shellfish, flaxseed, hemp oil, soya oil, canola oil, chia seeds, pumpkin seeds, sunflower seeds, leafy vegetables, walnuts, sesame seeds, avocados, salmon and albacore tuna (Schagen *et al.*, 2012). Using nutrients such as omega-3 PUFAs for the promotion of skin health and treatment of skin disorders is a novel concept (Marini, 2011). Scientific studies have drawn attention to the anti-ageing properties of α-linolenic acid showing a link between inflammation and skin ageing (Morganti, 2012; Giacomoni, 2005) and its protective activity on these conditions (Kim *et al.*, 2006). The fatty acids have an anti-oxidant, free radical-scavenging effect. Therefore, eicosapentaenoic acid (omega-3 PUFA) may provide significant protection against UV radiation-induced erythema (Boelsma *et al.*, 2001). In a clinical study, 10 subjects enriched their diets daily with fish oil containing 2.8 g eicosapentaenoic acid (EPA) and 1.2 g docosahexaenoic acid (DHA) and 10 other subjects received a placebo (Orengo *et al.* 1992). After 4 weeks, a small but statistically significant increase in the MED was seen in the fish-oil group (Orengo *et al.* 1992). In line with this, dietary supplementation with 10 g/day fish oil (18% EPA and 12% DHA) increased MED (Rhodes *et al.*, 1994). The effect of fish oil on UV-induced inflammation may be partially explained by its ability to reduce prostaglandin E2 levels (Rhodes *et al.*, 1995).

9.5 Pre- and probiotics

Thanks to the recent advances in microbiology and immunology, immense progress has been made in our understanding of the cutaneous microflora (reviewed in Krutmann, 2009). Preservation of the microflora is a means of maintaining healthy skin functions, and because of their role in skin health and disease, the maintenance or restoration of healthy skin microbiota has become the aim of modern therapies (Krutmann, 2009). Pre- and probiotics have been suggested as important applications of such therapies and in the last few years have achieved scientific popularity as safe and effective agents to regulate the body's micro-environment and skin health (Marini & Krutmann, 2012). A constantly growing body of literature exists concerning their relevance in cosmetic and dermatology (reviewed in Marini & Krutmann, 2012). Most of these examples deal with the oral administration of food-grade products, but recently their use in cosmetic products applied directly to the skin has been proposed. While prebiotics rebalance the skin microflora, probiotic topic treatments consist of applying an inactivated microbial biomass to the skin (Marini & Krutmann, 2012).

Gibson and Roberfroid in 1995 introduced the concept and defined prebiotics as "non-digestible food ingredients that beneficially affect the host by selectively stimulating the growth and/or activity of one, or a limited number of, bacteria in the colon" (Gibson & Roberfroid, 1995). Traditional dietary sources of prebiotics include soybeans, inulin sources (such as Jerusalem artichoke and chicory root), raw oats, unrefined wheat, unrefined barley and yacon (Marini & Krutmann, 2012). In line with the concept of a prebiotic, it is believed that some of the oligosaccharides that naturally occur in breast milk play an important role in the development of a healthy immune system in infants (Marini & Krutmann, 2012).

Probiotics are defined as "live organisms which upon administration in adequate amounts confer a health benefit to the host" by improving the characteristics of the intestinal microflora (Krutmann, 2009). Probiotics can be consumed in various forms of fermented or nonfermented food products. Food vehicles include live yoghurts, fermented dairy drinks, freeze-dried supplements (capsules, pills, liquid suspensions and sprays), cheese, fromage frais and fruit juices (Marini & Krutmann, 2012). Over the years, a wide range of bacteria have been proposed and used as probiotics (Marini & Krutmann, 2012). However, only those classified as lactic acid bacteria have received major consideration with regard to food and nutrition (Marini & Krutmann, 2012). Most probiotics currently used are microbes typical of healthy gastrointestinal microbiota, with the aim of promoting gut health and improving immune system function (discussed in Chapter 5). They include *Lactobacillus* (*L. casei, L. rhamnosus, L. Johnonii*) and *Bifidobacterium* species (*B. breve, B. longum, B. bifidum*), which belong to the lactic acid bacteria group, as well as *Enterococcus, Propionibacterium, Bacillus* and some yeast (Marini & Krutmann, 2012). Nutritional supplementation of hairless mice with *L. johnsonii* provided protection of the skin immune system against UVB radiation-induced immunosuppressive effects (Guéniche *et al.*, 2006). Oral supplementation with *L. johnsonii* has been shown to accelerate the recovery of human skin immune homeostasis after UV-induced immunosuppression (Leclaire *et al.*, 2008). In a human study it has been shown that oral consumption of a probiotic (*L. johnsonii*) with carotenoids (β-carotene, 4.8 mg/day; lycopene, 2 mg) increases MED and counteracts UV-induced decrease of Langerhans cell density; therefore, this combination may represent a novel approach to protecting the skin immune system against UV radiation (Bouilly-Gauthier *et al.*, 2010). Probiotics improve gut barrier function, restore healthier gut microecology, stimulate the host immune system and antagonize the inflammatory alterations (Marini & Krutmann, 2012). A study demonstrated that, after 43 days of supplementation, a specific probiotic called *L. paracasei* significantly decreased skin sensitivity compared with placebo, and also increased the recovery rate of the skin barrier function induced by mechanical disruption (Benyacoub *et al.*, 2008). The regular consumption of fermented dairy products is likely to improve the natural skin barrier function and improve its cosmetic appearance. In the case of diseases that result from imbalance of microorganisms, such as impure skin/mild acne or dry skin/mild atopic dermatitis, pre- and probiotic concepts represent an effective alternative to strictly antibacterial products (Marini & Krutmann, 2012). Nutritional interventions using probiotics are described in some studies as exerting beneficial effects in the treatment and/or prevention of atopic dermatitis (Betsi *et al.*, 2008). Additionally, Koch *et al.* (2008) reported the decrease of SCORAD (SCORing Atopic Dermatitis) after DHA supplementation in atopic eczema.

Although carotenoids, vitamins, polyphenols and PUFAs are used in various cosmeceutical products, many other emerging ingredients are gaining in popularity (Chaudary, 2010) such as ectoin, which protects the skin from the effects of UVA-induced cell damage (Buenger & Driller, 2004), melatonin, a powerful anti-oxidant (Biagini *et al.*, 2006), coenzyme Q_{10}, which is a naturally occurring compound that has both energizing and anti-oxidative properties (Puizina-Ivic *et al.*, 2010), French maritime pine bark extract, which was found to improve skin hydration and elasticity (Marini *et al.*, 2012), and several ingredients known for their anti-oxidative activity, such as glucosamine, pomegranate (Chaudary, 2010), vitamin K2 (Geleijnse *et al.*, 2004), polyglucosides, such as chitin and chitosan (Janak *et al.*, 2011), ferulic acid (Wu *et al.*, 2012), glutathione (Wu *et al.*, 2012) and others.

9.6 Conclusions

To conclude, there is clear evidence of the link between nutrition and skin condition. A diverse and well-balanced healthy diet rich in fruit and vegetables definitely helps to preserve the healthy and youthful appearance of skin. A balanced diet associated with cosmetic and/or oral supplementation at nutritional doses and/or drugs could represent a globalized approach for improving skin health and beauty. A promising strategy for enhancing skin protection from oxidative stress is to support the endogenous system with anti-oxidant-containing products that are normally present in the skin and are capable of promoting skin health and beauty. However, it is important to note that this does not include the permanent intake of nonphysiological high dosages of isolated anti-oxidants. We have briefly illustrated the beneficial effects of some interesting substances used as functional foods; however, further research is essential to confirm their benefits and their use in clinical practice.

Appropriate nutritional supplementation is beneficial in preventing the harmful effects of UV exposure and managing skin ageing. It is important to note that endogenous photoprotection is complementary to topical photoprotection, and that these two forms of prevention clearly should not be considered mutually exclusive.

References

Alaluf, S., U. Heinrich, W. Stahl, H. Tronnier, and S. Wiseman. 2002. Dietary carotenoids contribute to normal human skin color and UV photosensitivity. *J. Nutr.* 132:399–403.

Baumann, L. (ed.). 2009. *Cosmetic Dermatology: Principles and Practice*, 2nd edn. New York: McGraw-Hill.

Benyacoub, J., A. Gueniche, I. Bureau-Franz, and I. Castiel. 2008. Probiotiques et peau. *In*: M. Roberfroid, V. Coxam, and N. Delzenne (eds) *Aliments Fonctionnels*, 2nd edn. Paris: Lavoisier, pp. 633–643.

Betsi, G. I., E. Papadavid, and M. E. Falagas. 2008. Probiotics for the treatment or prevention of atopic dermatitis: a review of the evidence from randomized controlled trials. *Am. J. Clin. Dermatol.* 2:93–103.

Biagini, G., F. Gabbanelli, G. Lucarini, K. Kyrikidou, M. Mattioli-Belmonte, and P. Morganti. 2006. The green chemistry. Activity of an antioxidant network melatonin rich. *SOFW-J.* 132:16–26.

Bikle, D. D. 2012. The skin and vitamin D. *In*: V. R. Preedy (ed.) *Handbook of Diet, Nutrition and the Skin*. Wageningen: Academic, pp. 93–113.

Bilski, P., M. Y. Li, M. Ehrenshaft, M. E. Daub, C. F. and Chignell. 2000. Vitamin B_6 (pyridoxine) and its derivatives are efficient singlet oxygen quenchers and potential fungal antioxidants. *Photochem. Photobiol.* 71:129–134.

Boelsma, E., H. F. Hendriks, and L. Roza. 2001. Nutritional skin care: health effects of micronutrients and fatty acids. *Am. J. Clin. Nutr.* 73:853–864.

Bouilly-Gauthier, D., C. Jeannes, Y. Maubert, L. Duteil, C. Queille-Roussel, N. Piccardi, C. Montastier, P. Manissier, G. Piérard, and J. P. Ortonne. 2010. Clinical evidence of benefits of a dietary supplement containing probiotic and carotenoids on ultraviolet-induced skin damage. *Br. J. Dermatol.* 163:536–543.

Brigelius-Flohe, R. and M. G. Traber. 1999. Vitamin E: function and metabolism. *J. FASEB* 13:1145–1155.

Buenger, J. and H. Driller. 2004. Ectoin: an effective natural substance to prevent UVA-induced premature photoaging. *Skin Pharmacol. Physiol.* 17:232–237.

Burton, J. L. 1989. Diet and dermatology. *BMJ.* 298:770–771.

Camera, E., A. Mastrofrancesco, C. Fabbri, F. Daubrawa, M. Picardo, H. Sies, and W. Stahl. 2009. Astaxanthin, canthaxanthin and beta-carotene differently affect UVA-induced oxidative damage and expression of oxidative stressresponsive enzymes. *Exp. Dermatol.* 18:222–231.

Cassano, R. 2012. Vitamin E chemistry, biological activity and benefits on the skin. *In*: V. R. Preedy (ed.) *Handbook of Diet, Nutrition and the Skin*. Wageningen: Academic, pp. 145–163.

Cesarini, J. P., L. Michel, J. M. Maurette, H. Adhoute, and M. Béjot. 2003. Immediate effects of UV radiation on the skin: modification by an antioxidant complex containing carotenoids. *Photodermatol. Photoimmunol. Photomed.* 19:182–189.

Chaudary, R. 2010. Good nutrition for healthy skin. *NBT* 6:12–17.

De Haes, P., M. Garmyn, A. Verstuyf, P. De Clercq, M. Vandewalle, H. Degreef, K. Vantieghem, R. Bouillon, and S. Segaert. 2005. 1,25-Dihydroxyvitamin D3 and analogues protect primary human keratinocytes against UVB-induced DNA damage. *J. Photochem. Photobiol. B.* 78:141–148.

Dixon, K. M., S. S. Deo, G. Wong, M. Slater, A. W. Norman, J. E. Bishop, G. H. Posner, S. Ishizuka, G. M. Halliday, V.E. Reeve, and R. S. Mason. 2005. Skin cancer prevention: a possible role of 1,25 dihydroxyvitamin D3 and its analogs. *J. Steroid Biochem. Mol. Biol.* 97:137–143.

Dréno, B. 2003. New assessment methods applied to a patented lacto-lycopene, soy isoflavones and vitamin C in the correction of skin aging. *Nouv. Dermatol.* 22:1–6.

Duarte, T. L. and I. F. Almeida. 2012. Vitamin C, gene expression and skin health. *In*: V. R. Preedy (ed.) *Handbook of Diet, Nutrition and the Skin*. Wageningen: Academic, pp. 115–127.

Eberlein-König, B. and M. Placzek. 1998 Protective effect against sunburn of combined systemic ascorbic acid (vitamin C) and D-α-tocopherol (vitamin E). *J. Am. Acad. Dermatol.* 38:45–48.

Fisher, G. J., Z. Q. Wang, S. C. Datta, J. Varani, S. Kang, and J. J. Voorhees. 1997. Pathophysiology of premature skin aging induced by ultraviolet light. *New Engl. J. Med.* 337:1419–1428.

Fisher, G. J., S. Datta, Z. Wang, X. Y. Li, T. Quan, J. H. Chung, S. Kang, and J. J. Voorhees. 2000. c-Jun-dependent inhibition of cutaneous procollagen transcription following ultraviolet irradiation is reversed by all-*trans* retinoic acid. *J. Clin. Invest.* 106:663–670.

Fuchs, J. 1998. Potentials and limitations of the natural antioxidants RRR-α-tocopherol, L-ascorbic acid and beta-carotene in cutaneous photoprotection. *Free Radic. Biol. Med.* 25:848–873.

Fuchs, J. and H. Kern. 1998. Modulation of UV-light-induced skin inflammation by D-α-tocopherol and L-ascorbic acid: a clinical study using solar simulated radiation. *Free Radic. Biol. Med.* 25:1006–1012.

Gärtner, C., W. Stahl, and H. Sies. 1997. Lycopene is more bioavailable from tomato paste than from fresh tomatoes. *Am. J. Clin. Nutr.* 66:116–122.

Geleijnse, J. M., C. Vermeer, D. E. Grobbee, L. J. Schurgers, M. H. Knapen, I. M. van der Meer, A. Hofman, and J. C. Witteman. 2004. Dietary intake of menaquinone is associated with a reduced risk of coronary heart disease: the Rotterdam study. *ASN* 34:3100–3108.

Giacomoni, P. U. 2005. Aging science and the cosmetics industry. The micro-inflammatory model serves as a basis for developing effective anti-aging products for the skin. *EMBU Report* 6:545–548.

Gibson, G. R. and M. B. Roberfroid. 1995. Dietary modulation of the human colonic microbiota: introducing the concept of prebiotics. *J. Nutr.* 125:1401–1412.

Guéniche, A., J. Benyacoub, T. M. Buetler, H. Smola, and S. Blum. 2006. Supplementation with oral probiotic bacteria maintains cutaneous immune homeostasis after UV exposure. *Eur. J. Dermatol.* 16:511–517.

Heinrich, U., K. Neukam, H. Tronnier, H. Sies, and W. Stahl. 2006. Long-term ingestion of high flavanol cocoa provides photoprotection against UV-induced erythema and improves skin condition in women. *J. Nutr.* 36:1565–1569.

Heng, M. C. 2010. Curcumin targeted signaling pathways: basis for anti-photoaging and anti-carcinogenic therapy. *Int. J. Dermatol.* 49:608–622.

Humbert, P., D. Binda, S. Robin, and J. Krutmann. 2011. Beauty from Inside: Nutrition-Based strategies in cosmetic dermatology. *In*: J. Krutmann and P. Humbert (eds) *Nutrition for Healthy Skin*. Berlin: Springer, pp. 189–196.

Janak, K., J. K. Vidanarachchi, Maheshika, S. Kurukulasuriya, and K. Se-Kwon. 2011. Chitin, chitosan and their oligosaccharides in food industry. *In*: K. Se-Kwon (ed.) *Chitin, Chitosan and their Oligosaccharides and their Derivatives*. New York: CRC Press, pp. 543–560.

Kannan, K. and S. K. Jain. 2004. Effect of vitamin B_6 on oxygen radicals, mitochondrial membrane potential, and lipid peroxidation in H_2O_2-treated U937 monocytes. *Free Radic. Biol. Med.* 36:423–428.

Karajiannis, H. and C. Fish. 2011. Legal aspects. *In*: J. Krutmann and P. Humbert (eds) *Nutrition for Healthy Skin*. Berlin: Springer, pp. 167–180.

Kato, N. 2012. Role of vitamin B_6 in skin health and diseases. *In*: V. R. Preedy (ed.) *Handbook of Diet, Nutrition and the Skin*. Wageningen: Academic, pp. 59–66.

Kim, H. H., S. Cho, S. Lee, K. H. Kim, K. H. Cho, H. C. Eun, and J. H. Chung. 2006. Photoprotective and anti-skin-aging effects of eicosapentaenoic acid in human skin in vivo. *J. Lipid. Res.* 47:921–930.

Kim, J. and J. S. Hwang. 2001. Protective effects of (−)-epigallocatechin-3-gallate on UVA- and UVB-induced skin damage. *Skin Pharmacol. Appl. Skin Physiol.* 14:11–19.

Kitazawa, M., Y. Ishitsuka, M. Kobayashi, T. Nakano, K. Iwasaki, K. Sakamoto, K. Arakane, T. Suzuki, and L. H. Kligman. 2005. Protective effects of an antioxidant derived from serine and vitamin B_6 on skin photoaging in hairless mice. *Photochem. Photobiol.* 81:970–974.

Kligmann, L. H. and A. M. Kligmann. 1986. The nature of photoaging: its prevention and repair. *Photodermatology* 3:215–227.

Koch, C., S. Dölle, M. Metzger, C. Rasche, H. Jungclas, R. Rühl, H. Renz, and M. Worm. 2008. Docohexaenoic acid (DHA) supplementation in atopic eczema: a randomized, double-blind, controlled trial. *Br. J. Dermatol.* 158:786–792.

Köpcke, W. and J. Krutmann. 2008. Protection from sunburn with beta-carotene – a meta-analysis. *Photochem. Photobiol.* 84:284–288.

Krutmann, J. 2000. Ultraviolet A radiation-induced biological effects in human skin: relevance for photoaging and photodermatosis. *J. Dermatol. Sci.* 23 Suppl 1:22–26.

Krutmann, J. 2009. Pre- and probiotics for human skin. *J. Dermatol. Sci.* 54:1–5.

Krutmann, J. 2011. Skin Aging. *In*: J. Krutmann and P. Humbert (eds) *Nutrition for Healthy Skin*. Berlin: Springer, pp. 15–24.

Krutmann, J. and P. Humbert (eds). 2011. *Nutrition for Healthy Skin*. Berlin: Springer,

Krutmann, J. and D. Yarosh. 2006. Modern photoprotection of human skin. *In*: B. A. Gilchrest and J. Krutmann (eds) *Skin Aging*. New York: Springer, pp. 103–112.

Liebler, D. C. 1993. The role of metabolism in the antioxidant function of vitamin E. *Crit. Rev. Toxicol.* 23:147–169.

Lu, T., Y. Xu, E. S. Monttinen, and N. Kato. 2008. Supplementing vitamin B_6 to a low vitamin B_6 diet exaggerates UVB-induced skin tumorigenesis in DMBA-treated hairless mice. *J. Nutr. Sci. Vitaminol. (Tokyo)* 54:262–265.

Lyons, N. M. and N. M. O'Brien. 2002. Modulatory effects of an algal extract containing astaxanthin on UVA-irradiated cells in culture. *J. Dermatol. Sci.* 30:73–84.

Manach, C., A. Scalbert, C. Morand, C. Rémésy, and L. Jiménez. 2004. Polyphenols: food sources and bioavailability. *Am. J. Clin. Nutr.* 79:727–747.

Marini, A. 2011. Beauty from the inside. Does it really work? *Hautarzt* 62:614–617.

Marini, A. 2012. Nahrungsergänzungspräparate in der Dermatologie. *Dermatologie Praxis* 4:14–18.

Marini, A. and J. Krutmann. 2012. Pre- and probiotics for human skin. *In*: V. R. Preedy (ed.) *Handbook of Diet, Nutrition and the Skin*. Wageningen: Academic, pp. 319–331.

Marini, A., S. Grether-Beck, T. Jaenicke, M. Weber, C. Burki, P. Formann, H. Brenden, F. Schönlau, and J. Krutmann. 2012. Pycnogenol® effects on skin elasticity and hydration coincide with increased gene expressions of collagen type I and hyaluronic acid synthase in women. *Skin. Pharmacol. Physiol.* 25:86–92.

McArdle, F., L. E. Rhodes, R. Parslew, C. I. Jack, P. S. Friedmann, and M. J. Jackson. 2002. UVR-induced oxidative stress in human skin in vivo: effects of oral vitamin C supplementation. *Free Radic. Biol. Med.* 33:1355–1362.

McVean, M. and D. C. Liebler. 1999. Prevention of DNA photodamage by vitamin E compounds and sunscreens: roles of ultraviolet absorbance and cellular uptake. *Mol. Carcinog.* 24:169–176.

Middelkamp-Hup, M. A., M. A. Pathak, C. Parrado, D. Goukassian, F. Rius-Díaz, M. C. Mihm, T. B. Fitzpatrick, and S. González. 2004. Oral polypodium leucomotos extract decreases ultraviolet-induced damage of human skin. *J. Am. Acad. Dermatol.* 51:910–918.

Moore, J. O., Y. Wang, W. G. Stebbins, D. Gao, X. Zhou, R. Phelps, M. Lebwohl, and H. Wei. 2006. Photoprotective effect of isoflavone genistein on ultraviolet B-induced pyrimidine dimer formation and PCNA expression in human reconstituted skin and its implications in dermatology and prevention of cutaneous carcinogenesis. *Carcinogenesis.* 27:1627–1635.

Morganti, P. 2012. Skin photoprotection and nutraceuticals: an overview. *In*: V. R. Preedy (ed.). *Handbook of Diet, Nutrition and the Skin*. Wageningen: Academic, pp. 217–231.

Morganti, P., C. Bruno, F. Guarneri, A. Cardillo, P. Del Ciotto, and F. Valenzano. 2002. Role of topical and nutritional supplement to modify the oxidative stress. *Int. J. Cosmet. Sci.* 24:331–339.

Nichols, J. A. and S. K. Katiyar. 2010. Skin photoprotection by natural polyphenols: anti-inflammatory, antioxidant and DNA repair mechanisms. *Arch. Dermatol. Res.* 302:71–83.

Omenn, G. S., G. E. Goodman, M. D. Thornquist, J. Balmes, M. R. Cullen, A. Glass, J. P. Keogh, F. L. Meyskens, B. Valanis, J. H. Williams, S. Barnhart, and S. Hammar, S. 1996. Effects of a combination of beta carotene and vitamin A on lung cancer and cardiovascular disease. *New Engl. J. Med.* 334: 1150–1155.

Orengo, I. F., H. S. Black, and J. E. Wolf. 1992. Influence of fish oil supplementation on the minimal erythema dose in humans. *Arch. Dermatol. Res.* 284:219–221.

Pelz, R., B. Schmidt-Faber, and H. Heseker. 1998. Carotenoid intake in the German National Food Consumption Survey. *Z. Ernährungswissenschaft.* 37:319–327.

Piccardi, N. and P. Manissier. 2009. Nutrition and nutritional supplementation. *Dermatoendocrinology* 5:271–274.

Placzek, M., S. Gaube, U. Kerkmann, K. P. Gilbertz, T. Herzinger, E. Haen, and B. Przybilla. 2005. Ultraviolet B-induced DNA damage in human epidermis is modified by the antioxidants ascorbic acid and D-α-tocopherol. *J. Invest. Dermatol.* 124:304–307.

Preedy, V. R. (ed.). 2012. *Handbook of Diet, Nutrition and the Skin.* Wageningen: Academic,

Puizina-Ivic, N., L. Miric, A. Carija, D. Karlica, and D. Marasović. 2010. Modern approach to topical treatment of aging skin. *Coll. Antropol.* 34:1145–1153.

Reagan-Shaw, S., F. Afaq, M. H. Aziz, and N. Ahmad. 2004. Modulations of critical cell cycle regulatory events during chemoprevention of ultraviolet B-mediated responses by resveratrol in SKH-1 hairless mouse skin. *Oncogene* 23:5151–5160.

Rhodes, L. E., S. O'Farrell, M. J. Jackson, and P. S. Friedmann. 1994. Dietary fish-oil supplementation in humans reduces UVB-erythemal sensitivity but increase epidermal lipid peroxidation. *J. Invest. Dermatol.* 103:151–154.

Rhodes, L. E., B. H. Durham, W. D. Fraser, and P. S. Friedmann. 1995. Dietary fish oil reduces basal and ultraviolet B-generated PGE2 levels in skin and increases the threshold to provocation of polymorphic light eruption. *J. Invest. Dermatol.* 105:532–535.

Ribaya-Mercado, J. D., M. Garmyn, B. A. Gilchrest, and R. M. Russell. 1995. Skin lycopene is destroyed preferentially over beta-carotene during ultraviolet irradiation in humans. *J. Nutr.* 125:1854–1859.

Rona, C. and E. Berardesca. 2008. Aging skin and food supplements: the myth and the truth. *Clin. Dermatol.* 26:641–647.

Schagen, S. K., V. A. Zampeli, E. Evgenia Makrantonaki, and C. C. Zouboulis. 2012. Discovering the link between nutrition and skin aging. *Dermatoendocrinol.* 4:298–307.

Sies, H. and W. Stahl. 2004. Nutritional protection against skin damage from sunlight. *Annu. Rev. Nutr.* 24:173–200.

Stahl, W. 2011a. Systemic photoprotection by carotenoids. *In*: J. Krutmann and P. Humbert (eds): *Nutrition for Healthy Skin*. Berlin: Springer, pp. 65–70.

Stahl, W. 2011b. Flavonoid-rich nutrients for the skin. *In*: J. Krutmann and P. Humbert (eds): *Nutrition for Healthy Skin*. Berlin: Springer, pp. 85–90.

Stahl, W. and H. Mukhtar. 2006. Vitamins and polyphenols in systemic photoprotection. *In*: B. A. Gilchrest and J. Krutmann (eds): *Skin Aging*. Springer Verlag, New York. pp. 113–121.

Stahl, W. and H. Sies. 2002. Carotenoids and protection against solar UV radiation. *Skin Pharmacol. Appl. Skin Physiol.* 15:291–296.

Stahl, W., U. Heinrich, H. Jungmann, H. Sies, and H. Tronnier. 2000. Carotenoids and carotenoids plus vitamin E protect against ultraviolet light-induced erythema in humans. *Am. J. Clin. Nutr.* 71:795–798.

Stahl, W., U. Heinrich, S. Wiseman, O. Eichler, H. Sies, and H. Tronnier. 2001. Dietary tomato paste protects against ultraviolet light-induced erythema in humans. *J. Nutr.* 131:1449–1451.

Suganuma, K., H. Nakajima, M. Ohtsuki, and G. Imokawa. 2010. Astaxanthin attenuates the UVA-induced up-regulation of matrix-metalloproteinase-1 and skin fibroblast elastase in human dermal fibroblasts. *J. Dermatol. Sci.* 58:136–142.

Toklu, H. Z., T. Tunali-Akbay, G. Erkanli, M. Yüksel, F. Ercan, and G. Sener. 2007. Sylmarin, the antioxidant component of Sylibum marianum, protects against burn-induced oxidative skin injury. *Burns* 33:908–916.

Traber, M. G. and H. Sies. 1996. Vitamin E in humans: demand and delivery. *Annu. Rev. Nutr.* 16:321–347.

Tsai, S. H., S. Y. Lin-Shiau, and J. K. Lin. 1999. Suppression of nitric oxide synthase and the down-regulation of the activation of NFkappaB in macrophages by resveratrol. *Br. J. Pharmacol.* 126:673–680.

Vayalil, P. K. and A. Mittal. 2004. Green tea polyphenols prevent ultraviolet light-induced oxidative damage and matrix metalloproteinases expression in mouse skin. *J. Invest. Dermatol* 122:1480–1487.

Vierkötter, A. and J. Krutmann. 2012. Environmental influences on skin aging and ethnic-specific manifestations. *Dermatoendocrinology* 4:227–231.

Wagner, H., P. Diesel, and M. Seitz. 1974. The chemistry and analysis of silymarin from *Silybum marianum* Gaertn. *Arzneimittelforschung.* 24:466–471.

Wang, S. Q., U. Osterwalder, and K. Jung. 2011. Ex vivo evaluation of radical sun protection factor in popular sunscreens with antioxidants. *J. Am. Acad. Dermatol.* 65:525–530.

Wondrak, G. T., M. J. Roberts, M. K. Jacobson, and E. L. Jacobson. 2004. 3-Hydroxypyridine chromophores are endogenous sensitizers of photooxidative stress in human skin cells. *J. Biol. Chem.* 279: 30009–30020.

Wu, Y., H. D. Chen, Y. H. Li, X. Y. Gao, and V. H. Preedy. 2012. Antioxidant and skin: an overview. *In*: V.R. Preedy (ed.) *Handbook of Diet, Nutrition and the Skin*. Wageningen: Academic, pp. 69–90.

Yamada, Y., M. Obayashi, T. Ishikawa, Y. Kiso, Y. Ono, and K. Yamashita. 2008. Dietary tocotrienol reduces UVB-induced skin damage and sesamin enhances tocotrienol effects in hairless mice. *J. Nutr. Sci. Vitaminol. (Tokyo)*. 54:117–123.

CHAPTER 10

Retarding brain ageing and cognitive decline

José Paulo Andrade
Department of Anatomy, Faculty of Medicine, University of Porto, Porto, Portugal

10.1 Ageing and brain

Ageing is a process that results in progressive accumulation of morphological and physiological changes that occur as a result of time. It is accompanied by a diminished ability to maintain homeostasis with a progressive loss of performance of organs and systems, increasing susceptibility to disease and terminating with the death of the organism (Harman, 2006; Troen, 2003). No unifying theory exists to explain the cause and the mechanisms of ageing in different organisms, tissues and cells. While some theories explain ageing by genetic factors, others regard the molecular lesions caused by environmental factors as the main cause (Esiri, 2007; Troen, 2003). One of the basic chemical processes that can motivate ageing was first proposed in 1956 by Denham Harman and is known as the free radical/oxidative stress theory (discussed in Chapter 1). It states that the reaction of active free radicals normally produced in organisms, and greatly increased in aged cells owing to mitochondria functional decline, initiates the changes associated with ageing (Harman, 2006).

The different systems of the human body present different degrees of vulnerability to oxidative stress, and the central nervous system is one of the most affected (Andrade & Assunção, 2012; Wang *et al.*, 2010). Neurons have to manage the delicate equilibrium between pro-oxidant and anti-oxidant systems to have optimal efficiency. When an "imbalance between the production of reactive species and the available antioxidant defense" (Halliwell, 2006) occurs, oxidative stress emerges in the central nervous system. Oxidative stress can be due to the disruption of redox signaling and control and, contrary to the notion of a global organic imbalance, seems to be relatively discreet and compartmentalized in neurons, offering a new conceptual framework to study the functions of free radicals (Jones, 2006).

The peculiar susceptibility of the brain to oxidative stress is due to several factors, such as the great demand of neurons for oxidative metabolism to maintain a large surface membrane, the presence of an active system of transport and the ion gradients involved in impulse transmission (Floyd & Hensley, 2002). This need for oxygen (20% of the total amount used in humans) explains the high quantity of oxygen per unit weight of the brain. Equally important and contributing to the unbalancing of the equilibrium between anti-oxidant and pro-oxidant factors are the elevated content of easily peroxidizable

Anti-Ageing Nutrients: Evidence-Based Prevention of Age-Associated Diseases, First Edition. Edited by Delminda Neves.

unsaturated fatty acids, the high content of iron and other metals, and the relatively low anti-oxidant capacity of the brain, that is, 10–20% when compared with the liver or heart, resulting in low anti-oxidant protective defenses (Esiri, 2007). Finally, the postmitotic nature of neurons and the reduced capacity for cellular regeneration compared with other organs allied to all of the previous factors can result in oxidative stress (Floyd & Hensley, 2002; Esiri, 2007).

This vulnerability is not uniform in the brain; some neuronal populations are more vulnerable than others, depending on factors such as high intrinsic oxidative stress, elevated demand of reactive species signaling, decreased ATP production and inflammatory response (Wang *et al.*, 2010). It should be remembered that oxygen and nitrogen reactive species can be used physiologically in the brain as signals to mediate intracellular responses, including the modulation of synaptic plasticity (Wang *et al.*, 2010). However, the redox steady state can easily revert to pro-oxidant conditions during ageing, resulting in oxidative stress that is involved in premature lesions of various cellular compounds, increases in metabolic processes related to senescence, and involvement in the etiopathogeny of some neurodegenerative diseases, namely Parkinson and Alzheimer diseases (Esiri, 2007; Halliwell, 2006).

10.2 From "healthy ageing" to dementia

The terms "healthy ageing" or "successful ageing" have been used to describe the process of ageing without serious diseases throughout the lifespan (Rowe and Khan, 1997). It is also called "vital ageing" or "active ageing", suggesting freedom, life satisfaction and independence (Rowe & Kahn, 1997; Daffner, 2010). Rowan and Kahn included three main components in "successful ageing": (a) low probability of disease and disease-related disability; (b) high cognitive and physical functional capacity; and (c) active engagement with life (Rowe & Kahn, 1997).

Ageing affects the central nervous system from the cellular to the functional levels (Caracciolo *et al.*, 2014). Changes associated with the advancing age result in a decline in several abilities, including sensory, motor and higher cognitive functions. Cognitive decline is the paradigm of evolution from age-related changes to age-associated diseases in older people (Caracciolo *et al.*, 2014).

Dementia is a clinical syndrome caused by neurodegeneration and characterized by inexorably progressive deterioration in multiple cognitive domains and capacity for independent living (Prince *et al.*, 2013). Dementia among the elderly seems to be a geriatric syndrome caused by numerous factors including cortical loss, alterations in cerebral circulation, nutritional deficiencies and probably many other factors (Strandberg & O'Neill, 2013). Alzheimer disease, vascular dementia, Lewy body and frontotemporal dementia are the most common underlying pathologies of dementia in the elderly (Prince *et al.*, 2013). Alzheimer disease is characterized by the presence neurofibrillary tangles and senile plaques in the brain, and is the most common cause of dementia in aged people, accounting for 60–70% of all cases when applying diagnostic criteria for dementia subtypes (Caracciolo *et al.*, 2014; Blennow *et al.*, 2006). Vascular dementia is the second most common cause of dementia in elderly people and is defined as a loss of cognitive function resulting from ischemic, hypoperfusive or hemorrhagic brain lesions owing to cerebrovascular disease or cardiovascular pathology (Román, 2003). Mixed dementia, combining these two main dementias, is probably the most common type of dementia in older individuals (Caracciollo *et al.*, 2014)

The prevalence of dementia increases exponentially with age, doubling with every 5.5–6.7 year increment in age depending on the world region. In 2010 there were an estimated 35.6 million people worldwide living with dementia (Prince *et al.*, 2013). As the number of people over the age of 60 is expected to double between 2000 and 2050 (Prince *et al.*, 2013), the incidence of cognitive decline and age-associated neurodegenerative disease will rise significantly, as well as the inherent healthcare costs, representing a heavy burden to governments. For example, as the mean age of populations increases worldwide, the prevalence of dementia, Parkinson disease and Alzheimer disease will also increase. The number of people who will be affected by dementia worldwide will double every 20 years, reaching 65.7 million in 2030 and 115.4 million in 2050 (Barnes & Yaffe, 2011).

Concomitantly, there is increasing interest in the prevention of mild cognitive impairment (Sofi *et al.*, 2013), a mental disorder that refers to the grey zone between the normal cognitive changes of "healthy ageing" and early dementia (Petersen, 2011). These individuals suffer a decline of cognitive functions greater than expected for their age. Mild cognitive decline was reported to be an independent risk factor for Alzheimer disease (Sofi *et al.*, 2013). Individuals suffering from this mild cognitive decline are a high-risk group because they develop dementia at a rate 2–7% per year higher when compared with the general population (Palmer *et al.*, 2008). Cognitive decline can be described as a continuum that ranges from intact cognition in "healthy ageing" through mild cognitive impairment, and finally, dementia.

Neurodegenerative diseases do not have an effective therapy and present treatments have limited efficacy (Sofi *et al.*, 2013), but the projections of future incidence of this group of age-associated diseases may be modified substantially by preventive interventions, improvements in treatment and care, and disease progression-modifying interventions. For example, interventions that could delay the onset of dementia by just 5 years have the power to reduce by 50% the number of affected individuals. In the particular case of Alzheimer disease, there are several known potentially modifiable risk factors (diabetes, midlife hypertension, midlife obesity, smoking, depression, cognitive inactivity or low educational attainment, and physical inactivity) and a 10–25% reduction in some of the modifiable risk factors could potentially prevent as many as 1.1–3.0 million cases worldwide (Barnes & Yaffe, 2011).

Therefore, the prevention and even improvement of neurodegenerative disorders related to ageing and dementia with modification of lifestyle and diet have become vital as critical determinants of "healthy ageing" (González-Sarrías *et al.*, 2013). The concept of "healthy ageing" includes the notion that it can be dependent on individual choice and effort (Rowe & Kahn, 1997), although genetics also have a role to play (Masoro, 2001). As development of a therapeutic weapon is not likely, physicians and researchers are trying to act on the modifiable risk factors that can be changed in prevention strategies. Some of those possibilities include the use of nutraceuticals, modification of the diet and multidomain interventions. In this chapter we will review some of these possibilities for building a route for active ageing, with a particular focus on green tea, curcumin and the Mediterranean diet.

10.3 Green tea as a functional food and source of nutraceuticals

There are numerous dietary supplements, medical foods, nutraceuticals and functional foods that have come onto the market of food and health products with the objective of maintaining health during ageing contributing for neurodegenerative disease prevention or even therapy (for a review see González-Sarrías *et al.*, 2013). Only a few can be really considered useful for prevention or treatment of age-associated neurodegenerative diseases. Green tea is one of those that may have real effects and contribute to "healthy ageing". Green tea can be considered a "functional food" and a source of polyphenolic flavonoids, mainly catechins. On the other hand, catechins may be used as a nutraceutical or a model for future synthetic pharmacological compounds with similar characteristics.

Tea is the most consumed drink following water, with a worldwide per capita consumption of approximately 120 ml/day, and possesses a very high content of powerful anti-oxidant compounds (Macready *et al.*, 2009). Among the several types of tea, green tea is a major source of catechins, constituting 30–40% of the solid extracts (Manach *et al.*, 2004; Mandel *et al.*, 2006; Andrade & Assunção, 2012). Green tea is produced by using young tea leaves of the *Camellia sinensis* and is packed for consumption without fermentation. As such, it has approximately four times more catechins than black tea owing to the reduction in the time of exposure to oxidation in the treatment of the leaves. Tea catechins modulate cellular and molecular mechanisms associated with oxidative stress and inflammation (Manach *et al.*, 2004; Mandel *et al.*, 2006).

Although for a long time there was only empirical evidence linking the improvement of human health with tea or green tea consumption, scientific papers studying the effects of intake of this beverage are now steadily growing (for a review see Andrade & Assunção, 2012). A review of observational and interventional studies related to green tea or the main component of the catechin fraction, (−)-epigallocatechin-3-gallate (EGCG), including PubMed and Cochrane Library, indicated that clinical evidence is not conclusive but chronic green tea ingestion may give some protection against prostate and breast cancers but not against others (Clement, 2009). Green tea may also reduce the incidence of cardiovascular disease and stroke owing to its action on risk factors associated with atherosclerosis (Clement, 2009). Epidemiological studies have demonstrated that drinking tea is associated with a better memory performance and a lower prevalence of cognitive impairment. For example, in China, a longitudinal examination showed that men who drank tea almost every day had a 10–20% lower risk of death and better health longevity compared with their counterparts who rarely drink tea (Qiu *et al.*, 2012). The same study demonstrated that high frequency of tea consumption was significantly associated with reduced disability of daily activities, cognitive impairment and health deficits, or in other words, healthy ageing (Qiu *et al.*, 2012).

Human interventional studies concerning the anti-oxidant effects of green tea have shown that its moderate consumption (one to six cups per day) increased plasma anti-oxidant capacity and reduced oxidative damage in DNA and lipids (McKay & Blumberg, 2002; Higdon & Frei, 2003; Rietveld & Wiseman, 2003). The consumption of two cups of green tea per day for 42 days increased anti-oxidant status and reduced plasma peroxides in a randomized controlled study (Erba *et al.*, 2005). In another controlled study, drinking green tea for 7 days increased plasma glutathione, increased ferric reducing/anti-oxidant power and improved the postexercise increase in lipid hydroperoxidase (Panza *et al.*, 2008). Concerning alterations in cognition and/or neurodegenerative diseases, just nine of the 156 studies involving green tea or EGCG were listed at clinicaltrials.gov in May 2014. Despite this lack of systematic clinical trials of the actions of green tea in the brain, some epidemiological data suggest that prolonged consumption of green tea can be linked to lower prevalence of cognitive impairment in Japanese aged ≥70 years of age (Kuriyama *et al.*, 2006). Also, a reduction of the risk of Parkinson disease was associated with the ingestion of two to three cups of tea per day in epidemiological studies in Finland and the USA (Hu *et al.*, 2007; Checkoway *et al.*, 2002). A study in Singapore Chinese was not conclusive (Tan *et al.*, 2008).

10.3.1 Bioavailability of the catechins of green tea

Catechins have been found to be powerful anti-oxidants *in vitro*, where they are tested generally in high concentrations (Halliwell, 2006). On the other hand, studies related to the bioavailability of catechins of green tea and their actions *in vivo* present divergent results (Scheepens *et al.*, 2010). This is understandable as the catabolism of the polyphenols present in green tea in the human body is complex because flavonoids are metabolized as xenobiotics and therefore rapidly removed from circulation (Halliwell, 2006; Scheepens *et al.*, 2010). In the gastrointestinal tract there are fractions of catechins not absorbed in the small intestine and metabolized in the liver and kidneys that undergo further microbial chemical changes in the large intestine and are decomposed into smaller molecules (Halliwell, 2006; Scheepens *et al.*, 2010). These molecules, mainly ring-fission metabolites were found in high concentrations in urine and plasma of human after ingestion of green tea (Del Rio *et al.*, 2010). More importantly, catechins are able to modify the composition and metabolism of gut bacteria known to determine the status of global health (Caracciolo *et al.*, 2014). After passing through the liver, these low-molecular-weight metabolites reach systemic circulation and are distributed to the major organs of the human body, including the brain.

The central nervous system is protected by the blood–brain barrier and the access of green tea biocompounds to the brain is also a subject for debate (Spencer *et al.*, 2001; Youdim & Joseph, 2001; Zini *et al.*, 2006). To reach brain cells, polyphenols must be very lipid-soluble or subject to active transport processes (Scheepens *et al.*, 2010). In addition, the blood–brain barrier contains efflux pumps known as ATP-binding cassette (ABC) transporters that constitute an additional problem to be overcome (Zini *et al.*, 2006). In an *in vivo* experiment in human, flavan-3-ols or their metabolites were detected in blood but did not pass through the blood–brain barrier, although the authors theorize that the beneficial action of polyphenols may be systemic and, therefore, effective throughout the body (Zini *et al.*, 2006). On the other hand, *in vitro* studies showed that some flavonoids or their metabolites cross the blood–brain barrier and that the potential for permeation is consistent with compound lipophilicity (Youdim *et al.*, 2003). In another report (+)-catechin crossed RBE-4 cells, an immortalized cell line of the rat cerebral capillary endothelial cells, in a time-dependent manner (Faria *et al.*, 2010). In a conscious and freely moving rat, EGCG penetrated the blood–brain barrier and the calculated bioavailability of this compound in the brain was approximately 5% (Lin *et al.*, 2007). Finally, minimal concentrations of EGCG and epicatechin or their metabolites were found in the brain after oral administration and accumulated on several brain regions (Abd El Mohsen *et al.*, 2002). Epicatechin, another catechin present in green tea and/or its metabolites administered orally (3 or 30 mg per day for 13 days) crossed the blood–brain barrier and were detected and quantified in perfused brain tissue from mice, stimulating neurogenesis and retention of spatial memory (Van Praag *et al.*, 2007). Therefore, these minimal concentrations found in the central nervous system appear to be biologically active and able to exert neuroprotective and neuromodulatory effects.

Extrapolation of these results to humans is not linear owing to differences in flavonoid absorption and metabolism and differences in the structure of the blood–brain barrier (Faria *et al.*, 2010, 2011). A simple extrapolation of *in vitro* and animal data to humans is misleading: "what happens in a Petri dish or preclinical assays may not happen to people" (Bjelakovic & Gluud, 2007). Therefore, it is not surprising that a human study found that, after oral intake of a cup of green tea, several catechin metabolites did not pass through the blood–cerebrospinal fluid barrier, although they were present in the blood (Zini *et al.*, 2006). Nonetheless, Schaffer and Halliwell note that, as the ascorbic acid brain concentration in rat brain is 3000–4000 times higher than that of catechins, it is unlikely that polyphenols exert direct anti-oxidant actions in basal conditions and *in vivo*, despite their potent and high anti-oxidant activity *in vitro* (Schaffer & Halliwell, 2012).

10.3.2 Direct and indirect actions of catechins

In spite of the erratic bioavailability of catechins and the opinion of the above-mentioned authors (Schaffer & Halliwell, 2012), the direct actions such as free radical scavenging, chelation of heavy metals and modulation of anti-oxidant enzymes should be considered as the aged central nervous system needs an increased supply of anti-oxidants and dietary catechins may be necessary (Andrade & Assunção, 2012). Protection against oxidative reactions, generally seen as an initiator of the oxidative damage to lipids and proteins, can be one of the mechanisms by which catechins can protect neurons in the aged brain. Other mechanisms such as an increase in the intracellular glutathione redox status and interaction with nitric oxide regulatory pathways are probably shielding mechanisms that protect neurons during ageing (Andrade & Assunção, 2012).

Another hypothesis to consider is the activation of a hormetic response, that is, the exposure to a low dose of a toxic element gives rise to a beneficial effect (Calabrese *et al.*, 2010). Catechins can be considered hormetic stressors and in low concentrations act upon signaling cascades in neurons and glia, which can generate pleiotropic beneficial effects, including neuroprotection (Davinelli *et al.*, 2012; Schaffer & Halliwell, 2012). For example, pre-treatment with oral epicatechin reduced the brain infarcts in stroke-induced wild-type mice and decreased neurological deficit scores when compared with a control group (Shah *et al.*, 2010). However, this neuroprotection was absent in mice lacking the enzyme heme oxygenase 1 or the transcription factor nuclear factor-erythroid 2 p45-related factor 2, regulators of the induction of anti-oxidant and neuroprotective genes, respectively (Shah *et al.*, 2010).

Finally, catechins can act upon peripheral targets and, in turn, these peripheral targets may have influence on the central nervous system. As an example, a meta-analysis demonstrated that moderate consumption of tea substantially enhanced endothelial-dependent vasodilation in humans. This vasodilation, providing more oxygen and glucose, can be related to the reduced risk of cardiovascular events and stroke observed among green tea and black tea drinkers (Ras *et al.*, 2011). Obviously, this indirect effect provides the brain with more oxygen and glucose owing to improved blood flow. On the other hand, endothelial dysfunction was correlated with decreased cerebral perfusion and dementia (Ras *et al.*, 2011).

10.3.3 Action of catechins in brain

The small quantities of polyphenols that reach the brain may possess local neuroprotective activity and potential molecular targets of the catechins of the green tea have indeed been proposed: (a) action in calcium homeostasis modulation (Ishige *et al.*, 2001); (b) influence on the activity of mitogen-activated protein kinases/extracellular signal-regulated kinase (Schroeter *et al.*, 2002) and protein kinase C (Kalfon *et al.*, 2007); (c) regulation of anti-oxidant enzymes and the anti-oxidant response element (Chen *et al.*, 2000); (d) modulation of cell death and cell survival genes and proteins associated with mitochondrial function (Weinreb *et al.*, 2003); and (f) modulation of iron sensors and regulators (Ishige *et al.*, 2001; Schroeter *et al.*, 2002; Weinreb *et al.*, 2003; Davinelli *et al.*, 2012; Andrade & Assunção, 2012). In line with this belief, it was demonstrated that the intraperitoneal injection of EGCG inhibited L-DOPA methylation, improved the bioavailability of L-DOPA and protected against oxidative hippocampal neurodegeneration (Kang *et al.*, 2010). Catechin also had a neuroprotective effect against glutamate-induced oxidative toxicity *in vitro* and protected against kainic acid-induced hippocampal neurodegeneration *in vivo* after intraperitoneal injection (Kang *et al.*, 2013).

Additionally, EGCG inhibited catechol-*O*-methyltransferase and averted depletion of dopamine in the striatum, prevented dopaminergic neuron loss in the substantia nigra, and increased the activity of superoxide dismutase and catalase in brain tissue and the levels of glutathione and protein kinase C on the hippocampal formation while reducing neurotoxicity and memory deficits induced by amyloid β-peptide (Levites *et al.*, 2001; Kim *et al.*, 2009). In 19-month-old rats consuming green tea from 12 months of age, this beverage was able to reverse most of the impairments associated with ageing to levels similar to those found in 12-month-old control rats (Assunção *et al.*, 2010, 2011). These improvements were observed in the levels of lipid peroxidation, protein carbonyls, anti-oxidant enzymes, deposition of neuronal lipofuscin in the hippocampal region and spatial memory related to the morphological integrity of the hippocampal formation (Assunção *et al.*, 2010, 2011). Using the same model, green tea was also shown to increase the activation of the transcription factor cAMP response element-binding protein and the levels of brain-derived neurotrophic factor and anti-apoptotic protein B cell-lymphoma 2 in the hippocampal formation when compared with age-matched controls (Assunção *et al.*, 2010, 2011).

10.3.4 Catechins and neurodegenerative diseases

Protein misfolding and aggregation are a hallmark of aged cells (discussed in Chapters 1 and 2) and have been directly implicated in Alzheimer and Parkinson diseases and familial amyloid polyneuropathy. Catechins have been shown to have positive effects in transgenic mice models of Alzheimer disease. EGCG decreased β-amyloid levels and plaques associated with the promotion of the α-secretase-proteolytic pathway, which is known to be nonamyloidogenic (Rezai-Zadeh *et al.*, 2005). Further, it was shown to be effective in the prevention of aggregation and remodeling of amyloid fibrils comprising different amyloidogenic proteins (Palhano *et al.*, 2013). Another possible pathway is the induction of cellular neutral endopeptidase activity, as demonstrated in the neuroblastoma cell line SK-N-SH treated with green tea extract, through a mechanism related to the increase of cyclic adenosine monophosphate (cAMP) levels (Ayoub & Melzig, 2006). This enzyme degrades β-amyloid complexes, preventing the accumulation of senile plaques in the central nervous system (Ayoub & Melzig, 2006). In this regard, it was also shown that both EGCG and green tea extracts inhibited the enzyme cholinesterase, improving the cholinergic system (Okelo *et al.*, 2004; Lee *et al.*, 2009).

To date, there are no clinical data confirming these laboratory studies. There is an ongoing clinical trial (Clinicaltrials.gov identifier NCT00951834) entitled "Sunphenon EGCG (epigallocatechin-gallate) in the early stage of Alzheimer's disease (SUN-AK)", investigating whether EGCG (daily dose from 200 to 800 mg) in the early stages of dementia positively affects the course of Alzheimer disease when co-medicated with acetylcholinesterase inhibitors.

As stated previously, green tea can be considered a functional food, that is, a product consumed in the regular diet that can provide health benefits beyond nutritional functions. Therefore, we can advance with the support of some laboratory scientific evidence validated by observational studies that moderate consumption of green tea not only may improve global health, but may also have a positive effect on the cognition of the elderly with improvement of the quality of life, contributing to a healthy ageing. In addition to the tea itself, the method of making the drink also influences the effects of tea consumption (Song *et al.*, 2012). For example, the addition of milk to green tea can probably affect the availability of the catechins owing to their interaction with β-casein, the main milk protein (Song *et al.*, 2012). Also, the addition of sugar to green tea is not advisable as there is a direct interaction between polyphenols and sugars, as has been described, and this complexation may hamper their intestinal absorption (Williamson & Manach, 2005; Carneiro *et al.*, 2008). In addition, the existence of direct pro-oxidant effects of the carbohydrates not efficiently counterbalanced by anti-oxidant compounds cannot be excluded (Carneiro *et al.*, 2008).

In addition to the polyphenols, L-theanine, an amino-acid present in tea, also has neuroprotective effects (Song *et al.*, 2012). Caffeine, likewise found in tea, has been associated in epidemiological studies with a reduced risk of dementia (Song *et al.*, 2012).

Concerning the use of isolated catechins or combination of catechins and their use as nutraceuticals, health statements should not be based only on basic scientific evidence. In fact, concerning the effects of complex mixtures of catechins it is not known if these biocompounds act independently, synergistically, additively or even in an antagonistic manner. Further investigations are required to understand the effects of catechins and to identify biomarkers that can respond to simultaneous active and physiological concentrations of catechins. Only then will it be possible to perform pharmacodynamic and clinical studies in humans with levels of evidence that are still not available. This data must be obtained from randomized clinical trials and complete with details of the biological mechanisms. However, at present, knowledge is still limited, and many questions remain. For example, the pharmacologically active dose of catechins is not known. In the clinical trials found in clinicaltrials.gov, the daily intake of catechins varied from 200 mg to a maximum of 1200 mg and most of the trials used a median dose of 600 mg daily in capsules twice a day.

There are also potential safety issues if megadoses of catechins are consumed daily. There is a biphasic performance and a catechin can become pro-oxidant and cytotoxic depending on the dose (Andrade & Assunção, 2012). Other reasons for concern are the possible interactions with drug-metabolizing enzymes and potential hepatotoxicity (Andrade & Assunção, 2012). In old rats, the oral consumption of green tea significantly decreased the plasma testosterone levels owing probably to the presence of phytoestrogens in the complex biological matrix and the increase in the levels of aromatase, the enzyme that converts testosterone to estrogen (Neves *et al.*, 2008; Andrade & Assunção, 2012). Human clinical trials need to be performed as there are no studies concerning human sexual health and prolonged consumption of green tea.

10.3.5 Other polyphenols

Two other polyphenols have received attention owing to their potential to modulate several intracellular processes and pleiotropic effects leading to neuroprotection: curcumin and resveratrol (Kim *et al.*, 2010; Davinelli *et al.*, 2012). Curcumin is a yellow pigment present in the rhizome of *Curcuma longa*. Curiously, the prevalence of Alzheimer disease in India is 4.4-fold less that in the USA, and some authors suggest that the diet rich in curcumin might be responsible for this reduced risk in aged Indians (Ganguli *et al.*, 2010). This biocompound has anti-oxidant, anti-inflammatory and anti-amyloidogenic properties (Ramsewak *et al.*, 2000; Ferreira *et al.*, 2013; Ringman *et al.*, 2005). Laboratory studies *in vitro* demonstrated that curcumin inhibits Aβ fibril formation, a strategy useful for treatment or prevention of Alzheimer disease (Ono *et al.*, 2004). In animals, low doses of curcumin reduced the levels of Aβ plaques in the brain of a mouse model of Alzheimer disease (Tg2576; Lim *et al.*, 2001)

Still, curcumin has poor water solubility (Davinelli *et al.*, 2012) and consequent low bioavailability following administration orally or via parental route (Sharma *et al.*, 2005). To circumvent this fact, there is a solid lipid curcumin particle named Longvida, that is being evaluated in a Phase II Alzheimer clinical trial (NCT01001637). This formulation was able to maintain the curcumin concentration in plasma above the level required for biological activity (Dadhaniya *et al.*, 2011).

Resveratrol is another polyphenol with pleiotropic actions (Kim *et al.*, 2010; Davinelli *et al.*, 2012). It is a phytoalexin compound with low bioavailability present in very small amounts in grapes and other plants (Davinelli *et al.*, 2012). Resveratrol modulates various systems, providing neuroprotection, as demonstrated in several *in vitro* and *in vivo* models of Alzheimer disease, owing to strong anti-oxidant radical scavenging functions, anti-inflammatory activity and activation of sirtuins, mimicking energy restriction (discussed in Chapter 2; Baur & Sinclair, 2006). In a mouse model of Alzheimer disease, an energy-restricted diet reduced Alzheimer disease pathogenesis through an increase in sirtuin 1 activity (Saiko *et al.*, 2008; Davinelli *et al.*, 2012). *Trans*-resveratrol prevented cognitive impairment and spatial memory deficits (Kumar *et al.*, 2007).

However, in human an observational study showed that, in 800 individuals 65 years or older, an increased consumption of foods rich in resveratrol did not affect long-term health over 9 years, which may be explained by the low quantities present in foods and the low bioavailability (Semba *et al.*, 2014). There was a Phase III clinical trial (NCT00678431) to evaluate the effects of resveratrol in mild to moderate Alzheimer disease in combination with glucose and malate, with no report of results.

10.4 Modulatory effect of diet pattern on age-associated cognitive decline

Accumulating evidence supports the hypothesis that, rather than single nutrients, what is most beneficial for the brain is a balanced diet with an ideal combination of different vital compounds (Caracciolo *et al.*, 2014). Even among randomized clinical trials on the effect of anti-oxidant vitamin supplementation and cognitive decline, the outcomes of tests that included supplementation that consisted of a mixture of anti-oxidants were the most successful (Kesse-Guyot *et al.*, 2012; Summers *et al.*, 2010).

In the same line of thought, epidemiological studies focused on consumption of groups of anti-oxidant-rich foods such as vegetables and fruit were far more successful than studies that focused on single compounds (Caracciolo *et al.*, 2014). A systematic review (Loef & Walach, 2012) identified nine longitudinal studies that investigated the correlation between the development of mild cognitive impairment, dementia or cognitive decline and the consumption of fruit and vegetables. A total of 44,004 participants were followed over time and in eight out of nine of the studies there was found a negative association of intake of fruit and vegetables, or of vegetables alone, with the development of cognitive decline, dementia or mild cognitive impairment. However, one report that exposed a decline in executive functioning in individuals with the highest category of vegetable intake (Loef & Walach, 2012).

These apparent protective effects of the vegetables toward cognitive decline may be mediated by the polyphenolic compounds. The PAQUID Study (meaning "Personnes Agées QUID"), was one of the first epidemiological studies (3777 individuals aged 65 years or older who have been studied since 1988 in southwestern France) to suggest that flavonoids may have a protective role against cognitive decline and Alzheimer disease (Commenges *et al.*, 2000; Letenneur *et al.*, 2007; Schaffer *et al.*, 2012). More recent findings from the SU.VI.MAX (Supplementation with Vitamins and Mineral Antioxidants) study confirm earlier results, showing an association between total polyphenol intake and better performance in language and verbal memory tasks (Kesse-Guyot *et al.*, 2012). However, other studies, in particular the Rotterdam study, have reported that dietary intake levels of vitamin C, β-carotene and flavonoids are not associated with dementia risk or Alzheimer disease (Devore *et al.*, 2010). In addition to the anti-oxidant abundance, vegetables may also have a neuroregulatory role owing to the induction of satiety, leading to reduction of the risk of obesity (Panickar, 2013), a major risk factor for cognitive decline and dementia. Vegetables could also influence gut microbiota, which have been found to be associated with insulin regulation and obesity and ultimately with cognitive decline progression (Caracciolo *et al.*, 2014).

Specific dietary patterns may be even more beneficial than high consumption of individual food items. The Mediterranean diet is by far the most studied dietary pattern in relation to the maintenance of brain health (Valls-Pedret & Ros, 2013; Sofi *et al.*, 2013; Caracciolo *et al.*, 2014; Gotsis *et al.*, 2014). In fact, this pattern of diet includes most of the individual nutrients and food items that have been associated with reduced rates of cognitive decline and mild cognitive impairment and dementia, that is, fruit and vegetables (rich in anti-oxidants, including polyphenols), olive oil (rich of unsaturated fatty acids, vitamin E and polyphenols) and fish (rich in fatty acids and also vitamin B_{12} and selenium). Moreover, the components of a diet may be involved in numerous synergistic and antagonist interactions (Gotsis *et al.*, 2014). In the last few years the tendency for epidemiological studies has been to evaluate the adherence of populations to the Mediterranean diet using diet indices (Milá-Villarroel *et al.*, 2011). The Mediterranean diet indices summarize the diet by means of a single score that results from a function of different components, such as food, food groups or a combination of foods and nutrients (Bach *et al.*, 2006). Moreover, these indices are also useful tools to measure food consumption trends and to identify the factors involved (Bach *et al.*, 2006). The indices are further used to define the associations between the Mediterranean diet and health parameters (Behrens *et al.*, 2013).

Concerning the effects in brain health, higher adherence to a Mediterranean diet was associated with reduced cognitive decline (Caracciolo *et al.*, 2014). A recent meta-analysis, the EPIC-Greece cohort (European Prospective Investigation into Cancer and Nutrition), analyzed the association between adherence to the Mediterranean diet and cognitive impairment, Parkinson disease and depression (Psaltopoulos *et al.*, 2013). In a total of 732 men and women, 60 years or older, residing in the Attica region of Greece, sociodemographic, anthropometric, medical, dietary and lifestyle variables were ascertained at enrolment (1993–99). Six to 13 years later, cognitive function was evaluated and partial data analysis showed that a high adherence to the Mediterranean diet significantly reduced the risk of ischemic stroke, cognitive impairment, dementia and Alzheimer disease. Adherence to this diet pattern also protected against depression, independently of age, but the benefits of moderate adherence have a tendency to reduce with the advancement of age (Psaltopoulos *et al.*, 2013). A similar result was found in the Predimed-Navarra, a randomized trial (Martínez-Lapiscina *et al.*, 2013). The results of this primary prevention nutrition interventional trial conducted in older subjects living in Spain ($n=7477$) at high risk of cardiovascular disease demonstrated that diets supplemented with extra-virgin olive oil or mixed nuts during almost 5 years reduced the incidence of cardiovascular disease by 30%, compared with a low-fat control diet. Stroke risk was reduced by 34% (with the olive oil diet) and by 49% (mixed nuts diet). A subgroup of subjects who were asymptomatic but at high vascular risk ($n=522$) subjected to the diets enhanced with either olive oil or mixed nuts appeared to have improved cognition when examined after 6.5 years of nutritional intervention compared with counterparts on the control diet. Also, urinary polyphenols metabolite excretion in these individuals was associated with better scores in immediate verbal memory (Valls-Pedret *et al.*, 2012; Martínez-Lapiscina *et al.*, 2013).

Part of the InCHIANTI Study (Invecchiare in Chianti, aging in the Chianti area), a prospective population-based study of older persons in Tuscany, Italy, including 935 men and women aged 65 years and older, demonstrated that adherence to the Mediterranean diet resulted in a slower decline of mobility over time in community-dwelling older persons (Milaneschi *et al.*, 2011). In this cohort, cognition was evaluated in several studies (Harries *et al.*, 2012).

Lourida *et al.* (2013) performed a review of 12 published studies associating the Mediterranean diet and cognitive outcome: eight concerning cognitive functions; four related to mild cognitive impairment; and seven concerning dementia, particularly Alzheimer disease. Despite the heterogeneity of the studies and some contradictory findings, the results show that the Mediterranean Diet may have no effect on mild cognitive impairment but may decrease the cognitive decline and reduce the risk of developing Alzheimer disease (Lourida *et al.*, 2013; Valls-Pedret *et al.*, 2012). More recently, an observational study from Samieri *et al.* (2013) showed no association of the Mediterranean diet and cognitive scores, or their changes over 4 years, in a large sample of US elderly women. However, as usual in non-Mediterranean countries, the use of olive oil was minimal (Samieri *et al.*, 2013). In a French study with 3083 middle-aged subjects (participants of the SU.VI.MAX study), it was found that midlife adherence to a Mediterranean diet pattern was not associated with improved global cognitive performance assessed 13 years later (Kesse-Guyot *et al.*, 2013). Sofi *et al.* (2013) performed two meta-analyses, demonstrating the protective effect of adherence to the Mediterranean diet in relation to neurodegenerative diseases. The first analysis demonstrated that adherence to this type of diet resulted in a 13% reduction in the risk of suffering from these diseases (Sofi *et al.*, 2008), confirmed two years later in an updated meta-analysis (Sofi *et al.*, 2010).

A large randomized controlled trial of dietary patterns and health based on the Mediterranean diet called NU-AGE [acronym for "New dietary strategies addressing the specific needs of elderly population for a healthy ageing in Europe (Nutrition)"] is ongoing. It is an ambitious 9 million euro European multicenter study, involving 30 partners from 16 European Union countries, focused on aged adults and including in-depth molecular and cognitive assessments (Santoro *et al.*, 2014). The rationale of this study is that one year of the Mediterranean whole diet will reduce inflammation and will have beneficial effects on physical and cognitive health of fully characterized subjects aged 65–79 years (Santoro *et al.*, 2014).

The inconsistencies of the various outcomes may be due to methodological issues, as the dietary composition is heterogeneous across studies. Several methodological challenges should be overcome to provide a higher level of evidence supporting the development of nutritional policies to prevent cognitive decline and Alzheimer disease. All of these results, mostly from observational studies, claim the necessity of additional randomized clinical trials. Meanwhile, there is enough scientific evidence to recommend the Mediterranean diet "to anybody who wishes to age in good health while enjoying their food" (Valls-Pedret & Ros, 2013).

10.5 Multidomain interventions

The inconsistent findings and the difficulty of finding strong effects in single intervention trials may be due partially to limitations of the methodology. Another hypothesis is that the isolated interventions approaches are too simplistic with regard to the complex and multifactorial nature of cognitive impairment and dementia (Schneider & Yvon, 2013). In fact, genetic, biological and psychosocial risk factors interact with protective factors in lifelong cumulative effects, but age emerges as the strongest risk factor for dementia (Schneider & Yvon, 2013).

There have been three completed trials that included diet-related interventions associated with exercise, social programs or program weight management (Schneider & Yvon, 2013). De Jong *et al.* (2001) found no effect on cognition following enriched food (containing multiple micronutrients: 25–100% of the Dutch recommended dietary allowances), associated with exercise or a social program. In line with this, Cetin *et al.* (2010) found no effect of vitamin E supplementation on cognitive outcomes and exercise based on event-related brain potentials and P3 latency evaluation. The Dietary Approaches to Stop Hypertension (DASH) trial studied a subgroup from the Exercise and Nutrition Interventions for Cardiovascular Health (ENCORE) study (Smith *et al.*, 2010). A total of 124 overweight individuals with elevated blood pressure received the DASH intervention diet or DASH diet plus behavioral weight management intervention, including exercise and energy restriction (1600 calories per day) for a period of 4 months. The study results demonstrated improved executive function memory and learning results and improved psychomotor speed for DASH plus weight management intervention, while the DASH diet alone did not show improvement when compared with usual care patients, used as controls (Schneider & Yvon, 2013; Smith *et al.*, 2010). Eight multidomain intervention trials targeting cognition including nutritional guidance, cognitive training and several types of exercise are ongoing (Schneider & Yvon, 2013). However, there are many challenges to this type of intervention as individuals willing to modify their lifestyle factors are likely to have a higher level of education than the general population and better overall health, and behavioral changes cannot be evaluated with precision (Schneider & Yvon, 2013). In addition, it is difficult to define a good control group regarding physical and cognitive interventions. Finally, double-blind interventions are not possible. Changes in lifestyle and nutritional habits are difficult, requiring high levels of individual effort, but they may be a cost-effective, safe and sustainable solution for the prevention of age-associated diseases, and in particular cognitive impairment (Schneider & Yvon, 2013).

More importantly, because behavioral adherence is more important than diet composition, the best approach would be to counsel patients to choose a dietary plan that they find easy to adhere to in the long term (Pagoto & Appelhans, 2013).

10.6 Conclusions

The risk of developing chronic illness, poor mental health and neurodegenerative diseases tends to increase in the ageing population of the world. The consumption of functional foods such as green tea or some related nutraceuticals may be advised. However, compared with single-food methods, the whole-diet or dietary pattern approach is more interesting for several reasons. In particular, dietary quality, focused on healthful foods and dietary patterns rather than single nutrients, presents an important role in the prevention of cognitive decline. The available data suggest that the Mediterranean diet could be used as a preventive strategy in early intervention schemes. In fact, this diet may improve cognitive functions, lower the risk of disabilities and provide better mental and physical health in elderly people. The multidomain approach has also shown some promising results, but more studies are needed and adherence to a change of lifestyle should be emphasized and obtained to achieve the best effects of this intervention.

Acknowledgment

This work was supported by National Funds through Fundação para a Ciência e a Tecnologia within the scope of the Strategic Project Centro de Morfologia Experimental (CME/FM/UP) – 2011-2012, Project PEst-OE/SAU/UI0121/2011 and Center for Health Technology and Service Research (CINTESIS).

References

Abd El Mohsen, M. M., G. Kuhnle, A. R. Rechner, H. Schroeter, S. Rose, P. Jenner, and C. A. Rice-Evans. 2002. Uptake and metabolism of epicatechin and its access to the brain after oral ingestion. *Free Radic. Biol. Med.* 33:1693–1702.

Andrade, J. P. and M. Assunção. 2012. Protective effects of chronic green tea consumption on age-related neurodegeneration. *Curr. Pharma Des.* 18:4–14.

Assunção, M., M. J. Santos-Marques, F. Carvalho, and J. P. Andrade. 2010. Green tea averts age-dependent decline of hippocampal signaling systems related to antioxidant defenses and survival. *Free Radic. Biol. Med.* 48:831–838.

Assunção, M., M. J. Santos-Marques, F. Carvalho, N. V. Lukoyanov, and J. P. Andrade. 2011. Chronic green tea consumption prevents age-related changes in rat hippocampal formation. *Neurobiol. Aging* 32:707–717.

Ayoub, S. and M. F. Melzig. 2006. Induction of neutral endopeptidase (NEP) activity of SK-N-SH cells by natural compounds from green tea. *J. Pharm. Pharmacol.* 58:495–501.

Bach, A., L. Serra-Majem, J. L. Carrasco, B. Roman, J. Ngo, I. Bertomeu, and B. Obrador. 2006. The use of indexes evaluating the adherence to the Mediterranean diet in epidemiological studies: a review. *Public Health Nutr.* 9(1A):132–146.

Barnes, D. E. and K. Yaffe. 2011. The projected effect of risk factor reduction on Alzheimer's disease prevalence. *Lancet Neurol.* 10:819–828.

Baur, J. A. and D. A. Sinclair. 2006. Therapeutic potential of resveratrol: the in vivo evidence. *Nat. Rev. Drug Discov.* 5:493–506.

Behrens, G., B. Fischer, S. Kohler, Y. Park, A. R. Hollenbeck, and M. F. Leitzmann MF. 2013. Healthy lifestyle behaviors and decreased risk of mortality in a large prospective study of U.S. women and men. *Eur. J. Epidemiol.*28:361–372.

Bjelakovic, G. and C. Gluud. 2007. Surviving antioxidant supplements. *J. Natl Cancer Inst.* 99:742–743.

Blennow, K., M. J. de Leon, H. Zetterberg. 2006. Alzheimer's disease. *Lancet* 368:387–403.

Calabrese, V., C. Cornelius, A. T. Dinkova-Kostova, E. J. Calabrese, and M. P. Mattson MP. 2010. Cellular stress responses, the hormesis paradigm, and vitagenes: novel targets for therapeutic intervention in neurodegenerative disorders. *Antioxid. Redox Signal.* 13:1763–1811.

Caracciolo, B., W. Xu, S. Collins, and L. Fratiglioni. 2014. Cognitive decline, dietary factors and gut–brain interactions. *Mech. Ageing Dev.* 136–137:59–69.

Carneiro, A., M. Assunção, V. De Freitas, M. M. Paula-Barbosa, and J. P. Andrade. 2008. Red Wine, but not port wine, protects rat hippocampal dentate gyrus against ethanol-induced neuronal damage – relevance of the sugar content. *Alcohol Alcohol.* 43:408–415.

Cetin, E., E. C. Top, G. Sahin, Y. G. Ozkaya, H. Aydin, and F. Toraman. 2010. Effect of vitamin E supplementation with exercise on cognitive functions and total antioxidant capacity in older people. *J. Nutr. Health Aging* 14:763–769.

Checkoway, H., K. Powers, T. Smith-Weller, G. M. Franklin, W. T. Longstreth Jr, and P. D. Swanson. 2002. *Am. J. Epidemiol.* 155:732–738.

Chen, C., R. Yu, E. D. Owuor, and A. N. Kong. 2000. Activation of antioxidant-response element (ARE), mitogen-activated protein kinases (MAPKs) and caspases by major green tea polyphenol components during cell survival and death. *Arch. Pharm. Res.* 23:605–612.

Clement, Y. 2009. Can green tea do that? A literature review of the clinical evidence. *Prev. Med.* 49: 83–87.

Commenges, D., V. Scotet, S. Renaud, H. Jacqmin-Gadda, P. Barberger-Gateau, and J. F. Dartigues. 2000. Intake of flavonoids and risk of dementia. *Eur. J. Epidemiol.* 16:357–363.

Dadhaniya, P., C. Patel, J. Muchhara, N. Bhadja, N. Mathuria, K. Vachhani, and M. G. Soni. 2011. Safety assessment of a solid lipid curcumin particle preparation: acute and subchronic toxicity studies. *Food Chem. Toxicol.* 49:1834–1842.

Daffner, K. R. 2010. Promoting successful cognitive aging: a comprehensive review. *J. Alzheimers Dis.* 19:1101–1122.

Davinelli, S., N. Sapere, D. Zella, R. Bracale, M. Intrieri, and G. Scapagnini. 2012. Pleiotropic protective effects of phytochemicals in Alzheimer's disease. *Oxid. Med. Cell. Longev.* 2012:386527.

de Jong, N., M. J. Chin A Paw, and L. C. de Groot. 2001. Nutrient-dense foods and exercise in frail elderly: effects on B vitamins, homocysteine, methylmalonic acid, and neuropsychological functioning. *Am. J. Clin. Nutr.* 73:338–346.

Del Rio, D., L. Calani, C. Cordero, S. Salvatore, N. Pellegrini, and F. Brighenti. 2010. Bioavailability and catabolism of green tea flavan-3-ols in humans. *Nutrition* 26:1110–1116.

Devore, E. E., F. Grodstein, F. J. van Rooij, A. Hofman, M. J. Stampfer, J. C. Witteman, and M. M. Breteler. 2010. Dietary antioxidants and long-term risk of dementia. *Arch. Neurol.* 67:819–825.

Erba, D., P. Riso, A. Bordoni, P. Foti, P. L. Biagi, and G. Testolin. 2005. Effectiveness of moderate green tea consumption on antioxidative status and plasma lipid profile in humans. *J. Nutr. Biochem.* 16:144–149.

Esiri, M. M. 2007. Ageing and the brain. *J. Pathol.* 211:181–187.

Faria, A., D. Pestana, D. Teixeira, J. Azevedo, V. De Freitas, N. Mateus, and C. Calhau. 2010. Flavonoid transport across RBE4 cells: a blood–brain barrier model. *Cell Mol Biol Lett* 15:234–241.

Faria, A., D. Pestana, D. Teixeira, P. O. Couraud, I. Romero, B. Weksler, V. de Freitas, N. Mateus, and C. Calhau. 2011. Insights into the putative catechin and epicatechin transport across blood–brain barrier. *Food Funct.* 2:39–44.

Ferreira, N., S. A. Santos, M. R. Domingues, M. J. Saraiva, and M. R. Almeida. 2013. Dietary curcumin counteracts extracellular transthyretin deposition: insights on the mechanism of amyloid inhibition. *Biochim. Biophys. Acta* 1832:39–45.

Floyd, R. A. and K. Hensley. 2002. Oxidative stress in brain aging. Implications for therapeutics of neurodegenerative diseases. *Neurobiol. Aging* 23:795–807.

Ganguli, M., V. Chandra, M. I. Kamboh, J. M. Johnston, H. H. Dodge, B. K. Thelma, R. C. Juyal, R. Pandav, S. H. Belle, and S. T. DeKosky. 2000. Apolipoprotein E polymorphism and Alzheimer disease: the Indo-US Cross-National Dementia Study. *Arch. Neurol.* 57:824–830.

González-Sarrías, A., M. Larrosa, M. T. García-Conesa, F. A. Tomás-Barberán, and J. C. Espín. 2013. Nutraceuticals for older people: facts, fictions and gaps in knowledge. *Maturitas* 75:313–334.

Gotsis, E. P. Anagnostis, A. Mariolis, A. Vlachou, N. Katsiki, and A. Karagiannis. 2014. Health benefits of the Mediterranean diet: an update of research over the last 5 years. *Angiology*, in press.

Halliwell, B. 2006. Oxidative stress and neurodegeneration: where are we now? *J. Neurochem.* 97:1634–1658.

Harman, D. 2006. Free radical theory of aging: an update: increasing the functional life span. *Ann. NY Acad. Sci.* 1067:10–21.

Harries, L. W., R. M. Bradley-Smith, D. J. Llewellyn, L. C. Pilling, A. Fellows, W. Henley, D. Hernandez, J. M. Guralnik, S. Bandinelli, A. Singleton, L. Ferrucci, and D. Melzer. 2012. Leukocyte CCR2 expression is associated with mini-mental state examination score in older adults. *Rejuvenation Res.* 15:395–404.

Higdon, J. V. and B. Frei. 2003. Tea catechins and polyphenols: health effects, metabolism, and antioxidant functions. *Crit. Rev. Food Sci. Nutr.* 43:89–143.

Hu, G., S. Bidel, P. Jousilahti, R. Antikainen, and J. Tuomilehto. 2007. Coffee and tea consumption and the risk of Parkinson's disease. *Mov. Disord.* 22:2242–2248.

Ishige, K., D. Schubert, and Y. Sagara. 2001. Flavonoids protect neuronal cells from oxidative stress by three distinct mechanisms. *Free Radic. Biol. Med.* 30:433–446.

Jones, D. P. 2006. Redefining oxidative stress. *Antioxid. Redox Signal.* 8:1865–1879.

Kalfon, L., M. B. Youdim, and S. A. Mandel. 2007. Green tea polyphenol (−)-epigallocatechin-3-gallate promotes the rapid protein kinase C- and proteasome-mediated degradation of Bad: implications for neuroprotection. *J. Neurochem.* 100:992–1002.

Kang, K. S., Y. Wen, N. Yamabe, M. Fukui, S. C. Bishop, and B. T. Zhu. 2010. Dual beneficial effects of (−)-epigallocatechin-3-gallate on levodopa methylation and hippocampal neurodegeneration: in vitro and in vivo studies. *PloS One* 5(8): e11951.

Kang, KS, N. Yamabe, Y. Wen, M. Fukui, and B. T. Zhu. 2013. Beneficial effects of natural phenolics on levodopa methylation and oxidative neurodegeneration. *Brain Res.* 1497:1–14.

Kesse-Guyot, E., L. Fezeu, A. Andreeva, M. Touvier, A. Scalbert, S. Hercberg, and P. Galan. 2012. Total and specific polyphenol intakes in midlife are associated with cognitive function measured 13 years later. *J. Nutr.* 142:76–83.

Kesse-Guyot, E., V. A. Andreeva, C. Lassale, M. Ferry, C Jeandel, S. Hercberg S, P. Galan, and SU.VI.MAX 2 Research Group. 2013. Mediterranean diet and cognitive function: a French study. *Am. J. Clin. Nutr.* 97:369–376.

Kim, C. K., C. Lee, G. H. Park, and J. H. Jang. 2009. Neuroprotective effect of (−)-epigallocatechin-3-gallate against β-amyloid-induced oxidative and nitrosative cell death via augmentation of antioxidant defense capacity. *Arch. Pharm. Res.* 32:869–881.

Kim, J., H. J. Lee, and K. W. Lee. 2010. Naturally occurring phytochemicals for the prevention of Alzheimer's disease. *J. Neurochem.* 112:1415–1430.

Kumar, A., P. S. Naidu, N. Seghal, and S. S. Padi. 2007. Neuroprotective effects of resveratrol against intracerebroventricular colchicine-induced cognitive impairment and oxidative stress in rats. *Pharmacology* 79:17–26.

Kuriyama, S., A. Hozawa, K. Ohmori, T. Shimazu, T. Matsui, S. Ebihara, S. Awata, R. Nagatomi, H. Arai, and I. Tsuji. 2006. Green tea consumption and cognitive function: a cross-sectional study from the Tsurugaya Project 1. *Am. J. Clin. Nutr.* 83:355–361.

Lee, J. W., Y. K. Lee, J. O. Ban, T. Y. Ha, Y. P. Yun, S. B. Han, K. W. Oh, and J. T. Hong. 2009. Green tea (−)-epigallocatechin-3-gallate inhibits β-amyloid-induced cognitive dysfunction through modification of secretase activity via inhibition of ERK and NF-κB pathways in mice. *J. Nutr.* 139:1987–1993.

Letenneur, L., C. Proust-Lima, A. Le Gouge, J. F. Dartigues, and P. Barberger-Gateau. 2007. Flavonoid intake and cognitive decline over a 10-year period. *Am. J. Epidemiol.* 165:1364–1371.

Levites, Y., O. Weinreb, G. Maor, M. B. Youdim, and S. Mandel. 2001. Green tea polyphenol (−)-epigallocatechin-3-gallate prevents *N*-methyl-4-phenyl-1,2,3,6-tetrahydropyridine-induced dopaminergic neurodegeneration. *J. Neurochem.* 78:1073–1082.

Lim, G. P., Chu T., Yang F., W. Beech, S. A. Frautschy, and G. M. Cole. 2001. The curry spice curcumin reduces oxidative damage and amyloid pathology in an Alzheimer transgenic mouse. *J. Neurosci.* 21: 8370–8377.

Lin, L. C., M. N. Wang, T. Y. Tseng, J. S. Sung, and T. H. Tsai. 2007. Pharmacokinetics of (−)-epigallocatechin-3-gallate in conscious and freely moving rats and its brain regional distribution. *J. Agric. Food Chem.* 55:1517–1524.

Loef, M. and H. Walach. 2012. Fruit, vegetables and prevention of cognitive decline or dementia: a systematic review of cohort studies. *J. Nutr. Health Aging* 16:626–630.

Lourida, I., M. Soni, J. Thompson-Coon, N. Purandare, I. A. Lang, O. C. Ukoumunne, and D. J. Llewellyn. 2013. Mediterranean diet, cognitive function, and dementia: a systematic review. *Epidemiology* 24:479–489.

Macready, A. L., O. B. Kennedy, J. A. Ellis, C. M. Williams, J. P. Spencer JP, and T. L. Butler. 2009. Flavonoids and cognitive function: a review of human randomized controlled trial studies and recommendations for future studies. *Genes Nutr.* 4:227–242.

Manach, C., A. Scalbert, C. Morand, C. Rémésy, and L. Jiménez. 2004. Polyphenols: food sources and bioavailability. *Am. J. Clin. Nutr.* 79:727–747.

Mandel, S., T. Amit, L. Reznichenko, O. Weinreb, M. B. Youdim. 2006. Green tea catechins as brain-permeable, natural iron chelators-antioxidants for the treatment of neurodegenerative disorders. *Mol. Nutr Food Res.* 50:229–234.

Martínez-Lapiscina, E. H., P. Clavero, E. Toledo, R. Estruch, J. Salas-Salvadó, B. San Julián, A. Sanchez-Tainta, E. Ros, C. Valls-Pedret, and M. Á. Martinez-Gonzalez. 2013. Mediterranean diet improves cognition: the PREDIMED-NAVARRA randomised trial. *J. Neurol. Neurosurg. Psychiatry* 84:1318–1325.

Masoro, E. J. 2001. Physiology of aging. *Int. J. Sport Nutr. Exerc. Metab.* 11 Suppl:S218–222.

McKay, D. L. and J. B. Blumberg. 2002. The role of tea in human health: an update. *J. Am. Coll. Nutr.* 21:1–13.

Milaneschi, Y., S. Bandinelli, A. M. Corsi, F. Lauretani, G. Paolisso, L. J. Dominguez, R. D. Semba, T. Tanaka, A. M. Abbatecola, S. A. Talegawkar, J. M. Guralnik, and L. Ferrucci. 2011. Mediterranean diet and mobility decline in older persons. *Exp. Gerontol.* 46:303–308.

Milà-Villarroel, R., A. Bach-Faig, J. Puig, A. Puchal, A. Farran, L. Serra-Majem, and J. L. Carrasco. 2011. Comparison and evaluation of the reliability of indexes of adherence to the Mediterranean diet. *Public Health Nutr.* 14:2338–2345.

Neves, D., M. Assunção, F. Marques, J. P. Andrade, and H. Almeida. 2008. Does regular consumption of green tea influence expression of vascular endothelial growth factor and its receptor in aged rat erectile tissue? Possible implications for vasculogenic erectile dysfunction progression. *Age (Dordr.)* 30:217–228.

Okello, E. J., S. U. Savelev, and E. K. Perry. 2004. *In vitro* anti-β-secretase and dual anti-cholinesterase activities of *Camellia sinensis L.* (tea) relevant to treatment of dementia. *Phytother. Res.* 18:624–627.

Ono, K., K. Hasegawa, H. Naiki, and M. Yamada. 2004. Curcumin has potent anti-amyloidogenic effects for Alzheimer's β-amyloid fibrils *in vitro*. *J. Neurosci. Res.* 75:742–750.

Pagoto, S. L. and B. M. Appelhans. 2013. A call for an end to the diet debates. *JAMA* 310:687–688.

Palhano, F. L., J. Lee, N. P. Grimster, and J. W. Kelly. 2013. Toward the Molecular Mechanism(s) by which EGCG treatment remodels mature amyloid fibrils. *J. Am. Chem. Soc.* 135:7503–7510.

Palmer, K., L. Bäckman, B. Winblad, and L. Fratiglioni. 2008. Mild cognitive impairment in the general population: occurrence and progression to Alzheimer disease. *Am. J. Geriatr. Psychiatry* 16:603–611.

Panickar, K. S. 2013. Effects of dietary polyphenols on neuroregulatory factors and pathways that mediate food intake and energy regulation in obesity. *Mol. Nutr. Food Res.* 57:34–47.

Panza, V. S., E. Wazlawik, G. Ricardo Schutz, L. Comin, K. C. Hecht, and E. L. da Silva. 2008. Consumption of green tea favorably affects oxidative stress markers in weight-trained men. *Nutrition* 24:433–442.

Petersen, R. C. 2011. Clinical practice. Mild cognitive impairment. *New Engl. J. Med.* 364:2227–2234.

Prince, M., R. Bryce, E. Albanese, A. Wimo A, W. Ribeiro, and C. P. Ferri. 2013. The global prevalence of dementia: a systematic review and metaanalysis. *Alzheimers Dement.* 9:63–75 e2.

Psaltopoulou, T., T. N. Sergentanis, D. B. Panagiotakos, I. N. Sergentanis, R. Kosti, and N. Scarmeas. 2013. Mediterranean diet, stroke, cognitive impairment, and depression: a meta-analysis. *Ann. Neurol.* 74:580–591.

Qiu, L., J. Sautter, and D. Gu. 2012. Associations between frequency of tea consumption and health and mortality: evidence from old Chinese. *Br. J. Nutr.* 108:1686–1697.

Ramsewak, R. S., D. L. DeWitt, and M. G. Nair. 2000. Cytotoxicity, antioxidant and anti-inflammatory activities of curcumins I–III from *Curcuma longa*. *Phytomedicine* 7:303–308.

Ras, R. T., P. L. Zock, and R. Draijer. 2011. Tea consumption enhances endothelial-dependent vasodilation; a meta-analysis. *PloS One* 6:e16974.

Rezai-Zadeh, K., D. Shytle, N. Sun, T. Mori, H. Hou, D. Jeanniton, J. Ehrhart, K. Townsend, J. Zeng, D. Morgan, J. Hardy, T. Town, and J. Tan. 2005. Green tea epigallocatechin-3-gallate (EGCG) modulates amyloid precursor protein cleavage and reduces cerebral amyloidosis in Alzheimer transgenic mice. *J. Neurosci.* 25:8807–8814.

Rietveld, A. and S. Wiseman. 2003. Antioxidant effects of tea: evidence from human clinical trials. *J. Nutr.* 133:3285S–3292S.

Ringman, J. M., S. A. Frautschy, G. M. Cole, D. L. Masterman, and J. L Cummings. 2005. A potential role of the curry spice curcumin in Alzheimer's disease. *Curr. Alzheimer Res.* 2:131–136.

Román, G. C. 2003. Vascular dementia: distinguishing characteristics, treatment, and prevention. *J. Am. Geriatr. Soc.* 51(5 Suppl Dementia):S296–304.

Rowe, J. W. and R. L. Kahn. 1997. Successful aging. *Gerontologist* 37:433–440.

Saiko, P., A. Szakmary, W. Jaeger, and T. Szekeres. 2008. Resveratrol and its analogs: defense against cancer, coronary disease and neurodegenerative maladies or just a fad? *Mutat. Res.* 658:68–94.

Samieri, C., F. Grodstein, B. A. Rosner, J. H. Kang, N. R. Cook, J. E. Manson, J. E. Buring, W. C. Willett, and O. I. Okereke. 2013. Mediterranean diet and cognitive function in older age. *Epidemiology* 24:490–499.

Santoro, A., E. Pini, M. Scurti, G. Palmas, A. Berendsen, A. Brzozowska, B. Pietruszka, A. Szczecinska, N. Cano, N. Meunier, C. P. de Groot, E. Feskens, S. Fairweather-Tait, S. Salvioli, M. Capri, P. Brigidi, C. Franceschi, and NU-AGE Consortium. 2014. Combating inflammaging through a Mediterranean whole diet approach: the NU-AGE project's conceptual framework and design. *Mech. Ageing Dev.* 136–137:3–13.

Schaffer, S. and B. Halliwell. 2012. Do polyphenols enter the brain and does it matter? Some theoretical and practical considerations. *Genes Nutr.* 7:99–109.

Schaffer, S., H. Asseburg, S. Kuntz, W. E. Muller, and G. P. Eckert. 2012. Effects of polyphenols on brain ageing and Alzheimer's disease: focus on mitochondria. *Mol. Neurobiol.* 46:161–178.

Scheepens, A., K. Tan, and J. W. Paxton. 2010. Improving the oral bioavailability of beneficial polyphenols through designed synergies. *Genes Nutr.* 5:75–87.

Schneider, N. and C. Yvon. 2013. A review of multidomain interventions to support healthy cognitive ageing. *J. Nutr. Health Aging* 17:252–257.

Schroeter, H., C. Boyd, J. P. Spencer, R. J. Williams, E. Cadenas, and C. Rice-Evans. 2002. MAPK signaling in neurodegeneration: influences of flavonoids and of nitric oxide. *Neurobiol. Aging* 23:861–880.

Semba, R. D., L. Ferrucci, B. Bartali, M. Urpí-Sarda, R. Zamora-Ros, K. Sun, A. Cherubini, Bandinelli, and C. Andres-Lacueva. 2014. Resveratrol levels and all-cause mortality in older community-dwelling adults. *JAMA Intern. Med.*, 174:1077–1084.

Shah, Z. A., R. C. Li, A S. Ahmad, T. W. Kensler, M. Yamamoto, S. Biswal, and S. Doré. 2010. The flavanol (−)-epicatechin prevents stroke damage through the Nrf2/HO1 pathway. *J. Cereb. Blood Flow Metab.* 30:1951–1961.

Sharma, R. A., A. J. Gescher, and W. P. Steward. 2005. Curcumin: the story so far. *Eur. J. Cancer* 41:1955–1968.

Smith, P. J., J. A. Blumenthal, M. A. Babyak, L. Craighead, K. A. Welsh-Bohmer, J. N. Browndyke, T. A. Strauman, and A. Sherwood. 2010. Effects of the dietary approaches to stop hypertension diet, exercise, and caloric restriction on neurocognition in overweight adults with high blood pressure. *Hypertension* 55:1331–1338.

Sofi, F., F. Cesari, R. Abbate, G. F. Gensini GF, and A. Casini. 2008. Adherence to Mediterranean diet and health status: meta-analysis. *BMJ* 337:a1344.

Sofi, F., R. Abbate, G. F. Gensini, and A. Casini. 2010. Accruing evidence on benefits of adherence to the Mediterranean diet on health: an updated systematic review and meta-analysis. *Am. J. Clin. Nutr.* 92:1189–1196.

Sofi, F., C. Macchie, and A. Casini. 2013. Mediterranean diet and minimizing neurodegeneration. *Curr. Nutr. Rep.* 2:75–80.

Song, J., H. Xu, F. Liu, and L. Feng. 2012. Tea and cognitive health in late life: current evidence and future directions. *J. Nutr. Health Aging* 16:31–34.

Spencer, J. P., H. Schroeter, A. R. Rechner, and C. Rice-Evans. 2001. *Antioxid. Redox Signal.* 3:1023–1039.

Strandberg, T. E. and D. O'Neill. 2013. Dementia – a geriatric syndrome. *Lancet* 381:533–534.

Summers, W. K., R. L. Martin, M. Cunningham, V. L. DeBoynton, and G. M. Marsh. 2010. Complex antioxidant blend improves memory in community-dwelling seniors. *J. Alzheimers Dis.* 19:429–439.

Tan, L. C., W. P. Koh, J. M. Yuan, R. Wang, W. L. Au, J. H. Tan, E. K. Tan, and M. C. Yu. 2008. Differential effects of black versus green tea on risk of Parkinson's disease in the Singapore Chinese Health Study. *Am. J. Epidemiol.*167:553–560.

Troen, B. R. 2003. The biology of aging. *Mt. Sinai J. Med.* 70:3–22.

Valls-Pedret, C. and E. Ros. 2013. Commentary: Mediterranean diet and cognitive outcomes: epidemiological evidence suggestive, randomized trials needed. *Epidemiology* 24:503–506.

Valls-Pedret, C., R. M. Lamuela-Raventós, A. Medina-Remón, M. Quintana, D. Corella, X. Pintó, M. Á. Martínez-González, R. Estruch, and E. Ros. 2012. Polyphenol-rich foods in the Mediterranean diet are associated with better cognitive function in elderly subjects at high cardiovascular risk. *J. Alzheimers Dis.* 29:773–782.

van Praag, H., M. J. Lucero, G. W. Yeo, K. Stecker, N. Heivand, C. Zhao, E. Yip, M. Afanador, H. Schroeter, J. Hammerstone, and F. H. Gage. 2007. Plant-derived flavanol (−)epicatechin enhances angiogenesis and retention of spatial memory in mice. *J. Neurosci.* 27:5869–5878.

Wang, X., M. L. Michaelis, and E. K. Michaelis. 2010. Functional genomics of brain aging and Alzheimer's disease: focus on selective neuronal vulnerability. *Curr. Genom.* 11:618–633.

Weinreb, O., S. Mandel, and M. B. Youdim. 2003. Gene and protein expression profiles of anti- and pro-apoptotic actions of dopamine, *R*-apomorphine, green tea polyphenol (−)-epigallocatechine-3-gallate, and melatonin. *Ann. NY Acad. Sci.* 993:351–361.

Williamson, G. and C. Manach. 2005. Bioavailability and bioefficacy of polyphenols in humans. II. Review of 93 intervention studies. *Am. J. Clin. Nutr.* 81:243S–255S.

Youdim, K. A. and J. A. Joseph. 2001. A possible emerging role of phytochemicals in improving age-related neurological dysfunctions: a multiplicity of effects. *Free Radic. Biol. Med.* 30:583–594.

Youdim, K. A., M. S. Dobbie, G. Kuhnle, A. R. Proteggente, N. J. Abbott, and C. Rice-Evans. 2003. Interaction between flavonoids and the blood–brain barrier: in vitro studies. *J. Neurochem.* 85:180–192.

Zini, A., D. Del Rio, A. J. Stewart, J. Mandrioli, E. Merelli, P. Sola, P. Nichelli, M. Serafini, F. Brighenti, C. A. Edwards, and A. Crozier. 2006. Do flavan-3-ols from green tea reach the human brain? *Nutr. Neurosci.* 9:57–61.

PART III

Evidence-based retardation of ageing

CHAPTER 11

Science-based anti-ageing nutritional recommendations

Inês Tomada[1] and José Paulo Andrade[2]

[1] *Department of Experimental Biology, Faculty of Medicine, and Institute for Molecular and Cell Biology, University of Porto, Porto, Portugal*

[2] *Department of Anatomy, Faculty of Medicine, University of Porto, Porto, Portugal*

11.1 Introduction

Ageing is a normal biological process that leads to a general and progressive deterioration of many tissues and organs, accompanied by the increased incidence and severity of a wide variety of chronic, incurable and often fatal diseases. Despite the inevitable nature and complexity of the process, the possibility of reducing or alleviating the manifestations of ageing, and improving the quality of life in old age, has renewed the interest of the scientific world in anti-ageing therapies. In effect, anti-ageing medicine strives to redefine ageing as a target for biomedical and scientific intervention, challenging the way ageing has been understood until now (Flatt *et al.*, 2013).

Elderly people are one of the fastest growing segments of the world population. Despite improvements in the quality of diet and nutrition, and advancements in biology, chemistry and medicine, most elderly people suffer from noncommunicable diseases, such as degenerative and cardiovascular diseases (CVD), cancer and diabetes (Pan *et al.*, 2012). Therefore, as the number of older people increases, the role of diet quality in reducing the progression of chronic diseases will become increasingly important.

While some parts of the world experience food shortages, chronic metabolic diseases have emerged from food overconsumption in other parts of the world. Both situations can result in shorter life expectancy and represent a major global health problem. Several epidemiological studies suggest not only that diet plays an important role in the treatment of different diseases, but also that the right choice of foods can help in the prevention of illness. In addition, recent scientific research provides evidence that many dietary factors have potential effects in slowing the ageing process by modulating the molecular causes of cell senescence. Thus, considering that health is under the influence of several nutrient-sensing pathways (Fontana *et al.*, 2010), the adoption of healthy nutrition throughout the lifespan is crucial for a healthy ageing. Even in old age, dietary changes should be encouraged, in order to ameliorate or improve the health status of the elderly.

Older adults tend to have more healthful and more satisfactory nutrition behaviors than do youths (Estaquio *et al.*, 2009; Knowler *et al.*, 2009). Regardless of this, the natural

Anti-Ageing Nutrients: Evidence-Based Prevention of Age-Associated Diseases, First Edition. Edited by Delminda Neves.

process of ageing influences how nutrients are used, may reduce nutrient absorption, increases the urinary nutrient loss and alters normal pathways of nutrient metabolism (Shatenstein, 2008). Although these changes can be compensated for to some extent by a nutrient-dense diet that remains within energy needs, a substantial portion of the aged population fails to meet the recommended intakes of food groups and/or specific nutrients (Dabhade & Kotwal, 2013). Despite the need to target recommendations for nutrient supplements to certain segments of the population (e.g. the elderly), there are insufficient data to justify an alteration in public health policy from one that emphasizes food and diet to one that highlights nutritional supplements (Lichtenstein & Russell, 2005). Indeed, the most promising data in the area of nutrition and positive health outcomes relate to dietary patterns, and not to nutritional supplements (Marra & Boyar, 2009).

11.2 The relevance of nutraceuticals and functional nutrients in anti-ageing medicine

The distinction between food and medicines is becoming increasingly blurred. In the last few years knowledge of the relation between diet and health has increased and a new trend in the anti-ageing industry has emerged. The terms "nutraceutical", "designer foods" and "pharmafoods" have appeared in the general society and ordinary food stores and these are considered to be the "foods of the future" (Vainio & Mutanen, 2000). The term "nutraceutical" was first introduced by Stephen Defelice, combining "nutrition" and "pharmaceutical", being defined as "a food (or part of a food) that provides medical or health benefits, including the prevention and/or treatment of a disease" (Kalra, 2003). Afterwards, more definitions appeared, but always considering nutraceuticals as food, food components or nutrients, providing health or physiological benefits beyond the basic nutritional value of the product (González-Sarrías *et al.*, 2013).

In a recent paper, González-Sarrías *et al.* (2013) tried to characterize more precisely what is a "nutraceutical" after a revision of the different definitions provided by the European Nutraceutical Association, American Nutraceutical Association, Health Canada, European Food Safety Authority (EFSA) and the US Food and Drug Administration (FDA). Also they attempted to differentiate these from similar concepts such as "functional foods". In this view, "functional foods" are those "that exert a scientifically proven specific health benefit (health claim) beyond their nutritional properties", presented as a food or fortified beverages, juices, milk, etc. (González-Sarrías *et al.*, 2013).

"Dietary (food) supplements" are defined as products consumed in a pharmaceutical format (pill, tablet, powder, etc.) to complement the diet. Dietary or food supplements can be further divided into medical foods, botanicals and nutraceuticals. "Medical foods" are formulated specifically to provide certain nutrients to patients under medical supervision. They are used in cancer or metabolic disorder treatment, for example. "Botanicals" are from nonfood origin and are not essential to human life, but have some possible actions on human health. Ginseng and gingko extracts are examples of these. Finally, "nutraceutical" is a product that delivers a concentrated form (extract, purified compounds or combinations) of a presumed bioactive agent or bioactive agents from food origin. The dose of these compounds must be superior to that one obtained from normal foods in a balanced diet (González-Sarrías *et al.*, 2013). In addition, nutraceuticals are used with the objective of enhancing health, including the prevention, delay or improvement of diseases, or complementing pharmacological therapy under medical supervision. A caveat is that nutraceuticals should not be used to treat diseases. Capsules of grape extract with high doses of resveratrol, tomato extract rich in lycopene or purified lutein are some examples of nutraceuticals (González-Sarrías *et al.*, 2013).

This definition, although complete, needs further considerations (a) the bioactive agent in a nutraceutical can be present in a dose achieved through diet, but it must present features to enhance the absorption and/or the physiological effect; (b) isolated compounds can be used in nutraceuticals only if they are present in foods; and (c) vitamins, minerals, amino acids and other nutrients or micronutrients only will become nutraceuticals when dosage superior to the recommended daily allowance (RDA) is related to a beneficial effect (González-Sarrías *et al.*, 2013).

The difference between "functional food" and "nutraceutical" may be not very clear in some cases (Espín *et al.*, 2007). For example, a phytochemical dissolved in a certain amount of juice is a potential "functional food". However, the same amount of the phytochemical in a pill or capsule can be considered a "nutraceutical" (Espín *et al.*, 2007).

The main strength of the nutraceuticals is the idea that they may provide protection from ageing and diseases associated with the advance of ageing. CVD, neurodegenerative disease, type 2 diabetes mellitus and several types of cancer are associated with advancing age and dietary patterns (Espín *et al.*, 2007). Manufacturers of food are sensitive to consumers' interest in maintaining their health and somehow preventing the effects of ageing. There is increasing pressure from consumers interested in the benefits of a healthy diet and at the same time reluctant to use pharmacological aid (Scheepens *et al.*, 2010), which is more expensive and presents negative secondary effects (Nicoletti, 2012). Also, in the mind of consumers and patients there is the false and dangerous perception that "all natural medicines are good" (Nicoletti, 2012).

Many products that can be classified as "nutraceuticals" are already commercially available and marketed to prevent, improve or even treat a plethora of age-associated diseases. A query arises: can a manufacturer claim that a certain nutraceutical is safe? This is followed by another important question: are the nutraceuticals effective in improving health or preventing a specific disease? In fact, concerning nutraceuticals, very few have been subjected to clinical trials and most of them are sold only on the basis of laboratory and *in vitro* evidence (Scheepens *et al.*, 2010). The health claims of most of these products available in shops and supermarkets are not approved by the FDA or EFSA. As a consequence, good science in this area of nutrition has been misinterpreted or even overstretched for commercial purposes (Schmitt & Ferro, 2013). Notwithstanding this, such products are always perceived in a much more favorable light than the highly regulated pharmaceuticals. A 2001 poll by Harris Interactive (Rochester, NY, USA) showed that 72% of the surveyed American population used supplements. The reasons given were to feel better, to live longer, to build muscle strength and to maintain weight, and approximately one-third followed the advice of a physician (Brower, 2005). Almost all were satisfied with the supplements and more than half said they offered benefits similar to drugs but with fewer side effects (Brower, 2005).

However, the functional and anti-ageing claims of any nutraceutical product should be evidence-based and supported by strong and convincing scientific data. Human studies, well executed and well designed should be the ultimate proof of efficacy. However, even this "gold standard" may present limitations such as the feasibility of translating the interventions to practice (Daffner, 2010). Other lines of evidence are available for evaluating whether a proposed nutraceutical promotes successful ageing, namely: (a) epidemiological/cohort studies, where the major limitation is that findings can only establish the presence of an association between a nutraceutical and the improvement of the health status; (b) animal/basic science studies, where the translation from animal studies or *in vitro* results to humans can fail; and (c) human "proof-of-concept" studies, which allow a preclinical hypothesis to be tested and provide a rationale for further hypothesis and testing, but results may not be very clear (Daffner, 2010).

Studies are very difficult to execute and the design of clinical trials and epidemiological/cohort studies needs special consideration. For example, populations are difficult to characterize owing to self-medication and variability in the effects may occur. The different lifestyles of individuals, particularly exercise or the lack of it, may also influence the outcomes of the clinical trials. For example, individuals who exercise often are more health conscious and tend to follow healthier habits, confounding the outcomes of clinical trials (Scarmeas *et al.*, 2009; Gillete-Guyonnet *et al.*, 2013). Furthermore, when studying complex biological matrices such as green tea or red wine, the exact bioactive compounds are not well defined owing to the natural variations in the composition (Carneiro *et al.*, 2008; Assunção *et al.*, 2010). Also, the different compounds within a particular nutraceutical or within the diet may have unexpected antagonistic, agonistic or synergistic effects, complicating the interpretation of eventual findings (Carneiro *et al.*, 2008). If added to the diet, these effects may vary depending on the composition of this diet. If not added to the diet, but replacing another component, the eventual effects may be due to the newly introduced compound or the removal of the other or even both factors. The stability of the bioactive compounds in the gastrointestinal tract, symbiotic bacteria and their influence on metabolization, and interindividual variability are additional factors that may impact the final outcome of the trials (Espín *et al.*, 2007, 2013; Berger *et al.*, 2012).

Finally, it appears that most nutraceuticals have real effects in a cumulative fashion, that is, only after prolonged periods of consumption – months or even years. The design of experiments is obviously a challenge taking into account these many caveats (Schmitt & Ferro, 2013). Very few trials have been carried out in individuals more than 65 years old (Gonzáles-Sarrías *et al.*, 2013). Long-term studies are needed with large cohorts of elderly subjects to evaluate whether a certain nutraceutical can have a role in the prevention of age-associated diseases.

A more radical view is defended by Ioannidis (2013), claiming that most of the results of research in human nutrition are implausible. He states that almost every nutrient has a peer-reviewed publication with an association with almost any outcome. He further adds that the observational results tested afterwards in randomized trials generally fail to be confirmed (Ioannidis, 2013). To complicate matters further, there are many papers that are passion-driven owing to cultural or emotional issues concerning food, diets and nutraceuticals. The hard truth is that reliable knowledge on the effects of nutraceuticals remains very limited (Berger *et al.*, 2012).

It is obvious that the most convincing benefits in favor of a certain nutraceutical should be supported through converging lines of evidence. Major efforts should be made to ensure transparency about what is known vs what is speculative (Daffner, 2010). Unfortunately, this transparency is rarely seen in the nutraceuticals market, which tends to state only the most favorable information while disregarding the sometimes obvious limitations of available data. There is a hype of the benefits of nutraceuticals, and older individuals are the targets of strong campaigns from the nutraceutical industry. Although some of these nutraceuticals are promising, others have claims that are not supported by research in humans (Berger *et al.*, 2012; Halliwell, 2013). More well-designed studies to obtain strong evidence are needed. Owing to the dearth of hard scientific evidence, consumers are left to rely on their own knowledge and the internet to assess the deluge of promises that are present in the packaging of most nutraceutical and functional nutrients.

In Europe, since 2007, evaluation of the efficacy of foodstuffs has been covered by the provisions of the European Nutrition and Health Claims Regulation (NHCR). This is entrusted to the EFSA, the European Union's food safety advisory body. The NHCR does not specify the criteria for such assessments, and thus a rigorous methodology was developed by the EFSA based on work that has been developed in the framework of two EU-funded projects: Functional Food Science in Europe (FUFOSE) and the Process for the Assessment of Scientific Support for Claims on Foods (PASSCLAIM). The results of human randomized controlled trials are based on the establishment of cause–effect relationships between the intake of a food component and an effect on health (Williamson *et al.*, 2011). On the other hand, observational trials, experimental and animal studies are only seen as complementary support. The EFSA has already published opinions on numerous claim submissions and in the vast majority of cases it has indicated that the proposed effect had not been demonstrated by the evidence provided (Williamson *et al.*, 2011). The European Parliament (regulation no. 1169/2011) and the Council of 25 October 2011 on Nutrition and Health Claims Made on Foods indicates the necessity of scientific support for health interventions, the nature of labelling, the presentation of foodstuffs and publicity. The publicity must not attribute to any food the property of preventing, treating or curing a human disease. Also, it must not mislead the consumer about the characteristics and properties or the effects of the foodstuff. The cornerstone of this legislation is the safety of the consumer and it will be effective in December 2014. However, nutraceuticals, owing to their definition, may avoid this legislation.

There are numerous challenges to performing research concerning the effect of nutraceuticals on the elderly. The funding of the studies is an important issue as the nutraceutical industry can sell its products without being required to substantiate claims through rigorous scientific investigation. Therefore, many manufacturers are not willing to pay for research and clinical trials.

The risks of many proposed nutraceuticals with anti-ageing properties are relatively low and are directed at old but healthy individuals, not persons with diseases. However, the precaution should be taken of holding these compounds to the same high standards of evidence as other kinds of drugs in the field of medicine. In other words, the exact compound that exerts the effect in the nutraceutical and its bioavailability and metabolism must be properly characterized (González-Sarrías *et al.*, 2013). This is important for understanding the mechanism of action and establishing the ideal dose for the elderly population and to reduce potential adverse effects from toxicity (Espín *et al.*, 2007). Although most nutraceuticals available in the market present a recommended dose, the scientific basis of this recommendation is absent in most cases (Espín *et al.*, 2007). It is also important to remember that the effects of nutraceuticals and functional nutrients are generally very subtle (Williamson *et al.*, 2011). Dietary interventions generally constitute chronic intervention and, in order to be safe, they ideally should be less biologically active than pharmacological drugs (Williamson *et al.*, 2011).

There is a wide gap between the scientists who have the most up-to-date knowledge on nutraceuticals and functional nutrients and the healthcare professionals who must give a response to their patients. Given the persistent desire of individuals not only to live longer, but also to age successfully, healthcare professionals need to be in a position to recognize the relevant issues, deliver thoughtful recommendations on nutraceuticals and functional nutrients, and instruct and safeguard the public. We will shed light on some of these important issues in the following pages and narrow the gap between research and healthcare professionals.

11.3 Nutrition from food vs from supplements

Food is of major importance in our daily life and most individuals want to know how to improve their health by consuming the proper foods. Natural dietary compounds possess a broad range of biological activities, including anti-oxidant, anti-inflammatory and regulation of several signaling pathways. Many natural dietary substances have protective actions against age-associated pathologies by targeting specific signaling molecules, such as those involved in cellular metabolism, nutrition sensing, mitochondrial biogenesis, cell survival/death, senescence and stress resistance. Data from several animal models of ageing clearly support the idea that multiple food compounds may prevent, retard or improve age-associated diseases, thereby contributing to increased longevity.

The consumption of adequate levels and a proper balance of essential nutrients is critical for maintaining health. Nutrition-related epidemiological studies investigating the relationship between diet and health often focus on a particular food, or a nutrient, and its association with a chronic disease. The results from these studies coupled with the identification, isolation and purification of nutrients have raised the possibility that optimal health outcomes could be realized through nutrient supplementation. However, it is now recognized that other factors in food, or the relative abundance of some foods and the absence of others, are more important than the levels of individual nutrients consumed (Lichtenstein & Russell, 2005).

The existence of dietary patterns that relate to future chronic disease development supports the food synergy perspective, further discussed later (Jacobs & Tapsell, 2007). The identification of bioactive components in food is helpful to explain the health effects of nutrients, but such information is likely to be limited owing to interactions between naturally occurring nutrients in foods (Estaquio *et al.*, 2009). Thus, food should be seen as a whole integrated system, and not merely as a collection of individual nutrients. The term "food synergy", defined as additive or more than additive influences of dietary patterns, foods and food constituents on health, is commonly used to denote the effects of the food matrix on human biological processes (Jacobs *et al.*, 2012). In turn, the concept of the food matrix points to the fact that the nutrients contained in foods interact on different time scales with the components and structures of the medium, whether of cellular origin or a structure produced by processing (Aguilera, 2005). Recent scientific data demonstrate that, *in vivo*, the state of the food matrix may favor or hinder the nutritional response of certain nutrients. Hence, supported by the increased belief that foods, and not nutrients, are the fundamental unit of nutrition (Jacobs & Tapsell, 2007), there is an emerging interest in the impact of food structure on human nutritional status, health and wellness (Lundin *et al.*, 2008). Nevertheless, observational studies and randomized controlled trials are still required to identify which dietary patterns or foods have the greatest impact on disease (Jacobs *et al.*, 2012).

The more scientists learn about nutrition and the human body, the more they realize the importance of eating foods in their most intact forms without added solid fats, sugars, starches or sodium. For example, some studies have shown that people who eat a diet rich in β-carotene have a lower rate of several kinds of cancer. In contrast, others have shown that taking β-carotene in pill form does not decrease the risk of cancer in healthy individuals and that, indeed, supplemental nutrients may be harmful (Bjelakovic *et al.*, 2007). In addition to clinical trials focused on the effects of β-carotene supplementation, trials testing the outcomes of total fat reduction and complex B vitamin supplementation have also failed to show a reduction in chronic disease risk, and in some cases have even shown increased risk (Jacobs & Tapsell, 2007). The failure of trials to demonstrate the expected benefits of supplements suggests that the number of variables in the original food might be greater than estimated by food component. In fact, it is possible that β-carotene and other nutrients are most beneficial to health when they are consumed in their natural form and in combination with each other, as occurs in vegetables, fruit and whole grains. These foods contain not only the essential vitamins and minerals that are often targeted in nutrient supplement pills, but also hundreds of naturally occurring phytonutrients and other substances, such as carotenoids, flavonoids, isoflavones and protease inhibitors that may not only protect against cancer, but also be protective of heart disease, osteoporosis and other chronic health conditions (discussed in Chapters 4–10).

All staple foods contain naturally occurring nutrients at variable levels, but a number of food products have both naturally occurring nutrients and nutrients added through fortification and/or enrichment. Although the current dietary guidance advises that individuals may achieve the recommended nutrient intakes from food sources while not exceeding their energy requirements (USDA Center for Nutrition Policy and Promotion, 2010), many people, in addition to obtaining nutrients from foods, also use nutrient-containing dietary supplements in the form of pills, capsules or syrups, often without any clinical prescription and/or supervision (Rock, 2007; Bailey *et al.*, 2011).

Although nutritional supplements may provide an optimal amount of a specific nutrient (or nutrients) in a highly absorbable form, individuals should be warned that any nutritional supplement should be taken cautiously, as it may not be free from harmful effects (Buhr & Bales, 2009; Maraini *et al.*, 2009). For that reason, health professionals must be aware of the contributions that the intake of conventional, enriched and/or fortified foods and the use of nutritional supplements make to nutritional status and health (Fulgoni *et al.*, 2011).

In this context, obtaining essential micronutrients from foods, when possible, is the optimal approach and reliance on multivitamin–mineral supplements is discouraged. At present, people are encouraged to meet overall nutrient requirements within energy levels that balance daily energy intake with expenditure. This can be accomplished through a variety of food intake patterns that include nutrient-dense forms of foods.

11.3.1 Food enrichment and fortification

The addition of nutrients to foods, either by enrichment (replacing essential nutrients in foods lost during its processing, storage or handling) or by fortification (adding nutrients at higher levels than naturally occur in the food), enhances the levels of one or more nutrients in certain foods that are widely consumed, raising the intakes to more desirable levels with a minimal risk of toxicity (Allen *et al.*, 2006). Broadly, most grain products are enriched and a variety of other food products are fortified. For example, in some countries, bread is enriched with thiamin, niacin, riboflavin and iron; and most milk is fortified with vitamin D. Whole-grain products are typically not fortified or enriched, as many of these nutrients are naturally present in the whole grain, but most ready-to-eat cereals are fortified with iron and complex B vitamins, such as folate and vitamin B_{12}.

Albeit it is possible to add a mixture of vitamins and minerals to relatively inert and dry foods, such as cereals, interactions that occur between them and the fortificant nutrients can adversely affect the organoleptic qualities of the food and/or the stability of the nutrients. For example, the addition of calcium to foods is limited by many technological issues, from taste to solubility troubles (Richardson, 2007); nevertheless, when these are overcome, and large amounts of calcium are added, this can inhibit the absorption of iron from a fortified food. Conversely, the presence of vitamin C increases iron absorption. However, considering that ascorbic acid is very unstable when exposed to an alkaline environment or to oxygen, light and heat, the use of ascorbic acid as a food additive deserves particular attention, as substantial amounts of it can be lost during food storage and preparation. In this area, knowledge about the quantitative impact of interactions among nutrients added as a mixture on the absorption of the individual nutrients is still lacking, which makes the estimation of the proper amount of each nutrient to be added difficult.

Another novel approach that is currently being considered is the biofortification of staple foods, that is, the breeding and genetic modification of plants to improve their nutrient content and/or absorption (Allen *et al.*, 2006). Plant modification technologies include: (a) increasing the concentration of certain trace minerals (iron or zinc) and vitamins (β-carotene); (b) enhancing the bioavailability of micronutrients by reducing the concentration of antinutrient factors (inhibitors of absorption) such as phytic acid; and (c) increasing the concentration of promoters of absorption (for example, raising the levels of sulfur-containing acids, which can promote the absorption of zinc). The strategy of breeding plants that enrich themselves and load high amounts of minerals and vitamins into their edible parts has the potential to substantially reduce the recurrent costs associated with fortification and supplementation. Although this area is promising, much more research still needs to be done before the efficacy and effectiveness of these foods are definitively proven (Bawa & Anilakumar, 2013).

In the European Union, where the fortification and enrichment practices are lower than in the USA, fortified foods do not contribute significantly to increasing the intakes of any nutrient (Flynn *et al.*, 2009). Despite the regular consumption of fortified foods allowing the maintenance of body stores of selected micronutrients more efficiently and more effectively than intermittent nutritional supplements, it should never replace the consumption of a good quality diet that supplies adequate amounts of energy, protein, essential fatty acids and other constituents required for optimal health (Allen *et al.*, 2006). Indeed, naturally nutrient-dense foods, such as fruit and vegetables, whole grains and nuts, milk and lean meats, are more likely to help individuals to meet their nutritional needs and age healthily.

11.3.2 Nutritional supplements

The most commonly used categories of nutritional supplements include multivitamin–mineral combinations (providing most of the known essential micronutrients in amounts approximating recommended Dietary Reference Intake levels), products combining two or more nutrients that target a specific health function (such as anti-oxidants to reduce cardiovascular risk, or vitamin D plus calcium for bone health), and single-nutrient supplements. In addition, nutrient fortification of foods is increasingly widespread, as is the use of alternative supplemental products such as herbal and botanical compounds, all of which can add to or interact with the effects of nutritional supplements (Buhr & Bales, 2009).

11.3.2.1 Nutritional compounds as drugs delivered via food

Many nutritional supplements, despite being isolated substances from foods, could be classified as drugs. Plant sterols/stanols are available as dietary supplements in pill form, like drugs, but they can also be added to foods. The same is true for whole food extracts, such as soy protein or cod liver oil. Thus, it can be said that these substances fall between foods and drugs (Jacobs & Tapsell, 2007). In this categorization, and where the intended health outcomes are defined in prophylactic or therapeutic terms, foods enriched with an isolated substance, such as some plant phytochemicals and marine lipids added to dairy products, can be seen as drugs delivered via a food.

Margarines enriched in β-sitostanol, a phytostanol with cholesterol-lowering properties, are a good example (Lin *et al.*, 2010). At this point, β-sitostanol is a natural plant substance provided in excess of what would be obtained from foods, and the observed health benefit can be specifically attributed to the added substance (Weststrate & Meijer, 1998). However, the added substance (β-sitostanol) is not a natural part of the food vehicle (margarine), and therefore not naturally part of the given food matrix. Thus, the added substance (whether β-sitostanol, β-carotene, calcium or something else) may not have the same biological action as if it was naturally occurring and integrated with the rest of the food constituents. A question in the practice of nutrition is whether obtaining a similar and adequate amount of a food component in a naturally occurring food matrix is achievable and, if not, what the health effect of a strategy that encompasses the use of an alternative vehicle would be (Jacobs & Tapsell, 2007).

The real benefit of bioactive compounds added to foods is dependent on their bioaccessibility and bioavailability, that is, the bioactive agent should be released from the food matrix in its active form by the time it reaches the gastrointestinal tract (bioaccessibility), where it can be adsorbed and reach the systemic circulation (bioavailability). For that reason, considering the potential effect of the food matrix on the nutritional properties, the food to which the compound is added should be judiciously selected to be a good vector. In recent years, food scientists have performed amazing feats to develop new ways to incorporate, stabilize and deliver these bioactive molecules (water- or lipid-soluble substances, suspensions, colloidal particles, etc.; Turgeon & Rioux, 2011).

11.3.2.1.1 Multivitamin–mineral supplements

Many people recognize that nutrient intake should come mostly from foods, but others believe that a daily multivitamin–mineral pill will substitute for eating the foods that they know are good for them. Regardless, it must be taken into consideration that nutritional status at baseline strongly modifies the long-term health effects of nutritional supplements, as well as the age at which nutritional supplements are initiated, and the duration of the treatment (Fairfield & Stampfer, 2007).

Typical users of multivitamin–mineral supplements are older, have a high level of education and physical activity, low body mass index and good nutrient adequacy of dietary intake (Rock, 2007; Sebastian *et al.*, 2007). These demographic and physical characteristics are also positively correlated with an overall healthy lifestyle, including healthcare screening and self-efficacy in primary prevention of chronic disease. Distinguishing the contribution of a single-nutrient or combined-nutrient supplement to long-term health outcomes is difficult in a healthy population (Coates *et al.*, 2007). The results of large-scale randomized trials in the past two decades have shown that, for the majority of the population, multivitamin–mineral supplements are not only ineffective, but that they may be deleterious to health (Kamangar & Emadi, 2012). In fact, there is no evidence to support the recommendation for the use of multivitamin–mineral supplements in the primary prevention of chronic diseases (National Institutes of Health State-of-the-Science Panel, 2007).

Recent meta-analysis, authoritative reviews and expert panel reports, clearly conclude that, for the general population, and for prevention of chronic diseases such as cancer and CVD: (a) treatment with β-carotene, vitamin A and vitamin E may increase mortality (Bjelakovic *et al.*, 2007); (b) the potential roles of vitamin C and selenium on mortality need further clarification (Bjelakovic *et al.*, 2007); (c) dietary supplementation with folic acid to lower homocysteine levels has modest or any effects on cardiovascular events, and may have a negative impact with respect to specific developmental and degenerative disorders, including colorectal, prostate and breast cancers, cognitive decline and a range of other conditions (Smith *et al.*, 2008; Ebbing *et al.*, 2009; Figueiredo *et al.*, 2009; Hirsch *et al.*, 2009; Lucock & Yates, 2009; Clarke *et al.*, 2010; Miller *et al.*, 2010; Yang *et al.*, 2012); (d) folic acid supplementation with or without additional B-vitamins in adult men and women with pre-existing vascular disease does not appear to reduce risk of CVD, and may even increase risk slightly (Bønaa *et al.*, 2006; Ray *et al.*, 2007; Albert *et al.*, 2008; Ebbing *et al.*, 2008); and (e) calcium supplements with or without vitamin D increase the risk of cardiovascular events, particularly myocardial infarction (Bolland *et al.*, 2011). Despite calcium and vitamin D supplements having been linked to a lower risk and even prevention of many chronic conditions such as osteoporosis, colon cancer and hypertension (Dabhade & Kotwal, 2013), some research indicates that too much of these nutrients may be harmful (Bernstein & Munoz, 2012).

In spite of the substantial evidence of lack of any health benefit from multivitamin–mineral supplement use for the majority of the adult population, these products are widely marketed. This arises from the desire of many people to take an active role in improving their health and living longer. Avoiding tasty but unhealthy food may be difficult for many reasons, but taking a pill once a day is relatively easy. As others have discussed, prescription is always more convenient than proscription (Kamangar & Emadi, 2012).

Although a daily multivitamin–mineral supplement may not offer health benefits for the general healthy population, and perhaps for those with already established disease, it can greatly help people with diagnosed nutritional deficiencies (characterized by specific symptoms that can be prevented, and often reversed, by giving the shortfall nutrient in an isolated or pure form) and in population groups at risk of deficit, such as pregnant and perimenopausal women, and the elderly (Jacobs *et al.*, 2012).

Concerning pregnant and perimenopausal women, there is strong evidence for the beneficial use of some nutritional supplements: (a) the use of periconceptional folate supplements substantially reduces the risk of neural tube defects (Wolff *et al.*, 2009; Blencowe *et al.*, 2010); (b) during pregnancy iron supplements can reduce the risk of anemia and perinatal complications in mothers (Yakoob & Bhutta, 2011); and (c) calcium supplements (preferably in combination with vitamin D to optimize calcium absorption) have been recommended for postmenopausal women to prevent osteoporotic fractures (Maraini *et al.*, 2009; Spangler *et al.*, 2011).

A number of studies have demonstrated a remarkable impact of vitamin status on health benefit and disease prevention in elderly people. Although subject to debate, vitamins with anti-oxidant properties such as vitamins E and C have been suggested to have a beneficial effect on the pathogenesis of atherosclerosis (Kritharides & Stocker, 2002). Moreover, B vitamins, including folate and vitamins B_6 and B_{12}, have a remarkable effect on lowering plasma levels of the cardiovascular risk factor homocysteine (Kahn *et al.*, 2008) and improve cognitive performance and functions such as memory and information processing (Aisen *et al.*, 2008; Kennedy *et al.*, 2010). It is interesting to note that, when the intake of foods naturally rich in folic acid (e.g. deep green leafy vegetables, citrus fruit and dried beans and peas) and/or folic acid-fortified foods is combined with supplements containing folic acid, excessive levels may be consumed. Folic acid intake in excess may mask the diagnosis of a vitamin B_{12} deficiency. Even at subclinical levels of deficiency, older adults may have changes in their mental status, which can be overlooked or attributed to normal ageing (Bernstein & Munoz, 2012).

Vitamin D has a significant role in bone health by regulating bone mass. The health effects of this vitamin are not confined to the reduction of risk of osteoporosis and bone fracture prevention (discussed in Chapter 7) (Bischoff-Ferrari, 2009). It may have a role in CVD, glucose tolerance, dental health, hypertension and certain cancers (Buhr & Bales, 2009). An adequate supply of vitamin D is of particular relevance for the elderly, for the following reasons: (a) aged skin produces less vitamin D (owing to a reduced concentration of the precursor 7-dehydrocholesterol) (Mithal *et al.*, 2009); (b) renal conversion of 25-hydroxyvitamin-D (25-hydroxycholecalciferol or calcidiol) to the active form is impaired; and (c) gut responsiveness to 1,25(OH)2D (calcitriol) is reduced (Buhr & Bales, 2009). Thus, it is recommended to increase the intake of vitamin D-rich foods (although vitamin D is naturally present in very few foods, such as oily fish and egg yolk, it is added to many others by fortification processes). Concerning vitamin D supplementation, it remains an area of considerable debate, and further work is still needed to determine the requirement for health and the relative contribution from diet to assess whether supplementation would be of benefit (Mensink *et al.*, 2013). For now, since the most physiologically active form of this vitamin is perhaps that which is dependent on exposure to UV light, cautious sunlight exposure should be part of a healthful lifestyle (Wolpowitz & Gilchrest, 2006).

In brief, when dietary selection is limited, nutrient supplementation with low-dose multivitamin and mineral supplements can be helpful for older adults to meet recommended intake levels (Sebastian *et al.*, 2007). Of specific concern for older adults are the nutrients consistently found to be deficient in the diet, such as anti-oxidants, calcium and vitamin D, and those for which the digestion, absorption or metabolism declines with age, such as vitamin B_{12} (Bernstein & Munoz, 2012).

11.3.2.1.2 Anti-oxidant supplements

The production of free radicals increases with age, while some of the endogenous defense mechanisms decrease (discussed in Chapter 1). This imbalance leads to progressive damage of cellular structures, presumably resulting in the ageing phenotype (Poljsak *et al.*, 2013). After the genesis of reactive oxygen species, free radicals react with adjacent molecules, such as lipids, proteins or nucleic acids, resulting in their functional impairment. The anti-oxidative network, which includes vitamins (A, C, D and E), enzymes (superoxide dismutase, catalase, glutathione peroxidase, etc.), carotenoids (α- and β-carotene, lycopene, lutein, zeaxanthin, etc.) and other substances (such as flavonoids, lipoic acid, uric acid, selenium, coenzyme Q10, etc.), acts as a protective chain, in which various anti-oxidants possess a synergistic effect and protect each other from direct destruction in the processes of neutralizing free radicals (Lademann *et al.*, 2011b; Poljsak *et al.*, 2013).

The inappropriate use of dietary supplements may lead to "anti-oxidative stress", a term used to describe the negative effects of anti-oxidants (Villanueva & Kross, 2012). In fact, both "anti-oxidative" and oxidative stresses leading to anti-oxidative defenses imbalance can be dangerous to the organism and can result in carcinogenesis and ageing phenotype (Poljsak *et al.*, 2013). Indeed, anti-oxidant nutrient supplementation in healthy subjects has not always been successful. Although a number of studies have revealed some positive effects after anti-oxidant supplementation, others, such as the Selenium and Vitamin E Cancer Prevention Trial (SELECT Trial), have shown that vitamin E supplementation could increase the risk of prostate cancer among healthy men (Klein *et al.*, 2011). Even more alarming results were those provided by the studies where healthy people were supplemented with high doses of β-carotene or vitamins A, C or E (Hennekens *et al.*, 1996; Omenn *et al.*, 1996; Pryor *et al.*, 2000; Goodman *et al.*, 2004; Gallicchio *et al.*, 2008; Sesso *et al.*, 2008; Gaziano *et al.*, 2009). Many of these trials had to be suspended owing to an increased mortality rate from lung cancer and ischemic cardiac disease.

Considering that the biological anti-oxidant network in healthy subjects already contains adequate amounts of water- and fat-soluble anti-oxidants working in an interactive manner, further increases of single or combinations of anti-oxidants within a physiological range might not affect the overall *in vivo* anti-oxidant network and might lead to imbalance (Li *et al.*, 2010). The elegant study from Cornelli *et al.* (2001) depicts well that, after exceeding a critical concentration, the anti-oxidants exhibit pro-oxidant properties instead of acting as radical quenchers. The researchers showed that a combination of low doses of anti-oxidants (close to or less than the RDA), taken during one week in a liquid form decreased oxidative stress in healthy volunteers. Higher doses did not result in such an effect, while very large doses resulted in a pro-oxidative effect. Therefore, the authors concluded that it is not desirable to use a high dose of just one anti-oxidant, since it is possible that its pro-oxidative activity supersedes its anti-oxidative effect. Since a balanced mixture is important for the formation of the protective chains, that is, for the stability of the anti-oxidants in tissues, optimum results can be expected from studies using lower doses of anti-oxidants isolated or in association. The best example of this is the French study Supplémentation en Vitamines et Minéraux Antioxydants (SU.VI.MAX), a double-blind randomized clinical study that enrolled more than 13,000 healthy volunteers monitored since 1994. A lower incidence of CVD and cancer was observed in men who received an anti-oxidant preparation of vitamin C (120 mg), vitamin E (30 mg), β-carotene (6 mg), selenium (100 µg) and zinc (20 mg) for eight years (Galan *et al.*, 2005).

Among the experts, there is a continuing discussion on the pros and cons of natural anti-oxidant application via food or supplements. Furthermore, the optimal concentration and composition of anti-oxidant supplements are still a matter of debate (Lademann *et al.*, 2011b). Hence, while there are no consistent recommendations in this area, the best strategy against the harmful action of free radicals is a well-regulated lifestyle with low stress conditions and balanced nutritional habits, including the ingestion of anti-oxidant-rich foods, such as fruit, vegetables, extra-virgin olive oil, oilseeds, nuts, spices, green tea, red wine, coffee and cocoa (Cornelli, 2009). These foods may follow or substitute for supplements, since they are able to increase the anti-oxidant level of the body, and have a positive influence on the prevention and medical treatment of various chronic diseases, including various types of cancer (Darvin *et al.*, 2006; Aune *et al.*, 2009).

In particular conditions, such as the case of individuals who are not able or willing to adopt such a lifestyle, the use of anti-oxidant supplements at physiological concentrations, in the form of tablets or juice extracts, may be an alternative. However, at the moment, assessing whether a chosen product contains the right levels of anti-oxidants is difficult for consumers. The development of suitable standards and the clear labeling of such products is an essential project that should be undertaken (Lademann *et al.*, 2011b).

Presently, the use of supplemental anti-oxidants can be advised only in cases of well-known conditions, where the depletion of anti-oxidants is known and can be predicted. Exercise is a good example. Although physical activity has many well-established health benefits, ageing and strenuous exercise are both associated with increased free radical generation in the skeletal muscle. Recent studies suggested a beneficial relationship between anti-oxidant vitamin (e.g. vitamin C) intake and physical performance in elderly people (Saito *et al.*, 2012). It has been also shown that intake of resveratrol, together with habitual exercise, is beneficial for suppressing the ageing-related decline in physical performance (Murase *et al.*, 2009). However, there are conflicting results concerning the effects of exercise training combined with anti-oxidant supplementation in the elderly (Gomez-Cabrera *et al.*, 2013). More research for a better clarification of the field is required. Hence, daily use of synthetic supplements has not been proven to be beneficial, and excessive use may be harmful. Balanced food still seems to be the best option (Poljsak *et al.*, 2013).

11.3.2.1.3 Omega-3 polyunsaturated fatty acids supplements

Omega-3 long-chain polyunsaturated fatty acids, including eicosapentaenoic acid (EPA) and docosahexaenoic acid (DHA), are dietary fats with an array of health benefits throughout life. Low intake of dietary EPA and DHA is thought to be associated with increased inflammatory processes as well as poor fetal development, poor general cardiovascular health and risk of the development of Alzheimer disease (Swanson *et al.*, 2012). Conversely, an adequate intake of omega-3 fatty acids from oily fish (salmon, mackerel, tuna, etc.) and plant sources (nuts and vegetable oils, such as canola, soybean and flaxseed oils), or even from supplements, has a positive impact on a variety of critical biological functions (Buhr & Bales, 2010; Swanson *et al.*, 2012). Beyond their immunomodulatory effects and their role in vision and cognition, prospective cohort studies and secondary prevention trials provide strong evidence that consumption of omega-3 fatty acids may prevent CVD (Calder, 2009; Mozaffarian, 2008; Abete *et al.*, 2011; Oken *et al.*, 2012).

The cardioprotective effects of omega-3 fatty acids are ascribed to improvements in various cardiovascular risk factors, including reduction in blood triglycerides, platelet aggregation, blood pressure and inflammation, and enhanced endothelial function (Bloomer *et al.*, 2009; Prasad, 2009; Phang *et al.*, 2012), health benefits that arise from their ability to reduce the production of inflammatory eicosanoids, cytokines and reactive oxygen species (Calder, 2009). These fatty acids also modulate the activity of transcription factors related to the expression of many genes involved in inflammatory and atherogenesis-related pathways, such as nuclear transcription factor κB signaling, eicosanoid synthesis, scavenger receptor activity, adipogenesis and hypoxia signaling (Bouwens *et al.*, 2009; Cicero *et al.*, 2009). In spite of increased intakes of fatty fish or supplements of omega-3 marine fatty acids possibly playing a positive role in insulin sensitivity, this is still a highly controversial issue (Abete *et al.*, 2008; Mostad *et al.*, 2009).

Although the bioavailability of fatty acids is appreciably higher when ingested from fish (Sirtori *et al.*, 2009), equal health benefits may be derived from omega-3 fatty acids supplied by dietary supplements (Oken *et al.*, 2012). Currently, the Nutrition Committee of the American Heart Association recommends that patients without documented coronary heart disease should eat oily fish, high in EPA and DHA, twice weekly. These two servings of fish per week would make an average intake of 250–500 mg of EPA and DHA per day. Conversely, patients with documented coronary heart disease are advised to consume about 1 g of EPA plus DHA daily, preferably from oily fish. For these patients, EPA plus DHA supplements could be considered in consultation with their physician. Individuals with hypertriglyceridemia are recommended 2–4 g daily of EPA plus DHA, provided as capsules under a physician's care (Eckel *et al.*, 2013).

The use of fish oil capsules is not only useful in the prevention and treatment of coronary diseases (Sirtori *et al.*, 2009), but also assumes particular relevance considering the concerns about the regular consumption of some species of fish and the resulting exposure to toxic substances, such as heavy metals (particularly methylmercury), dioxins and polychlorinated biphenyls (Kris-Etherton *et al.*, 2009; Oken *et al.*, 2012). Although most studies that have looked at reputable brands of fish-oil supplements have not found significant levels of contamination, it should be noted that these supplements may retain some of the above-mentioned contaminants unless they have undergone molecular distillation to purify them (Kris-Etherton *et al.*, 2009).

It should be pointed out that fish-oil supplements are not free from adverse effects. One potential side effect is the increased risk of immunosuppression and bleeding (the risk of hemorrhagic stroke is increased, especially at high doses). Fish oils are known to cause a variety of digestive problems, including flatulence, bloating, acid reflux, nausea and diarrhea (Kris-Etherton *et al.*, 2002), conditions that can be prevented by taking fish-oil supplements with meals. These supplements cannot be indicated for individuals who have already low blood pressure, owing to their blood pressure-lowering effects. Attempts should be made to establish an optimal omega-3 dosage to maximize the reward-to-risk ratio of supplementation.

11.3.2.1.4 Amino acids and amino acid mixture supplements

Protein and its constituent amino acids are key components of any healthy diet. Maintenance of body protein stores is key to survival, it being well accepted that loss of body protein is associated with increased morbidity and mortality. Loss of skeletal muscle (sarcopenia), osteopenia, reduced immunity and impaired wound healing are all effects of the ageing process, as well as imbalance of body protein status and amino acid availability (Fukagawa, 2013).

Adequate protein intake is needed for the maintenance of muscle and bone mass and is important to counter the development of sarcopenia and osteoporosis (discussed in Chapter 7). The recommended daily intake value of 0.8 g/kg body weight may not be adequate for the maintenance of muscle mass for adults aged 55–77 (Woo, 2011). The PROT-AGE Study Group also advocates that older people need more dietary protein than do younger people; older people should consume an average daily intake at least in the range of 1.0–1.2 g/kg body weight. The requirements are greater for older adults who have an acute or chronic disease, and those with severe illness or injury or with marked malnutrition. Protein quality, timing of intake and amino acid supplementation may be considered so as to achieve the greatest benefits from protein intake (Bauer *et al.*, 2013).

Since amino acids are reported to have unique physiological effects, over the past decade, increasing knowledge about the role of specific amino acids in the regulation of physiological processes has stimulated interest in whether specific amino acid-containing supplements or amino acids mixtures (specifically designed to mimic the amino acids pattern seen in an ideal protein, most often egg) may help to mitigate, or even treat, age-associated disorders (Fukagawa, 2013). Below, the health benefits of some of the best studied amino acids supplements are briefly described.

The most studied group of essential amino acids with respect to human health, are branched-chain amino acids, which include leucine, isoleucine and valine. Among them, leucine has been heavily investigated as a potential pharmaconutrient, owing to its role in muscle protein synthesis and its insulin secretagogue action (Leenders & van Loon, 2011; Valerio *et al.*, 2011). Although short-term studies suggest that single leucine supplementation can stimulate muscle mass accretion in the elderly (Leenders & van Loon, 2011), prolonged leucine supplementation does not modulate body composition, muscle mass, strength, glycemic control and/or lipidemia in elderly patients who consume adequate levels of dietary protein (Leenders *et al.*, 2011). Conversely, leucine co-ingestion with a bolus of pure dietary protein further stimulates postprandial muscle protein synthesis rates in elderly men. As a result, it has been suggested that fortifying meals with free leucine may represent an effective strategy to increase the muscle protein synthetic response to food intake in the elderly and, as such, may be used to attenuate the loss of muscle mass with ageing (Wall *et al.*, 2013).

Branched-chain amino acids supplementation may have other implications for the overall health management of older individuals. For instance, Qin *et al.* (2011) found an inverse relationship between higher intakes of branched-chain amino acids mixtures and the prevalence of overweight and obesity in middle-aged individuals. Positive effects of branched-chain amino acids on mood, perceived exertion and mental fatigue have also been described (Fernstrom, 2013). The ingestion of large neutral amino acids, notably tryptophan and tyrosine, concomitantly with branched-chain amino acids, modifies tryptophan and tyrosine uptake into the brain, and their conversion to serotonin and catecholamine neurotransmitters (dopamine, norepinephrine and epinephrine), respectively. Owing to the competitive nature of the transporter for large neutral amino acids at the blood–brain barrier, the rise in branched-chain amino acids levels in blood lowers tryptophan and tyrosine uptake, leading to a parallel decline in serotonin and catecholamine synthesis. Even though branched-chain amino acids may prevent serotonin-related central fatigue, it is likely that they may fail to increase physical performance because dopamine is also reduced. For that reason, it was hypothesized that branched-chain amino acids should be co-administered with tyrosine, in order to prevent the decline in dopamine. Regardless, a balanced large neutral amino acids mixture might be an effective enhancer of physical performance (Fernstrom, 2013).

Concerning age-related reduction in muscle mass and consequent muscle weakness and functional limitations, supplementation with creatine has been used owing to its ergogenic effects with minimal side effects. Evidence of benefits from this supplement has also been reported in a broad range of diseases, including cancer, myopathies, rheumatic diseases and type 2 diabetes (Gualano *et al.*, 2012). Interestingly, creatine supplementation can improve cognitive performance in young subjects as well as in elderly people (McMorris *et al.*, 2007), and may also have a role in neurodegenerative disorders, such as Alzheimer and Parkinson diseases, since creatine might alleviate cerebral energy depletion, exacerbated oxidative stress and mitochondrial dysfunction, conditions that characterize these disorders (Andres *et al.*, 2008).

Cysteine is now recognized as a conditionally essential sulfur amino acid. It plays a key role in the metabolic pathways involving methionine, taurine and glutathione, and may help fight chronic inflammation by boosting anti-oxidant status. In stressed and inflammatory states, sulfur amino acid metabolism adapts to meet the increased requirements for cysteine as a rate-limiting substrate for glutathione synthesis – the main endogenous anti-oxidant in the body, important in the maintenance of redox status, including the balance of reduced and oxidized forms of dietary anti-oxidants such as vitamins E and C. For this reason, dietary cysteine has been recognized as a potential nutraceutical. Despite cysteine supplements possibly having a role in respiratory and neurodegenerative disorders prevention, as well as in heart and liver diseases, there are concerns related to the stability, toxicity and absorption of both glutathione and cysteine, alone or combined, when administered orally. Cysteine is easily oxidized to its insoluble dimeric form, cystine, and both are toxic at high concentrations (McPherson & Hardy, 2012). Hence, consumption of naturally occurring cysteine-rich proteins, whey or keratin, may have advantages over the simple amino acid or its derivatives, to safely and beneficially improve anti-oxidant status in health and disease (McPherson & Hardy, 2011).

Taurine, one of the few amino acids not incorporated into proteins, is formed from cysteine and involved in the conjugation of bile acids, osmoregulation, retinal and neurological development, regulation of cellular calcium levels and immune function (Ripps & Shen, 2012). Oral taurine administration has been proposed for disorders ranging from diabetes to CVD, retinal degeneration, and skeletal muscle dysfunction, with little evidence of adverse effects (Ito *et al.*, 2012).

A recent systematic review and meta-analysis of randomized clinical trials confirmed that in severely ill patients, that is, patients with severe inflammatory state or sepsis, or traumatized or burn patients, enterally administered glutamine supplementation reduced infections and length of stay in hospital, but the meta-analysis did not demonstrate a significant reduction in mortality (Bollhalder *et al.*, 2013). Many healthy individuals consume large quantities of glutamine supplement in the belief that it will aid in muscle building, enhance athletic performance, boost immunity or improve memory. In this regard, while short-term intake of high amounts of glutamine may be safe, there are still unanswered questions concerning the chronic consumption of a glutamine-enriched diet (Holecek, 2013). Glutamine enhances brain function as it fuels two of the brain's most important neurotransmitters: glutamic acid and γ-aminobutyric acid (Andrews & Griffiths, 2002). Promising data from animal models of Alzheimer disease support the hypothesis that glutamine supplementation may protect neurons against DNA damage, β-amyloid protein and oxidative stress (Chen & Herrup, 2012).

Arginine is one of the most versatile amino acids and is known to have many anti-ageing benefits, including the prevention and treatment of CVD by increasing nitric oxide bioavailability in the body, which improves blood circulation, cognitive function and the performance of activities of daily living, and reduces the risk of clot formation (Heffernan *et al.*, 2010). Furthermore, arginine is also able to stimulate the release of human growth hormone, secretion of which declines with ageing, a primary reason for decreased muscle mass and for the slower rate of skin growth, leading to thinner and less flexible skin (de Castro-Barbosa *et al.*, 2006). Unfortunately, the beneficial effects of arginine supplementation are not uniform across the studies and there remains controversy about whether long-term supplementation would be helpful. Furthermore, the effects of arginine differ according to the concentration range achieved in plasma by oral supplementation. For instance, doses of 3–8 g daily are associated with fewer untoward effects, but higher intakes are reportedly associated with gastrointestinal symptoms (Luiking *et al.*, 2012).

11.3.3 Pills, capsules, powders and syrups

Dietary supplements are available in many forms, including tablets, capsules, powders, energy bars and liquids. They include, among others, vitamin and mineral products, botanical or herbal products (plant materials, algae, macroscopic fungi or a combination of these), amino acid products and enzyme supplements.

Gabriels and Lambert (2013) analyzed how consumers of nutritional supplement products acquire information to assist their purchasing decisions. The authors found that the majority of nutritional supplement users are strongly influenced by the ingredient information on the container label, and only one-fifth point out that dosage and directions for use influence the purchase. In this setting, it is interesting to note that the term "multivitamin" currently encompasses hundreds, if not thousands, of products with varied content and dose of vitamins and minerals. Owing to the lack of standardization, this tremendous heterogeneity is a serious obstacle to informative labeling and guidance to consumers, and constitutes a significant challenge for research on how this distinct group of products is used by the public (Rosenberg, 2007).

Randomized placebo-controlled trials reduce the confounding effects on the main outcomes of multivitamin–mineral supplement use on chronic disease endpoints; however, a common limitation of other types of study is the insufficient standardization of preparation procedures, compositions and characteristics of the products. Indeed, some discrepancies exist between the real content of nutrients in supplements and the amounts reported on product labels, along with differences in chemical formulations and dosing regimens that affect bioavailability, bioequivalency and, ultimately, biological effects. Although for some nutrients bioequivalence is closely related to bioavailability, for others, equal absorption does not mean equal biological effects because the nutrient sources are chemically different, resulting in differences in nutrient activity (Yetley, 2007). Many studies have been lacking in adequate recognition that the effectiveness of these substances is not binary (present or absent) but, as in the rest of biology, is dependent on dose (Rosenberg, 2007).

In the last decade, Hoag and Hussain (2001) identified two categories of factors that affect bioavailability and bioequivalence of product formulation: (a) factors that affect product dissolution or release (different chemical forms of nutrients and nutrient–nutrient interactions may affect bioavailability); and (b) factors related to excipients or inactive ingredients that may affect stability, absorption and metabolic processes.

As previously described, folate status is of utmost importance in the periconceptional period. Considering that 50–95% of the native dietary folate can be destroyed by cooking, owing to the high sensitivity of this molecule to heat, pH, metal ions and anti-oxidant levels (Lucock, 2004), the prescription of folate supplements is demanded. Currently, it is commercially available a synthetic form of folic acid, the fully oxidized pteroylmonoglutamic acid, which does not occur in nature, whose bioavailability is up to 100% compared with an estimated 50% for naturally occurring folate in foods (in the form of reduced folylmono- or folylpolyglutamic acids; Lucock *et al.*, 2013). Furthermore, up to half of the women taking iron supplements during pregnancy or in postmenopausal phase experience adverse gastrointestinal effects, such as nausea, epigastric discomfort and constipation, particularly if taken without food (Flynn *et al.*, 2009). In accordance with Nguyen *et al.* (2008) findings, the ensuing limited adherence to supplementation during pregnancy can be further exacerbated by morning sickness and may also be related to tablet size. For such cases, a powdered form was designed of iron and folic acid packaged in single-serve sachets, which are sprinkled over any semi-solid foods just before consumption. This formulation seems to improve adherence by reducing the side-effects of the iron through the use of microencapsulated ferrous fumarate as the iron source, as well as the buffering effect of the food to which the fortificant is added. The encapsulate is an edible vegetable-based lipid that dissolves in the low-pH environment of the stomach, which is able to mask the metallic taste of the iron and possibly protects the gastric epithelium from local irritation by the iron salt. A disadvantage of microencapsulated ferrous fumarate is its limited solubility, thus it is not readily suitable for use in beverages.

One of the vitamins that is often added to foods is B_{12}. Since the ability to absorb naturally occurring vitamin B_{12} from food decreases with age, whereas the absorption of the crystalline form (the form that is used as a fortificant) is maintained by most individuals, the consumption of B_{12} vitamin-fortified foods may represent an important approach to ensuring a reasonable status of this vitamin, particularly in older people (Allen, 2009). Interestingly, clinical trials, either among free-living or institutionalized elderly, demonstrated that oral vitamin B_{12} supplements either alone or as multivitamin–mineral supplements could improve vitamin B_{12} status. A systematic review of oral vs intramuscular administration of vitamin B_{12} in the treatment of vitamin B_{12} deficiency demonstrated that oral doses may be more effective in short-term hematological and neurological responses (Butler *et al.*, 2006).

11.3.4 Factors that affect the bioavailability of nutrients

Foods constitute a complex chemical and biological mix, resulting from the interaction of natural constituents, industrial processing and household preparation. All of these factors cause marked changes in the physicochemical properties of a meal, and thus determine the amount and the bioavailability of nutrients. Moreover, diet constituents continue to interact along the gastrointestinal tract and at the level of intermediary metabolism. There is a consensus that the release of nutrients from the food matrix as well as the interactions between food components and restructuring phenomena during transit in the digestive system are far more important than the original content of nutrients (Troncoso & Aguilera, 2009).

11.3.4.1 Food processing and cooking methods

Nearly every food preparation process reduces the amount of nutrients in food. The greatest nutrient loss is caused by processes that expose foods to high levels of heat, light and/or oxygen. Nutrients can also be lost from foods by fluids that are introduced during the cooking process, as well as when foods are broiled, roasted or fried in oil.

The amount of nutrient loss caused by cooking has encouraged some health-conscious consumers to eat more raw foods. In general, this is a positive step; however, cooking can be advantageous in many ways, as it improves the organoleptic characteristics of foods (taste, flavor, appearance and texture), and ensures food safety, as it inactivates pathogenic and spoilage microorganisms and endogenous enzymes, leading to improved quality and shelf-life of the product (Rawson *et al.*, 2011). Furthermore, food processing modifies physical and chemical properties of food, which influences the rate and the extent of digestion, as well as the rate of absorption of nutrients in the digestive tract (Jacobs & Tapsell, 2007; Turgeon & Rioux, 2011).

Usually, solid foods with strong tissue structure, such as fresh whole fruit and vegetables, breads containing whole grains, and whole meat products, are digested more slowly and are more satiating than foods that have soft, overripe or a highly processed structure. As a result, processing is an important factor because it influences the food matrix structure. For example, the impact of freezing, defrosting and toasting on the glycemic response of white bread was studied (Burton & Lightowler, 2008). Breads that were frozen and defrosted, fresh and toasted, and toasted after freezing and defrosting, showed a lower incremental area under the glucose response curve compared with fresh white bread. This could be explained by the increased resistant starch content after the cooling and freezing steps, limiting its enzyme susceptibility.

Extrusion cooking is a high-temperature, short-time process of intense mechanical shear, which is utilized in the industrial production of ready-to-eat cereals, salty and sweet snacks, and croutons for soups and salads. This process is also used for weaning foods, dietetic foods and meat replacers, in which the nutritional quality is important. Mild extrusion conditions (high moisture content, low residence time and low temperature) can improve the nutritional quality of food. Better retention of amino acids and vitamins as well as higher protein and starch digestibility is observed under this process. Moreover, there is an increase in the soluble dietary fiber content, a decrease in lipid oxidation and a better absorption of minerals (Singh *et al.*, 2007).

Grilling and barbecuing meats are very popular cooking methods. In addition to the wonderful taste these methods impart on meats, they can be considered healthy alternatives to other cooking practices, because some of the meat's saturated fat content is reduced by grilling process. However, depending on the type of meat, cooking method and preferred level of browning or doneness, red and white meats cooked at high temperature (i.e. grilling, barbecuing, broiling and pan-frying) may have high levels of meat mutagens: heterocyclic amines and polycyclic aromatic hydrocarbons. The first group of compounds is produced by the reaction of creatine and amino acids from proteins, when meats are directly exposed to a flame or very high-temperature surface, while polycyclic aromatic hydrocarbons derive from incomplete burning of organic substances, mainly from meat grilling or broiling. Furthermore, *N*-nitroso compounds can be formed in meats preserved with nitrates or nitrites (e.g. cured meats or sausages) and can also be endogenously produced by the reaction of amines and amides from red meat with nitrosating agents in the intestines (John *et al.*, 2011).

Although recent studies reported an increased risk of esophageal, colorectal, prostatic, breast and endometrial cancers for elevated red meat consumption, irrespective of cooking methods (Carruba *et al.*, 2006; Xu *et al.*, 2006; Fu *et al.*, 2011; Punnen *et al.*, 2011; De Stefani *et al.*, 2012; Di Maso *et al.*, 2013), pancreatic cancer has been consistently associated not only with high red meat consumption but particularly with high intake of dietary heterocyclic amines and polycyclic aromatic hydrocarbons (Stolzenberg-Solomon *et al.*, 2007; Polesel *et al.*, 2010; John *et al.*, 2011; Larsson & Wolk, 2012). These results were consistent with the findings from animal models, showing carcinogenic effects of several heterocyclic amines and polycyclic aromatic hydrocarbons (Wei *et al.*, 2003).

The amount of these carcinogenic compounds formed in meats can be considerably reduced by slight alterations in cooking methods, as follows: (a) selecting leaner meats; (b) marinating meats before grilling (the marinade forms a protective barrier for the meat juices that prevents the formation of heterocyclic amines up to 90%); (c) cooking at lower temperatures; (d) prevent flare-ups; and (e) not overcooking meats, as the formation of harmful compounds increases not only with temperature but also with the duration of cooking (Di Maso *et al.*, 2013).

Nutrient losses for common processing methods for vegetables also depend on cooking time and temperature. Vegetables provide a major dietary source of phytochemicals with potential anti-ageing properties. However, the levels of these substances not only vary between species, but are also strongly influenced by climatic, agronomic and harvest conditions (Tiwari & Cummins, 2013). Post-harvest operations, that is, food processing and storage, also play a determinant role in the total amount of phytochemicals that are ingested. In fact, these compounds can be extensively degraded by conventional (or thermal), nonthermal (high pressure, ultrasound, irradiation), industrial (canning, drying) and domestic (washing, peeling, cutting) processes (Rawson *et al.*, 2011), and also during storage. For example, it was recently found that phytostanols and phytosterols, included in several commercial spreadable fats, margarines, milk and yoghurts, undergo degradation during storage, curiously, at low temperatures. At the end of 18 weeks, one-third of phytostanols have disappeared from stored margarines (Rudzińska *et al.*, 2014).

Vitamins, carotenoids, flavonoids and fiber are more concentrated in the peel than in the pulp. Thus, the simple trimming or peeling of fruit and vegetables can discard appreciable amounts and significantly reduce the levels of these substances in the portions utilized. Alkaline treatments to facilitate peeling can also cause losses, although relatively small, of labile vitamins such as folate, ascorbic acid and thiamin at the surface of the product (Francis *et al.*, 2012).

Vitamins and bioactive compounds are naturally protected in plant tissues. The cutting, chopping, shredding and pulping of fruit and vegetables destroy this protection, increase exposure to oxygen and release enzymes that catalyze their degradation. Enzymatic degradation may be a more serious problem than thermal decomposition in many foods. Thus, thermal processing of vegetables and fruit should be carried out immediately after peeling and cutting operations (Pasha *et al.*, 2014).

As a general rule, whatever the processing method is chosen, the retention of phytochemicals in vegetables decreases exponentially with increases in cooking duration and magnitude (Patras *et al.*, 2010; Tiwari & Cummins, 2013; Singhal *et al.*, 2012). Boiling results in the greatest losses of water-soluble phytochemicals, such as the polyphenols, through leaching, thermal degradation and oxidation. In contrast, gentle stir-frying appears to result in the least losses (Patras *et al.*, 2010). Nevertheless, there are reports showing that mechanical disruption of the food matrix or heat treatment aid the extractability of phytochemicals, such as carotenoids, leading to increased concentrations (Ruiz-Rodriguez *et al.*, 2008), and therefore to higher bioavailability. For example, the absorption of β-carotene from a raw carrot is about 42.0%, but it can reach 66.0% if the carrot is cooked (van Boekel *et al.*, 2010). Similarly, the bioavailability of lycopene, of which the major dietary sources are tomato and tomato products, has been shown to be much higher from processed tomato products (e.g. tomato paste) as compared with fresh tomato (Mordente *et al.*, 2011). However, the influence of food matrix on carotenoid bioavailability is not the same among carotenoids. Indeed, the relative bioavailability of lutein from spinach is greater than that of β-carotene (i.e. 67.0 and 14.0%, respectively) and less affected by the food matrix (van Boekel *et al.*, 2010).

Nutrients can also be lost from foods by fluids that are introduced during the cooking process. For example, boiling a potato causes the migration of a considerable proportion of its water-soluble vitamins (B group and C) to the boiling water. People may still benefit from those nutrients if the boiling liquid is consumed (e.g. if the potato and its cooking water are being turned into potato soup). Similar losses also occur when foods are broiled or fried in oil. Conversely, alternative cooking methods such as grilling, roasting, steaming, stir-frying or microwaving generally preserve a greater proportion of vitamins and other nutrients.

11.3.4.2 Competitive interactions between nutrients

Virtually any nutrient can cause adverse effects if ingested in excessive amounts. Such undesirable effects may depend on the inherent toxicity of the excess intake, but often they are caused by the antagonistic effect of the excess nutrient on the bioavailability of other dietary components. Likewise, non-nutritional substances, such as drugs, can interfere with nutrient utilization, as discussed later.

Although the term "interaction" denotes a bidirectional effect, many interactions are unidirectional, that is, one nutrient affects the biological disposition of another, which remains more or less passive. Bidirectional interactions are most common among nutrients with similar physicochemical properties and sharing a common mechanism of absorption or metabolism; finally, some unidirectional or bidirectional interactions could be affected by the presence of a third dietary constituent. Nutrient interactions are not usually additive.

From the physiological standpoint, nutrient interactions can occur at different levels: (a) in the diet, the mode of preparation of foods may be as important as diet composition in determining nutrient interactions (e.g. cooking in an alkaline medium may decrease the interaction between ascorbic acid and iron by destroying the vitamin); (b) in the intestinal lumen, interactions at this level have received the most attention, because they determine the real availability of a nutrient for translocation through the enterocyte; most luminal interactions consist of direct nutrient–nutrient interactions, but certain nutrients can indirectly affect the absorption of others by modifying gastrointestinal physiological activities (e.g. certain dietary fibers can stimulate gastrointestinal hormone secretion or inhibit micellar formation, thus indirectly affecting nutrient absorption); and (c) in the postabsorptive phase, many interactions take place after the process of absorption has been completed; these interactions may be in the form of physiological synergism, such as that of vitamin A and zinc on the visual process, or between vitamin

A and iron mobilization; conversely, negative interactions may affect circulating or storage levels of nutrients (e.g. it has been reported that 1.5 g of vitamin C for 2 months significantly lowers ceruloplasmin levels and serum copper concentration in blood; Finley & Cerklewski, 1983).

Competitive interactions can occur between nutrients that have similar physicochemical properties. An example is the interaction of iron and copper with zinc. Zinc absorption is strongly reduced when iron and copper are present in large amounts, such as in the form of supplements or in aqueous solution. In line with this, high levels of dietary calcium (>1 g/day) can inhibit zinc absorption, particularly in the presence of phytates. Unlike iron, zinc absorption is neither inhibited by phenolic compounds nor enhanced by vitamin C.

Dietary fiber has been a focus of interest in the past decade, mainly because of epidemiological data suggesting a protective effect against chronic diseases of the gastrointestinal tract. Fibers modulate several gastrointestinal physiological functions, such as motility, acid secretion and hormone release. Although dietary fiber may have a significant inhibitory effect on the absorption of nutrients, some of its actions on nutrient absorption can, therefore, be beneficial in the dietary prevention or management of diseases such as diabetes and hypercholesterolemia (Gunness & Gidley, 2010; Parada & Aguilera, 2011).

The bioavailability of many nutrients, besides being influenced by the amount that is consumed, may be compromised by the consumption of foods rich in phytate (present in large amounts in legumes and whole grain cereals), oxalate (high in spinach, sweet potatoes, beans and soy products) and phenolic compounds (present in coffee and tea) (Allen *et al.*, 2006). Once again, the bioavailability of iron and zinc is reduced by this group of compounds. Concerning iron, the main risk factors for its poor nutritional status include the low intake of heme-iron (which is present in meat, poultry and fish), an inadequate intake of vitamin C from fruit and vegetables (a natural enhancer of iron absorption), and also a reduced absorption of iron from diets that are high in phytate or phenolic compounds. Similarly, the amount of phytates in diet also inhibits the absorption of zinc. Zinc supplementation has been reported to influence the development and function of immune cells and the activity of stress-related proteins and anti-oxidant enzymes, and to help in maintaining genomic integrity and stability (Haase & Rink, 2009). The inclusion of animal proteins in the diet improves the total zinc intake and the efficiency of zinc absorption even from a high-phytate diet.

In fact, among all the antinutritional components, phytic acid is considered the most powerful antinutrient for human nutrition and health management. Phytate is abundant in legumes, cereals and nuts, and its unique structure offers it the ability to strongly chelate divalent and trivalent mineral cations, such as calcium, magnesium, zinc, copper, iron and manganese, to form large insoluble salts that are not readily absorbed by the human gastrointestinal tract, reducing the bioavailability of these minerals (Scheers, 2013). In addition, phytate has also been reported to form complexes with proteins at both low and high pH values. These complex formations alter the protein structure, which may result in decreased protein solubility, enzymatic activity and proteolytic digestibility (Kumar *et al.*, 2010).

In the context of high-phytate diets and impaired bioavailability of nutrients, it should be noted that the phytic acid content of cereals and legumes can be substantially reduced by several methods, such as milling (removes about 90% of the phytic acid from cereal grains), fermentation (activates naturally occurring cereal phytases, necessary to phytate degradation) and the addition of natural phytases to foods (the addition of whole wheat or whole rye to other cereals to completely degrade phytic acid) (Kumar *et al.*, 2010).

In spite of the many negative aspects on human health, the favorable effects of phytate-rich food consumption were recently revised by Kumar *et al.* (2010). These authors compiled evidence describing how phytate consumption may prevent a variety of cancers through mechanisms that involve anti-oxidation properties, interruption of cellular signal transduction, cell cycle inhibition and enhancement of natural killer cell activity. Phytates may also have a role in the prevention of diabetes, since they lower the blood glucose response by reducing the rate of starch digestion and slowing gastric emptying, and regulate insulin secretion via its effect on calcium channel activity (Barker & Berggren, 1999). It is also believed that phytates reduce blood clots, cholesterol and triglycerides and thus prevent CVD (Onomi *et al.*, 2004). Despite a series of studies on the positive and negative features of phytate, information on the dosage for humans is limited and the optimal dosage for clinical therapies is yet to be determined (Kumar *et al.*, 2010).

11.3.4.3 Drug–food and drug–nutrients interactions

A drug–food interaction is defined as a physical, chemical, physiological or pathophysiological relationship between a drug and a nutrient (Chan, 2013). These interactions may lead to changes in the kinetic or dynamic profile of a drug or a nutrient, or even to nutritional status (Genser, 2008). The term "kinetics" (pharmaco- or nutrikinetics) refers to the quantitative disposition of a drug or nutrient in the human body along time, which includes absorption, distribution, metabolism and excretion of the compound. The term "dynamics" (pharmaco- or nutridynamics) relates to clinical or physiological effects of the drug or nutrient, and often involves antagonism between them at the site of action (Chan, 2013).

Drug treatment can have detrimental effects on nutritional status, since it can adversely impair food intake through a variety of mechanisms, such as disturbance of the sense of taste and smell, anorexia and impairment of the absorption, metabolism and excretion of nutrients (Ortolani *et al.*, 2013). In fact, several drugs affect appetite by either central or peripheral mechanisms, inducing sedation or evoking an adverse response when food is ingested. Centrally acting drugs include catecholaminergic or dopaminergic (L-dopa) modulators, which act to suppress appetite. Drugs that affect peripheral mechanisms lead to a reduction in nutrient ingestion or absorption directly by inhibition of gastric emptying (L-dopa) or indirectly by causing nausea and vomiting (e.g. antibiotics, cytotoxic agents, iron preparations, levodopa, nicotine, opiates, selective serotonin reuptake inhibitors), diarrhea (e.g. broad-spectrum antibiotics, colchicin-related drugs, digoxin, erythromycin, lithium, metformin, metoclopramide, domperidone), xerostomia (e.g. amitryptiline, atropine, captopril, chlorphenamine, citalopam, codeine, diazepam, enalapril, fluoxetine, levodopa, paroxetine), hypogeusia/ageusia (e.g. ampicillin, benzodiazepines, clopidogrel, diltiazem, levodopa, metformin, nifedipine, spironolactone, tricyclic antidepressants) or olfactory disturbance (Van Zyl, 2011). In addition, several drugs have been associated clinically with taste complaints such as loss of taste (e.g. angiotensin-converting-enzyme inhibitors, cephalosporins, clopidogrel, metformin), bitter taste (e.g. aspirin, L-dopa, carbamazepine) or metallic taste (e.g. allopurinol, captopril, nifedipine) (Toffanello *et al.*, 2013).

The nutritional effects of several commonly used drugs are summarized in Table 11.1. Broadly, therapeutic agents may modify nutrient status at several levels: (a) by decreasing nutrient availability in the intestinal lumen (e.g. antibacterial agents of the tetracyclin group inhibit the absorption of several minerals owing to their chelating action; other

Table 11.1 Nutritional effects of some commonly used drugs

Antacids
- ↓ Bioavailability of thiamine
- ↓ Intestinal absorption of iron
- ↓ Phosphorus and vitamin A absorption (aluminum-containing antacids)
- Calcium carbonate antacids may cause steatorrhea

Antibiotics

Chloramphenicol
- ↑ Iron serum levels, and total iron binding capacity
- ↓ Physiological action of folic acid, increasing its requirements
- ↑ Vitamin B_{12} requirements; may cause peripheral neuropathy

Gentamicin
- ↑ Urinary losses of magnesium and potassium

Kanamicin
- Malabsorption of fats, vitamins A, D, K, and B_{12}

Neomycin
- Malabsorption of fats, vitamins A, D, K, and B_{12}
- ↓ Plasma vitamin B_{12} levels
- ↓ Intestinal absorption of iron, calcium, potassium and sodium

Penicillin
- At high doses may cause hypokalemia by ↑ urinary potassium losses
- Causes steatorrhea (oxacillin)

Sulfas
- ↓ Folic acid intestinal synthesis, absorption and serum levels
- Impairs response to folic acid supplements, increasing its requirements

Tetracycline
- Inhibits intestinal absorption of iron, calcium, zinc and magnesium
- Acts as chelating agent and ↓ synthesis of transport proteins at the enterocyte
- ↓ Intestinal absorption of fats
- ↓ Availability of vitamin K from intestinal bacteria
- ↑ Urinary losses of vitamin C and ↓ its concentration in plasma and leukocytes

Anticonvulsants *(phenobarbital, phenylhidantoin, phensuximide)*
- ↓ Serum vitamin D levels by activating the P450 oxidative system in the liver
- May cause osteomalacia and hypocalcemia
- ↓ Absorption and serum levels of folate
- ↓ Vitamin B_{12} transport; may cause neuropathy and megaloblastic anemia
- ↑ Copper serum levels

Antihyperlipidemic
- ↓ Absorption of fat-soluble vitamins and niacin

Antihypertensive drugs

Angiotensin-converting enzyme inhibitors (captopril, enalapril, lisinopril, ramipril)
- ↑ Potassium levels
- ↑ Sodium excretion

Atropine
- ↓ Intestinal absorption of iron

Barbiturates
- ↑ Vitamin D requirements by increasing its degradation
- ↑ Bone reabsorption of calcium and may cause osteomalacia
- ↓ Thiamine intestinal absorption
- ↑ vitamin C urinary losses
- ↓ Serum levels of vitamin B_{12}; prolonged use may lead to megaloblastic anemia

Continued

Table 11.1 Continued

Corticosteroids *(dexamethasone, hydrocortisone, prednisone)*
- ↓ Intestinal absorption of calcium and phosphorus and ↑ their urinary excretion
- High doses and chronic use may ↓ serum 1,25-$(OH)_2$-D_3 levels and cause osteoporosis
- May lead to negative nitrogen balance by ↑ urinary nitrogen losses of zinc
- ↑ Total cholesterol serum levels
- ↑ Glycemia and is associated with glucose tolerance impair

Indomethacin
- ↓ Vitamin C levels in plasma and platelets
- ↓ Intestinal absorption of amino acids

Laxatives
- ↓ Absorption of many vitamins (A, D, K and carotenes) and minerals
- Bisacodyl laxatives ↓ absorption of calcium, sodium, potassium and amino acids

Levodopa
- ↓ Absorption of amino acids

Oral contraceptives
- ↓ Ascorbic acid concentration in plasma, platelets, and leukocytes
- ↓ Serum levels of folic acid and vitamin B_{12}; may cause megaloblastic anemia
- Impair tryptophan metabolism and may change the plasma amino acid profile
- ↑ Serum levels of vitamin A and E, and copper
- ↑ Vitamin B_6 requirements

Proton pump inhibitors
- ↓ Absorption of calcium, iron, magnesium and vitamin B_{12}

Salycilates
- ↓ Vitamin C concentration in serum and platelets
- Antagonize vitamin K action on the coagulation system
- ↓ Intestinal absorption of many amino acids, particularly tryptophan, increasing their urinary excretion

Thiazide diuretics
- In combination with calcium and vitamin D supplements may cause hypercalcemia

Akamine *et al.* (2007); Genser, (2008); Ito & Jensen (2010); Teramura-Grönblad *et al.* (2010); Fabian *et al.* (2011); Van Zyl (2011); Brewer & Williams (2013); Chan (2013); Ortolani *et al.* (2013).

antibiotics may decrease the availability of vitamins by eliminating the local bacterial flora that synthesize them); (b) by inhibiting nutrient transport across the intestinal wall (a common mechanism of drugs that inhibit protein synthesis, such as chloramphenicol); (c) by antagonizing the physiological actions of nutrients in the postabsorptive phase (e.g. salycilates antagonize the anticoagulant action of vitamin K); (d) by enhancing nutrient catabolism (e.g. anti-epileptic drugs may lead to catabolism of vitamin D and hypocalcemia); and (e) by increasing nutrient losses (a large number of drugs increase fecal or urinary excretion of nutrients and non-nutrient circulating substances, e.g. gentamicin and barbiturates increase electrolyte and ascorbic acid losses, respectively). Additionally, some drug–nutrient interactions occur only when the nutrient and drugs such as those that change the intestinal pH are ingested concomitantly (Brewer & Williams, 2013).

Proton pump inhibitors are widely used in older people to treat acid peptic disorders and to reduce the risk of gastrointestinal bleeding related to the use of nonsteroidal anti-inflammatory drugs and low-dose aspirin. However, long-term therapy with proton pump inhibitors is associated with several nutritional risks, as its use seems to affect iron, magnesium and calcium absorption and increase the risk of hip fractures. It also diminishes vitamin B_{12} serum levels, a phenomenon that is not reduced by oral supplementation of this vitamin (Ito & Jensen, 2010). Furthermore, treatment with these drugs induces a clinical state similar to atrophic gastritis with markedly reduced gastric acid production, which inhibits pepsin activity because of augmented gastric pH. This condition is frequently associated with bacterial overgrowth, which may result in the malabsorption of fat, carbohydrate, protein, micronutrients and clinical manifestations of abdominal pain, diarrhea and even malnutrition (Teramura-Grönblad *et al.*, 2010).

Owing to the extensive media coverage of the potential health benefits of vitamin D supplementation over recent years that resulted in increased intakes of supplements, the potential for drug–vitamin D interactions deserves particular attention. Although there is insufficient evidence to determine whether lipase inhibitors, antimicrobial agents, antiepileptic drugs, highly active antiretroviral agents or histamine type 2 receptor antagonists alter serum vitamin D concentrations, the interaction with other common drugs, such as atorvastatin and thiazide diuretics, has been established. Atorvastatin, a widely used cholesterol-lowering drug, appears to increase vitamin D concentrations in blood, while concurrent vitamin D supplementation decreases circulating levels of the drug (Schwartz, 2009; Sathyapalan *et al.*, 2010). Concerning thiazide diuretics, their use in combination with calcium and vitamin D supplements may cause hypercalcemia in elderly individuals and in those with hyperparathyroidism or compromised renal function (Robien *et al.*, 2013).

Elderly patients are at particular high risk of suffering from adverse events associated with drug–nutrient interactions (Akamine *et al.*, 2007; Fabian *et al.*, 2011). This occurs because older people often receive chronic medications, usually more than one drug to manage different disease states, but mainly because ageing itself modifies several physiological functions that could affect the bioavailability, volume of distribution, clearance and half-life of drugs (Ortolani *et al.*, 2013). In older adults, nutrient–drug interactions may lead to a serious increase in morbidity and mortality, which may be misdiagnosed by the symptoms of the underlying disease process. In addition, the extent or consequences of nutrient–drug interaction may require a relatively long period of exposure to observe an effect. Furthermore, it should be noted that poor nutritional status, often observed in aged people, may also compromise drug metabolism by impairing absorption, and therefore limiting efficacy (Genser, 2008).

The growing knowledge of the potential for interaction between commonly ingested foods and prescribed medications should make prescribers and patients more aware of the possibility of (clinically meaningful) drug–food interactions, but without necessarily compromising a normal healthy diet (Brewer & Williams, 2013). Regular intake of several drugs may create submarginal nutrient deficiencies, such as vitamin deficiencies, with serious consequences in the elderly. Hence, the medication schedules and nutritional status of these subjects should be monitored closely to ensure that daily micronutrient requirements are met (Fabian *et al.*, 2012).

11.4 Favorable combinations of nutrients in food

Moving from a single food to food combinations, the concept of food synergy is of utmost importance. It results from the combination of foods within diet patterns, and of food components in single foods that are often the basis for diet and health relationship.

The food synergy argument is supported by studies focused on combinations of foods and from analyses of parts of certain foods, such as the investigations of Liu (2004) and Eberhardt *et al.* (2000). The first author demonstrated that the combination of orange, apple, grape and blueberry displayed a synergistic effect in anti-oxidant activity. The median effective dose (EC_{50}, the dose exhibiting 50% of total anti-oxidant activity) of the combination of fruit was one-fifth of the EC_{50} of each fruit alone (Liu, 2004). In addition, Eberhardt *et al.* (2000) studied the diversity and differential distribution of biochemical activity throughout the apple. They found that 100 g of apple with peel contained 290 mg of total phenolics and 143 mg of total flavonoids, compared with 220 and 98 mg, respectively, in the same amount of fruit without the peel. It was also verified that apple with peel contains 5.7 mg of vitamin C per 100 g, which contrasts with the 4.0 mg present in 100 g of peeled apples. Correspondingly, the total anti-oxidant activity was nearly double in the apples with peel than in those peeled.

The food synergy concept gains even more credence when effects observed under laboratory conditions are also verified in the everyday use of food, such as in salad preparation. Ninfali *et al.* (2005) reported that, when marjoram is added to salad, it can increase the anti-oxidant capacity of the dish by 200%. This might explain, in part, the apparent superior effects of certain cuisines and cultural dishes that involve combinations of foods, in particular herbs and spices.

The cell signaling pathways that control the initiation and development of many age-associated diseases are complex and interconnected. It has been shown that appropriate combinations of dietary phytochemicals can interact positively with these pathways. The consumption of vegetables that are rich in a wide variety of phytochemicals (phenolic acids, flavonols, carotenoids and organosulfurs) and which are cooked to best maintain the levels of these agents (see Section 11.3.3.1) may assist in the prevention and dietary control of many chronic diseases through additive or even synergistic mechanisms.

Extra-virgin olive oil is richer than regular or light olive oil in many beneficial compounds and nutrients, such as oleocanthal, a phenolic compound with anti-oxidant, anti-inflammatory and neuroprotective properties (Estruch *et al.*, 2013; Ibarrola-Jurado *et al.*, 2013). In order to maximize the benefits of oleocanthal present in extra-virgin olive oil, it should be consumed crude, since its biological activity and concentration diminish significantly with heat (Cicerale *et al.*, 2009; Lucas *et al.*, 2011). Interestingly, a further benefit of olive oil consumption might be related to its peculiar aroma, which seems to increase the feeling of satiety after a meal. The addition of an aromatic extract of olive oil to food reduces the amount of calories consumed and improves the blood sugar response. As compared with canola oil or lard, olive oil may also produce an increase in levels of blood serotonin, a monoamine neurotransmitter that is involved in satiety (O'Connor, 2013). Thus, the regular use of olive oil may represent an interesting approach in weight control management.

The need to encourage increased dietary intake of foods that are sources of heme-iron (meat, poultry and fish), and nonheme-iron (ready-to-eat fortified cereals and whole grains), is of great importance to attain and/or maintain a good iron status. However, foods containing nonheme-iron should be consumed along with enhancers of iron absorption, such as vitamin C-rich foods. The addition of ascorbic acid (vitamin C) to iron-fortified foods, reducing the effect of the inhibitors, can be an effective way of increasing the total amount of iron absorbed. Furthermore, ascorbic acid helps in reducing the risk of most cancers by inhibiting the production of cancer-causing nitrosamines formed as a result of the ingestion of cured meats (preserved with nitrates or nitrites) and/or endogenously produced by the reaction of amines and amides from red meat (John *et al.*, 2011).

Non-nutrient-dense foods supply relatively few micronutrients and more calories than their nutrient-dense counterparts. The regular consumption of diets that are high in energy but low in nutrients can paradoxically leave a person overweight but undernourished and thus at higher risk of CVD, type 2 diabetes, hypertension, hyperlipidemia, osteoporosis and certain types of cancers. In this setting, numerous studies demonstrate that the avoidance of high-energy/high-fat diets in favor of the daily ingestion of nutrient-dense foods, such as high-fiber whole grains, olives, nuts, fruit and vegetables, low-fat forms of milk, seafood, lean meat and poultry, prepared without (or minimal) added fats and/or sugars, protects against CVD and reduces the risk of coronary heart disease, all-cause mortality, ischemic strokes, breast and colorectal cancers (Chedraui & Pérez-López, 2013). These foods provide a full range of essential nutrients, and are found in a variety of forms (e.g. intact, minimally processed, sliced, diced, frozen, canned or cooked). The nutrient-dense diet should also be prepared using the best practices for food safety and quality. A balanced variety of foods among all the food groups, consumed in moderation, that are culturally appealing will offer pleasurable eating experiences and promote healthy ageing (Pérez-López *et al.*, 2009).

Notwithstanding the pernicious effects of high-fat diets, foods that contain high-quality fat have a positive impact on health. Dietary recommendations advise reduction of saturated and *trans* fatty acids intake in favor of mono- and polyunsaturated fats (Elmadfa & Kornsteiner, 2009). Considering this, over recent decades, the food industry has endeavored to adapt many high-fat products, such as margarines, to contain less *trans* fatty acids and saturated fat, and more essential polyunsaturated fats (fatty acids of the omega-3 and -6 families). At the same time, these products preserve natural beneficial minor components like vitamin E, and are often fortified with fat-soluble vitamins A and D (Zevenbergen *et al.*, 2009).

It is also important to note that the ingestion of foods that are rich in fats, preferably high-quality fats, contributes to the required intake of fat-soluble vitamins. Concerning vitamin A, the best sources are animal foods, in particular, liver, eggs and dairy products, which contain vitamin A in the form of retinol, the form that is readily used by the organism. Hence, it is not surprising that the risk of vitamin A deficiency is related to diets low in animal source foods, especially in those low in fat. Fruit and vegetables also contain vitamin A in the form of carotenoids, the most important of which is β-carotene. However, since carotenoids are powerful lipophilic anti-oxidants (Lademann *et al.*, 2011a), their bioavailability is much higher when ingested in a denatured form together with a lipid-containing carrier substance in comparison to the bioavailability of carotenoids obtained from raw fruit and vegetables (Gartner *et al.*, 1997). Various food preparation techniques, such as cooking, grinding and the addition of oil, can improve the absorption of food carotenoids. In a mixed diet, the conversion rate of β-carotene to retinol is approximately 12:1, whereas the conversion of other provitamin-A carotenoids to retinol is less efficient (24:1). Synthetic β-carotene in oil, which is widely used in vitamin A supplements, has a conversion rate to retinol of 2:1, and the synthetic forms of β-carotene that are commonly used to fortify foods have a conversion rate of 6:1 (Allen *et al.*, 2006).

Considering the research findings on the effects of processing and storage of foods on micronutrients and bioactive compounds, in recent years, several recommendations have emerged to maximize the retention of health-promoting food components. Fruits and vegetables should be stored intact, protected from direct sunlight and at low temperatures (for prolonged storage refrigeration is recommended). When the peel of fruit and vegetables is edible, they should not be peeled, otherwise they should be washed just before peeling or cutting, not after. Cutting the fruit and vegetables into very small pieces should also be avoided. They should be consumed or cooked immediately after peeling, cutting, chopping or pulping.

As previously described, nutrients can also be lost from foods during the cooking process in a temperature- and time-dependent fashion. Thus, alternative cooking methods such as grilling, roasting, steaming, stir-frying and microwaving generally preserve a greater proportion of vitamins and other nutrients, particularly in vegetables, in comparison to boiling or frying.

11.5 Lifestyle strategies for successful ageing

The Dietary Guidelines for Americans are designed to improve the health of all individuals aged 2 years and older (USDA Center for Nutrition Policy and Promotion, 2010). There are only a few age-specific recommendations regarding lower sodium, higher vitamin D and consumption of vitamin B_{12} from fortified foods or dietary supplements. Conversely, in Australia there is specific dietary guidance for older people – the Dietary Guidance for Older Australians – in which the nutritional requirements for older adults are divided into two groups: older adults in the third age and in the fourth age of life (Truswell, 2009). This is a very interesting perspective as the third age of life is considered a time of active healthy ageing when age-related conditions such as diabetes, hypertension and hyperlipidemia can be managed through diet and medication. In contrast, the fourth age is a time of declining and fragile health, weight loss and potential malnutrition. In the fourth age, advice to limit energy and consume a low-fat and low-sugar diet may no longer apply, because the focus should be on maintaining weight and strength. The American Academy of Nutrition/American Dietetic Association also supports less restrictive diets for very old adults (Dorner *et al.*, 2010).

Optimal nutrient intakes are those that, while minimizing the risk of excess, promote health and reduce risk for chronic disease. The Institute of Medicine's Dietary Reference Intakes (DRIs) are the best available evidence-based nutrient standards to assess adequate and excess nutrient intakes and plan diets for individuals or groups. The DRIs include the Estimated Average Requirements (EARs, values that meet the requirements of 50% of people in their target group within a given life stage and for a particular sex), RDA values, which are set to meet the needs of 97–98% of healthy population (RDAs are not individual nutritional requirements), Adequate Intakes (AIs, when there is insufficient and consistent scientific evidence to set an EAR for the entire population; the value is based on observed intakes of the nutrient by a group of healthy persons), and Tolerable Upper Intake Levels (UL, the maximum level of daily nutrient intake that is likely to pose no risks of toxicity for almost all individuals). The current DRIs for adults are summarized in Table 11.2. In this context, it should be emphasized that, in clinical practice, RDAs and AIs may not be adequate for malnourished individuals, as well as those with specific health conditions or who take medications that alter their requirement for a nutrient. Furthermore, usual intakes that fall below recommended levels should not be

Table 11.2 Dietary Reference Intakes for adults, from Food and Nutrition Board, Institute of Medicine, National Academies

		Males				Females			
		19–30 years	31–50 years	51–70 years	>70 years	19–30 years	31–50 years	51–70 years	>70 years
Total water and macronutrients									
Total water[a] (l/day)	AI* or RDA	3.7*	3.7*	3.7*	3.7*	2.7*	2.7*	2.7*	2.7*
Carbohydrate (g/day)	EAR	100	100	100	100	100	100	100	100
	AI* or RDA	130	130	130	130	130	130	130	130
	AMDR	45–65	45–65	45–65	45–65	45–65	45–65	45–65	45–65
Total fiber (g/day)	AI* or RDA	38*	38*	30*	30*	25*	25*	21*	21*
Total fat (g/day)	AI* or RDA	ND	ND	ND	ND	ND	ND	ND	ND
	AMDR	20–35	20–35	20–35	20–35	20–35	20–35	20–35	20–35
Linoleic acid (g/day)	AI* or RDA	17*	17*	14*	14*	12*	12*	11*	11*
	AMDR	5–10	5–10	5–10	5–10	5–10	5–10	5–10	5–10
α-Linolenic acid (g/day)	AI* or RDA	1.6*	1.6*	1.6*	1.6*	1.1*	1.1*	1.1*	1.1*
	AMDR	0.6–1.2	0.6–1.2	0.6–1.2	0.6–1.2	0.6–1.2	0.6–1.2	0.6–1.2	0.6–1.2
Protein[b] (g/kg/day)	EAR	0.66	0.66	0.66	0.66	0.66	0.66	0.66	0.66
	AI* or RDA	0.8	0.8	0.8	0.8	0.8	0.8	0.8	0.8
	AMDR	10–35	10–35	10–35	10–35	10–35	10–35	10–35	10–35
Essential amino acids									
Histidine (mg/kg/day)	EAR	11	11	11	11	11	11	11	11
	AI* or RDA	14	14	14	14	14	14	14	14
Isoleucine (mg/kg/day)	EAR	15	15	15	15	15	15	15	15
	AI* or RDA	19	19	19	19	19	19	19	19
Leucine (mg/kg/day)	EAR	34	34	34	34	34	34	34	34
	AI* or RDA	42	42	42	42	42	42	42	42
Lysine (mg/kg/day)	EAR	31	31	31	31	31	31	31	31
	AI* or RDA	38	38	38	38	38	38	38	38
Methionine plus cysteine (mg/kg/day)	EAR	15	15	15	15	15	15	15	15
	AI* or RDA	19	19	19	19	19	19	19	19
Phenylalanine plus tyrosin (mg/kg/day)	EAR	27	27	27	27	27	27	27	27
	AI* or RDA	33	33	33	33	33	33	33	33
Threonine (mg/kg/day)	EAR	16	16	16	16	16	16	16	16
	AI* or RDA	20	20	20	20	20	20	20	20

Tryptophan(mg/kg/	EAR	4	4	4	4	4	4	4	4
day)	AI* or RDA	5	5	5	5	5	5	5	5
Valine (mg/kg/day)	EAR	19	19	19	19	19	19	19	19
	AI* or RDA	24	24	24	24	24	24	24	24
Vitamins									
Vitamin A[c] (μg/day)	EAR	625	625	625	625	500	500	500	500
	AI* or RDA	900	900	900	900	700	700	700	700
	UL	3,000	3,000	3,000	3,000	3,000	3,000	3,000	3,000
Vitamin C (mg/day)	EAR	75	75	75	75	60	60	60	60
	AI* or RDA	90	90	90	90	75	75	75	75
	UL	2,000	2,000	2,000	2,000	2,000	2,000	2,000	2,000
Vitamin D[d] (μg/day)	EAR	10	10	10	10	10	10	10	10
	AI* or RDA	15	15	15	20	15	15	15	20
	UL	100	100	100	100	100	100	100	100
Vitamin E[e] (mg/day)	EAR	12	12	12	12	12	12	12	12
	AI* or RDA	15	15	15	15	15	15	15	15
	UL	1,000	1,000	1,000	1,000	1,000	1,000	1,000	1,000
Vitamin K (μg/day)	EAR	ND	ND	ND	ND	ND	ND	ND	ND
	AI* or RDA	120*	120*	120*	120*	90*	90*	90*	90*
	UL	ND	ND	ND	ND	ND	ND	ND	ND
Thiamin (mg/day)	EAR	1.0	1.0	1.0	1.0	0.9	0.9	0.9	0.9
	AI* or RDA	1.2	1.2	1.2	1.2	1.1	1.1	1.1	1.1
	UL	ND	ND	ND	ND	ND	ND	ND	ND
Riboflavin (mg/day)	EAR	1.1	1.1	1.1	1.1	0.9	0.9	0.9	0.9
	AI* or RDA	1.3	1.3	1.3	1.3	1.1	1.1	1.1	1.1
	UL	ND	ND	ND	ND	ND	ND	ND	ND
Niacin[f] (mg/day)	EAR	12	12	12	12	11	11	11	11
	AI* or RDA	16	16	16	16	14	14	14	14
	UL	35	35	35	35	35	35	35	35
Vitamin B_6 (mg/day)	EAR	1.1	1.1	1.4	1.4	1.1	1.1	1.3	1.3
	AI* or RDA	1.3	1.3	1.7	1.7	1.3	1.3	1.5	1.5
	UL	100	100	100	100	100	100	100	100
Folate[g] (μg/day)	EAR	320	320	320	320	320	320	320	320
	AI* or RDA	400	400	400	400	400	400	400	400
	UL	1,000	1,000	1,000	1,000	1,000	1,000	1,000	1,000

Continued

Table 11.2 Continued

Vitamin B_{12}[h] (µg/day)	EAR	2.0	2.0	2.0	2.0	2.0	2.0	2.0	2.0
	AI* or RDA	2.4	2.4	2.4	2.4	2.4	2.4	2.4	2.4
	UL	ND	ND	ND	ND	ND	ND	ND	ND
Minerals									
Calcium (mg/day)	EAR	800	800	800	1,000	800	800	1,000	1,000
	AI* or RDA	1,000	1,000	1,000	1,200	1,000	1,000	1,200	1,200
	UL	2,500	2,500	2,000	2,000	2,500	2,500	2,000	2,000
Phosphorus (mg/day)	EAR	580	580	580	580	580	580	580	580
	AI* or RDA	700	700	700	700	700	700	700	700
	UL	4	4	4	3	4	4	4	3
Iron (mg/day)	EAR	6	6	6	6	8.1	8.1	5	5
	AI* or RDA	8	8	8	8	18	18	8	8
	UL	45	45	45	45	45	45	45	45
Chromium (µg/day)	EAR	ND	ND	ND	ND	ND	ND	ND	ND
	AI* or RDA	35*	35*	30*	30*	25*	25*	20*	20*
	UL	ND	ND	ND	ND	ND	ND	ND	ND
Magnesium (mg/day)	EAR	330	350	350	350	255	265	265	265
	AI* or RDA	400	420	420	420	310	320	320	320
	UL**	350	350	350	350	350	350	350	350
Fluoride (mg/day)	EAR	ND	ND	ND	ND	ND	ND	ND	ND
	AI* or RDA	4*	4*	4*	4*	3*	3*	3*	3*
	UL	10	10	10	10	10	10	10	10
Copper (µg/day)	EAR	700	700	700	700	700	700	700	700
	AI* or RDA	900	900	900	900	900	900	900	900
	UL	10,000	10,000	10,000	10,000	10,000	10,000	10,000	10,000
Iodine (µg/day)	EAR	95	95	95	95	95	95	95	95
	AI* or RDA	150	150	150	150	150	150	150	150
	UL	1,100	1,100	1,100	1,100	1,100	1,100	1,100	1,100
Molybdenum (µg/day)	EAR	34	34	34	34	34	34	34	34
	AI* or RDA	45	45	45	45	45	45	45	45
	UL	2,000	2,000	2,000	2,000	2,000	2,000	2,000	2,000

Selenium (μg/day)	EAR	45	45	45	45	45	45	45	45
	AI* or RDA	55	55	55	55	55	55	55	55
	UL	400	400	400	400	400	400	400	400
Manganese (mg/day)	EAR	ND	ND	ND	ND	ND	ND	ND	ND
	AI* or RDA	2.3*	2.3*	2.3*	2.3*	1.8*	1.8*	1.8*	1.8*
	UL	11	11	11	11	11	11	11	11
Zinc (mg/day)	EAR	9.4	9.4	9.4	9.4	6.8	6.8	6.8	6.8
	AI* or RDA	11	11	11	11	8	8	8	8
	UL	40	40	40	40	40	40	40	40
Elements									
Potassium (g/day)	EAR	ND	ND	ND	ND	ND	ND	ND	ND
	AI* or RDA	4.7*	4.7*	4.7*	4.7*	4.7*	4.7*	4.7*	4.7*
	UL	ND	ND	ND	ND	ND	ND	ND	ND
Sodium (g/day)	EAR	ND	ND	ND	ND	ND	ND	ND	ND
	AI* or RDA	1.5*	1.5*	1.3*	1.2*	1.5*	1.5*	1.3*	1.2*
	UL	2.3	2.3	2.3	2.3	2.3	2.3	2.3	2.3
Chloride (g/day)	EAR	ND	ND	ND	ND	ND	ND	ND	ND
	AI* or RDA	2.3*	2.3*	2.0*	1.8*	2.3*	2.3*	2.0*	1.8*
	UL	3.6	3.6	3.6	3.6	3.6	3.6	3.6	3.6

Dietary Reference Intakes for Calcium, Phosphorous, Magnesium, Vitamin D, and Fluoride (1997); Dietary Reference Intakes for Thiamin, Riboflavin, Niacin, Vitamin B_6, Folate, Vitamin B_{12}, Pantothenic Acid, Biotin, and Choline (1998); Dietary Reference Intakes for Vitamin C, Vitamin E, Selenium, and Carotenoids (2000); Dietary Reference Intakes for Vitamin A, Vitamin K, Arsenic, Boron, Chromium, Copper, Iodine, Iron, Manganese, Molybdenum, Nickel, Silicon, Vanadium, and Zinc (2001); Dietary Reference Intakes for Energy, Carbohydrate, Fiber, Fat, Fatty Acids, Cholesterol, Protein, and Amino Acids (2002/2005); Dietary Reference Intakes for Water, Potassium, Sodium, Chloride, and Sulfate (2005); and Dietary Reference Intakes for Calcium and Vitamin D (2011). These reports may be accessed at www.nap.edu.

DRIs, Dietary Reference Intakes; EARs, Estimated Average Requirements; RDAs, Recommended Dietary Allowances; AIs, Adequate Intakes; ULs, Tolerable Upper Intake Levels; ND, not determinable; AMDR, Acceptable Macronutrient Distribution Range.

*AI; **the ULs for magnesium represent intake from a pharmacological agent only and do not include intake from food and water; ***as a percentage of energy.

[a] Total water includes all water contained in food, beverages and drinking water. [b] Based on grams protein per kilogram of body weight for the reference body weight, for example, for adults 0.8 g/kg body weight for the reference body weight. [c] As retinol activity equivalents (RAEs); 1 RAE = 1 μg retinol, 12 μg β-carotene, 24 μg α-carotene or 24 μg β-cryptoxanthin. The RAE for dietary provitamin A carotenoids is two-fold greater than the retinol equivalent (RE), whereas the RAE for preformed vitamin A is the same as RE. [d] As cholecalciferoL; 1 μg cholecalciferol = 40 IU vitamin D; under the assumption of minimal sunlight. [e] As α-tocopherol; α-tocopherol includes *RRR*-α-tocopherol, the only form of α-tocopherol that occurs naturally in foods, and the 2*R*-stereoisomeric forms of α-tocopherol (*RRR*-, *RSR*-, *RRS*- and *RSS*-α-tocopherol) that occur in fortified foods and supplements. It does not include the 2*S*-stereoisomeric forms of α-tocopherol (*SRR*-, *SSR*-, *SRS*- and *SSS*-α-tocopherol), also found in fortified foods and supplements. [f] As niacin equivalents (NE); 1 mg of niacin = 60 mg of tryptophan. [g] As dietary folate equivalents (DFE); 1 DFE = 1 μg food folate = 0.6 μg of folic acid from fortified food or as a supplement consumed with food = 0.5 μg of a supplement taken on an empty stomach. [h] Because 10–30% of older people may malabsorb food-bound B_{12}, it is advisable for those older than 50 years to meet their RDA mainly by consuming foods fortified with B_{12} or a supplement containing B_{12}.

interpreted as inadequate. Clinical status and biochemical indexes should be among the factors included with intake data to assess an individual's dietary adequacy and nutritional status. The complete information should be used to determine if a person is likely to benefit, or not, from nutrient supplementation (Marra & Boyar, 2009).

As reported before, a wide selection of nutrient-rich foods is generally the best strategy for meeting nutrient needs. Foods, particularly of vegetable origin, such as fruit, vegetables, whole grains, beans, nuts, seeds and teas, provide an array of other health-promoting substances beyond vitamins and minerals, including carotenoids and polyphenols. Data suggest that positive health outcomes are related more to dietary patterns, the types and amounts of foods consumed, than to intakes of individual nutrients (Lichtenstein & Russell, 2005; Murphy *et al.*, 2007). In line with this, notwithstanding the importance of dietary reference values or recommended nutrient intakes, in Europe, the Food-based Dietary Guidelin*es* were designed according to the principles of nutritional education mostly as foods (EFSA, 2010). They represent the form in which advice is provided to people to assist them in selecting a diet to meet their needs for health. In addition, in 2012, World Health Organization (WHO) published a user-friendly guide – Promoting a Healthy Diet for the WHO Eastern Mediterranean Region – in which information on individual nutrients and food components is provided (World Health Organization, 2012). The recommendations contained in this guide are compatible with the different cultures and eating patterns of consumers within the target population and are based on the availability of local and affordable foods that are widely consumed by the population.

11.5.1 The Mediterranean and Asian diets

The enjoyment of food has crucial importance in health-related quality of life and the ageing process progression (Bernstein & Munoz, 2012). Evidence shows that, besides a nutritious diet, maintaining an appropriate body weight and an active lifestyle are the key to avoiding the physical and cognitive degeneration associated with ageing (Bernstein & Munoz, 2012). Within this scope, a number of diets have received attention owing to their possible benefits for health (de Lorgeril, 2013). Two of these are the Mediterranean and Asian diets.

These diets are rich in fruit and, especially, in vegetables, thereby providing high amounts of bioactive compounds such as polyphenols. Furthermore, fish, which are rich in omega-3 fatty acids, are also present in both diets (Pallauf *et al.*, 2013). There are specific plant bioactive compounds that occur in the Mediterranean, like those found in red wine and olive oil. In the Asian diet there are also those found in soybean (isoflavones), green tea (catechins) and, in coastal Asia, seaweed (a source of anti-oxidant vitamins and polyunsaturated omega 3 fatty acids). In India and other Eastern Asia countries, curry spices are widely used for flavoring many food preparations and recipes. These include curcumin, which has anti-oxidant, anti-inflammatory and antiproliferative properties (Pallauf *et al.*, 2013).

From a nutritional point of view, there is a substantial overlap between Asian and Mediterranean diets (de Lorgeril, 2013; Pallauf *et al.*, 2013; Sofi *et al.*, 2013). Pallauf *et al.* (2013) even proposed adopting a "MediterrAsian" diet to describe a diet combining Asian and Mediterranean foods that could be an approach to improving human health. They advanced the concept and proposed denominating these diets "sirtfoods" owing to their likely sirtuin-activation properties (discussed in Chapter 2).

Interestingly, from a cultural point of view, but, and this is an important point to stress, not from that of the international health organizations, the Mediterranean Diet was nominated as the World's Intangible Cultural Heritage of Humanity by the United Nations Educational, Scientific and Cultural Organization (UNESCO) in December 2010, including Spain, Greece, Italy and Morocco, with the addition of Portugal, Cyprus and Croatia in December 2013. According to a prepared statement by UNESCO, "The Mediterranean diet is a set of traditional practices, knowledge and skills passed on from generation to generation and providing a sense of belonging and continuity to the concerned communities" (http://www.unesco.org/culture/ich/RL/00884). The traditional dietary culture of Japan (washoku), a typical Asian diet, was also inscribed in December 2013 on the Representative List of the Intangible Cultural Heritage of Humanity, reading that "washoku is a social practice based on a set of skills, knowledge, practice and traditions related to the production, processing, preparation and consumption of food", and also that it "favours the consumption of various natural, locally sourced ingredients such as rice, fish, vegetables and edible wild plants" (http://www.unesco.org/culture/ich/RL/00869).

From the scientific point of view, there is a marked contrast between these two diets and the "Western" diet. In fact, the INTERHEART and INTERSTROKE studies (Iqbal *et al.*, 2008; O'Donnell *et al.*, 2010) considered the existence of three dietary patterns, assessed by a simple dietary risk score: (a) "Western", with high intake of fried foods, salty snacks, eggs and meat; (b) "oriental", high in tofu, soy and other sauces; and (c) "prudent", with a high intake of fruit and vegetables. It was found that the "Western diet" increased the population risk for acute myocardial infarction and stroke by approximately 30%, whereas the "prudent diet", with some characteristics of the Mediterranean diet, lowered the same risk by 30%. Curiously, the "oriental diet" was neutral, probably because the high intake of fruit, fish and vegetables was offset by other factors, such as high salt intake (Iqbal *et al.*, 2008; O'Donnell *et al.*, 2010).

A subtype of Asian diet, the Okinawan diet, and its effects during ageing and on longevity, were described in Chapter 2. We will now analyze more deeply the Mediterranean diet, as there are more studies published regarding it.

The concept of the Mediterranean diet dates back to the middle of the 20th century. Ancel Keys, a nonphysician American scientist, observed that there was a low incidence of coronary heart disease in the region of Naples in Italy and associated this finding with the "Mediterranean diet", a term coined by him (Keys, 1995). This diet was essentially vegetarian and used fruit for dessert, contrary to the diet generally adopted in North America and North Europe, rich in high-sugar and high-fat foods, meat and dairy products (Key, 1995). These observations led to the "Seven Countries Study" (Keys, 1970). In this now famous study, data from countries of the Mediterranean region (Greece, former Yugoslavia and Italy) showed lower coronary heart disease incidence than those from the Netherlands and USA (Keys, 1970). The continuation of the "Seven Countries Study" also demonstrated that the slowly changing habits of the population of the Mediterranean region from a "healthy" diet and active life to a less active lifestyle and changes in the diet have resulted in an increase in the risk of CVD in Greece and Italy (Menotti *et al.*, 1996; Kafatos *et al.*, 1997).

There are many "Mediterranean diets" (Noah & Truswell, 2001) and even travesties of Mediterranean diets (Keys, 1995). Defining a Mediterranean-style diet is challenging considering that the geographical region includes more than 17 countries. In addition, there are several types of diet within each country, for example in Italy and France. There is no single ideal Mediterranean diet and when the concept is utilized it would be more correct to identify not only the country, but also the region of the country (Noah & Truswell, 2001, 2006). Furthermore, between the early 1950s and 1960s and the present time, there have been great changes in food consumption patterns in the Mediterranean countries (Noah & Truswell, 2001, 2006). Owing to these changes, the time in history is also relevant when defining a Mediterranean diet (Noah & Truswell, 2001, 2006). Many differences in culture, ethnic background, religion, economy and agricultural production result in different diets. According to de Lorgeril (2013), an acceptable definition of Mediterranean diet is the following: "a modern nutritional recommendation inspired by the traditional dietary patterns of Greece and South Italy". This common Mediterranean dietary pattern is based in the following characteristics: (a) high consumption of fruit, legumes and vegetables, bread and other cereals, potatoes, beans, nuts and seeds; (b) olive oil as the main monounsaturated fat source; (c) dairy products, fish and poultry consumed in low to moderate amounts, and little red meat; and (d) wine consumed in low to moderate amounts and generally during meals (de Lorgeril, 2013).

Striking benefits in the secondary prevention of CVD from a Mediterranean diet supplemented with margarine containing the essential omega-3 fatty acid α-linolenic acid in comparison with the typically recommended low-fat diet, were reported as early as 1994 and known as the Lyon Diet–Heart Study (de Lorgeril *et al.*, 1994). This randomized controlled trial tested a modern version of the Mediterranean diet, according to the authors but disputed by others (Appel & van Horn, 2013), in patients who had already survived prior acute myocardial infarction (de Lorgeril *et al.*, 1994, 1999; de Lorgeril, 2013). In this Lyon study, after a mean follow-up of 27 months, there was a 50% reduction in the risk of cardiovascular events, fewer cancers and a significant reduction of overall mortality that was much lower in the group given the diet enriched with acid α-linolenic acid (de Lorgeril *et al.*, 1994).

In 2003, Trichopoulou *et al.* published a large prospective study using a Mediterranean diet-score, the first modern epidemiological study concerning the health effects of the Mediterranean diet (Trichopoulou *et al.*, 2003). After adjustment for confounders (physical activity, several socio-economic factors, etc.) the authors verified that deaths from coronary heart disease and cancer were inversely associated with greater adhesion with the diet. The Mediterranean diet was demonstrated to be highly protective and not associated with major adverse effects as shown by the lower all-cause mortality in adherents. Also noteworthy is that only the whole dietary pattern was protective, that is, the associations between the individual food groups were generally not significant when total mortality was considered (Trichopoulou *et al.*, 2003). This study involving more than 22,000 adults in Greece confirmed the findings of the Lyon study.

Following this Greek study, several other research groups analyzed population groups in a large number of observational studies that have suggested that subjects following a "Mediterranean-type diet" tend to have lower levels of cardiovascular risk factors, fewer diseases and lower mortality. As observational studies, they fail, however, to demonstrate a cause–effect relationship. However, summarizing the prospective observational studies, a meta-analysis was published by Sofi *et al.* in 2008 and updated in 2010 (Sofi *et al.*, 2008, 2010). The studies analyzed prospectively the association between adherence to a Mediterranean diet, mortality and incidence of diseases, with a total of more than 2 million subjects followed for a time ranging from 3 to 18 years.

Greater adherence to a Mediterranean diet is associated with a significant improvement in health status, as seen by a significant reduction in overall mortality (9%), mortality from CVD (9%), incidence of or mortality from cancer (6%), and incidence of Parkinson and Alzheimer diseases (13%), denoting a consistent protection related to the adherence to diet for the occurrence of major chronic degenerative diseases associated with ageing (Sofi *et al.*, 2008, 2010).

One of the latest pieces of evidence concerning the Mediterranean diet outcomes was published in 2013 in the New England Journal of Medicine, focused on the Prevención con Dieta Mediterránea (PREDIMED) trial, a multicenter randomized clinical trial (Estruch *et al.*, 2013). The PREDIMED results showed that relatively small changes in diet can have powerful and beneficial effects (Estruch *et al.*, 2013). The clinical trial in Spain was carried out among 7447 subjects at risk of CVD (on the basis of the presence of diabetes, hypertension, dyslipidemia and other risk factors). The clinical trial compared the effects of two versions of a Mediterranean-type diet, without any energy restriction. One version of the Mediterranean-type diet contained large amounts of extra-virgin olive oil and the other was supplemented with mixed nuts. There was a "control group", made up of subjects who were advised to follow a low-fat, low-cholesterol diet, typically recommended for reducing the risk of CVD (Estruch *et al.*, 2013; Ros *et al.*, 2014).

Both of the groups advised to consume a Mediterranean diet showed an increase in total ingested fat, from an average of 39.3% of total energy provided from fat to an average of more than 41%; on the other hand, the group advised to decrease their total fat lowered their intake from 39 to 37% of energy provided from fat. All three groups showed slight decreases in saturated fat and slight decreases in dietary cholesterol intake (but blood cholesterol levels were not reported). Only the group with added nuts showed an increase in α-linolenic acid, the fatty acid related to the lowest risk of CVD in the Cretan cohort of the Seven-Countries Study and in the Lyon Diet-Heart Study (Keys, 1970, 1995; de Lorgeril *et al.*, 1994). The work of Renaud *et al.* (1995) also repeatedly showed that higher levels of α-linolenic acid, and lower levels of linoleic acid, are key factors in reducing cardiovascular risk. On the basis of interim results, the study was stopped earlier than initially planned by a monitoring board after a median follow-up of just under 5 years. The conclusions showed that the adoption of a Mediterranean style diet reduced the risk of cardiovascular complications by 30%, including a reduction of the risk of stroke by 40% over a follow-up of approximately 5 years (Estruch *et al.*, 2013). The number of recorded complications was very small in the three experimental groups. In other words, even the "low-fat" control group had a low rate of cardiovascular complications, probably because they also followed a Mediterranean diet (de Lorgeril, 2013).

What were the key elements of the Mediterranean diet leading to the better health outcomes? When reviewing the nutrient data provided, better results were obtained from a diet that was higher in total fat and with slightly more fish and legumes than the typical "low-fat diet" that was advised for the control group. However, the main contributors to the effects observed appear to be the supplements provided to subjects: rather large amounts of extra-virgin olive oil or several helpings per week of nuts. The authors agreed, as they stated, that: "extra virgin olive oil and nuts were probably responsible for most of the observed benefits of the Mediterranean diets". More likely, the interaction between various nutrients is probably the source of biological protection, confirming the data from the Lyon Study and the Greek population studied by Trichopoulou and collaborators (de Lorgeril, 2013).

In the Editorial of the same issue of the *New England Journal of Medicine*, Appel and Van Horn, remarked that the PREDIMED trial was not a pure test of a Mediterranean diet or a pure test of extra-virgin oil and nuts (Appel & Van Horn, 2013). They also note that both the PREDIMED and Lyon studies are very similar in their complexity (Appel & Van Horn, 2013). In the same issue, in another paper, Tracy writes that "the Mediterranean diet has become the standard of healthy eating" (Tracy, 2013) and points to a dietary template that may be of particular value as chronic diseases become a particular issue during ageing (de Lorgeril, 2013; Tracy, 2013). De Lorgeril (2013) also claims that now "in terms of evidence-based medicine, the full adoption of a modern version of the Mediterranean diet pattern can be considered one of the most effective approaches for the prevention of fatal and nonfatal cardiovascular complications". Contrary to the pharmacological approach of cardiovascular prevention, the adoption of the Mediterranean diet was associated with a significant reduction in new cancers and overall mortality (de Lorgeril, 2013).

However, there are many criticisms of the PREDIMED trial and other studies related to the Mediterranean diet. According to Ioannidis, many favorable reports, including PREDIMED and Lyon trials, studying the Mediterranean diet are implausible (Ioannidis, 2013). This author claims that observational studies and even some randomized trials are not valid owing to the presence of many confounding factors and other types of bias creating noise and not giving safe conclusions. In addition, he argues that, although the Lyon Diet Heart Study and the PREDIMED trial showed enormous relative risk reductions in clinical outcomes with Mediterranean diets, effect sizes are exaggerated owing to early termination of the trials and the selection of high-risk populations (heart disease in the first study; metabolic syndrome in the second study; Ioannidis, 2013). Patients in the PREDIMED study were already under treatment with multiple cardiovascular drugs like statins and there were many other confounders. In addition, there was only a significant reduction in death from stroke and the reduction of mortality of cardiovascular causes was only significant when considering the pool of deaths from stroke.

However, Ioannidis concedes that these two randomized trials represent a big step and probably they are the path to identifying nutrition-related interventions capable of lowering the relative risk in overall mortality by 5–10% in the general population, not just in high-risk individuals. He considers, however, that this would require more than 10 times the sample size of PREDIMED, long-term follow-up, good adherence and good death registry. Preferably, sponsoring and conduct should be free of conflicts and allegiance bias should be minimized. Ioannidis stresses this latter point, given that fanatical opinions are very frequent in nutrition research (Ioannidis, 2013).

Also in 2013, a review was published by the Cochrane Heart Group concerning the "Mediterranean" dietary pattern for the primary prevention of CVD (Rees *et al.*, 2013). The Mediterranean dietary pattern was defined and should have at least two of the following characteristics to be included in the review: (a) high monounsaturated/saturated fat ratio (olive oil used for cooking); (b) low to moderate red wine consumption; (c) high consumption of legumes; (d) high consumption of grains and cereals; (e) high consumption of fruit and nuts; (f) low consumption of meat and meat products, with increased consumption of fish; and (g) moderate consumption of milk and dairy products (Rees *et al.*, 2013).

This systematic review included 11 random controlled trials of 15 papers and 52,044 randomized participants. The PREDIMED trial was not included because it did not meet the strict inclusion criteria of the analysis as the comparison group was not minimal, for example, received face-to-face dietary advice (Rees *et al.*, 2013). The authors concluded that there is limited evidence to date, but the Mediterranean diet may reduce some cardiovascular risk factors (total cholesterol levels, low-density-lipoprotein cholesterol levels). As usual, they point to the necessity of more trials to verify the effects of the participants recruited and different dietary interventions for analysis of which interventions might work best. Nevertheless, they concede that the available evidence is promising and supportive of the favorable effects of this diet. There is also a strong biological plausibility supported by numerous other studies. Mechanisms that can explain these effects include a reduction in blood pressure and insulin resistance, an improvement in the lipid profile and anti-inflammatory effects (Rees *et al.*, 2013). Other mechanisms may result from polyphenols and omega-3 action, but further studies are necessary to confirm all of these hypotheses (de Lorgeril, 2013).

Even more recently, it was published that adherence to a Mediterranean diet-style pattern was associated with a 7% reduction in all-cause mortality in 6137 men and 11,278 women with myocardial infarction, stroke, angina pectoris, coronary bypass and coronary angioplasty (Lopez-Garcia *et al.*, 2014). A systematic review and meta-analysis of observational studies found that adherence to Mediterranean diet is associated with a significant reduction of overall of cancer mortality (10%), colorectal cancer (14%), prostate cancer (4%) and aerodigestive cancer (56%) (Schwingshackl & Hoffmann, 2014). No significant risk reduction was observed for breast, gastric and pancreatic cancer. Again, there are biological explanations for these observational findings related to cancer. For example, the phenolic content of extra-virgin and virgin oil is able to affect cancer-regulated oncogenes (Sotiroudis & Kyrtopoulos, 2008; Schwingshackl & Hoffmann, 2014). The lower risk of cancer may be due to the multiple and pleiotropic effects of the flavonoids in the high consumption of fruit and vegetables, including antioxidant activity, anti-inflammatory action, antimutagenic and antiproliferative properties as well as regulation of cell signaling and cell cycle, and angiogenesis (Arts & Hollman, 2005; Schwingshackl & Hoffmann, 2014).

Most of the studies are conducted on Mediterranean populations but one paper studied the effects of adherence to the Mediterranean-style diet on CVD biomarkers, metabolic syndrome and body composition in a homogeneous cohort of active male firefighters of the US Midwest, minimizing confounding factors such as gender or socioeconomic differences. They found that a greater adherence to this dietary pattern had inverse associations with metabolic syndrome features including low-density-lipoprotein cholesterol and reported weight gain, and on the other hand, was associated with higher high-density-lipoprotein (HDL) cholesterol (Yang *et al.*, 2014).

With this accumulated evidence the question that arises is: should health professionals recommend the Mediterranean diet? The authors of the Cochrane Review concluded that there is no reason for such advice, owing to the limitations and variables of the study populations and the partial adherence to the Mediterranean dietary patterns (Rees *et al.*, 2013). However, we cannot disregard the fact that there is some consensus, and based on the persuasive body of evidence from observational studies, some policymakers already recommend some aspects and components of a Mediterranean-style diet (Appel & van Horn, 2013). For example, there are the clinical guidelines for the prevention of CVD such as the DASH (Dietary Approaches to Stop Hypertension) diet (Appel *et al.*, 2006) and the advice to eat at least five portions of fruit and vegetables per day by the US Dietary Guidelines for Americans (USDA Center for Nutrition Policy and Promotion, 2010). However, the position of the American Heart Association is more cautious. They assume that Mediterranean-style diets are close to their own dietary recommendations, but they stress that the high percentages of energy derived from fat in the diet can lead to obesity. They also write that lifestyle factors, such as physical activity and extended social support systems, may also play a part in the lower number of deaths from CVD in some of the populations of the Mediterraneum (www.heart.org/HEARTORG/GettingHealthy/NutritionCenter/MediterraneanDiet_UCM_306004_Article.jsp). As customary, they conclude that more studies are needed. In the same line of thought, The European Society of Cardiology mentions the Mediterranean diet in CVD guidelines, stating that this pattern of diet has gained interest in recent years. Again, they write that it is not yet clear which specific nutrients cause protective effects; therefore they recommend eating a varied diet based on some general principles (www.escardio.org/guidelines-surveys/esc-guidelines/Pages/cvd-prevention.aspx).

The holistic turn in nutrition science related to dietary patterns where nutrients in food can interact synergistically is a paradigm shift. At the beginning of the 20th century, research was centered on the roles of micronutrients, such as specific vitamins, and the prevention of deficiency diseases such as beriberi, pellagra and scurvy (Tracy, 2013). During the 1950s and 1960s atherosclerosis, hypertension and cancer were the dominant health threats and macronutrients were considered the potential contributors to CVD. Cholesterol was the focus of this research. The first dietary guidelines for the prevention of CVD were issued in 1957 based on the link between heart disease and dietary fat. By 1968, dietary cholesterol was considered the main culprit and the main advice was to limit dietary cholesterol and to adhere to the principles of good nutrition (Tracy, 2013). Since 1980, the Dietary Guidelines for Americans from the US Department of Agriculture (USDA) and Department of Health and Human Services have been revised every 5 years (USDA Center for Nutrition Policy and Promotion, 2010). The 2010 guidelines fill more than 95 pages and are somewhat difficult to understand for the general public. This is a reflection of dialogue between evidence-based dietary advice and the food industry lobby. In summary, they advise eating more fruit, vegetables and nuts; limiting dairy and red meat; consuming more fish and poultry; avoiding salt and sugar; using olive oil and other vegetable oils; and substituting refined grains for whole grains (Tracy, 2013). Concerning fruit and vegetable consumption, a paper was published in March 2014 concluding that it decreased all-cause mortality, cancer and CVD in England (Oyebode *et al.*, 2014). Those individuals eating seven or more portions of fruit and vegetables daily had the lowest risk of mortality from any cause (Oyebode *et al.*, 2014). The participants (65,226 aged more than 35 years) were representative of the noninstitutionalized English population, and physical activity was adjusted to avoid this important confounding factor. The main limitation of the study is that it relies on self-reports and the measurement of fruit and vegetables intake occurred at only one point, increasing the social desirability bias and random error (Cope & Allison, 2010).

Overall, summarizing all available data, there appears to exist a widespread agreement that the components of the Mediterranean diet are consistent with a healthy diet. If not entirely evidence-based, it can be endorsed with solid facts (Holt, 2014). However, in the same Mediterranean region, adhesion to this diet appears to be diminishing owing to the increased prices and the current financial crisis (Bonaccio *et al.*, 2014). Studies among children and adolescents in these countries indicate that they are abandoning their traditional diet (Bonaccio *et al.*, 2012a; Naska & Trichopoulou, 2014). These factors have led people to favor less expensive food, which allows them to save money but is unhealthy (Bonaccio *et al.*, 2012a, b, 2014). As usual, higher-quality diets are consumed by better educated and wealthier people while individuals from lower socioeconomic groups tend to eat low-quality diets (highly palatable and low-cost energy-dense foods composed of refined grains, sugars or fats) and therefore are exposed to nutrition-related disease (Bonaccio *et al.*, 2014; Naska & Trichopoulou, 2014).

An additional problem is that knowledge often is not easily translated to behavior. Media frenzy over health issues has given epidemiological research a bad reputation by causing uncertainty and confusion over what is healthy and what is not healthy. Studies reporting new associations of food ingredients or biocompounds with diseases are common, and sensational headlines appear almost daily in the media. Thus, in a recent provocative paper, Schoenfeld and Ioannidis (2013) randomly selected 50 common ingredients from a cookbook, and reported that 40 were apparently associated with increased cancer risk in peer-reviewed studies. However, most of these associations disappeared in subsequent meta-analyses. The final outcomes are increases in media profits and public anxiety and confused policy-makers and politicians. Indeed, oversaturation of contradictory evidence permeates nutritional epidemiology research. Despite mass media not representing a threat to public health, they can play a positive role in the promotion of healthy behaviors through propagating balanced information as reported by Bonaccio *et al.* (2012b) concerning the adherence to Mediterranean diet in an Italian adult population.

Related to the advice to adopt or not adopt to the Mediterranean diet is the presence of ethanol in the diet. Ethanol, consumed mostly in form of wine and during meals, was found to be one of the components of the Mediterranean diet responsible for the lower mortality (Trichopoulou *et al.*, 2009). Also in the PREDIMED subjects, about one-third of subjects in the Mediterranean diet groups reported consuming seven or more glasses of wine per week vs about one-quarter in the control group (Estruch *et al.*, 2013). This issue of ethanol consumption and the possible effects on health, mainly cardiovascular health, will be analyzed in the next section, the "French Paradox".

11.5.2 The French paradox

In June 1992, Renaud and collaborators published a paper entitled "Wine, alcohol, platelets, and the French paradox for coronary heart disease" (Renaud & de Lorgeril, 1992). It is written in the Abstract that "the consumption of wine by the French could explain their low death rates from heart disease" although they eat as much fat as individuals in other countries (Renaud & de Lorgeril, 1992). The term "French paradox" was first used in November 1991, in the CBS show "60 Minutes", where the apparently disagreeing evidence of regular high-fat diet consumption and very low incidence of heart disease in France was discussed (Mudry, 2010). This catchy term captured the mind of the general public, mainly in the USA, and following the broadcast, the sale of wines in this country increased by 40% (Mudry, 2010). The message spread by the mass media concerning the putative health benefits of drinking is confusing, contradictory or spurious. It is evident that the "French paradox" is not a straightforward story. There exists a great deal of influence of the mass media mixed with commercial interests. However, in the general press and society in general, wine has become scientized, rationalized and medicalized (Mudry, 2010), and sometimes described only as a matrix for active biocompounds such as phenols, anthocyanins, resveratrol and many others, which are probably (or not) responsible for the presumed beneficial effects on health. Owing to this, and the rise of probabilistic thinking in public health, the US government defined numeric guidelines characterizing a "healthy" and a "moderate" drinker (Mudry, 2010). This "healthy drinker", as opposed to an "alcoholic", is a self-restrained individual who possesses the rational ability to consume only the amount of wine necessary to supply adequate chemical compounds (Mudry, 2010).

In spite of the sociological considerations, numerous scientific papers studying ethanol and its effect in CVD and an increasing amount of circumstantial evidence show that wine can influence not only cardiovascular health but also other diseases (Alkerwi *et al.*, 2009; Di Castelnuovo *et al.*, 2010; Daviglus *et al.*, 2011). A meta-analysis of 84 clinical trials demonstrated a clear beneficial effect of moderate consumption of ethanol in the reduction of the incidence of coronary heart disease and stroke (Grigorakis, 2011; Ronskley *et al.*, 2011). The health benefits of moderate alcohol consumption can be attributed to several factors, among which are the increased plasma levels of high-density-lipoprotein cholesterol, effects on hemostatic factors and a significant content of anti-oxidant substances such as polyphenols and resveratrol in wine (Covas *et al.*, 2010). Concerning resveratrol, although it is present in very low amounts in wine, it was considered a promising molecule owing to its pleiotropic actions widely described *in vitro* and in experimental animals (Catalgol *et al.*, 2012; Cherniak &Troen, 2013). There are some limited human studies with no convincing results (Cherniak &Troen, 2013). Recently, a study showed that, in 800 individuals 65 years or older, an increased consumption of foods rich in resveratrol did not affect long-term health over 9 years (Semba *et al.*, 2014). In other words, dietary amounts of resveratrol did not translate into fewer deaths, cancer or CVD (Semba *et al.*, 2014). A placebo-controlled study would be more conclusive, but is difficult to justify with these results.

However, the real existence of the "French paradox" is not proven. It is not disputed that, in many Western populations, middle-aged and elderly people who drink moderately have a lower risk of death from CVD than either total abstainers or heavy drinkers. However, there is also evidence that the real explanation of this pattern is not that wine is protective, but simply that the average health status of people who drink low or moderate amounts of alcohol is better than that of abstainers (Hansel *et al.*, 2010). More recently Hansel *et al.* (2012) agreed that the results of observational studies and meta-analyses are largely concordant in suggesting the possibility of a beneficial effect of alcohol on CVD. However, they suggest that the findings of CVD protection by alcohol consumption may be partly owing to misclassification of numerous confounding factors, and on the other hand, that the drinking pattern is a crucial contributor to take into account when interpreting the results of every epidemiological study (Hansel *et al.*, 2012). In another paper, the same authors verified in a large French cohort of supermarket clients (more than 196,000 persons) that the ratio of healthy to unhealthy foods purchased is the highest in wine consumers, the lowest for consumers of other beverages (beer, aniseed-based alcoholic beverages, modern/aperitifs and whisky), and intermediate for nonalcohol consumers (Hansel *et al.*, 2013). They conclude that probably wine buyers display healthier dietary habits not only as compared with other categories of alcohol consumers, but also as compared with those who do not purchase alcohol (Hansel *et al.*, 2013).

As well-conducted randomized studies assessing the causal role of alcohol in cardioprotection are not feasible owing to ethical reasons and the absence of blind placebo

(Grigorakis *et al.*, 2011), future epidemiological studies evaluating this relationship should carefully choose the covariates in any multivariate analysis (Hansel *et al.*, 2012).

It is now considered more likely that the wine is not the sole protective factor in a diet with an apparent excess of fat consumption (Opie *et al.*, 2011). Even Renaud and collaborators in the *Lancet* paper of 1992, described a "Mediterranean-type diet" within which the consumption of wine had a place (Renaud & de Lorgeril, 1992). Therefore, regular modest wine with meals is an established component of the Mediterranean diet (Trichopoulou *et al.*, 2003). In addition, the diet is varied and diets with low diversity scores are associated with increased coronary heart disease (Kant *et al.*, 2009). This interaction between wine and meals in a context of an active lifestyle may have a positive interaction (Opie *et al.*, 2011). Furthermore, olive oil and wine consumed together have a synergistic postprandial hemodynamic response (Papamichael *et al.*, 2008; Opie *et al.*, 2011). Thus, it can be concluded that wine can confer health benefits as a part of a healthy lifestyle, and not in itself.

Should a doctor advise a patient to consume wine? Wine should not be consumed for its intended pharmacological properties. In an adequate diet and consumed moderately it can be an element of a healthy lifestyle. A simple common sense approach dictates that, concerning wine consumption: (a) Individuals who already drink should limit consumption to moderate amounts. In the USA, two drinks per day for men and one drink per day for women is considered moderate (<25 g/day) (Grigorakis *et al.*, 2011); (b) obviously, patients with liver disease and/or alcoholism or history of substance addiction should avoid alcohol consumption; and (c) physicians should not advise abstaining patients to drink wine (Grigorakis *et al.*, 2011). However, practices to direct heavy drinkers toward becoming low or moderate drinkers should be performed (Grigorakis *et al.*, 2011).

Concerning this last point, there is a percentage of individuals that may be prone to addiction or will fail to moderate consumption, and therefore the recommendation to drink alcohol is not advised. If there is abuse, these individuals may represent a hazard to society and it may have detrimental effects on their own health (Testino *et al.*, 2013). Furthermore, no benefits of moderate alcohol consumption have been found for nonvascular causes of death like different type of cancers, liver cirrhosis and chronic pancreatitis, for which there are increased risks with ethanol consumption (Corrao *et al.*, 2004; Mukamal & Rimm, 2008). In women, alcohol consumption, even moderate, is associated with increased risk of breast cancer (Fagherazzi *et al.*, 2014). Furthermore, alcohol drinking is related to mortality from hypertension, stroke, accidents and violence (Corrao *et al.*, 2004). These facts are reasons why some authors state that alcohol consumption should never be advised (Goldberg, 2003; Testino *et al.*, 2013, 2014), along with proved carcinogenicity. They state that the substitution of one medical condition for another, also potentially lethal, is not ethical (Goldberg, 2003; Testino *et al.*, 2013) and a total nonsense (Testino *et al.*, 2014).

The WHO has also a "zero tolerance" policy on alcohol consumption (Poli *et al.*, 2013; Testino *et al.*, 2013). The more reasonable option would be that the choice to consume alcohol should be based on individual considerations, taking into account several factors such as the influence on health and ageing, risk of abuse and other factors that may vary with age and lifestyle (Poli *et al.*, 2013). In short, the recognition of the likely benefits of light to moderate alcohol intake should not overshadow the problems associated with drinking and the possible burden to the individual and society.

It should be remembered that wine is a food to be enjoyed. It can never be considered a product to be consumed owing to the likely pharmacological properties. Its consumption should be moderate and responsible in the context of an adequate diet and an element of a healthy lifestyle.

To conclude, the most important measures to stay healthy during ageing are physical activity (Chin *et al.*, 2008) and nutritional interventions, in which some elements of the Mediterranean diet can be easily adopted without effort for years, owing to their relative ease of adherence. Stamler (2013) proposed a "modern" Mediterranean diet for the 21st century with an update to avoid the problematic aspects: high grain product intake from white flour; high wine intake; high energy intake leading to obesity; and high salt intake. In the same line, following the results of PREDIMED study, Estruch and Salas-Salvadó (2013) proposed a dietary pattern with extra-virgin olive oil, nuts, fatty fish and whole grain cereals, reduced sodium intake and moderate intake of wine with meals.

More simply, we can quote Barry Halliwell, who gives this advice after studying for many years the effects of dietary anti-oxidants: "So, eat well, including plenty of fruit, grains and vegetables, avoid obesity, don't smoke, exercise regularly" (Halliwell, 2013).

Acknowledgment

This work was supported by National Funds through the Fundação para a Ciência e a Tecnologia within the scope of the Strategic Project Centro de Morfologia Experimental (CME/FM/UP) – 2011-2012, Project PEst-OE/SAU/UI0121/2011 and Center for Health Technology and Service Research (CINTESIS).

References

Abete, I., D. Parra, A. B. Crujeiras, E. Goyenechea, and J. A. Martinez. 2008. Specific insulin sensitivity and leptin responses to a nutritional treatment of obesity via a combination of energy restriction and fatty fish intake. *J. Hum. Nutr. Diet.* 21:591–600.

Abete, I., E. Goyenechea, M. A. Zulet, and J. A. Martínez. 2011. Obesity and metabolic syndrome: potential benefit from specific nutritional components. *Nutr. Metab. Cardiovasc. Dis.* 21(Suppl. 2):B1–B15.

Aguilera, J. M. 2005. Why food microstructure? *J. Food Engineering* 67:3–11.

Aisen, P. S., L. S. Schneider, M. Sano, R. Diaz-Arrastia, C. H. van Dyck, M. F. Weiner, T. Bottiglieri, S. Jin, K. T. Stokes, R. G. Thomas, L. J. Thal; Alzheimer Disease Cooperative Study. 2008. Alzheimer Disease Cooperative Study. High-dose B vitamin supplementation and cognitive decline in Alzheimer disease: a randomized controlled trial. *JAMA* 300:1774–1783.

Akamine, D., M. K. Filho, and C. M. Peres. 2007. Drug–nutrient interactions in elderly people. *Curr. Opin. Clin. Nutr. Metab. Care.* 10:304–310.

Albert, C. M., N. R. Cook, J. M. Gaziano, E. Zaharris, J. MacFadyen, E. Danielson, J. E. Buring, and J. E. Manson. 2008. Effect of folic acid and B vitamins on risk of cardiovascular events and total mortality among women at high risk for cardiovascular disease: a randomized trial. *JAMA* 299:2027–2036.

Alkerwi, A., M. Boutsen, M. Vaillant, J. Barre, M. L. Lair, A. Albert, M. Guillaume, and M. Dramaix. 2009. Alcohol consumption and the prevalence of metabolic syndrome: a meta-analysis of observational studies. *Atherosclerosis* 204:624–635.

Allen, L. 2009. How common is vitamin B-12 deficiency? *Am. J. Clin. Nutr.* 89(Suppl.):693S–696S.

Allen, L., B. de Benoist, O. Dary, and R. Hurrell. 2006. *Guidelines on food fortification with micronutrients.* World Health Organization and Food and Agricultural Organization of the United Nations. Geneva: World Health Organization. Available from: http://www.who.int/nutrition/publications/guide_food_fortification_micronutrients.pdf (accessed 10 October 2013).

Andres, R. H., A. D. Ducray, U. Schlattner, T. Wallimann, and H. R. Widmer. 2008. Functions and effects of creatine in the central nervous system. *Brain. Res. Bull.* 76:329–343.

Andrews, F. J. and R. D. Griffiths. 2002. Glutamine: essential for immune nutrition in the critically ill. *Br. J. Nutr.* 87(Suppl. 1):S3–S8.

Appel, L. J. and L. Van Horn. 2013. Did the PREDIMED trial test a Mediterranean diet? *New Engl. J. Med.* 368:1353–1354.

Appel, L. J., M. W. Brands, S. R. Daniels, N. Karanja, P. J. Elmer, F. M. Sacks; American Heart Association. 2006. Dietary approaches to prevent and treat hypertension: a scientific statement from the American Heart Association. *Hypertension* 47:296–308.

Arts, I. C. and P. C. Hollman. 2005. Polyphenols and disease risk in epidemiologic studies. *Am. J. Clin. Nutr.* 81(Suppl. 1):317S–325S.

Assunção M., M. J. Santos-Marques, F. Carvalho, and J. P. Andrade. 2010. Green tea averts age-dependent decline of hippocampal signaling systems related to antioxidant defenses and survival. *Free Radic. Biol. Med.* 48:831–838.

Aune, D., E. De Stefani, A. Ronco, P. Boffetta, H. Deneo-Pellegrini, G. Acosta, and M. Mendilaharsu. 2009. Fruits, vegetables and the risk of cancer: a multisite case-control study in Uruguay. *Asian Pac. J. Cancer Prev.* 10:419–427.

Bailey, R. L., J. J. Gahche, C. V. Lentino, J. T. Dwyer, J. S. Engel, P. R. Thomas, J. M. Betz, C. T. Sempos, and M. F. Picciano. 2011. Dietary supplement use in the United States, 2003–2006. *J. Nutr.* 141:261–266.

Barker, C. J. and P. Berggren. 1999. Inositol hexakisphosphate and beta-cell stimulus secretion coupling. *Anticancer Res.* 19:3737–3742.

Bauer, J., G. Biolo, T. Cederholm, M. Cesari, A. J. Cruz-Jentoft, J. E. Morley, S. Phillips, C. Sieber, P. Stehle, D. Teta, R. Visvanathan, E. Volpi, and Y. Boirie. 2013. Evidence-based recommendations for optimal dietary protein intake in older people: a position paper from the PROT-AGE Study Group. *J. Am. Med. Dir. Assoc.* 14:542–559.

Bawa, A. S. and K. R. Anilakumar. 2013. Genetically modified foods: safety, risks and public concerns – a review. *J. Food Sci. Technol.* 50:1035–1046.

Berger, R. G., S. Lunkenbein, A. Ströhle, and A. Hahn. 2012. Antioxidants in food: mere myth or magic medicine? *Crit. Rev. Food Sci. Nutr.* 52:162–171.

Bernstein, M. and N. Munoz. 2012. Position of the Academy of Nutrition and Dietetics: food and nutrition for older adults: promoting health and wellness. *J. Acad. Nutr. Diet.* 112:1255–1277.

Bischoff-Ferrari, H. A. 2009. Vitamin D: What is an adequate vitamin D level and how much supplementation is necessary? *Best Pract. Res. Clin. Rheumatol.* 23:789–795.

Bjelakovic, G., D. Nikolova, L. L. Gluud, R. G. Simonetti, and C. Gluud. 2007. Mortality in randomized trials of antioxidant supplements for primary and secondary prevention: systematic review and meta-analysis. *JAMA* 297:842–857.

Blencowe, H., S. Cousens, B. Modell, and J. Lawn. 2010. Folic acid to reduce neonatal mortality from neural tube disorders. *Int. J. Epidemiol.* 39(Suppl. 1):i110–i121.

Bloomer, R. J., D. E. Larson, K. H. Fisher-Wellman, A. J. Galpin, and B. K. Schilling. 2009. Effect of eicosapentaenoic and docosahexaenoic acid on resting and exercise-induced inflammatory and oxidative stress biomarkers: a randomized, placebo controlled, cross-over study. *Lipids. Health Dis.* 8:36.

Bolland, M. J., A. Grey, A. Avenell, G. D. Gamble, and I. R. Reid. 2011. Calcium supplements with or without vitamin D and risk of cardiovascular events: reanalysis of the Women's Health Initiative limited access dataset and meta-analysis. *BMJ* 342:d2040.

Bollhalder, L., A. M. Pfeil, Y. Tomonaga, and M. Schwenkglenks. 2013. A systematic literature review and meta-analysis of randomized clinical trials of parenteral glutamine supplementation. *Clin. Nutr.* 32:213–223.

Bønaa, K. H., I. Njølstad, P. M. Ueland, H. Schirmer, A. Tverdal, T. Steigen, H. Wang, J. E. Nordrehaug, E. Arnesen, K. Rasmussen; NORVIT Trial Investigators. 2006. Homocysteine lowering and cardiovascular events after acute myocardial infarction. *New Engl. J. Med.* 354:1578–1588.

Bonaccio, M., A. E. Bonanni, A. Di Castelnuovo, F. De Lucia, M. B. Donati, G. de Gaetano, L. Iacoviello; Moli-sani Project Investigators. 2012a. Low income is associated with poor adherence to a Mediterranean diet and a higher prevalence of obesity: cross-sectional results from the Moli-sani study. *BMJ Open* 19;2. pii: e001685.

Bonaccio, M., A. Di Castelnuovo, S. Costanzo, F. De Lucia, M. Olivieri, M. B. Donati, G. de Gaetano, L. Iacoviello, and A. Bonanni. 2012b. Mass media information and adherence to Mediterranean diet: results from the Moli-sani study. *Int. J. Public Health* 57:589–597.

Bonaccio, M., A. Di Castelnuovo, A. Bonanni, S. Costanzo, F. De Lucia, M. Persichillo, F. Zito, M. B. Donati, G. de Gaetano, and L. Iacoviello. 2014. Decline of the Mediterranean diet at a time of economic crisis. Results from the Moli-sani study. *Nutr. Metab. Cardiovasc. Dis.* 2014. pii: S0939-4753(14)00085-4.

Bouwens, M., O. van de Rest, N. Dellschaft, M. G. Bromhaar, L. C. de Groot, J. M. Geleijnse, M. Muller, and L. A. Afman. 2009. Fish-oil supplementation induces antiinflammatory gene expression profiles in human blood mononuclear cells. *Am. J. Clin. Nutr.* 90:415–424.

Brewer, L. and D. Williams. 2013. Clinically relevant drug–drug and drug–food interactions. *Pharm. Med.* 27:9–23.

Brower, V. 2005. A nutraceutical a day may keep the doctor away. Consumers are turning increasingly to food supplements to improve well-being when pharmaceuticals fail. *EMBO Rep.* 6:708–711.

Buhr, G. and C. W. Bales. 2009. Nutritional supplements for older adults: review and recommendations – part I. *J. Nutr. Elder.* 28:5–29.

Buhr, G. and C. W. Bales. 2010. Nutritional supplements for older adults: review and recommendations – part II. *J. Nutr. Elder.* 29:42–71.

Burton, P. and H. J. Lightowler. 2008. The impact of freezing and toasting on the glycaemic response of white bread. *Eur. J. Clin. Nutr.* 62:594–599.

Butler, C. C., J. Vidal-Alaball, R. Cannings-John, A. McCaddon, K. Hood, A. Papaioannou, I. McDowell, and A. Goringe. 2006. Oral vitamin B_{12} versus intramuscular vitamin B_{12} for vitamin B_{12} deficiency: a systematic review of randomized controlled trials. *Fam. Pract.* 23:279–285.

Calder, P. C. 2009. Polyunsaturated fatty acids and inflammatory processes: new twists in an old tale. *Biochimie* 91:791–795.

Carneiro, A., M. Assunção, V. De Freitas, M. M. Paula-Barbosa, and J. P. Andrade. 2008. Red wine, but not port wine, protects rat hippocampal dentate gyrus against ethanol-induced neuronal damage – relevance of the sugar content. *Alcohol Alcohol.* 43:408–415.

Carruba, G., O. M. Granata, V. Pala, I. Campisi, B. Agostara, R. Cusimano, B. Ravazzolo, and A. Traina. 2006. A traditional Mediterranean diet decreases endogenous estrogens in healthy postmenopausal women. *Nutr. Cancer.* 56:253–259.

Catalgol, B., S. Batirel, Y. Taga, and N. K. Ozer. 2012. Resveratrol: French paradox revisited. *Front Pharmacol.* 3:141.

Chan, L. N. 2013. Drug–nutrient interactions. *JPEN.* 37:450–459.

Chedraui, P. and F. R. Pérez-López. 2013. Nutrition and health during mid-life: searching for solutions and meeting challenges for the aging population. *Climacteric.* 16(Suppl. 1):85–95.

Chen, J. and K. Herrup. 2012. Glutamine acts as a neuroprotectant against DNA damage, beta-amyloid and H_2O_2-induced stress. *PLoS One* 7:e33177.

Cherniack, E. P. and B. R. Troen. 2013. Resveratrol: effects on lipids and cardiovascular risk. *Curr. Cardiovasc. Risk Rep.* 7:9–16.

Chin A Paw, M. J., J. G. van Uffelen, I. Riphagen, and W. van Mechelen. 2008. The functional effects of physical exercise training in frail older people: a systematic review. *Sports Med.* 38:781–793.

Cicerale, S., X. A. Conlan, N. W. Barnett, A. J. Sinclair, and R. S. Keast. 2009. Influence of heat on biological activity and concentration of oleocanthal – a natural anti-inflammatory agent in virgin olive oil. *J. Agric. Food. Chem.* 57:1326–1330.

Cicero, A. F., S. Ertek, and C. Borghi. 2009. Omega-3 polyunsaturated fatty acids: their potential role in blood pressure prevention and management. *Curr. Vasc. Pharmacol.* 7:330–337.

Clarke, R., J. Halsey, S. Lewington, E. Lonn, J. Armitage, J. E. Manson, K. H. Bønaa, J. D. Spence, O. Nygård, R. Jamison, J. M. Gaziano, P. Guarino, D. Bennett, F. Mir, R. Peto, R. Collins; B-Vitamin Treatment Trialists' Collaboration. 2010. Effects of lowering homocysteine levels with B vitamins on cardiovascular disease, cancer, and cause-specific mortality: meta-analysis of 8 randomized trials involving 37,485 individuals. *Arch. Intern. Med.* 170:1622–1631.

Coates, P. M., J. T. Dwyer, and A. L. Thurn. 2007. Introduction to State-of-the-Science Conference: multivitamin/mineral supplements and chronic disease prevention. *Am. J. Clin. Nutr.* 85(Suppl. 1): 255S–256S.

Cope, M. B. and D. B. Allison. 2010. White hat bias: a threat to the integrity of scientific reporting. *Acta Paediatr.* 99:1615–1617.

Cornelli, U. 2009. Antioxidant use in nutraceuticals. *Clin. Dermatol.* 27:175–194.

Cornelli, U., R. Terranova, S. Luca, and M. Cornelli. 2001. Bioavailability and antioxidant activity of some food supplements in men and women using the d-Roms test as a marker of oxidative stress. *J. Nutr.* 131:3208–3211.

Corrao, G., V. Bagnardi, A. Zambon, and C. La Vecchia. 2004. A meta-analysis of alcohol consumption and the risk of 15 diseases. *Prev. Med.* 38:613–619.

Covas, M. I., P. Gambert, M. Fitó, and R. de la Torre R. 2010. Wine and oxidative stress: up-to-date evidence of the effects of moderate wine consumption on oxidative damage in humans. *Atherosclerosis* 208:297–304.

Dabhade, P. and S. Kotwal. 2013. Tackling the aging process with bio-molecules: a possible role for caloric restriction, food-derived nutrients, vitamins, amino acids, peptides, and minerals. *J. Nutr. Gerontol. Geriatr.* 32:24–40.

Daffner, K. R. 2010. Promoting successful cognitive aging: a comprehensive review. *J. Alzheimers Dis.* 19:1101–1122.

Darvin, M., L. Zastrow, W. Sterry, and J. Lademann. 2006. Effect of supplemented and topically applied antioxidant substances on human tissue. *Skin Pharmacol. Physiol.* 19:238–247.

Daviglus, M. L., G. A. Talavera, M. L. Avilés-Santa, M. Allison, J. Cai, M. H. Criqui, M. Gellman, A. L. Giachello, N. Gouskova, R. C. Kaplan, L. LaVange, F. Penedo, K. Perreira, A. Pirzada, N. Schneiderman, S. Wassertheil-Smoller, P. D. Sorlie, and J. Stamler. 2011. Prevalence of major cardiovascular risk factors and cardiovascular diseases among Hispanic/Latino individuals of diverse backgrounds in the United States. *JAMA* 308:1775–1784.

de Castro-Barbosa, T., L. Poyares, U. F. Machado, and M. T. Nunes. 2006. Chronic oral administration of arginine induces GH gene expression and insulin. *Life Sci.* 79:1444–1449.

de Lorgeril, M. 2013. Mediterranean diet and cardiovascular disease: historical perspective and latest evidence. *Curr. Atheroscler. Rep.* 15:370.

de Lorgeril, M., S. Renaud, N. Mamelle, P. Salen, J. L. Martin, I. Monjaud, J. Guidollet, P. Touboul, and J. Delaye. 1994. Mediterranean alpha-linolenic acid-rich diet in secondary prevention of coronary heart disease. *Lancet* 343:1454–1459.

de Lorgeril, M., P. Salen, J. L. Martin, I. Monjaud, J. Delaye, and N. Mamelle. 1999. Mediterranean diet, traditional risk factors, and the rate of cardiovascular complications after myocardial infarction: final report of the Lyon Diet Heart Study. *Circulation* 99:779–785.

De Stefani, E., H. Deneo-Pellegrini, A. L. Ronco, P. Boffetta, P. Correa, D. Aune, M. Mendilaharsu, G. Acosta, C. Silva, G. Landó, and M. E. Luaces. 2012. Meat consumption, cooking methods, mutagens, and risk of squamous cell carcinoma of the esophagus: a case–control study in Uruguay. *Nutr. Cancer* 64:294–299.

Di Castelnuovo, A., S. Costanzo, M. B. Donati, L. Iacoviello, and G. de Gaetano. 2010. Prevention of cardiovascular risk by moderate alcohol consumption: epidemiologic evidence and plausible mechanisms. *Intern. Emerg. Med.* 5:291–297.

Di Maso, M., R. Talamini, C. Bosetti, M. Montella, A. Zucchetto, M. Libra, E. Negri, F. Levi, C. La Vecchia, S. Franceschi, D. Serraino, and J. Polesel. 2013. Red meat and cancer risk in a network of case–control studies focusing on cooking practices. *Ann. Oncol.* 24:3107–3112.

Dorner, B., E. K. Friedrich, and M. E. Posthauer. 2010. Position of the American Dietetic Association: individualized nutrition approaches for older adults in health care communities. *J. Am. Diet Assoc.* 110:1549–1553.

Ebbing, M., Ø. Bleie, P. M. Ueland, J. E. Nordrehaug, D. W. Nilsen, S. E. Vollset, H. Refsum, E. K. Pedersen, and O. Nygård. 2008. Mortality and cardiovascular events in patients treated with homocysteine-lowering B vitamins after coronary angiography: a randomized controlled trial. *JAMA* 300:795–804.

Ebbing, M., K. H. Bønaa, O. Nygård, E. Arnesen, P. M. Ueland, J. E. Nordrehaug, K. Rasmussen, I. Njølstad, H. Refsum, D. W. Nilsen, A. Tverdal, K. Meyer, and S. E. Vollset. 2009. Cancer incidence and mortality after treatment with folic acid and vitamin B_{12}. *JAMA* 302:2119–2126.

Eberhardt, M. V., C. Y. Lee, and R. H. Liu. 2000. Antioxidant activity of fresh apples. *Nature* 405: 903–904.

Eckel, R. H., J. M. Jakicic, J. D. Ard, N. H. Miller, V. S. Hubbard, C. A. Nonas, J. M. de Jesus, F. M. Sacks, I. M. Lee, S. C. Smith Jr, A. H. Lichtenstein, L. P. Svetkey, C. M. Loria, T. W. Wadden, B. E. Millen, and S. Z. Yanovski. 2013. 2013 AHA/ACC Guideline on Lifestyle Management to Reduce Cardiovascular Risk. *J. Am. Coll. Cardiol.* 2013 Nov 7. pii: S0735-1097(13)06029-4.

EFSA Panel on Dietetic Products, Nutrition and Allergies (NDA). 2010. Scientific opinion on establishing food-based dietary guidelines. *EFSA Journal* 8:1460.

Elmadfa, I. and M. Kornsteiner. 2009. Dietary fat intake – a global perspective. *Ann. Nutr. Metab.* 54(Suppl. 1): 8–14.

Espín, J. C., M. T. García-Conesa, and F. A. Tomás-Barberán. 2007. Nutraceuticals: facts and fiction. *Phytochemistry* 68:2986–3008.

Espín, J. C., M. Larrosa, M. T. García-Conesa, and F. Tomás-Barberán. 2013. Biological significance of urolithins, the gut microbial ellagic acid-derived metabolites: the evidence so far. *Evid. Based Complement. Alternat. Med.* 2013:270418.

Estaquio, C., E. Kesse-Guyot, V. Deschamps, S. Bertrais, L. Dauchet, P. Galan, S. Hercberg, and K. Castetbon. 2009. Adherence to the French Programme National Nutrition Sante Guideline Score is associated with better nutrient intake and nutritional status. *J. Am. Diet. Assoc.* 109:1031–1041.

Estruch, R. and J. Salas-Salvadó. 2013. Towards an even healthier Mediterranean diet. *Nutr. Metab. Cardiovasc. Dis.* 23:1163–1166.

Estruch, R., E. Ros., J. Salas-Salvadó, M. I. Covas, D. Corella, F. Arós, E. Gómez-Gracia, V. Ruiz-Gutiérrez, M. Fiol, J. Lapetra, R. M. Lamuela-Raventos, L. Serra-Majem, X. Pintó, J. Basora, M. A. Muñoz, J. V. Sorlí, J. A. Martínez, M. A. Martínez-González; PREDIMED Study Investigators. 2013. Primary prevention of cardiovascular disease with a Mediterranean diet. *New Engl. J. Med.* 368:1279–1290.

Fabian, E., M. Bogner, A. Kickinger, K. H. Wagner, and I. Elmadfa. 2011. Intake of medication and vitamin status in the elderly. *Ann. Nutr. Metab.* 58:118–125.

Fabian, E., M. Bogner, A. Kickinger, K. H. Wagner, and I. Elmadfa. 2012. Vitamin status in elderly people in relation to the use of nutritional supplements. *J. Nutr. Health. Aging* 16:206–212.

Fagherazzi, G., A. Vilier, M. C. Boutron-Ruault, S. Mesrine, F. Clavel-Chapelon. 2014. Alcohol consumption and breast cancer risk subtypes in the E3N-EPIC cohort. *Eur. J. Cancer Prev.* 2014 Apr 16 [epub ahead of print].

Fairfield, K. and M. Stampfer. 2007. Vitamin and mineral supplements for cancer prevention: issues and evidence. *Am. J. Clin. Nutr.* 85(Suppl. 1):289S–292S.

Fernstrom, J. D. 2013. Large neutral amino acids: dietary effects on brain neurochemistry and function. *Amino Acids* 45:419–430.

Figueiredo, J. C., M. V. Grau, R. W. Haile, R. S. Sandler, R. W. Summers, R. S. Bresalier, C. A. Burke, G. E. McKeown-Eyssen, and J. A. Baron. 2009. Folic acid and risk of prostate cancer: results from a randomized clinical trial. *J. Natl Cancer Inst.* 101:432–435.

Finley, E. B. and F. L. Cerklewski. 1983. Influence of ascorbic acid supplementation on copper status in young adult men. *Am. J. Clin. Nutr.* 37:553–556.

Flatt, M. A., R. A. Settersten Jr., R. Ponsaran, and J. R. Fishman. 2013. Are "anti-aging medicine" and "successful aging" two sides of the same coin? Views of anti-aging practitioners. *J. Gerontol. B. Psychol. Sci. Soc. Sci.* 68:944–955.

Flynn, A., T. Hirvonen, G. B. Mensink, M. C. Ocké, L. Serra-Majem, K. Stos, L. Szponar, I. Tetens, A. Turrini, R. Fletcher, and T. Wildemann. 2009. Intake of selected nutrients from foods, from fortification and from supplements in various European countries. *Food Nutr. Res.* 53.

Fontana, L., L. Partridge, and V. D. Longo. 2010. Extending healthy life span – from yeast to humans. *Science* 328:321–326.

Francis, G. A., A. Gallone, G. J. Nychas, J. N. Sofos, G. Colelli, M. L. Amodio, and G. Spano. 2012. Factors affecting quality and safety of fresh-cut produce. *Crit. Rev. Food Sci. Nutr.* 52:595–610.

Fu, Z., S. L. Deming, A. M. Fair, M. J. Shrubsole, D. M. Wujcik, X. O. Shu, M. Kelley, and W. Zheng. 2011. Well-done meat intake and meat-derived mutagen exposures in relation to breast cancer risk: the Nashville Breast Health Study. *Breast. Cancer Res. Treat.* 129:919–928.

Fukagawa, N. K. 2013. Protein and amino acid supplementation in older humans. *Amino Acids* 44:1493–1509.

Fulgoni, V. L., D. R. Keast, R. L. Bailey, and J. Dwyer. 2011. Foods, fortificants, and supplements: where do Americans get their nutrients? *J. Nutr.* 141:1847–1854.

Gabriels, G. and M. Lambert. 2013. Nutritional supplement products: does the label information influence purchasing decisions for the physically active. *Nutr. J.* 12:133.

Galan, P., S. Briancon, A. Favier, S. Bertrais, P. Preziosi, H. Faure, J. Arnaud, N. Arnault, S. Czernichow, L. Mennen, and S. Hercberg. 2005. Antioxidant status and risk of cancer in the SUVIMAX study: is the effect of supplementation dependent on baseline levels? *Br. J. Nutr.* 94:125–132.

Gallicchio, L., K. Boyd, G. Matanoski, X. G. Tao, L. Chen, T. K. Lam, M. Shiels, E. Hammond, K. A. Robinson, L. E. Caulfield, J. G. Herman, E. Guallar, and A. J. Alberg. 2008. Carotenoids and the risk of developing lung cancer: a systematic review. *Am. J. Clin. Nutr.* 88:372–383.

Gartner, C., W. Stahl, and H. Sies. 1997. Lycopene is more bioavailable from tomato paste than from fresh tomatoes. *Am. J. Clin. Nutr.* 66:116–122.

Gaziano, J. M., R. J. Glynn, W. G. Christen, T. Kurth, C. Belanger, J. MacFadyen, V. Bubes, J. E. Manson, H. D. Sesso, and J. E. Buring. 2009. Vitamins E and C in the prevention of prostate and total cancer in men: The Physicians' Health Study II randomized controlled trial. *JAMA* 301:52–62.

Genser, D. 2008. Food and drug interaction: consequences for the nutrition/health status. *Ann. Nutr. Metab.* 52(Suppl. 1):29–32.

Gillette-Guyonnet, S., M. Secher, and B. Vellas. 2013. Nutrition and neurodegeneration: epidemiological evidence and challenges for future research. *Br. J. Clin. Pharmacol.* 75:738–755.

Goldberg, I. J. 2003. To drink or not to drink? *New Engl. J. Med.* 348:163–164.

Gomez-Cabrera, M. C., B. Ferrando, T. Brioche, F. Sanchis-Gomar, and J. Viña. 2013. Exercise and antioxidant supplements in the elderly. *J. Sport Health Sci.* 2:94–100.

González-Sarrías, A., M. Larrosa, M. T. García-Conesa, F. A. Tomás-Barberán, and J. C. Espín. 2013. Nutraceuticals for older people: facts, fictions and gaps in knowledge. *Maturitas* 75:313–334.

Goodman, G. E., M. D. Thornquist, J. Balmes, M. R. Cullen, F. L. Meyskens Jr., G. S. Omenn, B. Valanis, and J. H. Williams Jr. 2004. The Beta-Carotene and Retinol Efficacy Trial: incidence of lung cancer and cardiovascular disease mortality during 6-year follow-up after stopping betacarotene and retinol supplements. *J. Natl Cancer Inst.* 96:1743–1750.

Grigorakis, D., V. Bountziouka, and N. Kalogeropoulos. 2011. Alcohol Intake and Cardiovascular Disease Risk: Cheers, Tears, or Both? *Food Rev. Int.* 27:274–299.

Gualano, B., H. Roschel, A. H. Lancha Jr., C. E. Brightbill, and E. S. Rawson. 2012. In sickness and in health: the widespread application of creatine supplementation. *Amino Acids* 43:519–529.

Gunness, P. and M. J. Gidley. 2010. Mechanisms underlying the cholesterol-lowering properties of soluble dietary fibre polysaccharides. *Food Funct.* 1:149–155.

Haase, H. and L. Rink. 2009. The immune system and the impact of zinc during aging. *Immun. Ageing* 6:9.

Halliwell, B. 2013. The antioxidant paradox: less paradoxical now? *Br. J. Clin. Pharmacol.* 75:637–644.

Hansel, B., F. Thomas, B. Pannier, K. Bean, A. Kontush, M. J. Chapman, L. Guize, and E. Bruckert. 2010. Relationship between alcohol intake, health and social status and cardiovascular risk factors in the Urban Paris-Ile-de-France Cohort: is the cardioprotective action of alcohol a myth? *Eur. J. Clin. Nutr.* 64:561–568.

Hansel, B., A. Kontush, and E. Bruckert. 2012. Is a cardioprotective action of alcohol a myth? *Curr. Opin. Cardiol.* 27:550–555.

Hansel, B., R. Roussel, V. Diguet, A. Deplaude, M. J. Chapman, and E. Bruckert. 2013. Relationships between consumption of alcoholic beverages and healthy foods: the French supermarket cohort of 196,000 subjects. *Eur. J. Prev. Cardiol.* 2013 Sep 24 [epub ahead of print].

Heffernan, K. S., C. A. Fahs, S. M. Ranadive, and E. A. Patvardhan. 2010. Arginine as a nutritional prophylaxis against vascular endothelial dysfunction with aging. *J. Cardiovasc. Pharmacol. Ther.* 15:17–23.

Hennekens, C. H., J. E. Buring, J. E. Manson, M. Stampfer, B. Rosner, N. R. Cook, C. Belanger, F. LaMotte, J. M. Gaziano, P. M. Ridker, W. Willett, and R. Peto. 1996. Lack of effect of long-term supplementation with beta carotene on the incidence of malignant neoplasms and cardiovascular disease. *New Engl. J. Med.* 334:1145–1149.

Hirsch, S., H. Sanchez, C. Albala, M. P. de la Maza, G. Barrera, L. Leiva, and D. Bunout. 2009. Colon cancer in Chile before and after the start of the flour fortification program with folic acid. *Eur. J. Gastroenterol. Hepatol.* 21:436–439.

Hoag, S. W. and A. S. Hussain. 2001. The impact of formulation on bioavailability: summary of workshop discussion. *J. Nutr.* 131(Suppl. 4):1389S–1391S.

Holecek, M. 2013. Side effects of long-term glutamine supplementation. *J. Parenter. Enteral Nutr.* 37:607–616.

Holt, S. 2014. Cochrane corner: Mediterranean diet for the prevention of cardiovascular disease. *Adv. Integr. Med.* 1:61.

Ibarrola-Jurado, N., M. Bulló, M. Guasch-Ferré, E. Ros, M. A. Martínez-González, D. Corella, M. Fiol, J. Wärnberg, R. Estruch, P. Román, F. Arós, E. Vinyoles, L. Serra-Majem, X. Pintó, M. I. Covas, J. Basora,

J. Salas-Salvadó; PREDIMED Study Investigators. 2013. Cross-sectional assessment of nut consumption and obesity, metabolic syndrome and other cardiometabolic risk factors: the PREDIMED study. *PLoS One*. 8:e57367.

Ioannidis, J. P. 2013. Implausible results in human nutrition research. *BMJ* 347:f6698.

Iqbal, R., S. Anand, S. Ounpuu, S. Islam, X. Zhang, S. Rangarajan, J. Chifamba, A. Al-Hinai, M. Keltai, S. Yusuf; INTERHEART Study Investigators. 2008. Dietary patterns and the risk of acute myocardial infarction in 52 countries: results of the INTERHEART study. *Circulation* 118:1929–1937.

Ito, T. and R. T. Jensen. 2010. Association of long-term proton pump inhibitor therapy with bone fractures and effects on absorption of calcium, vitamin B_{12}, iron, and magnesium. *Curr. Gastroenterol. Rep.* 12:448–457.

Ito, T., S. W. Schaffer, and J. Azuma. 2012. The potential usefulness of taurine on diabetes mellitus and its complications. *Amino Acids* 42:1529–1539.

Jacobs, D. R. and L. C. Tapsell. 2007. Food, not nutrients, is the fundamental unit in nutrition. *Nutr. Rev.* 65:439–450.

Jacobs, D. R., L. C. Tapsell, and N. J. Temple. 2012. Food synergy: the key to balancing the nutrition research effort. *Public Health Rev.* 33:507–529.

John, E. M., M. C. Stern, R. Sinha, and J. Koo. 2011. Meat consumption, cooking practices, meat mutagens, and risk of prostate cancer. *Nutr. Cancer* 63:525–537.

Kafatos, A., A. Diacatou, G. Voukiklaris, N. Nikolakakis, J. Vlachonikolis, D. Kounali, G. Mamalakis, and A. S. Dontas. 1997. Heart disease risk-factor status and dietary changes in the Cretan population over the past 30 y: the Seven Countries Study. *Am. J. Clin. Nutr.* 65:1882–1886.

Kahn, R., R. Robertson, R. Smith, and D. Eddy. 2008. The impact of prevention on reducing the burden of cardiovascular disease. *Circulation*. 118:576–585.

Kalra, E. K. 2003. Nutraceutical – definition and introduction. *AAPS PharmSci*. 5:E25.

Kamangar, F. and A. Emadi. 2012. Vitamin and mineral supplements: do we really need them? *Int. J. Prev. Med.* 3:221–226.

Kant, A. K., M. F. Leitzmann, Y. Park, A. Hollenbeck, and A. Schatzkin. 2009. Patterns of recommended dietary behaviors predict subsequent risk of mortality in a large cohort of men and women in the United States. *J. Nutr.* 139:1374–1380.

Kennedy, D. O., R. Veasey, A. Watson, F. Dodd, E. Jones, S. Maggini, and C. F. Haskell. 2010. Effects of high-dose B vitamin complex with vitamin C and minerals on subjective mood and performance in healthy males. *Psychopharmacology* 211:55–68.

Keys, A. 1970. Coronary heart disease in seven countries. *Circulation* 41(Suppl. 1):1–211.

Keys, A. 1995. Mediterranean diet and public health: personal reflections. *Am. J. Clin. Nutr.* 61(6 Suppl.):1321S–1323S.

Klein, E. A., I. M. Thompson, C. M. Tangen, J. J. Crowley, M. S. Lucia, P. J. Goodman, L. M. Minasian, L. G. Ford, H. L. Parnes, J. M. Gaziano, D. D. Karp, M. M. Lieber, P. J. Walther, L. Klotz, J. K. Parsons, J. L. Chin, A. K. Darke, S. M. Lippman, G. E. Goodman, F. L. Meyskens Jr., and L. H. Baker. 2011. Vitamin E and the risk of prostate cancer: The Selenium and Vitamin E Cancer Prevention Trial (SELECT). *JAMA* 306:1549–1556.

Knowler, W. C., S. E. Fowler, R. F. Hamman, C. A. Christophi, H. J. Hoffman, A. T. Brenneman, J. O. Brown-Friday, R. Goldberg, E. Venditti, D. M. Nathan; Diabetes Prevention Program Research Group. 2009. 10-year follow-up of diabetes incidence and weight loss in the Diabetes Prevention Program Outcomes Study. *Lancet* 374:1677–1686.

Kris-Etherton, P. M., W. S. Harris, and L. J. Appel. 2002. Fish consumption, fish oil, omega-3 fatty acids, and cardiovascular disease. *Circulation* 106:2747–2757.

Kris-Etherton, P. M., J. A. Grieger, and T. D. Etherton. 2009. Dietary reference intakes for DHA and EPA. *Prostaglandins. Leukot. Essent. Fatty Acids* 81:99–104.

Kritharides, L. and R. Stocker. 2002. The use of antioxidant supplements in coronary heart disease. *Atherosclerosis*. 164:211–219.

Kumar, V., A. K. Sinha, H. P. S. Makkar, and K. Becker. 2010. Dietary roles of phytate and phytase in human nutrition: a review. *Food Chem.* 120:945–959.

Lademann, J., M. C. Meinke, W. Sterry, and M. E. Darvin. 2011a. Carotenoids in human skin. *Exp. Dermatol.* 20:377–382.

Lademann, J., A. Patzelt, S. Schanzer, H. Richter, M. C. Meinke, W. Sterry, L. Zastrow, O. Doucet, T. Vergou, and M. E. Darvin. 2011b. Uptake of antioxidants by natural nutrition and supplementation: pros and cons from the dermatological point of view. *Skin Pharmacol. Physiol.* 24:269–273.

Larsson, S. C. and A. Wolk. 2012. Red and processed meat consumption and risk of pancreatic cancer: meta-analysis of prospective studies. *Br. J. Cancer* 106:603–607.

Leenders, M. and L. J. van Loon. 2011. Leucine as a pharmaconutrient to prevent and treat sarcopenia and type 2 diabetes. *Nutr. Rev.* 69:675–689.

Leenders, M., L. B. Verdijk, L. van der Hoeven, F. Hartgens, W. K. Wodzig, W. H. Saris, and L. J. van Loon. 2011. Prolonged leucine supplementation does not augment muscle mass or affect glycemic control in elderly type 2 diabetic men. *J. Nutr.* 141:1070–1076.

Li, L., C. Y. O. Chen, G. Aldini, E. J. Johnson, H. Rasmussen, Y. Yoshida, E. Niki, J. B. Blumberg, R. M. Russell, and K. J. Yeum. 2010. Supplementation with lutein or lutein plus green tea extracts does not change oxidative stress in adequately nourished older adults. *J. Nutr. Biochem.* 21:544–549.

Lichtenstein, A. H. and R. M. Russell. 2005. Essential nutrients: food or supplements? Where should the emphasis be? *JAMA* 294:351–358.

Lin, X., S. B. Racette, M. Lefevre, C. A. Spearie, M. Most, L. Ma, and R. E. Ostlund Jr. 2010. The effects of phytosterols present in natural food matrices on cholesterol metabolism and LDL-cholesterol: A controlled feeding trial. *Eur. J. Clin. Nutr.* 64:1481–1487.

Liu, R. H. 2004. Potential synergy of phytochemicals in cancer prevention: mechanism of action. *J. Nutr.* 134(Suppl. 12):S3479–S3485.

Lopez-Garcia, E., F. Rodriguez-Artalejo, T. Y. Li, T. T. Fung, S. Li, W. C. Willett, E. B. Rimm, and F. B. Hu. 2014. The Mediterranean-style dietary pattern and mortality among men and women with cardiovascular disease. *Am. J. Clin. Nutr.* 99:172–180.

Lucas, L., A. Russell, and R. Keast. 2011. Molecular mechanisms of inflammation. Anti-inflammatory benefits of virgin olive oil and the phenolic compound oleocanthal. *Curr. Pharm. Des.* 17:754–768.

Lucock, M. 2004. Clinical review science, medicine, and the future: is folic acid the ultimate functional food component for disease prevention? *Br. Med. J.* 328:211–214.

Lucock, M. and Z. R. Yates. 2009. Folic acid fortification: a double edged sword. *Curr. Opin. Clin. Nutr. Metab. Care.* 12:555–564.

Lucock, M., Z. Yates, L. Boyd, C. Naylor, J. H. Choi, X. Ng, V. Skinner, R. Wai, J. Kho, S. Tang, P. Roach, and M. Veysey. 2013. Vitamin C-related nutrient–nutrient and nutrient–gene interactions that modify folate status. *Eur. J. Nutr.* 52:569–582.

Luiking, Y. C., G. A. Ten Have, R. R. Wolfe, and N. E. Deutz. 2012. Arginine de novo and nitric oxide production in disease states. *Am. J. Physiol. Endocrinol. Metab.* 303:E1177–E1189.

Lundin, L., M. Golding, and T. J. Wooster. 2008. Understanding food structure and function in developing foods for appetite control. *Nutr. Diet.* 65: S79–S85.

McMorris, T., G. Mielcarz, R. C. Harris, J. P. Swain, and A. Howard. 2007. Creatine supplementation and cognitive performance in elderly individuals. *Neuropsychol. Dev. Cogn. B. Aging Neuropsychol. Cogn.* 14:517–528.

McPherson, R. A. and G. Hardy. 2011. Clinical and nutritional benefits of cysteine-enriched protein supplements. *Curr. Opin. Clin. Nutr. Metab. Care* 14:562–568.

McPherson, R. A. and G. Hardy. 2012. Cysteine: the Fun-Ke nutraceutical. *Nutrition* 28:336–337.

Maraini, G., S. L. Williams, R. D. Sperduto, F. L. Ferris, R. C. Milton, T. E. Clemons, F. Rosmini, and L. Ferrigno. 2009. Effects of multivitamin/mineral supplementation on plasma levels of nutrients. Report No. 4 of the Italian-American clinical trial of nutritional supplements and age-related cataracts. *Ann. Ist. Super. Sanita.* 45:119–127.

Marra, M. V. and A. P. Boyar. 2009. Position of the American Dietetic Association: nutrient supplementation. *J. Am. Diet. Assoc.* 109:2073–2085.

Menotti, A., A. Keys, H. Blackburn, D. Kromhout, M. Karvonen, A. Nissinen, J. Pekkanen, S. Punsar, F. Fidanza, S. Giampaoli, F. Seccareccia, R. Buzin, I. Mohacek, S. Nedeljkovic, C. Aravanis, A. Dontas, H. Toshima, and M. Lanti. 1996. Comparison of multivariate predictive power of major risk factors for coronary heart diseases in different countries: results from eight nations of the Seven Countries Study, 25-year follow-up. *J. Cardiovasc. Risk* 3:69–75.

Mensink, G. B., R. Fletcher, M. Gurinovic, I. Huybrechts, L. Lafay, L. Serra-Majem, L. Szponar, I. Tetens, J. Verkaik-Kloosterman, A. Baka, and A. M. Stephen. 2013. Mapping low intake of micronutrients across Europe. *Br. J. Nutr.* 110:755–773.

Miller, E. R., S. Juraschek, R. Pastor-Barriuso, L. A. Bazzano, L. J. Appel, and E. Guallar. 2010. Meta-analysis of folic acid supplementation trials on risk of cardiovascular disease and risk interaction with baseline homocysteine levels. *Am. J. Cardiol.* 106:517–527.

Mithal, A., D. A. Wahl, J. P. Bonjour, P. Burckhardt, B. Dawson-Hughes, J. A. Eisman, G. El-Hajj Fuleihan, R. G. Josse, P. Lips, J. Morales-Torres; IOF Committee of Scientific Advisors (CSA) Nutrition Working Group. 2009. Global vitamin D status and determinants of hypovitaminosis. *Osteoporos. Int.* 20:1807–1820.

Mordente, A., B. Guantario, E. Meucci, A. Silvestrini, E. Lombardi, G. E. Martorana, B. Giardina, and V. Böhm. 2011. Lycopene and cardiovascular diseases: an update. *Curr. Med. Chem.* 18:1146–1163.

Mostad, I. L., K. S. Bjerve, S. Basu, P. Sutton, K. N. Frayn, and V. Grill. 2009. Addition of n-3 fatty acids to a 4-hour lipid infusion does not affect insulin sensitivity, insulin secretion, or markers of oxidative stress in subjects with type 2 diabetes mellitus. *Metabolism* 58:1753–1761.

Mozaffarian, D. 2008. Fish and n-3 fatty acids for the prevention of fatal coronary heart disease and sudden cardiac death. *Am. J. Clin. Nutr.* 87:1991S–1996S.

Mudry, J. 2010. The Poison is in the Dose. The French Paradox, the Healthy Drinker, and the Medicalization of Virtue. *Food Culture Soc.* 13:91–114.

Mukamal, K. J. and E. B. Rimm. 2008. Alcohol consumption: risks and benefits. *Curr. Atheroscler. Rep.* 10:536–543.

Murase, T., S. Haramizu, N. Ota, and T. Hase. 2009. Suppression of the aging-associated decline in physical performance by a combination of resveratrol intake and habitual exercise in senescence-accelerated mice. *Biogerontology* 10:423–434.

Murphy, S. P., K. K. White, S. Park, and S. Sharma. 2007. Multivitamin–multimineral supplements' effect on total nutrient intake. *Am. J. Clin. Nutr.* 85(Suppl. 1):280–284.

Naska, A. and A. Trichopoulou. 2014. Back to the future: the Mediterranean diet paradigm. *Nutr. Metab. Cardiovasc. Dis.* 24:216–219.

National Institutes of Health State-of-the-Science Panel. 2007. National Institutes of Health State-of-the-Science Conference Statement: multivitamin/mineral supplements and chronic disease prevention. *Am. J. Clin. Nutr.* 85:257S–264S.

Nguyen, P., A. Nava-Ocampo, A. Levy, D. L. O'Connor, T. R. Einarson, A. Taddio, and G. Koren. 2008. Effect of iron content on the tolerability of prenatal multivitamins in pregnancy. *BMC Pregnancy Childbirth* 8:17.

Nicoletti, M. 2012. Nutraceuticals and botanicals: overview and perspectives. *Int. J. Food Sci. Nutr.* 63(Suppl. 1):2–6.

Ninfali, P., G. Mea, S. Giorgini, M. Rocchi, and M. Bacchiocca. 2005. Antioxidant capacity of vegetables, spices and dressings relevant to nutrition. *Br. J. Nutr.* 3:257–266.

Noah, A. and A. S. Truswell. 2001. There are many Mediterranean diets. *Asia Pac. J. Clin. Nutr.* 10:2–9.

Noah, A. and A. S. Truswell. 2006. Changes in food supply in Mediterranean countries from 1961 to 2001. *Public Health Nutr.* 9:661–662.

O'Connor, A. 2013. Is the secret to olive oil in its scent? *The New York Times: Health*, 29 March 2013. http://well.blogs.nytimes.com/2013/03/29/is-the-secret-to-olive-oil-in-its-scent/?_r=0 Last accessed 10/10/13.

O'Donnell, M., D. Xavier, C. Diener, R. Sacco, L. Lisheng, H. Zhang, P. Pias, T. Truelsen, S. L. Chin, S. Rangarajan, L. Devilliers, A. Damasceno, C. Mondo, F. Lanas, A. Avezum, R. Diaz, J. Varigos, G. Hankey, P. Teal, M. Kapral, D. Ryglewicz, A. Czlonkowska, M. Skowronska, P. Lopez-Jaramillo, T. Dans, P. Langhorne, S. Yusuf; INTERSTROKE investigators. 2010. Rationale and design of INTERSTROKE: a global case–control study of risk factors for stroke. *Neuroepidemiology* 35:36–44.

Oken, E., A. L. Choi, M. R. Karagas, K. Mariën, C. M. Rheinberger, R. Schoeny, E. Sunderland, and S. Korrick. 2012. Which fish should I eat? Perspectives influencing fish consumption choices. *Environ. Health. Perspect.* 120:790–798.

Omenn, G. S., G. E. Goodman, M. D. Thornquist, J. Balmes, M. R. Cullen, A. Glass, J. P. Keogh, F. L. Meyskens, B. Valanis, J. H. Williams, S. Barnhart, and S. Hammar. 1996. Effects of a combination of beta carotene and vitamin A on lung cancer and cardiovascular disease. *New Engl. J. Med.* 334:1150–1155.

Onomi, S., Y. Okazaki, and T. Katayama. 2004. Effect of dietary level of phytic acid on hepatic and serum lipid status in rats fed a high-sucrose diet. *Biosci. Biotechnol. Biochem.* 68:1379–1381.

Opie, H., K. Lamont, and S. Lecour. 2011. Wine and heart health: learning from the French paradox. *SA Heart* 8:172–176.

Ortolani, E., F. Landi, A. M. Martone, G. Onder, and R. Bernabei. 2013. Nutritional status and drug therapy in older adults. *J. Gerontol. Geriat. Res.* 2:123.

Oyebode, O., V. Gordon-Dseagu, A. Walker, and J. S. Mindell. 2014. Fruit and vegetable consumption and all-cause, cancer and CVD mortality: analysis of Health Survey for England data. *J. Epidemiol. Community Health* 2014 Mar 31. doi: 10.1136/jech-2013-203500 [epub ahead of print].

Pallauf, K., K. Giller, P. Huebbe, and G. Rimbach. 2013. Nutrition and healthy ageing: calorie restriction or polyphenol-rich "MediterrAsian" diet? *Oxid. Med. Cell. Longev.* 2013:707421.

Pan, M. H., C. S. Lai, M. L. Tsai, J. C. Wu, and C. T. Ho. 2012. Molecular mechanisms for anti-aging by natural dietary compounds. *Mol. Nutr. Food Res.* 56:88–115.

Papamichael, C. M., K. N. Karatzi, T. G. Papaioannou, E. N. Karatzis, P. Katsichti, V. Sideris, N. Zakopoulos, A. Zampelas, and J. P. Lekakis. 2008. Acute combined effects of olive oil and wine on pressure wave reflections: another beneficial influence of the Mediterranean diet antioxidants? *J. Hypertens.* 26:223–229.

Parada, J. and J. M. Aguilera. 2011. Review: Starch Matrices and the Glycemic Response. *Food Sci. Technol. Int.* 17:187–204.

Pasha, I., F. Saeed, M. T. Sultan, M. R. Khan, and M. Rohi. 2014. Recent developments in minimal processing: a tool to retain nutritional quality of food. *Crit. Rev. Food Sci. Nutr.* 54:340–351.

Patras, A., N. P. Brunton, C. O'Donnell, and B. K. Tiwari. 2010. Effect of thermal processing on anthocyanin stability in foods, mechanisms and kinetics of degradation. *Trends Food Sci. Technol.* 21:3–11.

Pérez-López, F. R., P. Chedraui, J. Haya, and J. L. Cuadros. 2009. Effects of the Mediterranean diet on longevity and age-related morbid conditions. *Maturitas* 64:67–79.

Phang, M., A. J. Sinclair, L. F. Lincz, and M. L. Garg. 2012. Gender-specific inhibition of platelet aggregation following omega-3 fatty acid supplementation. *Nutr. Metab. Cardiovasc. Dis.* 22:109–114.

Polesel, J., R. Talamini, E. Negri, C. Bosetti, G. Boz, E. Lucenteforte, S. Franceschi, D. Serraino, and C. La Vecchia. 2010. Dietary habits and risk of pancreatic cancer: an Italian case–control study. *Cancer Causes Control* 21:493–500.

Poli A., F. Marangoni, A. Avogaro, G. Barba, S. Bellentani, M. Bucci, R. Cambieri, A. L. Catapano, S. Costanzo, C. Cricelli, G. de Gaetano, A. Di Castelnuovo, P. Faggiano, F. Fattirolli, L. Fontana, G. Forlani, S. Frattini, R. Giacco, C. La Vecchia, L. Lazzaretto, L. Loffredo, L. Lucchin, G. Marelli, W. Marrocco, S. Minisola, M. Musicco, S. Novo, C. Nozzoli, C. Pelucchi, L. Perri, F. Pieralli, D. Rizzoni, R. Sterzi, R. Vettor, F. Violi, and F. Visioli. 2013. Moderate alcohol use and health: a consensus document. *Nutr. Metab. Cardiovasc. Dis.* 23:487–504.

Poljsak, B., D. Šuput, and I. Milisav. 2013. Achieving the balance between ROS and antioxidants: when to use the synthetic antioxidants. *Oxid. Med. Cell Longev.* 2013:956792.

Prasad, K. 2009. Flaxseed and cardiovascular health. *J. Cardiovasc. Pharmacol.* 54:369–377.

Pryor, W. A., W. Stahl, and C. L. Rock. 2000. Beta carotene: from biochemistry to clinical trials. *Nutr. Rev.* 58:39–53.

Punnen, S., J. Hardin, I. Cheng, E. A. Klein, and J. S. Witte. 2011. Impact of meat consumption, preparation and mutagens on aggressive prostate cancer. *Plos One* 6:e27711.

Qin, L. Q., P. Xun, D. Bujnowski, M. L. Daviglus, H. L. Van, J. Stamler, and K. He. 2011. Higher branched-chain amino acid intake is associated with a lower prevalence of being overweight or obese in middle aged East Asian and western adults. *J. Nutr.* 141:249–254.

Rawson, A., A. Patras, B. K. Tiwari, F. Noci, T. Koutchma, and N. Brunton. 2011. Effect of thermal and non thermal processing technologies on the bioactive content of exotic fruits and their products: Review of recent advances. *Food Res. Int.* 44:1875–1887.

Ray, J. G., C. Kearon, Q. Yi, P. Sheridan, and E. Lonn. 2007. Homocysteine-lowering therapy and risk for venous thromboembolism: a randomized trial. *Ann. Intern. Med.* 146:761–767.

Renaud, S. and M. de Lorgeril. 1992. Wine, alcohol, platelets, and the French paradox for coronary heart disease. *Lancet* 339:1523–1526.

Renaud S., M. de Lorgeril, J. Delaye, J. Guidollet, F. Jacquard, N. Mamelle, J. L. Martin, I. Monjaud, P. Salen, and P. Toubol. 1995. Cretan Mediterranean diet for prevention of coronary heart disease. *Am. J. Clin. Nutr.* 61(6 Suppl.):1360S–1367S.

Rees, K., L. Hartley, N. Flowers, A. Clarke, L. Hooper, M. Thorogood, and S. Stranges. 2013. "Mediterranean" dietary pattern for the primary prevention of cardiovascular disease. *Cochrane Database Syst. Rev.* 2013 Aug 12;8:CD009825.

Richardson, D. P. 2007. Risk management of vitamins and minerals: a risk categorisation model for the setting of maximum levels in food supplements and fortified foods. *Food Sci. Tech. Bull.* 4:51–66.

Ripps H. and W. Shen. 2012. Review taurine: a "very essential" amino acid. *Mol. Vis.* 18:2673–2686.

Robien, K., S. J. Oppeneer, J. A. Kelly, and J. M. Hamilton-Reeves. 2013. Drug–vitamin D interactions: a systematic review of the literature. *Nutr. Clin. Pract.* 28:194–208.

Rock, C. L. 2007. Multivitamin–multimineral supplements: who uses them? *Am. J. Clin. Nutr.* 85:S277–S279.

Ronksley, P. E., S. E. Brien, B. J. Turner, K. J. Mukamal, and W. A. Ghali. 2011. Association of alcohol consumption with selected cardiovascular disease outcomes: a systematic review and meta-analysis. *BMJ* 342:d671.

Ros, E., M. A. Martínez-González, R. Estruch, J. Salas-Salvadó, M. Fitó, J. A. Martínez, and D. Corella. 2014. Mediterranean Diet and cardiovascular health: teachings of the PREDIMED Study. *Adv. Nutr.* 5:330S–336S.

Rosenberg, I. H. 2007. Challenges and opportunities in the translation of the science of vitamins.*Am. J. Clin. Nutr.* 85(Suppl.):325S–327S.

Rudzińska, M., R. Przybylski, and E. Wąsowicz. 2014. Degradation of phytosterols during storage of enriched margarines. *Food Chem.* 142:294–298.

Ruiz-Rodriguez, A., F. R. Marín, A. Ocaña, and C. Soler-Rivas. 2008. Effect of domestic processing on bioactive compounds. *Phytochem. Rev.* 7:345–384.

Saito, K., T. Yokoyama, H. Yoshida, H. Kim, H. Shimada, Y. Yoshida, H. Iwasa, Y. Shimizu, Y Kondo, S. Handa, N. Maruyama, A. Ishigami, and T. Suzuki. 2012. A significant relationship between plasma vitamin C concentration and physical performance among Japanese elderly women. *J. Gerontol. A. Biol. Sci. Med. Sci.* 67:295–301.

Sathyapalan, T., J. Shepherd, C. Arnett, A. M. Coady, E. S. Kilpatrick, and S. L. Atkin. 2010. Atorvastatin increases 25-hydroxy vitamin D concentrations in patients with polycystic ovary syndrome. *Clin. Chem.* 56:1696–1700.

Scarmeas, N., J. A. Luchsinger, N. Schupf, A. M. Brickman, S. Cosentino, M. X. Tang, and Y. Stern. 2009. Physical activity, diet, and risk of Alzheimer disease. *JAMA* 302(6):627–637.

Scheepens, A., K. Tan, and J. W. Paxton. 2010. Improving the oral bioavailability of beneficial polyphenols through designed synergies. *Genes Nutr.* 5:75–87.

Scheers, N. 2013. Regulatory effects of Cu, Zn, and Ca on Fe absorption: the intricate play between nutrient transporters. *Nutrients* 5:957–970.

Schmitt, J. and A. Ferro. 2013. Nutraceuticals: is there good science behind the hype? *Br. J. Clin. Pharmacol.* 75:585–587.

Schoenfeld, J. D. and J. P. Ioannidis. 2013. Is everything we eat associated with cancer? A systematic cookbook review. *Am. J. Clin. Nutr.* 97:127–134.

Schwartz, J. B. 2009. Effects of vitamin D supplementation in atorvastatin-treated patients: a new drug interaction with an unexpected consequence. *Clin. Pharmacol. Ther.* 85:198–203.

Schwingshackl, L. and G. Hoffmann. 2014. Mediterranean dietary pattern, inflammation and endothelial function: A systematic review and meta-analysis of intervention trials. *Nutr. Metab. Cardiovasc. Dis.* 2014 Apr 2. pii: S0939-4753(14)00109-4.

Sebastian, R. S., L. E. Cleveland, J. D. Goldman, and A. J. Moshfegh. 2007. Older adults who use vitamin/mineral supplements differ from nonusers in nutrient intake adequacy and dietary attitudes. *J. Am. Diet. Assoc.* 107:1322–1332.

Semba, R. D., L. Ferrucci, B. Bartali, M. Urpí-Sarda, R. Zamora-Ros, K. Sun, A. Cherubini, S. Bandinelli, and C. Andres-Lacueva. 2014. Resveratrol levels and all-cause mortality in older community-dwelling adults. *JAMA Intern. Med.* 2014 May 12. doi: 10.1001/jamainternmed.2014.1582 [epub ahead of print].

Sesso, H. D., J. E. Buring, W. G. Christen, T. Kurth, C. Belanger, J. MacFadyen, V. Bubes, J. E. Manson, R. J. Glynn, and J. M. Gaziano. 2008. Vitamins E and C in the prevention of cardiovascular disease in men: The Physicians' Health Study II randomized controlled trial. *JAMA* 300:2123–2133.

Shatenstein, B. 2008. Impact of health conditions on food intakes among older adults. *J. Nutr. Elder.* 27:333–361.

Singh, S., S. Gamlath, and L. Wakeling. 2007. Nutritional aspects of food extrusion: a review. *Int. J. Food Sci. Technol.* 42:916–929.

Singhal, R. S., A. B. Pandit, J. B. Joshi, S. B. Patel, S. P. Danao, Y. H. Shinde, A. S. Gudekar, N. P. Bineesh, and K. M. Tarade. 2012. Development of efficient designs of cooking systems. III. Kinetics of cooking and quality of cooked food, including nutrients, anti-nutrients, taste, and flavor. *Ind. Eng. Chem. Res.* 51:1923–1937.

Sirtori, C. R., C. Galli, J. W. Anderson, E. Sirtori, and A. Arnoldi. 2009. Functional foods for dyslipidaemia and cardiovascular risk prevention. *Nutr. Res. Rev.* 22:244–261.

Smith, D. A., Y. I. Kim, and H. Refsum. 2008. Is folic acid good for everyone? *Am. J. Clin. Nutr.* 87:517–533.

Sofi, F., F. Cesari, R. Abbate, G. F. Gensini, and A. Casini. 2008. Adherence to Mediterranean diet and health status: meta-analysis. *BMJ* 337:a1344.

Sofi, F., R. Abbate, G. F. Gensini, and A. Casini. 2010. Accruing evidence on benefits of adherence to the Mediterranean diet on health: an updated systematic review and meta-analysis. *Am. J. Clin. Nutr.* 92:1189–1196.

Sofi F., C. Macchi, R. Abbate, G. F. Gensini, and A. Casini. 2013. Mediterranean diet and health. *Biofactors* 39:335–342.

Sotiroudis, T. G. and Kyrtopoulos S A. 2008. Anticarcinogenic compounds of olive oil and related biomarkers. *Eur. J. Nutr.* 47(Suppl. 2):69–72.

Spangler, M., B. B. Phillips, M. B. Ross, and K. G. Moores. 2011. Calcium supplementation in postmenopausal women to reduce the risk of osteoporotic fractures. *Am. J. Health. Syst. Pharm.* 68: 309–318.

Stamler, J. 2013. Toward a modern Mediterranean diet for the 21st century. *Nutr. Metab. Cardiovasc. Dis.* 23:1159–1162.

Stolzenberg-Solomon, R. Z., A. J. Cross, D. T. Silverman, C. Schairer, F. E. Thompson, V. Kipnis, A. F. Subar, A. Hollenbeck, A. Schatzkin, and R. Sinha. 2007. Meat and meat-mutagen intake and pancreatic cancer risk in the NIH-AARP cohort. *Cancer Epidemiol. Biomarkers Prev.* 16:2664–2675.

Swanson, D., R. Block, and S. A. Mousa. 2012. Omega-3 fatty acids EPA and DHA: health benefits throughout life. *Adv. Nutr.* 3:1–7.

Teramura-Grönblad, M., H. Hosia-Randell, S. Muurinen, and K. Pitkala. 2010. Use of proton-pump inhibitors and their associated risks among frail elderly nursing home residents. *Scand. J. Prim. Health Care* 28:154–159.

Testino, G., V. Patussi, E. Scafato, O. Ancarani, and P. Borro. 2013. Alcohol, cardiovascular disease and cancer. *Alcohol Alcohol.* 48:627–628.

Testino, G., V. Patussi, S. Leone, E. Scafato, and P. Borro. 2014. Moderate alcohol use and health: a nonsense. *Nutr. Metab. Cardiovasc. Dis.* 24:e4–5.

Tiwari, U. and E. Cummins. 2013. Factors influencing levels of phytochemicals in selected fruit and vegetables during pre- and post-harvest food processing operations. *Food Res. Int.* 50:497–506.

Toffanello, E. D., E. M. Inelmen, A. Imoscopi, E. Perissinotto, A. Coin, F. Miotto, L. M. Donini, D. Cucinotta, M. Barbagallo, E. Manzato, and G. Sergi. 2013. Taste loss in hospitalized multimorbid elderly subjects. *Clin. Interv. Aging* 8:167–174.

Tracy, S. W. 2013. Something new under the sun? The Mediterranean diet and cardiovascular health. *New Engl. J. Med.* 368:1274–1276.

Trichopoulou, A., T. Costacou, C. Bamia, and D. Trichopoulos. 2003. Adherence to a Mediterranean diet and survival in a Greek population. *New Engl. J. Med.* 348:2599–2608.

Trichopoulou, A., C. Bamia, and D. Trichopoulos. 2009. Anatomy of health effects of Mediterranean diet: Greek EPIC prospective cohort study. *BMJ* 338:b2337.

Troncoso, E. and J. M. Aguilera. 2009. Food microstructure and digestion. *Food Sci. Technol. J.* 23: 30–33.

Truswell, A. S. 2009. Dietary guidance for older Australians. *Nutr. Diet.* 66:243–248.

Turgeon, S. L. and L. E. Rioux. 2011. Food matrix impact on macronutrients nutritional properties. *Food Hydrocoll.* 25:1915–1924.

USDA Center for Nutrition Policy and Promotion. 2010. The Report of the Dietary Guidelines Advisory Committee on the Dietary Guidelines for Americans. Alexandria, VA: USDA Center for Nutrition Policy and Promotion [cited 28 October 2010]. Available from: http://www.cnpp.usda.gov/DGAs2010-DGACReport.htm (accessed June 30, 2013).

Vainio, H. and M. Mutanen. 2000. Functional foods – blurring the distinction between food and medicine. *Scand. J. Work Environ. Health* 26:178–180.

Valerio, A., G. D'Antona, and E. Nisoli. 2011. Branched-chain amino acids, mitochondrial biogenesis, and healthspan: an evolutionary perspective. *Aging* 3:464–478.

van Boekel, M., V. Fogliano, N. Pellegrini, C. Stanton, G. Scholz, S. Lalljie, V. Somoza, D. Knorr, P. R. Jasti, and G. Eisenbrand. 2010. A review on the beneficial aspects of food processing. *Mol. Nutr. Food Res.* 54:1215–1247.

Van Zyl, M. 2011. The effect of drugs on nutrition. *S. Afr. J. Clin. Nutr.* 24:S38–S41.

Villanueva, C. and R. D. Kross. 2012. Antioxidant-induced stress. *Int. J. Mol. Sci.* 13:2091–2109.

Wall, B. T., H. M. Hamer, A. de Lange, A. Kiskini, B. B. Groen, J. M. Senden, A. P. Gijsen, L. B. Verdijk, and L. J. van Loon. 2013. Leucine co-ingestion improves post-prandial muscle protein accretion in elderly men. *Clin. Nutr.* 32:412–419.

Wei, D., H. Q. Xiong, J. L. Abbruzzese, and K. Xie. 2003. Experimental animal models of pancreatic carcinogenesis and metastasis. *Int. J. Gastrointest. Cancer* 33:43–60.

Weststrate, J. A. and G. W. Meijer. 1998. Plant sterol-enriched margarines and reduction of plasma total- and LDL-cholesterol concentrations in normocholesterolaemic and mildly hypercholesterolaemic subjects. *Eur. J. Clin. Nutr.* 52:334–343.

Williamson, G., P. Coppens, L. Serra-Majem, and T. Dew. 2011. Review of the efficacy of green tea, isoflavones and aloe vera supplements based on randomised controlled trials. *Food Funct.* 2:753–759.

Wolff, T., C. T. Witkop, T. Miller, S. B. Syed, and US Preventive Services Task Force. 2009. Folic acid supplementation for the prevention of neural tube defects: an update of the evidence for the U.S. Preventive Services Task Force. *Ann. Intern. Med.* 150:632–639.

Wolpowitz, D. and B. A. Gilchrest. 2006. The vitamin D questions: how much do you need and how should you get it? *J. Am. Acad. Dermatol.* 54:301–317.

Woo, J. 2011. Nutritional strategies for successful aging. *Med. Clin. N. Am.* 95:477–493.

World Health Organization. 2012. WHO Regional Office for the Eastern Mediterranean. Promoting a healthy diet for the WHO Eastern Mediterranean Region: user-friendly guide. Copenhagen: WHO, Europe. Available from: http://www.who.int/nutrition/publications/nutrientrequirements/healtydietguide2012_emro/en/index.html (accessed 27 December 2013).

Yakoob, M. Y. and Z. A. Bhutta. 2011. Effect of routine iron supplementation with or without folic acid on anemia during pregnancy. *BMC Public Health* 11(Suppl. 3):S21.

Yang, H. T., M. Lee, K. S. Hong, B. Ovbiagele, and J. L. Saver. 2012. Efficacy of folic acid supplementation in cardiovascular disease prevention: an updated meta-analysis of randomized controlled trials. *Eur. J. Intern. Med.* 23:745–754.

Yang, J., A. Farioli, M. Korre, and S. N. Kales. 2014. Modified mediterranean diet score and cardiovascular risk in a North American working population. *PLoS One* 9:e87539.

Yetley, E. A. 2007. Multivitamin and multimineral dietary supplements: definitions, characterization, bioavailability, and drug interactions. *Am. J. Clin. Nutr.* 85(Suppl. 1):269S–276S.

Xu, W. H., Q. Dai, Y. B. Xiang, G. M. Zhao, W. Zheng, Y. T. Gao, Z. X. Ruan, J. R. Cheng, and X. O. Shu. 2006. Animal food intake and cooking methods in relation to endometrial cancer risk in Shanghai. *Br. J. Cancer* 95:1586–1592.

Zevenbergen, H., A. de Bree, M. Zeelenberg, K. Laitinen, G. van Duijn, and E. Flöter. 2009. Foods with a high fat quality are essential for healthy diets. *Ann. Nutr. Metab.* 54(Suppl. 1):15–24.

Index

Note: Page numbers in *italics* refer to Figures; those in **bold** to tables.

Anti-Ageing Nutrients: Evidence-Based Prevention of Age-Associated Diseases, First Edition. Edited by Delminda Neves.